# Conversational Agents and Natural Language Interaction:

## Techniques and Effective Practices

Diana Perez-Marin
*Universidad Rey Juan Carlos, Spain*

Ismael Pascual-Nieto
*Universidad Autónoma de Madrid, Spain*

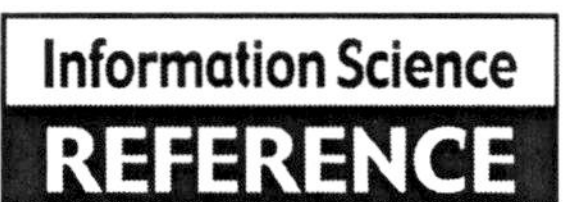

| | |
|---|---|
| Senior Editorial Director: | Kristin Klinger |
| Director of Book Publications: | Julia Mosemann |
| Editorial Director: | Lindsay Johnston |
| Acquisitions Editor: | Erika Carter |
| Development Editor: | Hannah Abelbeck |
| Production Editor: | Sean Woznicki |
| Typesetters: | Mike Brehm, Natalie Pronio, Milan Vracarich Jr., Deanna Jo Zombro |
| Print Coordinator: | Jamie Snavely |
| Cover Design: | Nick Newcomer |

Published in the United States of America by
Information Science Reference (an imprint of IGI Global)
701 E. Chocolate Avenue
Hershey PA 17033
Tel: 717-533-8845
Fax: 717-533-8661
E-mail: cust@igi-global.com
Web site: http://www.igi-global.com



Library of Congress Cataloging-in-Publication Data

Conversational agents and natural language interaction: techniques and effective practices / Diana Perez-Marin and Ismael Pascual-Nieto, editors.
p. cm.
Includes bibliographical references and index.
Summary: "This book is a reference guide for researchers entering the promising field of conversational agents, providing an introduction to fundamental concepts in the field, collecting experiences of researchers working on conversational agents, and reviewing techniques for the design and application of conversational agents"-- Provided by publisher.
ISBN 978-1-60960-617-6 (hardcover) -- ISBN 978-1-60960-618-3 (ebook) 1. Natural language processing (Computer science) 2. Computer-assisted instruction. 3. Discourse analysis--Data processing. 4. Speech therapy--Data processing. 5. Intelligent agents (Computer software) I. Perez-Marin, Diana, 1980- II. Pascual-Nieto, Ismael, 1981-
QA76.9.N38C674 2011
006.3--dc22

2011001310

British Cataloguing in Publication Data
A Cataloguing in Publication record for this book is available from the British Library.

# Editorial Advisory Board

# Table of Contents

**Preface** ........ xiv

**Acknowledgment** ........ xviii

**Section 1**
**Fundamental Concepts**

**Chapter 1**
From Chatbots to Dialog Systems ........ 1
*Tina Klüwer, DFKI GmbH, Germany*

**Chapter 2**
Designing and Evaluating Interactive Agents as Social Skills Tutors for Children with Autism Spectrum Disorder ........ 23
*Marissa Milne, Flinders University, Australia*
*Martin Luerssen, Flinders University, Australia*
*Trent Lewis, Flinders University, Australia*
*Richard Leibbrandt, Flinders University, Australia*
*David Powers, Flinders University, Australia*

**Section 2**
**Design of Conversational Agents**

**Chapter 3**
Designing ECAs to Improve Robustness of Human-Machine Dialogue ........ 50
*Beatriz López Mencía, Universidad Politécnica de Madrid, Spain*
*David D. Pardo, Universidad Politécnica de Madrid, Spain*
*Alvaro Hernández Trapote, Universidad Politécnica de Madrid, Spain*
*Luis A. Hernández Gómez, Universidad Politécnica de Madrid, Spain*

**Section 3**
**Practices**

**Section 4**
**Future Trends**

# Detailed Table of Contents

**Preface** ............ xiv

**Acknowledgment** ............ xviii

**Section 1**
**Fundamental Concepts**

**Chapter 1**
From Chatbots to Dialog Systems ............ 1
*Tina Klüwer, DFKI GmbH, Germany*

This chapter provides an introduction to the notion of dialog systems in contrast to chatbots, and the importance of applying Natural Language Processing (Computational Linguistics) methods to make more flexible human-agent dialogues possible.

**Chapter 2**
Designing and Evaluating Interactive Agents as Social Skills Tutors for Children with Autism Spectrum Disorder ............ 23
*Marissa Milne, Flinders University, Adelaide, Australia*
*Martin Luerssen, Flinders University, Adelaide, Australia*
*Trent Lewis, Flinders University, Adelaide, Australia*
*Richard Leibbrandt, Flinders University, Adelaide, Australia*
*David Powers, Flinders University, Adelaide, Australia*

Human-human communication is not just limited to verbal interaction, but it also includes non-verbal social communication. This chapter introduces the reader in how Embodied Conversational Agents are designed to attend the diversity, and teach social skills to children with autism.

## Section 2
## Design of Conversational Agents



In order to design a conversational agent, it is necessary to pay attention to the design of the human-machine dialogue. In this chapter, it is discussed the main features of non-verbal, visual communication that Embodied Conversational Agents (ECAs) bring 'into the picture' and which may be tapped into how to improve spoken dialogue robustness and the general smoothness and efficiency of the interaction between the human and the machine.



The authors of this chapter propose how automatic dialogue act recognition can be introduced in human-ECA interactions as a preliminary step in conversational analysis for modelling the users' attitudes in several domains. Some practical examples for English and Italian are also provided.



The chapter outlines the state-of-the-art systems and techniques for dialogue management in cognitive educational systems, and the underlying psychological, and social aspects. The authors present their framework for a dialogue manager aimed to reduce the uncertainty in users' sentences during the assessment of his/her requests.

Chapter 6 discusses some design challenges when developing a pedagogic conversational agent such as how to deal with the learners' expectations on the agent's knowledge profile and social profile, the learners' engagement in off-task conversation, and how to manage potential abuse of the agent.

**Chapter 7**
Design and Implementation Issues for Convincing Conversational Agents.................................... 156
*Markus Löckelt, German Research Center for Artificial Intelligence, Germany*

This chapter describes a selection of the experiences of the author from designing and implementing virtual conversational characters for multimodal dialogue systems. The chapter uses examples from the large interactive narrative VirtualHuman and some related systems of the task-oriented variety to identify and describe some issues that might also be relevant for the designer of a new system, to show how they can be addressed, and what problems still remain unresolved for future work.

**Chapter 8**
Extending Conversational Agents for Task-Oriented Human-Computer Dialogue........................... 177
*Pierre Andrews, University of Trento, Italy*
*Silvia Quarteroni, University of Trento, Italy*

Conversational agents can be designed to achieve complex tasks such as Interactive Question Answering and Persuasive Dialogue. In this chapter, the authors describe how agents combined with a planning infrastructure can help manage parts of the dialogue that cannot be planned a priori, are primordial to keep the system persuasive, as well as able to explicitly formulate queries adapted to the context.

**Chapter 9**
Affective Conversational Agents: The Role of Personality and Emotion in Spoken Interactions..........203
*Zoraida Callejas, University of Granada, Spain*
*Ramón López-Cózar, University of Granada, Spain*
*Nieves Ábalos, University of Granada, Spain*
*David Griol, Carlos III University of Madrid, Spain*

Affective conversational agents can be defined as conversational agents that take into account emotions and try to respond empathetically. Chapter 9 revisits the main theories of human emotion and personality and their implications for the development of this kind of agents, and their multiple applications in domains such as pedagogy, computer games, and computer-mediated therapy.

**Chapter 10**
Enhancement of Conversational Agents by Means of Multimodal Interaction................................ 223
*Ramón López-Cózar, University of Granada, Spain*
*Zoraida Callejas, University of Granada, Spain*
*Gonzalo Espejo, University of Granada, Spain*
*David Griol, Carlos III University of Madrid, Spain*

Multimodal conversational agents aim to provide a more engaged and participative communication by allowing users to employ more than one input methodologies and providing output channels that are different to exclusively using voice. This chapter presents a detailed study on the benefits, disadvantages, and implications of incorporating multimodal interaction in conversational agents.

## Section 3
## Practices



This chapter describes the architecture and application of conversational agents as virtual patients in the medical domain. These agents are designed to simulate a particular illness with a high degree of realism. That way, when novice clinicians interact with these agents, they are expected to improve their interpersonal skills, interviewing, and diagnosis.



Chapter 12 presents the experiences carried out with the conversational agent called Cassandra, which provides a way for senior users to perform tasks like managing reminders or appointments, medication schedules, shopping lists, and phone calls.



Companions are agents devised to accompany the users day by day building long-term relationships with them. That way, they do not only assist users for particular tasks in sporadic times, but they provide more support and have more information to adapt themselves to each time users' needs. Currently, these agents and their possibilities are being researched as a part of a European project, and the expectations for the future of these agents are outlined in chapter 17.

**Chapter 14**
Humanizing Conversational Agents: Indisys Practical Case Study in eHealth .................................. 312
*J. Gabriel Amores, Intelligent Dialogue Systems (Indisys), Spain*
*Pilar Manchón, Intelligent Dialogue Systems (Indisys), Spain*
*Guillermo Pérez, Intelligent Dialogue Systems (Indisys), Spain*

Maria is an e-health human-like conversational agent embedded in the web page of the Health Department of the Junta de Andalucía in Spain. In this chapter, Maria's creators describe her possibilities from a practical point of view to arrange doctor's appointments and provide assistance to the users.

**Chapter 15**
Design and Development of an Automated Voice Agent: Theory and Practice Brought Together......... 335
*Pepi Stavropoulou, University of Athens, Greece*
*Dimitris Spiliotopoulos, University of Athens, Greece*
*Georgios Kouroupetroglou, University of Athens, Greece*

This chapter constitutes a practical approach to spoken dialogue system development, comparing design methods and implementation tools highly suited for industry oriented spoken dialogue systems, and commenting on their interdependencies, in order to facilitate the developer's choice of the optimal tools and methodologies. The latter is done in the light of AVA, a real-life Automated Voice Agent that performs call routing and customer service tasks.

**Chapter 16**
Conversational Agents in Language and Culture Training ................................................................ 358
*Alicia Sagae, Alelo, USA*
*W. Lewis Johnson, Alelo, USA*
*Andre Valente, Alelo, USA*

This chapter describes the Virtual Role-Players (VRP), an agent architecture that relies on ontological models of world knowledge, language, culture, and agent state in order to achieve believable dialogue with learners. Authoring and user experiences are described, along with future directions for this work.

**Section 4**
**Future Trends**

**Chapter 17**
The Future of Companionable Agents ................................................................................................ 379
*Roberta Catizone, University of Sheffield, UK*
*Yorick Wilks, University of Sheffield, UK*

As commented in chapter 13, Companions are agents devised to accompany the users day by day building long-term relationships with them, instead of supporting users in sporadic moments or for specific moments. The expectations for the future of these agents are outlined in this chapter.

**Chapter 18**
Future Trends for Conversational Agents ........ 395
*Diana Pérez-Marín, Universidad Rey Juan Carlos, Spain*
*Ismael Pascual-Nieto, Universidad Autónoma de Madrid, Spain*

The chapter presents a summary of the main trends for future work in Conversational Agents. It is expected that the result of the research in this area fosters that in the next decades Conversational Agents become pervasive and natural in our daily lives.

**Compilation of References** ........ 401

**About the Contributors** ........ 439

**Index** ........ 451

# Preface

Human-Computer Interaction (HCI) can be understood as two potent information processors (a human and a computer) trying to communicate with each other using a highly restricted interface. Thus, it is important to study how to design the interface to overcome its limitations when interacting with the users.

Only using command-line interfaces could be adequate for expert users who are able to memorize the commands that they use every day. However, the rest of the users who are not experts, and they only need to interact with the computer from time to time, will not be able to memorize all the commands, and thus they are limited to the use of menus.

Any option that is not represented in the list of choices provided by the menus is ignored by those non-expert users, even being a valid option for the application. Moreover, any time that they want to use one of the options of the menus, they have to remember which tab is, and to click on it.

Natural Language (NL) Interaction, that is, to let the users express themselves, could be the solution to improve the communication between human and computers. By using NL interfaces, expert users can overcome the limits imposed by the use of keywords, and non-expert users can naturally interact with the application as they are used to interact with other humans, in their own language. The main difficulty to move from the current interfaces with command line or menus to NL interfaces is the lack of NL techniques to correctly and immediately process the language. NL is highly ambiguous, and to discover the exact meaning of a sentence uttered by a human is complex, even for another human being.

Therefore, the goal is not usually to perform a complete NL interaction, but to guide the interaction with a certain goal. That way, NL interfaces to databases have already proved their worth. Moreover, conversational agents have been developed to combine agent capabilities with computational linguistics.

Conversational agents exploit NL technologies to engage users in text-based information seeking and task-oriented dialogs for a broad range of applications such as:

- E-commerce: agents can answer the questions of the users about products and services, and finally guide the sell of the article and even order it from the company webpage.
- Help desk: agents can help with the doubts of users about certain technical problems with a product or device.
- Website navigation: agents can guide the users to navigate and find information in complex websites with a high number of links.
- Personalized service: agents can leverage internal and external databases to personalize interactions and provide specific data to each user. For instance, and as reported by Dr. Victoria Rubin, intelligent agents can be used libraries.

- Training or education: agents can teach or be taught by the students about a certain domain, and even to serve a leaner companions to avoid the so-called "isolation problem" of computer-based education.

Conversational agents have features which are quite similar to human intelligence such as the ability to learn, or adapt to new information. In fact, according to the Media Equation theory, people process technology-mediated experiences in the same way as they would do non-mediated experiences, because as Reeves and Nass claimed, "individual's interactions with computers, television, and new media are fundamentally social and natural, just like interaction in real life." Human users even tend to regard conversational agents as assistants to whom they can delegate work or be helped by them, instead of regarding conversational agents as computer programs to which they simply give orders. This feeling has been become deeper in the last decades with the introduction of embodied agents.

Embodied conversational agents differ from traditional conversational agents in the introduction of virtual characters with animated faces (sometimes even a complete body), which allows the agents to produce and respond not only to verbal communication, but also to non-verbal communication. The benefits of agent expressiveness have been highlighted both for verbal expressiveness and for non-verbal expressiveness. On the other hand, there are also studies indicating that when using conversational agents, mixed results can appear. These studies reveal the need to review the research in the field to identify the most effective practices when using conversational agents for different applications.

Some secondary objectives to fulfil the main goal are:

- To gather a comprehensive number of experiences in which conversational agents have been used for different applications.
- To review the current techniques used to design conversational agents.
- To encourage authors to publish not only successful results, but also non-successful results and a discussion of the reasons that may have caused them.

This book is intended to serve as a reference guide for people who want to start their research in the promising field of conversational agents. It will not be necessary that readers have previous knowledge on the topic, as the first part of the book will be devoted to the fundamental concepts. Similarly, readers are not expected to have technical knowledge as authors will be requested to write the chapters so that they can be understood by experts in non-technical domains, given the multidisciplinary nature of the field covered by the proposed book.

38 chapter proposals were received from 13 different countries (Argentina, Australia, Austria, Canada, France, Germany, Greece, Italy, Japan, Spain, The Netherlands, United Kingdom and United States of America). A double-blind review process was enforced with the help of 16 experts from the Editorial Advisory Boards, all of them with a PhD in topics related to the book and from 8 different countries (Australia, Bulgaria, Canada, Romania, Spain, Switzerland, The Netherlands and United States of America).

After reviewing the chapter proposals, 18 were accepted to be published (47% acceptance ratio). They have been distributed into four main sections. The first section comprises the chapters devoted to the fundamental concepts of conversational agents and Natural Language Interaction. The second section comprises the chapters devoted to the design of conversational agents. The third section comprises the chapters devoted to the experiences of use of conversational agents. Finally, the fourth section presents some insight about what the future of the field may be.

The first chapter entitled '*From ChatBots to Dialog Systems*' provides an introduction to the notion of dialog systems in contrast to chatbots, and the importance of applying Natural Language Processing (Computational Linguistics) methods to make more flexible human-agent dialogues possible.

The second chapter entitled '*Designing and Evaluating Interactive Agents as Social Skills Tutors for Children with Autism Spectrum Disorder*' ends the first block of fundamental concepts by introducing the notion of 'Embodied Conversational Agent', that is, agents with a body able to make gestures, and in some cases, agents that can be designed for non verbal social interaction to attend the diversity.

The second section on the design of conversational agents starts with the chapter entitled '*Designing ECAs to Improve Robustness of Human-Machine Dialogue*' giving a special attention to the possibility of spoken conversational agents. That is, the design of interaction no limited just to typing but for oral interaction.

The fourth chapter entitled '*Dialogue Act Classification Exploiting Lexical Semantics*' presents the use of automatic dialogue act recognition in human-ECA interactions as a preliminary step in conversational analysis for modelling the users' attitudes in several domains.

The fifth chapter entitled '*A Cognitive Dialogue Manager for Education Purposes*' focuses on the possibilities of applying dialogue management techniques to improve pedagogic conversational agents, that is, agents designed with educational purposes.

The sixth chapter, entitled '*Building a Social Conversational Pedagogical Agent: Design Challenges and Methodological Approaches*,' discusses the design challenges when developing a pedagogic conversational agent.

The seventh chapter, entitled '*Design and Implementation Issues for Convincing Conversational Agents*,' describes a selection of design experiences for multimodal dialogue systems.

The eight chapter, entitled '*Extending Conversational Agents for Task-Oriented Human-Computer Dialogue*,' presents the role of conversational agents for Interactive Question Answering and Persuasive Dialogue.

The ninth chapter, entitled '*Affective Conversational Agents: The Role of Personality and Emotion in Spoken Interactions*,' revisits the main theories of human emotion and personality and their implications for the development of affective conversational agents, which are conversational agents that take into account emotions and try to respond empathetically.

The tenth chapter, entitled '*Enhancement of Conversational Agents by Means of Multimodal Interaction*,' ends the second block of the book by providing a global overview of the design of multimodal interaction for conversational agents, that is, not only to interact by one channel (e.g. oral interaction), but also to provide alternative communication channels (e.g. typing / haptic interaction, etc.).

The eleventh chapter starts the third section of the book devoted to practical experiences of using conversational agents in several domains. In particular, this chapter, entitled '*Embodied Conversational Virtual Patients*,' is focused on the application of conversational agents as virtual patients in the medical domain.

The twelfth chapter, entitled '*A Conversational Personal Assistant for Senior Users*,' presents the experiences carried out with the conversational agent called Cassandra, which provides a way for senior users to perform tasks like managing reminders or appointments, medication schedules, shopping lists, and phone calls.

The thirteenth chapter, entitled '*A Companionable Agent*,' describes the 'Companion' system which is being developed and tested as part of an EU project, so that the agent can build a long-term relationship with the user.

The fourteenth chapter, entitled '*Humanizing Conversational Agents: Indisys Practical Case Study in eHealth*,' describes the eHealth human-like conversational agent called Maria and its use as embedded in the Web page of the Health Department of the Junta de Andalucía in Spain.

The fifteenth chapter, entitled '*Design and Development of an Automated Voice Agent: Theory and Practice Brought Together*,' presents the experiences in spoken dialogue systems and focuses on the AVA agent able to perform call routing and customer service tasks.

The sixteenth chapter, entitled '*Conversational Agents in Language and Culture Training*,' ends the practical experiences block by describing the work done on the domain of culture training.

The seventeenth chapter, entitled '*The Future of Companionable Agents*,' starts the fourth and last section of the book devoted on the future of conversational agents. In particular, this chapter provides the expectations for the Companiable Agents described in chapter 13.

Finally, the eighteenth chapter, entitled '*Future Trends for Conversational Agents*,' ends the book with a summary of the lines of future work that remain open for the next decades in which it is expected that Conversational Agents become pervasive and natural in our daily lives.

Building this book required the dedicated effort of many people. Firstly, we would like to thank the authors for their valuable contributions to the book. Secondly, we would like to thank the members of the Editorial Advisory Board for their diligence and expert reviewing. We would also wish to include here a word of appreciation for the excellent organization provided by IGI Global, who have smoothly and efficiently prepared the most appropriate environment for the book.

*Diana Perez-Marin*
*Universidad Rey Juan Carlos, Spain*

*Ismael Pascual-Nieto*
*Universidad Autónoma de Madrid, Spain*

# Acknowledgment

The book that you are about to read was devised in 2009, when IGI Global gave us the possibility of editing a book on the field of Conversational Agents and Natural Language Interaction from the most practical side with techniques and effective practices in use. We would like to express our most sincere gratitude to IGI Global for offering us this possibility.

The project of creating a book is a huge task which requires the effort of many people. This is the reason why we would like to thank the professionals of IGI Global who have helped us during the whole project, the authors who have answered our call and provided high quality chapters (the book would be nothing without your excellent contributions), and the Editorial Advisory Board who has promptly reviewed the assigned chapters and provided comments to assist the authors through the versions of their chapters.

We would also like to thank you as a reader of this book, which we hope you find interesting and useful for your research and studies.

*Diana Perez-Marin*
*Universidad Rey Juan Carlos, Spain*

*Ismael Pascual-Nieto*
*Universidad Autónoma de Madrid, Spain*

# Section 1
# Fundamental Concepts

# Chapter 1
# From Chatbots to Dialog Systems

**Tina Klüwer**
*DFKI GmbH, Germany*

## ABSTRACT

*This chapter provides an overview of the technologies used for chatbots on the one hand and research dialog systems on the other hand. By comparing the two, the main disadvantage of chatbots is shown: its dependency on huge amounts of inflexible language data. Methods originating from Computational Linguistics, which are frequently used in dialog systems, can provide a solution by offering further flexibility to the language processing part of the system.*

## INTRODUCTION

A common application field for conversational agents is web-based customer support, such as agents integrated into websites. These agents should provide additional ways to control and access information and functionality available beyond the traditionally offered interfaces. By giving the user the chance to interact with a machine via natural language, the provider also gives the user the possibility to come up with less restricted input. Therefore one of the most important requirements conversational agents in industrial applications have to meet is robustness in the face of unexpected input. Another one is an easy way to generate new language content; a task which presumably most of the time does not lie in the responsibility of linguists and therefore needs to be straightforward for content authors not experienced in linguistics. Because of these two demands, the dialog functionality of conversational agents is often based on pattern and/or keyword matching. This technique, which first gained popularity through Joseph Weizenbaum's chatbot "*ELIZA*" of the 1960s, fulfills the need of being easy to develop and assuring the understanding of at least a single part (e.g. simple keywords) of the user's input.

DOI: 10.4018/978-1-60960-617-6.ch001

Unfortunately, these techniques do not only carry the advantages of the idea, but also a lot of problems regarding the understanding of the user's utterance as well as a great dependency on huge amounts of pattern data. These disadvantages result in inflexible systems.

To overcome these problems several optimizations are possible, from which the integration of knowledge and methods originating from Linguistics and Computational Linguistics (CL) is especially useful. In this chapter, various techniques of Computational Linguistics used in research dialog systems are introduced and the advantage of a possible deployment in chatbot-like architectures is shown. The chapter presents how these technologies can preserve the robustness of a system and at the same time enhance the flexibility.

Firstly, a general overview of chatbot-like systems including their main benefits and disadvantages is given and the main differences between those and dialog systems developed in linguistic research are demonstrated. Afterwards a deeper insight into traditional chatbot systems is given using the chatbots "*ELIZA*" and "*ALICE*" as examples. Analogously, the chapter will supply a more detailed look into the work flow and architecture of dialog systems including their linguistic technologies, such as Part-of-Speech Tagging, Named Entity Recognition and Parsing, and shows some concrete examples of an integrated scenario giving an impression of how the different technologies can interact with and benefit from each other. Finally, the benefits and challenges with regard to an integrated architecture are summarized and discussed.

## COMPARISON OF CHATBOTS AND THEORY-BASED DIALOG SYSTEMS

There are several definitions of dialog systems and chatbots in the literature and parts of these definitions are similar or equal. This section presents a definition of "chatbots" and "dialog systems" as they are used in this chapter and describes how they differ. A detailed description of chatbots, dialog systems and their methods follows in the next two sections.

The terminology "chatterbot", also "chatbot", originates from the corresponding system CHATTERBOT, invented as a game character for a multiuser dungeon game (Mauldin, 1994). Its main task was to answer user questions regarding navigation through the dungeon, other gamers, and objects available in the game world. The system simulated conversational abilities via simple rules and some innovative tricks and successfully "fooled" the other players into thinking it was another user. They were unaware of the possibility of a bot in the game and hence were very cooperative.

In this respect it replicates the success of its ancestor ***ELIZA***, a program developed by the information scientist Joseph Weizenbaum (Weizenbaum, 1966). *ELIZA* is a small system which gained popularity by simulating a psychotherapist users can interact with via typed natural language conversation. Although Weizenbaum did not call his software a "chatbot", the chatbot genealogy indicated by this type of conversational system is generally assumed to start with *ELIZA*, and CHATTERBOT was developed directly based on the experience with the *ELIZA* program.

Both systems show the main characteristics of traditional chatbots as they are understood in this chapter: text-based interfaces and a stimulus-response pattern-matching algorithm constituting the basis for dialog functionality.

The stimulus-response algorithm is the core of the chatbot architecture. It determines the reaction to a user input via a database containing a fixed set of pattern-template pairs. The pattern can be seen as a surface string optionally enriched with regular expression syntax (in many systems this actually is the case) which can be matched to the user input. If an input was successfully matched against an existing pattern, the hard linked tem-

*Figure 1. The core of a traditional chatbot architecture*

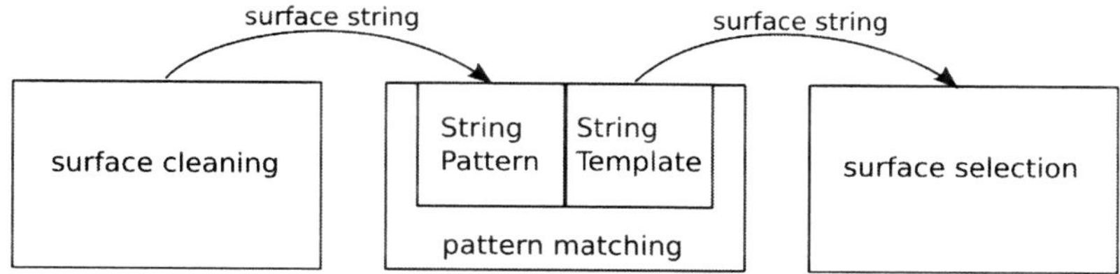


*Table 1. Example of a chatbot process sequence*

| Processing Step | Actions Done | Result |
|---|---|---|
| Input | The raw user input | *hey man, look at what I've found here ;)* |
| Input Cleaning | Removal and substitution of characters and words like smileys and contractions | *look at what I have found here* |
| Pattern Matching | Searches a pattern which matches the cleaned input in the database | <WHAT I HAVE FOUND HERE> |
| Pattern Matching | Get the matching answer templates | <WHAT DID YOU FIND?><br><THAT'S NOT INTERESTING!> |
| Output Selection | Select one of the answers and print it on the output device | *That's not interesting!* |

plate is delivered as answer to the user. Sometimes there are several answer possibilities to guarantee a minimum of variety in responses. Figure 1 shows the prototype architecture of a chatbot system, containing a small component for input analysis which does some string cleaning on the surface structures coming from the user, the dialog core which uses pattern matching to select the next utterance to say, and an output component which selects the next output and may provide further functionality such as the filling of variable slots in the template.

A typical process sequence may look like what is shown in Table 1.

"Dialog system" is a term deriving mainly from the field of Natural Language Processing and AI research and denotes a system which can conduct a conversation with another agent, usually a human.

McTear (2004) in particular notes the following differences between dialog systems and systems for "simulated conversation" (chatbots):

- Dialog systems make use of more theoretically motivated techniques.
- Dialog systems often are developed for a specific domain, whereas simulated conversational systems are aimed at open domain conversation.

The second difference, being more domain specific, is mainly caused by the first point: the use of more theoretically motivated and sophisticated methods. Because dialog systems often imply deep preparatory and development work, their use seems feasible only for a selected application domain.

The first feature is the one which shall serve as the base of definition for this chapter and can most easily be described by looking at the architecture of dialog systems. Dialog systems can be characterized by means of their components: they are at least equipped with an input processing and natural language understanding (NLU) functionality, one component which guides the

*Figure 2. A prototypical dialog system architecture*

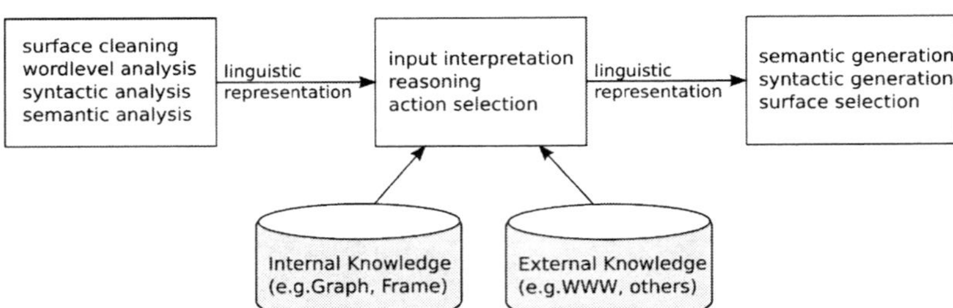


dialog flow, commonly named "dialog manager", and an output generation component.

This architecture sounds similar to the chatbot architecture discussed above, and for this reason chatbots are sometimes referred to as "dialog systems" too; but as we will see there are several crucial differences to a dialog system as it is developed in Computational Linguistics or Artificial Intelligence (AI) research.

Dialog systems usually incorporate into all of their three main units a lot of different processing components which provide additional knowledge to the system. This first of all includes linguistic processing components delivering sophisticated theory-based linguistic descriptions to the input and output modules, enriching the system's background about what actually has been said. Moreover, it includes further knowledge resources for the dialog manager. Those can be used to retrieve the next possible action or answer via real reasoning about the known facts regarding the world or the dialog context.

Figure 2 presents an example of a prototypical simplified dialog-system architecture, showing the similarities and differences to the chatbot architecture (a more detailed description is given in the section "Dialog Systems"). The input analysis is not limited to surface cleaning but runs through a whole linguistic processing chain from the surface to a linguistic representation. Similarly, the output generation uses a language-generation chain to derive a surface string from the linguistic description of the answer. Thus, it is able to provide several different surface strings originating from one single semantic description to the user.

The dialog manager selects a fitting linguistic output structure appropriate to the found linguistic input structure. This selection is not done by hard linking but by using several external knowledge bases keeping in mind the given information from the dialog plan (What has to be negotiated in the discourse?) and the dialog context (What has already been said?) to guarantee the most appropriate response of the system. Figure 2 refers to dialog context and dialog plan as "internal knowledge".

Keeping in mind the shown differences between dialog systems and chatbots, it becomes clear that chatbots are not able to "understand" the user's utterance like a dialog system may. As a result of this problem, they strongly depend on huge amounts of data. It is simply not possible to write a pattern for every input which may be said. To handle this shortcoming the authors of chatbot databases use regular expressions which in return lead to the problem of being overly permissive. Consider the following example:

```
(1)     User: My name is James and I
will wear you down!

Chatbot: It's a pleasure to meet you
James and I will wear you down!
```

Understandably, the authors did not want to write a pattern for every possible name which can be uttered by the user. They therefore wrote a pattern which searches only the surface "My name is" and remembers everything which was uttered afterwards to use it as part of the answer. While this may work very well for input such as "My name is James" or "My name is James Bond", it fails to generate the right response for input similar to (1) such as "My name is Bond, James Bond", which would result in the answer: "It's a pleasure to meet you Bond, James Bond."

## CHATBOT TECHNOLOGY

This section provides further insight into the technology used in pattern-matching chatbots showing the two popular chatbots *ELIZA* and *ALICE*.

### Eliza

*ELIZA* is a small, text-based stand-alone software running on two main technologies: pattern matching and keyword spotting. The general architecture consists of an input-processing component containing a set of decomposition rules and an output-generation component using a set of composition rules or "reassembly rules". Composition rules are assigned to the appropriate decomposition rules in a fixed way, called the "stimulus-response" method. The following interaction presents an example of a conversation which is possible via one pair of composition/decomposition rules.

```
(2)      User: I am feeling depressed.
ELIZA: How long are you feeling de-
pressed?
```

The rule generating the output in the example above would look like the following:

```
(3)      I am feeling *  => How long
are you feeling 4
```

This rule shows the way the *ELIZA* rules are working: the input string, or often a part of the input string, is matched against a decomposition rule. In the example the part "I am feeling" matches the string part of the rule and the regular expression * (asterisk) matches everything that follows after the first part of the rule, in this case "depressed". The composition rule generates a fixed answer as an output string for the matched rule and substitutes the "4" in the rule with the part of the input that was covered by the regular expression.

This simple analysis algorithm on the input's surface is called "pattern matching", because the input gets compared to all rules (patterns) in the database to find one that matches the input form. It is possible to write various reassembly rules for one decomposition rule. The system uses them sequentially to avoid repetition.

The most specific input rules are those which don't contain regular expressions but match a whole string. In addition to the asterisk, the plus character is the second possible regular expression operator matching exactly one or more tokens in the input, whereas the asterisk matches any number of tokens including zero.

To optimize the performance Weizenbaum incorporated the possibility of keywords into the rules. If a keyword was found in the input, only the rules which are indexed with this keyword are tested to find a matching rule. Multiple decomposition rules can be assigned to one keyword.

```
(4)   FATHER 6 (DecompositionRule1)
(Reassembly Rule 1, 1) (Reassembly
Rule 1, 2)
    (DecompositionRule1) (Reassembly
Rule 2, 1) (Reassembly Rule 2, 2)
```

If there are several keywords in the input a hierarchy is generated through the ranking numbers following every keyword and only the input rules belonging to the highest ranked keyword are processed. The keyword "FATHER" for example possesses a ranking value of "6".

It becomes clear that *ELIZA* simulates intelligent behavior without using much intelligence or knowledge about the world or language. Nevertheless the program was quite successful in gaining the users' enthusiasm. The experience with the users wanting to believe a computer being a human caused Weizenbaum to become an even heavier critic of the possibilities of computer science and the rationality of man.

Still, the shown mechanisms and comparable methods of natural language interaction were used in a large number of systems. Largely because of the growing popularity and availability of the WWW, commercial chatbots as well as free software gained new importance. One of the possibilities frequently used nowadays is based on the open source Artificial Intelligence Markup Language (AIML).

## Alice (AIML)

Similar to *ELIZA*, Artificial Intelligence Markup Language (AIML) bots are stimulus-response, pattern-matching machines, which map a pattern with or without regular expressions, to the input string and deliver a corresponding template answer saved in their database. These templates can likewise use matched pieces of the input as part of their output. Contrary to *ELIZA*, the most common AIML instance, the *ALICE* Bot, is an open source product with nearly 500 developers and content authors and an equally capacious database of over 40,000 pattern-template pairs. Due to their lack of explicit encoded intelligence or knowledge, pattern-matching bots are as intelligent as their database is extensive. This is the reason why you can have a funny conversation with *ALICE* at the beginning, but it gets confused and boring after a short time.

AIML is implemented as an XML dialect. Several AIML interpreters exist, mainly using a graph-based handling of the database. This effectively reduces the search space for the matching algorithm.

Comparable to *ELIZA*, the smallest possible unit in AIML is a single decomposition rule (pattern) combined with a reassembly rule (template). The example given above as (3) would look like (5) in AIML XML.

```
(5)  <category>
     <pattern>I AM FEELING *</pattern>
     <template>Why are you feeling </
star></template>
     </category>
```

But it is not just the big database which enables better conversations with *ALICE*. The developers included features such as recursion, topic annotation, variables and a short-term memory, which can make the conversation more flexible and cause different dialog states.

Each of these new features gets encoded in the AIML categories; for example, the short-term memory, which allows for at least three different states in the system, is integrated via the XML tag *<that>*.

```
(6)  <category>
     <pattern>YES</pattern>
     <that>DO YOU LIKE READING BOOKS?</
that>
     <template>Which one do you like
most?</template>
     </category>
```

The category in (6) shows a possibility to react to a yes-no answer in an expressive manner. If the pattern included only "yes", the bot would be forced to generate a really general answer, because it has already forgotten its own last utterance. In the "that" annotation the chatbot saves its last utterance and thus is able to give a meaningful reply.

Another context processing annotation is the *<topic>* tag. Topic should provide a handle for the actual topic of the conversation. This can be useful if the bot was not able to match any piece of the input: the chatbot is still able to support an informative answer if it remembers the last discussed topic, as you can see in the following example.

```
(7)  <topic name="POETRY"/>
     <category>
     <pattern>*</pattern>
     <template>Do you own any poetry
books?</template>
     </category>
```

This example shows the most general pattern possible: the single asterisk, which matches any input. It is the default pattern used as a final fallback option, if nothing was understood. The pattern in the example matches any input, if the last discussed topic was "poetry". Afterwards a topic specific response can be generated, in this case "Do you own any poetry books?"

The *<topic>* tag is not automatically inserted, but has to be set explicitly in the pattern which precedes the presented one. Topic is seen as a built-in variable to AIML which can be set via a getter and a setter method. The example below shows the initialization of a topic variable. Topics are set in the template part of a category.

```
(8)  <category>
     <pattern>DO YOU KNOW ANY POET-
RY?</pattern>
     <template>No, sorry. But you can
teach me some
       <set name="topic">POETRY</set>
     </template>
     </category>
```

Other built-in variables are slots for personal pronouns. They enable the system to remember who the referent of an appearing pronoun is.

Analogically, more variables can be created and retrieved by the AIML author through the tags:

```
<set name="XXX"> and
<get name="XXX">.
```

The context given via *<that>* and *<topic>* is regarded as a specification of the pattern side of a category. This implies that it influences the matching algorithm because some patterns are more concrete than others. Assuming that the algorithm is graph based, that would mean to insert the patterns in the following order to the search path:

Specific Pattern with Topic and That
Specific Pattern with Topic
Default Pattern with Topic and That
Default Pattern with Topic
Specific Pattern with That
Specific Pattern
Default Pattern with That
Default Pattern

AIML bots support a mechanism for recursive processing via the tag *<srai>*, which can be instantiated from inside a template. It forwards the input to another pattern. An example is shown in (9).

```
(9)  <category>
     <pattern>DO YOU KNOW WHAT POETRY
IS?</pattern>
     <template><srai>What is poetry</
srai></template>
     </category>
```

The pattern in (9) refers an input matching "Do you know what poetry is" to another pattern "What is poetry". This is especially useful for polysemantic patterns, i.e., patterns which may have the same or a very similar meaning but different input surfaces. Due to the *<srai>* tag it is not necessary to write the same answer twice; the author can use an already existing category. However, the author will still have to write a category for every surface form of the specific meaning which may occur.

Although the shown new features and even some more were added to the AIML bots, it is obvious that they still use the same basis as *ELIZA* in input analysis, operation method of their database (stimulus-response pattern matching) and output generation. While they continue to provide the benefits coming from *ELIZA* such as robustness and easy database development, they also carry with them the missing intelligence and limited knowledge.

## DIALOG SYSTEMS

So far we have looked at the techniques of chatbots including their benefits and disadvantages. This section continues with the description of dialog systems and their functionalities. The mentioned language technologies are shortly explained in the following subsection.

As we have seen, dialog systems are frequently classified according to their components. In particular, they are often clustered by means of their dialog model and the dialog management component, because the requirements of the dialog manager determine the results of the understanding and generation components.

Traditionally, dialog systems are understood as spoken dialog systems, which means the systems can understand speech input and deliver spoken output back to the user. Spoken dialog systems have their origin in telephone software, as it is used in call centers or for information hotlines (Allen et al., 2000; Peckham, 1993). Wahlster (2000) shows the use of spoken dialog technology embedded into a machine translation system.

In recent years these systems are being replaced more and more by multimodal systems, integrating more sensory information such as gesture identification and recognition of facial and/or body expressions (Wahlster, 2006). In addition, a lot of pure text-based systems are used, especially for applications in text-based environments such as the World Wide Web. Multimodal systems need additional modules which are able to handle the actual input (e.g. a camera for gestures and a component translating the shot images to a meaning) and combine different types of input to a merged representation. Furthermore, they need possibilities to plan and physically execute multimodal output.

For a better understanding of the linguistic processes, the following subsection first briefly describes the most common Natural Language Processing techniques and technical terms.

### Review of Natural Language Processing Techniques

This section very briefly introduces some of the main technologies developed and used in Computational Linguistics. For further information the reader is referred to Manning & Schütze (2003), Jurafsky & Martin (2008) or Cole (1997).

Several NLP techniques can be used to deliver helpful information belonging to a user input. Typically one or more of the following techniques is integrated into CL dialog systems: Part-of-Speech Analysis, Named Entity Recognition, Syntactic and Semantic Parsing.

Part-Of-Speech Tagging (POS Tagging) is the practice of retrieving lexical information belonging to the tokens in some data. This includes the classification of words to a part of speech, e.g., “noun”, “adj” or “verb”. (10) shows an example of a tagged sentence with the POS information following every word separated by a backslash:

```
(10)  Hi\UH my\PP name\NN is\VBZ Bond\NP.\SENT
```

Each word is labeled with the corresponding part of speech from the Penn Treebank[1] POS tag set. Punctuation marks are POS tagged, too. The Penn Treebank tag set is not the only possible POS set, several other tag sets are common. Tag sets may also depend on the language of the input data.

Some available POS taggers also derive morphological information such as inflection or lemma information. There are several POS taggers available on the net mostly working statistically, which achieve quite good results in accuracy between 96% and 97%. Due to the nature of the disambiguation task, the last 3% are still very complicated to solve[2]. Probabilistic systems naturally depend on their training data: a tagger trained on data from newspaper articles may lose accuracy when applied to data originating from another source.

POS tagging was found to be a useful intermediate level of processing, which is easier to solve than full parsing but already provides helpful language information according to the results of Francis & Kučera (1982).

Named Entity Recognition (NER) is a subtask of information extraction and similar to POS tagging, but it labels only those single words or sequences of words in a text which are names of things, such as people or company names. Such Named Entities (NE) constitute a significant part of natural language texts and their proper recognition is crucial for intelligent content extraction systems, as one can see from (11).

```
(11)  I know the world according to garp.
I know the world according to [garp] (NE_Person)
I know [the world according to garp] (NE_Movie)
```

The example in (11) shows one sentence with several possible readings, according to the recognized proper names. It is evident that the meaning of the sentence essentially depends on the recognition of the NEs.

Several approaches to NER are common. The easiest way is to create gazetteers (huge lists containing names), which are used for a comparison with either every token (or only every potential NE token) in the data. To avoid complicated and error-prone list manipulations, gazetteers can automatically be learned from annotated corpora containing named entities or semi-structured data sources like the Wikipedia. Generally, applications using NER do not solely rely on gazetteers but use integrated approaches including more sophisticated methods[3].

More advanced approaches determine the internal structure of a name via a language specific name grammar, including among others affixes and titles (Black et al., 1998; Drozdzynski et al., 2004). The occurrence of the suffix "son" in Icelandic, for example, shows that the person who bears that name is the son of somebody: "Gunnarsson" is the "son of Gunnar".

The task of Parsing can be considered as recognizing higher structural units than POS or chunks in the input data. The highest level traditional parsing gets applied to is the sentence level. Results of a parsing procedure are structural representations, which are often subdivided into syntax and semantics, where syntax is the grammar-like description of the structure in the sentence, describing which groups of words go together (as constituents) and which words are the subject or object of a verb. The semantics on the other hand represent the "meaning" of the sentence.

***Syntax***. For a successful assignment of a syntactic structure to a given sentence, a parser needs a grammar specifying valid structures. On the basis of the rules in this grammar the parser constructs one or more possible structures for the given input.

Most currently available parsers are probabilistic driven parsers, which use knowledge of language gained from hand-parsed sentences to produce the most likely analysis of a sentence. These statistical parsers commonly work rather well, regarding the actual possibilities of parsing. Parsing like most language technologies has to deal with a lot of problems inherent to natural language such as ambiguity, which is the capacity of single tokens and whole structures to denote different things with the same words. In addition to problems like lexical ambiguity (e.g. words with more than one meaning), which is crucial in tasks like POS tagging, parsing has to deal with ambiguity arising from structural variation. Structural Ambiguity can originate from multiple possible relations of constituents to one another. One example is the PP attachment ambiguity in sentences such as "The man looked at the woman with the spy-glass". This sentence has two different readings depending on which person is equipped with the spy-glass.

There are a lot of possibilities to encode the syntactic/semantic structure of a sentence, directly depending on what kind of grammar is chosen. For syntactic parsing one possibility is unification based grammar formalisms e.g., Head Driven Phrase Structure Grammar (HPSG) (Pollard & Sag, 1994), Lexical Functional Grammar (LFG) (Bresnan, 1982) or dependency parsing (see Kruijff (2002) for an overview of dependency grammar). Unification-based grammar formalisms are counted among the phrase structure grammars. Phrase structure grammars provide a formal description of sentences in terms of elementary grammatical constituents found in the data and their clustering to higher constituents named "phrases".

Consider the example sentence: "Colorless green ideas sleep furiously." The basal phrase structure of the sentence can be formulated in the bracketing notation below:

```
(12)   (ROOT
         (S
           (NP (JJ Colorless) (JJ green)
(NNS ideas))
           (VP (VBP sleep)
             (ADVP (RB furiously)))
           (..)))
```

The parser detects that the constituents "colorless", "green" and "ideas" are building one complex noun phrase, where "ideas" is the head of the constituent to which the two adjectives "colorless" and "green" are assigned. The other constituent recognized is a verb phrase containing the verb "sleep" and the adverb "furiously". These two constituents compose a sentence (S), which is the root element of the structure.

Besides the bracketing notation, sentence structure is often visualized as a tree or graph.

Dependency Structures on the other hand are based on the lexical items (words) of a sentence and the relationships (dependencies) between them. Unlike constituency grammar the origin of dependency grammar is not clearly known, but it is commonly accepted that there have been concepts of dependency grammar already in the medieval theories of grammar (Covington, 1984). The main idea of dependency grammar is that the words in a sentence depend on each other, except for one item which forms the root of the structure. In most cases the root of a dependency structure is the main or matrix verb of the sentence.

Semantics. Similarly to the syntactic structure, there are various ways to describe the semantic structure of a sentence, depending on what the underlying aim is and the theory framework used for the analysis. In general semantics deal with the "literal" meaning of a sentence, not regarding phenomena such as implied meanings (implicatures), humor or other context-dependent interpretations, which are dealt with in the field of pragmatics. The first analysis step executed by a semantic parser involves looking at the input's constituents, similar to the syntactic analysis. The elementary meaning comes from single words and morphemes, which then get combined into the meaning of the parent structure, i.e., the sentence or utterance. To connect atomic items (words), various operators are used, which provide different ways of relations (e.g. negation, logical conjunction) as you can see in the examples below.

Because of the large amount of different meaning encoding systems, it is impossible to survey all forms here. In the following paragraph we will shortly look at one example; for more information on how to encode meaning please see Poesio (2000).

A frequently used framework to represent the meaning of a sentence is first order predicate calculus (FOPC). Although there are a lot of shortcomings in traditional FOPC used as description language for natural language, it is still commonly utilized as a sort of inter-lingua representation level for a lot of semantic representations.

The basic concepts in FOPC are predicates and terms, where the predicates denote sets of objects with special characteristics and the terms represent single objects (e.g., a particular person). The FOPC description of the sentence "Mary is a pianist" would look like (13).

```
(13)  pianist(m)
```

In (13) "pianist" is the predicate referring to the set of objects which are pianists and "m" (Mary) is the atom term which this predicate is applied to. Other predicates do have a higher arity. This allows for the description of sentences such as "Mary loves Beethoven" in (14).

```
(14)  loves(m,b)
```

The term "m" denotes "Mary", whereas "b" stands for "Beethoven".

In addition to these main elements, FOPC offers operators which enable special functionality. The most popular ones are the quantifier "∃" and "∀". The universal quantifier "∀" is used to express that a set is a subset of another, as in "All pianos are musical instruments", which would look like (15) in FOPC and can be read as "For all x which are pianos it is the case that they are musical instruments".

```
(15)  ∀x piano(x) → musical_
instrument(x)
```

The existential quantifier "∃" on the other hand, permits the formalization of a set which has at least one member. Consider the example "Mary owns a piano" and its FOPC notation (16) meaning: there is at least one x existing which is a piano and it is the case that m (Mary) does own it.

```
(16)  ∃x piano(x) ∧ own(m, x)
```

Moreover, the example (16) shows the possibility to connect two statements via "∧", which is the FOPC connector and can be read as "and".

## Components of a Dialog System

The following section will focus on the three main components of dialog systems already mentioned: Natural Language Understanding, Dialog Management and Output Generation, and leave aside possible sensory components. Please, see Bui (2006) for more information on multimodal dialog systems and Chapter 10 of this book.

It is the task of the Natural Language Understanding (NLU) component to deliver a representation of the user's input which can be used by the other components of the system. This internal representation depends on the type of input the user enters into the system, e.g., typed text or an interim representation merging the results of different input components.

In nearly all systems working with free user input this component includes work on input cleaning, because a huge amount of given user input is ill-formed, containing for example typing errors or ungrammatical combinations.

The "understanding" of a user's utterance is a highly complicated task due to the properties of natural language being unrestricted in combinations and problems such as ambiguity. Ambiguity can occur on various levels of language: words can have several meanings and belong to more than one part of speech, pieces of utterances as well as whole sentences can be ambiguous in structure and meaning.

Furthermore, the NLU of a dialog system not only has to deal with problems occurring from word to sentence level, but also with all context phenomena appearing in natural language. Typical context phenomena that a discourse processing system such as a dialog system has to deal with are anaphoric expressions (e.g., the resolution of what is denoted with personal pronouns or definite nominal phrases), implicatures and challenges originating from the interaction character of a discourse, e.g., beliefs and interests of the participants.

A common way to encode an internal representation of the user's input on the pragmatic level are "dialog acts". Dialog acts are linguistic actions that incorporate participants' intentions and behavior originating from the theory of "speech acts" by Searle and Austin (Searle, 1969), which apply to all kinds of discourse. Speech and dialog acts provide an abstraction from the original input by detecting the intention of an utterance, which is not necessarily observable from the input's surface. Consider the following examples.

(17) `Can you show me a red car please?`
`Show me a red car!`

The intention behind the two utterances in (17) may be the same: The speaker wants the hearer to show a red car. While this is straightforward in the second sentence, a system may understand the first one as a real question regarding the system's ability to show a red car and answer with "yes" or "no". A dialog act recognition embedded in the system may detect that both utterances yield the same type of dialog act denoting a request from the speaker.

To detect the intention of an input, most systems use the step of NLU to enrich the user's input with linguistic metainformation. In the applied Computational Linguistics research this typically contains several steps of linguistic analysis. In a conventional dialog system the NLU module is implemented as a pipeline of linguistic analyses, proceeding from word level to the whole utterance, in which every element can be seen to deliver a more abstract representation of the input.

A traditional linguistic analysis pipeline could look like what is shown in Table 2.

Table 2 shows a schematic overview about a possible pipeline architecture, in which every module may consume the results of the preceding components. In modern systems, there are various components encapsulating multiple steps, for example a grammar can directly produce semantic output. Moreover, there are several tasks not mentioned here, and a dialog system may not necessarily pass every step of a processing pipeline, but use one of the lower level descriptions, e.g., the results of a syntactic analysis directly.

Dialog Management is the component which decides what the system should do next. This can include various different actions depending on the application scenario and the business domain of the actual system. The dialog manager is also responsible for triggering all necessary supplemental steps such as embedded reasoning. Moreover, it is the component which has access to the dialog context and the current dialog state.

Thus, the dialog manager needs to detect the next action(s) of the system according to the possibilities the system has in the current context of the conversation including the available knowledge bases. Usually, the model of a dialog consists of several different conversation states.

*Table 2. Linguistic analysis pipeline*

| *Processing Step* | *Tasks* |
|---|---|
| Input Cleaning | Deletion and substitution of unwanted characters, potentially correction of common typing and grammar errors. |
| Segmentation | Segmentation of the user input in single "utterances". |
| Word-Level Analysis | Processing of the words part of speech and morphological information, Named Entity Recognition (NER). |
| Syntactic Analysis | Detection of the constituents in an utterance and the relations between these constituents using knowledge about the structural characteristics of a language. |
| Semantic Analysis | Transfer of the given information into a description of the meaning of the utterance. |

Conversation states are context- and dialog-specific states of the system such as "offer an object" or "awaiting accept or reject". The active state can influence the reaction of the system according to the current situation. This is different to pattern-matching systems, in which an input gets directly mapped to an output without any further processing. Therefore pattern-matching systems resemble a question answering system, which can be developed using only two states, one meaning "waiting for question" and one "giving answer".

There are several ways to implement a dialog manager, which can guide a dialog flow with multiple states. Only three will be mentioned here to give an idea of dialog management, see also McTear (2004) for more information:

- Graph based: the dialog is controlled by a finite state graph. The graph encodes typical dialog states and possible transitions between them via edges. Edges can for example be of conditional type, which means that they can get traversed if the condition they are representing becomes true only. A possible condition could be that the system received an input from the user, or that a special meaning was contained in the input. A simple finite state graph has to be encoded beforehand. Every possible progress of a conversation is pre-encoded and the resulting dialog may lack flexibility. On the other hand, dialog modeling through finite state graphs is very robust, see Cohen (1997) for more information.
- Frame based: the dialog is controlled by a hidden electronic form, collecting information from the user (Aust et al., 1995; Constantinides et al., 1998; Klüwer et al., 2010). An example application could be a travel-support hotline, delivering information about train schedules to a user. One frame would be a "TrainTravel"-Frame with field for "origin", "destination", "date" and other information the system needs from the user to fulfill its task. At the beginning the system does not possess any information about the user's wishes, so all information slots are empty. During the conversation the system tries to get the missing information from the user. Every time the user provides missing information, it gets stored in the internal form. What the system asks or does is therefore led by the empty or filled slots in the form. The actions are not hard-coded, but the system's behavior depends on the form and may differ from use to use. Therefore, this approach provides much more flexibility than the graph-based technology. It is often combined with finite state graphs.
- Plan based: in contrast to the above mentioned methods the plan-based approach is very flexible and supports a greater complexity of conversations (Lesh et al., 2004; Rich & Sidner, 1998). The plan-based approach originates from AI research on planning methods and involves the detection of the plans, beliefs and desires of the users. These are then incorporated into rich descriptions, which can be used for further reasoning. See also BDI agents (Allen & Perrault, 1980), (Bratman et al., 1991). Due to the multiple reasoning steps the rich plan based approaches are nearly impossible to use in real-world applications without integrating further possibilities to reduce the search space for the next action.

Apart from deciding what action fits best to the actual state and triggering all the necessary subtasks (such as reasoning or a simple database query), the dialog component often first does an interpretation of the input. Since the dialog manager is the main component with access to the conversation context, the input analysis component may deliver only a semantic representation covering the meaning of a single utterance and the dialog manager tries to embed this representation into the context. A concrete example could be a mapping of a semantic description or a surface dialog act to a context aware dialog act.

If the system is based on intentions encoded by dialog acts, the dialog manager may also deliver such a dialog act as result to the output generator, which then generates an output action from this description.

After the system has decided on what information to present to the user, the output generator component has to construct a physical message encapsulating this information. The message may be implemented as speech- or text-based output, or in graphical form. If the system has a graphical interface at its disposal, for information such as a long list of options, showing a table or a map may be the most suitable response. In multimodal systems e.g., of an embodied agent, the output can also include gestures or other movements.

Common methods to generate output are:

- Pre-stored text. The easiest way to generate output is the selection of an appropriate canned-text snippet. This approach is comparable to the simple surface templates used in chatbots.
- Template filling. To gain some more flexibility, pre-encoded text snippets may contain variable slots in which different content can be inserted dynamically. These templates can produce one and the same output with slight variations and therefore provide more flexibility to the system. This method is equivalent to the more complex chatbot templates using variables.
- Language generation. In sophisticated research and industrial dialog systems, the output is planned at an abstracted level by the dialog manager and processed via a language generation pipeline similar to the language understanding pipeline (Kruijff et al., 2009; Reiter & Dale, 2000). The dialog component could decide on how to act on the intentional level, e.g., to react to a dialog act "REQUEST" with a dialog act "PROVIDE_INFO" and the appropriate information. The generation unit then has to calculate a possible semantic structure from this specification, which in turn can be transferred into multiple possible syntactic structures and, finally, surface structures. It is clear that this better protects the system from being repetitive, because one meaning may result in several surface structures. Moreover via language generation it is possible to insert anaphoric references such as personal pronouns or deictic expressions such as "here" and "there" to further enhance the natural effect.

## HOW TO APPLY NLP TO CHATBOTS

As shown in the comparison of chatbots and dialog systems, the architecture of chatbots can be seen as a very simple dialog system using only two different dialog states. The input analysis and the output generation component are minimized to the surface form and the dialog manager is limited to the look-up of matching templates to a given input.

One of the major problems of chatbots follows from this architecture, and it is the handling of surface variation. To be able to process one sentence with different structures, chatbots need as many patterns as there are syntactic and lexical alternatives, which leads to an exploding number of pattern-template pairs. To reduce the costs of the manual development, authors can use regular expression operators, which in turn leads to the problem of being overly permissive: there is no possibility to control what content the pattern is actually matching.

In general, optimization of chatbots can be applied to all three main units of the architecture: the amount of information processed in the input analysis, the approach to derive the next answer of the system in the dialog manager and the way the output is generated by the system.

Nevertheless, this chapter will just show the advantages of integrating NLP techniques into the linguistic components "NLU" and "output generator", disregarding the possibilities to change the actual dialog component of chatbots, because the author believes that the main characteristic and also the particular benefit of chatbots lies in the simple stimulus-response pattern-matching way of a dialog model. This approach is the main strength of the chatbot idea. Furthermore it is still an open challenge to implement needed knowledge resources and dialog skills completely linguistically when coming to open domain dialog. It may be an interesting step anyway, after the integration of more linguistic knowledge, to add more external knowledge to the dialog component, but this is not discussed here.

Instead some possibilities are shown to abstract from the surface level and still be able to control the structure by using information from syntactic and semantic analysis. In the previous section some of the most important language technology methods were introduced. This section should give an idea how these can be used to overcome the main problems of chatbot architectures by providing more flexibility. All examples presuppose the embedding of a language technology component which delivers the wanted information into the input analysis pipeline of a chatbot system and are explicitly presented via code examples inspired by the AIML XML. This should deliver the idea of enhancing pattern matching successfully enough for the reader to be able to transfer these examples to other chatbot systems.

## Abstraction from the Surface on the Word Level

Please examine the following pattern-template examples:

```
(18)  <category>
      <pattern>WHO IS ALBERT *</pattern>
     <template><srai>albert is a common
name</srai></template>
      </category>
      <category>
     <pattern>WHO IS CHRISTIAN *</pattern>
      <template><srai>christian is a
common name</srai></template>
      </category>
```

This pattern has a total number of 166 occurrences in the original *ALICE* data, differing only in the value of the actual name. To write that many patterns of the same style is not only unsatisfying and time consuming development work, it is theoretically never ending, because it is not possible to know all names which could occur in advance. The technology which can be used here is Named Entity Recognition. Computational Linguists have developed resources which are able to detect proper names in an input. Of course there should be concrete patterns in the *ALICE* data for special people such as Albert Einstein. Nevertheless, it is possible to write only one pattern handling all the 166 patterns mentioned and also all the unknown names which are not mentioned in a dynamic way via the integration of an NER module:

```
(19)   <category>
       <pattern>WHO IS NE_PERSON *</
pattern>
      <template>I don't know anybody
of that name.</template>
      </category>
```

The term "NE_PERSON" substitutes all kinds of person names which were found by a preceding Named Entity Recognizer and thus guarantees that only a proper person name can be matched at this location in the pattern. If the NER component has been integrated into the system in a reasonable way, the value of the encapsulating type "NE_PERSON" (e.g., "Albert" or "Christian") should be available also to the output generation, which can substitute the generic NE_PERSON with the original value and still produce output such as "Albert is a common name" via the shown template:

```
(20)   <category>
      <pattern>WHO IS NE_PERSON *</pattern>
       <template><srai>NE_PERSON is a
common name</srai></template>
       </category>
```

The same problem appears for patterns which are very similar but vary in single words within one part of speech. If these words are not distinctive for the meaning, authors could integrate the POS information into the pattern to allow for a matching without mentioning all lexical surface variations. Consider the following example:

```
(21)   <category>
       <pattern>I REALLY LIKE FLOWERS
</pattern>
       <template>Oh! Me too. Which one
do you like most?</template>
       </category>
```

Instead of "really" a user may also say "truly", "actually" or any other fitting adverb. If the AIML author wants to avoid writing a pattern for all possibilities, she may insert a regular expression to match anything between "I" and "LIKE FLOWERS". The pattern could look like:

```
(22)   <pattern>I + LIKE FLOWERS</pattern>
```

But the pattern in (22) may directly cause trouble for cases such as the following input "I DON'T LIKE FLOWERS". If the pattern with the regular expression exists, the "DON'T" will get matched against the wildcard and the negated meaning would be lost.

As a result of these issues, it may be desirable to write a pattern containing a regular expression but only for a special part of speech. This offers more flexibility to the pattern but keeps a fine-grained control over what can get matched, as in the example below.

```
(23)   <category>
       <pattern>I *\adv LIKE FLOWERS
</pattern>
       <template>Oh! Me too. Which one
do you like most?</template>
       </category>
```

This method could also handle the example (1) from, here repeated as (24), via the category in (25).

```
(24)       User: My name is James and I
will wear you down!
Chatbot: It's a pleasure to meet you
James and I will wear you down!
```

```
(25)   <category>
       <pattern>MY\PP$ NAME\NN IS\VBZ
*\NP</pattern>
       <template></template>
       </category>
```

(25) would match input such as "My name is James", and also the piece "My name is James" in the utterance "My name is James and I will wear you down", but it will prevent the whole piece "James and I will wear you down" from matching.

## Abstraction from the Surface on the Sentence Level

So far we have seen examples providing abstraction from the surface form on the word layer. The next step is to obtain abstraction on the level of the whole utterance (or sentence).

Basically, we have two alternative forms of abstraction: via the syntactic or the semantic structure of the sentence. As we recall from the introduction to the NLP technologies the syntactic structure is a formal description; for example, phrase structure descriptions. Other syntactic descriptions are so called "dependency structures". Dependency structures are based on the elementary grammatical constituents of a sentence and the relationships (dependencies) between them. Please have a look at the dependency structure in (26).

```
(26)  [ level_0 3-VB, give(null),
Char:7-10, ]
      [ level_1 2-MD, will(null),
Char:2-5, REL: dep(aux) ]
      [ level_1 1-PRP, I(null), Char:0-
0, REL: subj(nsubj) ]
      [ level_1 6-NN, book(null),
Char:20-23, REL: obj(dobj) ]
         [ level_2 5-DT, the(null),
Char:16-18, REL: mod(det) ]
         [ level_2 9-NN, tomorrow(null),
Char:33-40, REL: dep(prep_at) ]
            [ level_3 8-NN, work(null),
Char:28-31, REL: mod(nn) ]
      [ level_1 4-PRP, you(null),
Char:12-14, REL: obj(iobj) ]
```

This structure offers a syntactic-semantic abstraction from the surface form "I will give you the book at work tomorrow", insofar as it covers different possible surface variations which embed the same dependency structure (see also Adolphs et al. 2010).

(27) *I will give you the book at work tomorrow.*
*Tomorrow I will give you the book at work.*
*I will give you the book tomorrow at work.*

By making the dependency structure available to a chatbot system, the author can get rid of the necessity to write a pattern for each of the mentioned sentences. Instead the database author may write one pattern only containing the dependency structure of the sentence. For every matching process the system would then first try to retrieve the dependency structure belonging to the input and then match it to the given dependency patterns. It will be required to format the dependency structure in a way acceptable to the chatbot system, for example as flattened strings. This would include an additional step of post-processing of the dependency results.

A pattern including a simple flattened structure describing the dependencies of the sentence "I will give you the book at work tomorrow" could look like the following:

```
(28)  <category>
      <pattern>
      nsubj(give-1, I-1) aux(give-1,
will-1) iobj(give-1, you-1) det(book-1,
the-1) dobj(give-1, book-1)
prep(book-1, at-1) nn(tomorrow-1,
work-1) pobj(at-1, tomorrow-1)
      </pattern>
      <template>I don't want your
stupid book.</template>
      </category>
```

Some parsers also include generators, which are able to generate a surface string from a given grammatical description of a sentence. This is especially the case for bidirectional grammars such as the CCG. (see for example Steedman, 2001). Bidirectional grammars can be used to avoid manual work, if authors want to by-pass the repetition in system utterances. However, these resources are not very frequent even in research dialog systems (see Kruijff (2005) for an example of a dialog system using language generation via CCG). This is because of the complexity of deciding which linguistic structure should be the baseline for generation. Moreover, the existing components are often complicated to integrate.

The last possible abstraction step NLP can offer on the sentence level is a complete semantic analysis of the input; for example, a FOPC notation encodes the meaning of the sentence. At this level even syntactic variation such as an active or a passive construction will not afflict the analysis, because the upper level meaning, which may be of interest in a dialog system, is equal for the sentences. Given the example in (27) "I will give you the book at work tomorrow" a semantic description could also abstract from the examples in (29).

```
(29)  I will give you the book at
work tomorrow.
The book will be given to you by me
at work tomorrow.
```

Finally, it should be mentioned that most systems providing either syntactic or semantic descriptions can also deliver or at least automatically incorporate "lower level" information such as POS. Thus, it may be feasible to write patterns combining restrictions based on lower level information and syntactic/semantic structure as well.

## EVALUATION OF THE INTEGRATED SYSTEM

To estimate the actual benefit of the shown integration an evaluation is necessary. Unfortunately, the evaluation of conversational systems is a complicated task. Nevertheless, a lot of different possibilities for testing and evaluation of dialog systems were proposed (e.g., Walker, 1997).

In a task based system, which delivers an error message if no reply could be determined, the application can be tested in a functional test using a test suite. The test suite contains pairs of input data and correct output that the system necessarily should be able to handle. In a batch process every input gets fed into the system. Afterwards the output gets compared with the reply from the test suite. If the system's reply matches the given output possibility the system seems to work. That way it is possible to calculate the coverage in terms of well-known input.

This black-box testing is not very meaningful for the chatbot scenario, because the chatbot's answer is too difficult to predict. The *ALICE* chatbot for example will always answer something even if the answer makes no sense at all, because at least one of the default patterns will match the input. This means the coverage of the chatbot system will always be 100%, unless the author eliminates all default patterns. However, a chatbot system without default patterns is a completely different system that will lose the last bit of intelligence it ever possessed.

The same problem occurs in a unit test, in which the coverage and accuracy of individual system components are tested. This is in fact very interesting for the integration scenario. Before an evaluation of the whole system, the testing of single components can figure out the additional benefit of added NLP technologies. Interesting measures for component evaluation of a dialog system are "Sentence Accuracy" (the percentage of completely and correctly understood utterances) and "Sentence Understanding Rate" (the percentage of utterances correctly assigned to a meaning representation). See McTear (2004) for a detailed overview. The problem is that it is unclear, what the "correctly" understood or assigned meaning of an utterance in a chatbot system should be.

Therefore, the only reasonable way to evaluate a chatbot with integrated NLP versus one without NLP is by experiments with users. Common evaluation features originating from the user evaluation of task-based dialog systems are for example "Task Ease", "Perceived Completion" and "Expected Behavior" (Walker et al., 2001). Other measurement terms for the chatbot scenario should be appropriateness of the given reply as well as the naturalness of the system.

## CONCLUSION

In this chapter, the main differences between traditional stimulus-response pattern matching chatbots and theory-based dialog systems have been reviewed. Certain similarities between the two were shown, but also great differences, such as the simpler input understanding and output generation.

It was stated that the main benefit of chatbots lies in the simple dialog management and the simple database development. Unfortunately, this is also simultaneously the source of some of the problems which are inherent in the chatbot's architecture: a flexible handling of surface variations while keeping constant control over the matched structure is impossible. At this point the advantages of Natural Language Technology can be of great help, as was illustrated with some examples.

Of course the integration of NLP technologies is not always an easy task and the developer needs to have a good understanding of the methods used. For this reason a general overview over several linguistic components was given. Nevertheless, a chatbot developer wanting to integrate NLP into an existing system will probably face problems with the post-processing of the results of an embedded NLP component depending on the actual system and modules used. The integration of linguistic knowledge into a chatbot system may therefore reduce the advantage of simple pattern-template authoring. Particularly, if more than one kind of information should be used to achieve flexible patterns, the author may have to invest more thoughts on how to write the pattern.

Moreover, it has to be clear that Natural Language Processing is not an easy task; even the best parser will not detect a valid structure for an ungrammatical input and fragmentary and invalid input is very common in dialog systems. Besides, parsing in particular is still comparatively fragile when applied to longer sentences.

The technologies also suffer from problems such as ambiguity and it can happen that a component delivers the wrong information, e.g., the wrong part of speech for an ambiguous word.

Some of the technologies reviewed here have been successfully integrated into AIML chatbots systems in addition to the traditional surface patterns and templates (Klüwer, 2007; Klüwer, 2009). This ensures the original coverage of the chatbot and enables further flexibility through the added technologies.

## FUTURE TRENDS

Future work on bringing together dialog systems and chatbots will focus on two main aspects. Firstly, evaluation measures and methods for further experiments will be necessary to calculate the benefit of each integrated component on the one hand and the increased performance of the whole system on the other hand. The system should be measured in terms of chatbot specific attributes such as the naturalness of the conversation.

Furthermore, it would be interesting to change the point of view and integrate chatbot functionality into dialog systems to gain more naturalness and open domain ability. While this is easily done and actually very common for simple pattern matching, the main problem deriving from this approach is the question of data acquisition. In opposition to the integration of dialog system technology into chatbots, which can be provided additionally, the inverse integration contains the task of converting the chatbot data to a linguistically motivated format. This is a time-consuming and most probably manual work. Future research will focus on how to acquire the data in a more comfortable way.

## REFERENCES

Adolphs, P., Cheng, X., Klüwer, T., Uszkoreit, U., & Xu, F. (2010). (to appear). Question answering biographic information and social network powered by the Semantic Web. In. *Proceedings of the LREC*.

Allen, J. F., Ferguson, G., Miller, B. W., Ringger, E. K., & Zollo, T. S. (2000). Dialogue systems: From theory to practice in TRAINS-96. In Dale, R., Moisl, R., & Somers, H. (Eds.), *Handbook of natural language processing*. New York, NY: Marcel Dekker.

Allen, J. F., & Perrault, C. R. (1980). Analyzing intentions in dialogues. *Artificial Intelligence*, *15*(3), 143–178. doi:10.1016/0004-3702(80)90042-9

Aust, H., Oerder, M., Seide, F., & Steinbiss, V. (1995). The Philips automatic train timetable information system. *Speech Communication*, *17*, 3–4. doi:10.1016/0167-6393(95)00028-M

Black, W. J., Rinaldi, F., & Mowatt, D. (1998) Facile: Description of the ne system used for muc-7. In *Proceedings of Message Understanding Conference*, *7*.

Bratman, M. E., Israel, D., & Pollack, M. (1991). Plans and resource-bounded practical reasoning. In Cummins, R., & Pollock, J. L. (Eds.), *Philosophy and AI: Essays at the interface* (pp. 1–22). Cambridge, MA: The MIT Press.

Bresnan, J. (Ed.). (1982). *The mental representation of grammatical relations. MIT Press Series on Cognitive Theory and Mental Representation*. Cambridge, MA: MIT Press.

Bui, T. H. (2006). *Multimodal dialogue management - state of the art*. (Technical Report, TR-CTIT-06-01), Enschede, Centre for Telematics and Information Technology: University of Twente.

Cohen, P. (1997). Dialogue modeling. In Cole, R., Mariani, J., Uszkoreit, H., Zaenen, A., & Zue, V. (Eds.), *Survey the state of the art in human language technology*. New York, NY: Cambridge University Press.

Cole, R. (Ed.). (1997). *Survey of the state of the art in human language technology*. New York, NY: Cambridge University Press.

Constantinides, P., Hansma, S., Tchou, C., & Rudnicky, A. (1998). A schema-based approach to dialog control. In *Proceedings of the International Conference on Spoken Language Processing* (pp. 409-412). Sydney, Australia.

Covington, M. A. (1984). *Syntactic theory in the High Middle Ages*. Cambridge, UK: Cambridge University Press. doi:10.1017/CBO9780511735592

Drozdzynski, W., Krieger, H.-U., Piskorski, J., Schäfer, U., & Xu, F. (2004). Shallow processing with unification and typed feature structures – foundations and applications. In *German AI Journal KI-Zeitschrift, 1*(4). Bremen, Germany: Böttcher Verlag/ Gesellschaft für Informatik e.V.

Francis, W. N., & Kučera, H. (1982). *Frequency analysis of English usage: Lexicon and grammar*. Boston, MA: Houghton Mifflin.

Jurafsky, D., & Martin, J. H. (2008). *Speech and language processing*. New Jersey: Prentice Hall International.

Klüwer, T. (2007). *Semantische Auszeichnungen in sprachverarbeitenden Prozeskettensystemen*. Unpublished Master's thesis. University of Cologne, Germany.

Klüwer, T. (2009). RMRSBot - using linguistic information to enrich a Chatbot. In Z. Ruttkay, M. Kipp, A. Nijholt & H. H. Vilhjálmsson (Eds.) *Proceedings of the 9th international Conference on intelligent Virtual Agents. Lecture Notes in Artificial Intelligence, vol. 5773*. Berlin/ Heidelberg, Germany: Springer Verlag.

Klüwer, T., Adolphs, P., Xu, F., Uszkoreit, H., & Cheng, X. (2010). Talking NPCs in a virtual game world. In *Proceedings of the ACL 2010 System Demonstrations. Annual Meeting of the Association for Computational Linguistics (ACL-2010)*, Uppsala, Sweden.

Kruijff, G.-J. M. (2002). *Formal and computational aspects of dependency grammar: History and development of DG.* (Technical report, ESSLLI-2002).

Kruijff, G.-J. M. (2005). Context-sensitive utterance planning for CCG. In *Proceedings of the European Workshop on Natural Language Generation.* Aberdeen, Scotland.

Kruijff, G.-J. M., Lison, P., Benjamin, T., Jacobsson, H., Zender, H., & Kruijff-Korbayova, I. (2009). Situated dialogue processing for human-robot interaction. In Christensen, H. I., Sloman, A., Kruijff, G.-J. M., & Wyatt, J. (Eds.), *Cognitive systems: Final report of the CoSy project.* Berlin/Heidelberg, Germany: Springer Verlag.

Lesh, N., Marks, J., Rich, C., & Sidner, C. L. (2004). *Man-computer symbiosis revisited: Achieving natural communication and collaboration with computers. Transactions on Electronics.* IEICE.

Manning, C., & Schütze, H. (2003). *Foundations of statistical natural language processing.* Cambridge, MA: The MIT Press.

Mauldin, M. L. (1994). ChatterBots, TinyMuds, and the Turing test: Entering the Loebner Prize competition. In *Proceedings of the Twelfth National Conference on Artificial intelligence* (vol. 1) (pp. 16-21). Seattle, WA: American Association for Artificial Intelligence.

McTear, M. F. (2004). *Spoken dialogue technology – toward the conversational user interface.* London, UK: Springer Verlag.

Peckham, J. (1993). A new generation of spoken dialogue systems: Results and lessons from the SUNDIAL project. In *Proceedings of 3rd European Conference on Speech Communication and Technology (Eurospeech'93)* (pp. 33-40). Berlin, Germany: ESCA.

Poesio, M. (2000). Semantic analysis. In Dale, R., Moisl, H., & Somers, H. (Eds.), *Handbook of natural language processing.* New York, NY: Marcel Dekker.

Pollard, C., & Sag, I. A. (1994). *Head-driven phrase structure grammar. Studies in Contemporary Linguistics.* Chicago, IL: University of Chicago Press.

Reiter, E., & Dale, R. (2000). *Building applied natural language generation systems.* Cambridge, UK: University Press. doi:10.1017/CBO9780511519857

Rich, C., & Sidner, C. L. (1998). COLLAGEN: A collaboration manager for software interface agents. *An International Journal: User Modeling and User-Adapted Interaction, 8*(3/4), 315–350. doi:10.1023/A:1008204020038

Searle, J. R. (1969). *Speech acts: An essay in the philosophy of language.* Cambridge, UK: University Press.

Steedman, M. (2001). *The syntactic process.* Cambridge, MA: The MIT Press.

Wahlster, W. (2000) (Ed.). *Verbmobil: Foundations of speech-to-speech translation.* Berlin/Heidelberg, Germany; New York, NY; Barcelona, Spain; Hong Kong; London, UK; Milan, Italy; Paris, France; Singapore; Tokyo, Japan: Springer.

Wahlster, W. (2006) (Ed.). *SmartKom - foundations of multimodal dialogue systems.* Berlin/Heidelberg, Germany; New York, NY; Barcelona, Spain; Hong Kong; London, UK; Milan, Italy; Paris, France; Singapore; Tokyo, Japan: Springer Cognitive Technologies.

Walker, M. A., Litman, D., Kamm, C., & Abella, A. (1997). PARADISE: A framework for evaluating spoken dialogue agents. In *Proceedings of the 35th Annual Meeting of the Association of Computational Linguistics* (ACL 97) (pp. 271-280). Morristown, NJ: ACL Press.

Walker, M. A., Passonneau, R., & Boland, J. E. (2001). Quantitative and qualitative evaluation of Darpa communicator spoken dialogue systems. In *Proceedings of the 39th Annual Meeting of the Association for Computational Linguistics* (ACL/EACL-2001) (pp. 515-522). Morgan Kaufmann Publishers.

Weizenbaum, J. (1966). ELIZA - A computer program for the study of natural language communication between man and machine. *Communications of the ACM*, *9*(1), 36–45. doi:10.1145/365153.365168

## KEY TERMS AND DEFINITIONS

**Ambiguity:** The capacity of single tokens and whole structures to denote different things with the same words. Examples of common ambiguity types are "lexical ambiguity" (e.g. words with more than one meaning) or "structural ambiguity", which originates from multiple possible relations of constituents to one another.

**Chatbot:** A text-based system which incorporates pattern-matching methods to conduct a conversation with another agent.

**Dialog Acts:** A possibility to encode an abstracted meaning of an utterance in a dialog. Via dialog acts the intention of an utterance regarding the context of the conversation can be described.

**Dialog Manager:** The component of a dialog system which is responsible for the processing of the next step the system should do. This includes verbal answers as well as other actions the system is capable of.

**Dialog System:** A system which can conduct a conversation with another agent, for example a human or another dialog system. Dialog systems can use various forms of input and output (e.g. speech, gestures or text).

**Language Generation:** The Natural Language Processing technology which is used to generate surface strings from an abstract description of language data. For example, Language Generation could be used to generate a surface form from the dialog act description of an utterance.

**Natural Language Understanding:** The task to understand what a natural language utterance may mean. Technically, this means to assign a chosen formal linguistic description to given language input.

**Parsing:** The Natural Language Processing technology which aims at the structural description of language data, usually a sentence or an utterance. The basis of the parsing process is a grammar describing possible structures.

**Pattern Matching:** A method to check a token or sequence of tokens for the presence of the constituents of a pattern. In this chapter, it denotes the method that chatbot systems use to assign input to output.

**Utterance:** The term used in dialog research to denote the smallest contribution of a participant. An utterance may be a whole sentence or also fragmentary data.

## ENDNOTES

1 The Penn Treebank Project annotates naturally-occurring text for linguistic structure, for example POS and sentence structure. See http://www.cis.upenn.edu/~treebank/ for more information.

2 A list of open source, freeware and commercial taggers can be found at: http://www-nlp.stanford.edu/links/statnlp.html#Taggers

3 One Example is the NE Recognizer integrated into the popular GATE framework. The open source NLP framework can be applied to various NLP applications and comes with integrated gazetteers. (http://gate.ac.uk/).

# Chapter 2
# Designing and Evaluating Interactive Agents as Social Skills Tutors for Children with Autism Spectrum Disorder

**Marissa Milne**
*Flinders University, Australia*

**Martin Luerssen**
*Flinders University, Australia*

**Trent Lewis**
*Flinders University, Australia*

**Richard Leibbrandt**
*Flinders University, Australia*

**David Powers**
*Flinders University, Australia*

## ABSTRACT

*Autism spectrum disorder (ASD) makes communication and social interaction very difficult for those affected. Existing studies have reported positive results for teaching social skills to children with ASD using human-controlled virtual agents and language skills using autonomous agents. Here we combine these approaches and investigate the potential of autonomous agents as social skills tutors. A system for audio-visually synthesising an agent is developed towards this purpose and utilised together with two tutoring modules that we specifically designed for teaching conversation skills and how to deal with bullying. Following evaluation, children's thoughts about their experience with the virtual tutor were investigated through use of a survey. The positive feedback and the modest but significant improvements in test scores for both modules suggest that this strategy for teaching social skills has much potential and that further research and development in this area would be eminently worthwhile.*

DOI: 10.4018/978-1-60960-617-6.ch002

## 1. INTRODUCTION

Inter-human communication is not just about explicitly conveying facts and plans, but also about building friendship, authority, and other aspects of social relationships. Non-verbal signals play as important a role as verbal ones in this context, and learning how to correctly decipher and respond to them is essential to success in life.

People with autism spectrum disorder (ASD) find this more challenging than others, and therefore often struggle to participate successfully in society. Recent trends are pointing to a future in which we will be expected to also interact with computers in a more social way. Embodied conversational agents (ECAs) represent the ultimate form of this. ECAs are virtual anthropomorphic interface agents that emulate human face-to-face dialogue across all the natural modalities, including speech, intonation, gesture, gaze, and other verbal and non-verbal signals. Such virtual humans offer a new yet at the same time very familiar means of interacting with computers, and in attempting to create them we invariably also gain practical insights into human-to-human interaction.

ECAs constitute the ideal medium not just to explore but to convey knowledge in this domain; indeed, to act as tutors in social interaction. A computer cannot replace a human expert at this task, but any basic skills that can be taught in this way will allow the expert to spend more time on the difficult cases. Children with ASD are a promising target for this computer-aided approach, as they have the most to benefit from basic tutoring and also the greatest potential for improvement. This chapter shall hence be concerned with the creation and evaluation of an ECA that can assist such children in acquiring essential social skills.

We begin with an overview of ASD and consider the potential benefits and drawbacks of autonomous virtual agents as social skills tutors for children with ASD. Earlier software-based interventions are discussed and several ideas brought together to establish a new ECA-based approach towards bridging the gap between the theory and the practice of assisting these children. We establish an ECA synthesis framework that is customisable for this purpose and offer details on its implementation. Two lesson modules are then developed for the benefit of children with ASD; one focusing on conversation skills and the other on dealing with bullying. These lessons were chosen as they reflect common difficulties that children with autism face every day due to their communication difficulties and difficulties with reading body language. After testing the effectiveness of the lessons, children's thoughts about their experience with the virtual tutor are investigated through use of a survey. We finish with a view towards the future, examining the further prospects of effective intervention with ECAs and the technologies that will contribute to it.

## 2 BACKGROUND

### 2.1 The Nature of Autism

Autism is a pervasive developmental disorder characterised by the 'triad' of impairments, encompassing impairments of communication and social skills as well as a tendency towards repeated patterns of interest and behaviour (American Psychiatric Association [*DSM-IV-TR*], 2000). Affected individuals may interpret language very literally, causing misunderstanding when sarcasm and metaphors are involved (Rapin and Tuchman, 2008).

Children with Autism Syndrome Disorder (ASD) frequently have difficulties in using and understanding non-verbal cues such as body language, gaze and facial expression, which reduces their ability to develop friendships and other relationships. Individuals with ASD can also find changes to their routines and environment quite confronting and stressful, as they struggle to generalise their skills to new situations. New concepts need to be taught to them explicitly, step by step.

Implications of this 'triad' of impairments are vital in committing to appropriate training that can help a wide range of individuals on the spectrum. Conversation management, including initiation and turn-taking, constitutes a particular challenge to such individuals and can be taught directly. Furthermore, considering the atypical behaviours some individuals exhibit, social training can also be of value, especially since autistic children are easily exposed to bullying and therefore particularly vulnerable. Such training can be performed by a human tutor, but there is a substantial time cost to it. Technology could offer valuable assistance in this instance.

## 2.2 How Interactive Agents Can Help

There are many reasons to suggest that using interactive virtual agents for teaching skills to children with autism can be advantageous, not least of which is the affinity with computers that individuals on the autistic spectrum are reported to have (Putnam & Chong, 2008). Virtual tutors also have the benefit of being available to the learner whenever they wish to learn; they will never get tired or frustrated after extensive repetition, unlike even the best intentioned human tutor, and they can provide consistent and predictable feedback (Massaro, 2004).

Especially valuable is the direct control over the sensory stimulus that virtual agents offer. Sensory difficulties are often co-morbid with autism and can lead to very low or very high sensory tolerance and, associated with this, extreme sensory avoidance and seeking behaviours. For instance, some individuals report that they find looking directly at other people's faces confronting, even painful in some instances. This is thought to be due at least in part to the sheer amount of detail and non-verbal information being communicated and understandably can lead to anxiety in social situations. In order to prevent sensory overload and the consequent stress to the learner, a virtual tutor may simply display less detail or possibly reduce it dynamically. Likewise, by adjusting the subtlety and complexity of both verbal and non-verbal cues used by the tutor, any lesson content can evolve with the learner's capabilities. Working at their own pace has been found to be particularly important for ASD individuals, as it allows them to have a sense of control and security (Parsons et al., 2000).

The benefits of virtual tutors may also extend to others in the learner's environment. As interactive agents provide an automated means of reinforcing at least the more routine aspects of the learner's program, they can help ease the burden on caregivers, teachers and other professionals that work with the learner. Moreover, using agents to train social skills avoids some of the pitfalls of learning in a real world environment, such as disturbing other people in that environment or learning inappropriate responses from them (Kerr, 2002).

A very reasonable concern here is that interacting with virtual people rather than actual people may actually amplify the social isolation and tendency towards repetitive behaviours that affect many individuals with ASD. However, it is important to understand that virtual tutors are not intended to replace actual interaction. Instead, they are to be used as a teaching tool that can prepare the learner for real world situations, helping them to participate successfully in the complex task of human-to-human interaction.

# 3 EXISTING TECHNOLOGY-BASED INTERVENTIONS

A range of technology-based interventions have been designed with ASD in mind, targeting a variety of the known deficits and challenges that these individuals face, and with varying levels of effectiveness. Most notably, several software packages exist that aim to teach children on the autistic spectrum how to read emotions from faces – 'Gaining Face', 'FaceSay' and 'Emotion Trainer' are examples of such programs.

Silver and Oakes (2001) performed a randomised control trial to test the effectiveness of the 'Emotion Trainer' with eleven pairs of children with autism matched by age, gender and grade. One child in each pair was given the intervention and the other was not. It was found that all children involved in the intervention improved their skills, but there was much individual variation. Generalisation from using the computer to completing a paper based task was also found, which is promising as it is commonly accepted that generalisation of skills to the real world is a major challenge for individuals with ASD.

## 3.1 Virtual Environment Interventions

Recently, more cutting edge technologies such as virtual environments and virtual peers are emerging as possible avenues for investigation. Such environments have been used for some time to teach individuals with autism a whole range of skills including specific life skills such as crossing the road, how to find a seat in a crowded public area and social interaction skills (Strickland 1998; Kerr 2002; Parsons, Mitchell, & Leonard, 2005).

Individuals with autism often find it hard to learn from their own mistakes and need to be explicitly told what went wrong, why it went wrong and also need assistance in identifying alternative strategies to use if they encounter the situation again. It has been suggested that virtual environments, particularly collaborative ones where multiple people are interacting within the one environment, provide a means to role-play situations in a controlled manner (Kerr, 2002).

Additionally, imaginative play is an important aspect of social interaction for children with autism. Herrera et al. (2008) explored the effectiveness of a virtual environment game that used a scaffolding approach to take children from functional interaction to imaginative play. They observed significant improvements to the children's skills and strong generalisation of these skills.

## 3.2 Virtual Peer Interventions

Virtual peers can be broadly categorised as being either *authorable* or *autonomous*. Authorable peers are controlled by some external entity, such as a researcher pushing buttons on a control panel, whereas autonomous peers are self contained and interact independently. In the field of virtual peers for children with autism, two research teams are especially prominent: Tartaro and Cassell (2008), who have developed 'Sam', an authorable peer, and Bosseler and Massaro (2003), who have developed 'Baldi' and 'Timo', which are autonomous peers. 'Sam' has been used to improve nonverbal communication and other social skills in children with autism, while 'Baldi' and 'Timo' have been used to extend vocabulary and improve language skills.

Tartaro and Cassell (2008) designed Sam to be gender ambiguous so that both boys and girls would feel comfortable interacting with it. Sam is authorable in that its behaviour is fully defined and controlled (i.e. 'authored') by a researcher who observes the human participant's actions towards Sam. In this way, the researcher – through Sam – engages children with autism in collaborative storytelling in order to teach them appropriate social skills, particularly turn taking.

Sam is also able to display positive verbal and non-verbal behaviours, such as appropriate gaze, nodding, smiling and prompting. Tartaro and Cassell (2008) found that after a period of structured interaction with Sam children with ASD significantly improved their scores on the Test of Early Language Development. In an earlier case study, Tartaro and Cassell (2006) also established that children improved their gaze behaviour through interacting with 'Sam' and were able to use their new skills with their peers, thus demonstrating that the use of virtual peers can lead to the generalisation of acquired skills.

The virtual head Baldi is an autonomous virtual peer that can synthesise highly realistic speech movements and is mainly intended as a language tutor (Massaro, 2003). Baldi is autonomous in that it requires no researcher to be in control or even present; it is part of an educational computer program that children can use independently.

The software is aimed at increasing learners' vocabulary by presenting them with new words in a variety of ways, for example showing the text, an informative icon and having Baldi speak the word aloud, alone and in a sentence that gives the word context. Bosseler and Massaro (2003) discovered that children with autism improved their vocabulary significantly more if they watched Baldi while he spoke than when they just listened. Even after a month, 85% of the words learned were retained (Massaro, 2004). More importantly, children were able to use this new vocabulary in everyday situations, providing further evidence of generalisation (Bosseler & Massaro, 2003).

Sam and Baldi have both inspired the present study, which concerns the development of an autonomous social skills tutor for children with autism. Specifically, it implies that our software, like Baldi, is not controlled by a researcher or other adult, but can be used independently by the learner. However, we do not teach language skills as Baldi did, but skills applicable to human-human social situations, much like with Sam.

## 4 IMPLEMENTATION OF AN EMBODIED CONVERSATIONAL AGENT

Embodied conversational agents (ECAs) are defined as animated interface agents that engage the user in real-time, multimodal dialogue as observed in human-to-human interaction (Cassell, 2001). A complete implementation of such an agent must embrace a variety of technologies in the fields of computer vision, speech recognition, and conversation management.

However, it is the synthesis that makes the first and lasting impression, and we tend to have high expectations in this regard, as an abundance of sophisticated virtual characters exist in modern media. Yet while they are becoming increasingly photorealistic, this has no correspondence in our ability to actually interact with them – even games rely mainly on pre-recorded animation and speech. Conversely, ECAs need to respond in real-time to events and should be able to act in ways not anticipated in advance, e.g. speak the name of a new user.

Suitable ECA synthesis systems have been developed previously by assorted research teams. The aforementioned 'Baldi' is an example of this and belongs into a growing collection of animated agents that have been developed and evaluated in the pedagogical context, although most only offer very basic synthesis and interactivity (Moreno & Flowerday, 2006).

In contrast, a smaller number of agents include perceptual and reasoning capabilities; notable but very task-specific work includes MIT Media Lab's series of agents, such as REA, the virtual real estate agent (Bickmore & Cassell, 2005). A broader view towards studying interhuman communication is taken by the virtual body 'Greta' (Poggi, Pelachaud, de Rosis, Carofiglio, & De Carolis, 2005) and virtual head 'Ruth' (Oh & Stone, 2007), although the emphasis here is firmly on synthesis again. 'Max' is another noteworthy agent in this category, and it also offers gestural interaction capabilities within a virtual environment (Kopp, Sowa, & Wachsmuth, 2004).

The main issue with all of these agents is that they exhibit unique, unchangeable identities, which limit any prospects of employing them in other tasks, as users – especially children – can be quite particular about whom they wish to interact with (Gulz & Haakeb, 2006). It has certainly been our observation that a character's appearance and voice can easily overshadow any other qualities of the interaction.

Being able to customise the synthesis of a virtual character is therefore critical to the success of using such a character in an application. In light of this, we created "Head X", an audiovisual synthesis platform for ECAs that was developed with diversity in mind: diversity in what it can synthesise, but also in what it can be used for. This particularly, but not exclusively, incorporates the needs of the ECA's audience in this project. As the name suggests, Head X focuses on synthesising a head, as the face is generally the most expressive part of the body. The following sections will describe the essential technologies involved in this.

## 4.1 Face Synthesis

If you needed a custom 3D face, you would traditionally make use of the services of a 3D modelling artist, who would invest great manual effort into making it look natural and real. On a small budget, this is rarely practical, especially if your requirements frequently change or involve multiple different faces. Fortunately, humans look quite similar, so there is an easier way of accomplishing this. Elemental to this is a 3D parametric model whose parameters encode the natural variations of faces, so that even non-artists can produce a wide range of realistic characters by simply modifying these parameters.

A well-established process for obtaining such a parametric face model is to scan different faces of real people with a laser (Blanz & Vetter, 1999). With correct correspondence for the sampled geometry of a large enough face set, a statistical model can be fitted to the face distribution. New variations that lie within the bounds of this model will lead to new faces that still retain plausibility. The most important parameters of the face can be extracted using Principal Component Analysis (PCA), but these may not correspond to any intuitive facial attributes, such as gender or age. Instead, such attributes must be explicitly mapped to the parameter space of the model, using a hand-labelled set of example faces, with each label indicating the markedness of an attribute. The same process can be followed to distinguish facial expressions.

The above is a complex undertaking, but quality parametric models are readily available commercially. For our project, we acquired an academic license to the FaceGen SDK, a parametric face model that also includes basic blendshapes for facial expressions (Singular Inversions, 2009). Besides offering a large number of intuitive parameters, its 'PhotoFit' system simplifies creation of new faces by allowing 2D photos of a person to be semi-automatically converted into 3D models. Although its commercial nature restricts its use to licensed institutions, it is comparatively affordable for what it offers. The FaceGen Modeller tool permits easy customisation of faces and exports them into parametric face coordinates or full 3D models. As shown in Figure 1, these can subsequently be imported into our Head X software, which visualises and animates the face in real-time via the OpenGL graphics interface.

## 4.2 Speech Synthesis

In games and other media that involve virtual characters, speech is typically produced by a real human, and character animation must simply follow the recorded audio signal. A virtual character designed for flexible conversation, however, should just be able to take a text – e.g. from a conversation manager – and automatically convert it into audiovisual speech. A variety of software options exist for synthesising the audio component of speech, but they are rarely as freely configurable as the faces discussed above. Natural sounding voices generally follow a unit selection approach that picks speech fragments from a large database of speech of a single person. Due to the effort involved in collecting this data, the best voices tend to again be offered commercially.

Head X supports two text-to-speech (TTS) interfaces, MARY and SAPI, that provide access to free and commercial voices, respectively. MARY

*Figure 1. Head X animates a virtual head using a FaceGen 3D model and a corresponding face coordinate obtained from the freely available FaceGen Modeller. With a 3D modelling tool, additional head accessories can also be fitted to the animated head.*

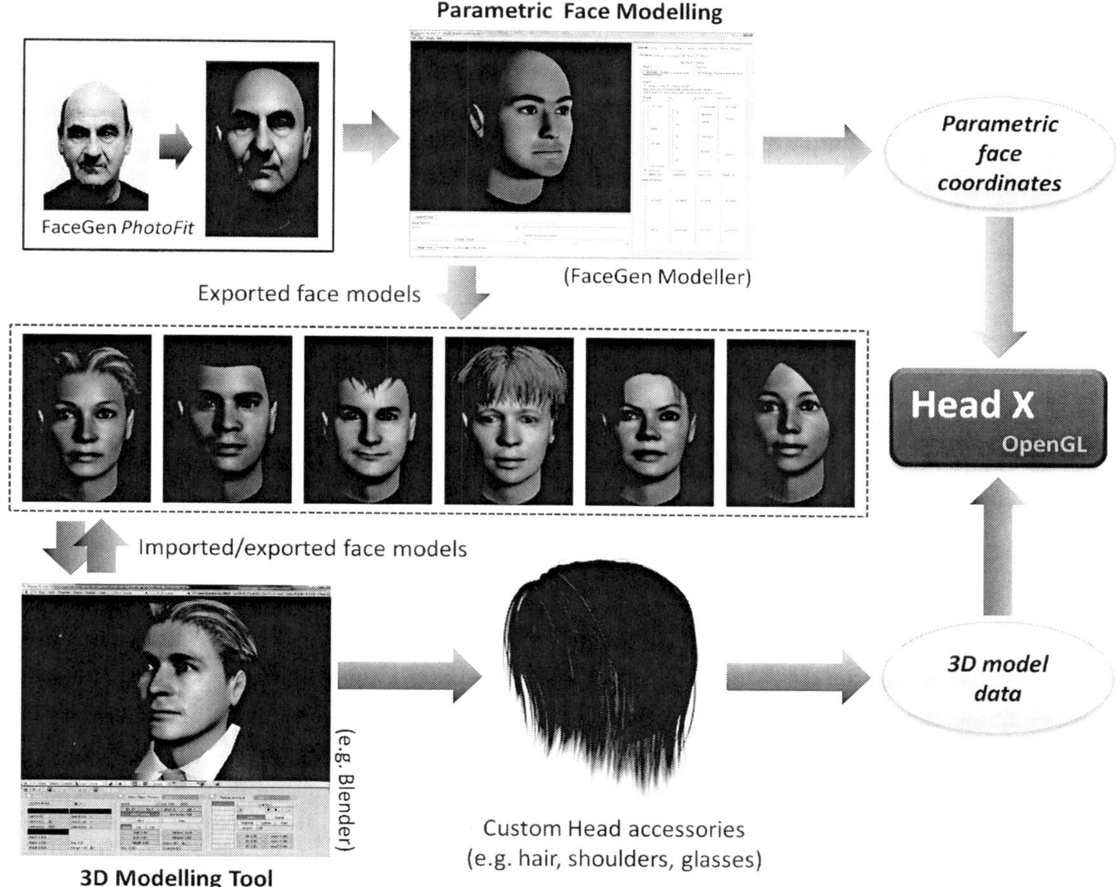


is open source and well-suited for research, but the availability of high-quality voices for it is limited (Schröder & Trouvain, 2003). In contrast, Microsoft's SAPI 5.3 Speech API is used by a vast library of voices from numerous companies in multiple languages and accents. SAPI also supports XML extensions, including SSML, that can be included in the text to be spoken and modify rate, pitch, and other aspects of the voice. For our tutors, we relied on Australian English SAPI voices, developed by Nuance Communications and offered as part of various screen reader packages.

## 4.3 Speech Animation

The FaceGen base model includes a comprehensive set of 39 blendshapes, 16 of which represent possible mouth shapes used during speech (so-called visemes). These need to be animated in synchrony with the synthesised audio output. Rather than analysing either the audio or the text, we rely on the SAPI (and the MARY) TTS system to supply the necessary information directly.

The SAPI interface affords real-time feedback from the voice engine by triggering viseme events whenever a viseme boundary is reached as it speaks. The SAPI 5 viseme set consists of 22 visemes that are based on the original 'Disney 13' set, which were chosen by Disney animators as being required to properly animate speech in their movies. Each SAPI event contains the current viseme code and its duration. Conversely, MARY does not support viseme events, but offers timed SAMPA phonemes for the outputted speech. Both the MARY phonemes and the SAPI visemes need to be mapped to the blendshapes of the 3D model, as neither exactly matches what is provided by FaceGen. We have established visually acceptable mappings for each, based on earlier work by Wang, Emmi, and Faloustos (2007).

The selected sequence of blendshapes needs to be blended into a smooth animation. For this purpose, we take a user-defined number of frames per second and weigh all the nearby blendshapes discretely for each frame. As depicted in step 4 of Figure 2, each viseme or morph is transitioned to and from by increasing and decreasing (or ramping) the weight associated with that morph's frame. The style of ramp is controlled by a customisable ramping function, which overlaps into the adjacent frames. However, even a smooth ramp and overlap is not safe from aliasing artefacts, so a final mixing of the current and adjacent frames is performed to overcome this. Individual frames are visualised when the corresponding position is reached in the audio stream; the process is illustrated in Figure 3.

### 4.4 Non-Verbal Animation

Speech is not the only means by which the Head can communicate with the user. The face is a source of many non-verbal signals that express emotion and intent, which are specifically relevant to the lesson plans for individuals with ASD.

FaceGen includes seven blendshapes for basic emotions, and further blendshapes for eye, eyelid, and eyebrow movements. Head X permits the user to define composites of all available blendshapes as facial expressions (or gestures), which can be triggered interactively and are animated in the same way that speech is.

However, when multiple blendshapes are applied simultaneously, unwanted results may appear because the blendshapes will stack. Our system is therefore designed to offer multiple expression channels, where expressions on separate channels only interact in restricted ways. By default, there is speech channel, an emotion channel, and an idle channel; expressions do not stack between these. The idle channel is automatically filled with randomly scheduled animations, such as head bobbing and blinking and subtle expressions that give the viewer the impression that the head is alive.

## 5 DESIGN CONSIDERATIONS FOR LEARNERS WITH ASD

Designing ECA-supported lessons for individuals with ASD brings with it a number of special considerations. Sensory overload is one of the most important issues, as individuals on the spectrum can have a very low to very high sensory tolerance. As a rule, any non-essential aspects should be omitted. For example, superfluous animations, sound effects or images can be distracting or cause fixation (Davis, Robins, Dautenhahn, Nehaniv, & Powell, 2005). Keeping with this, the teaching modules developed here use no sounds or animations outside of the ECA itself, and the display is uncluttered. Colour schemes need to be carefully considered; generally muted colours are best received. Low sensory tolerance or a lack of fine motor skills can mean that using a mouse is troublesome, so a touch screen or voice recognition implementation may be considered (Davis et al. 2005; Brown, Standen, Proctor, & Sterland, 2001).

As some children also suffer from low auditory tolerance, a set up that allows for choice between speaking, clicking or typing responses and having feedback presented visually, textually or verbally may ultimately be the best solution. For this prototype, participants were able to progress through

*Figure 2. Five steps to smoothly animating visemes over a sequence of image frames: visemes (phonemes with MARY) are mapped to the available blendshapes via a customisable ramping function (a sine curve by default), then discretised into frames, and finally again intermixed with neighbouring frames.*

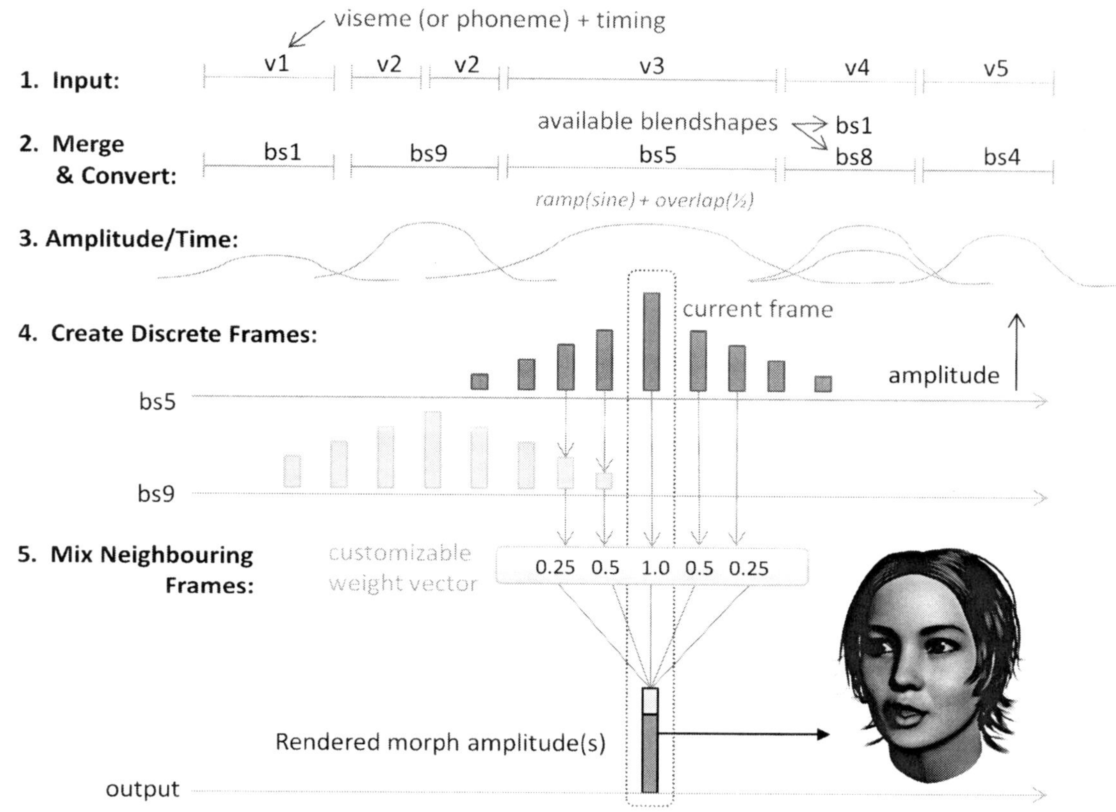


*Figure 3. Synchronisation of audiovisual speech is based upon either delaying frames if the audio needs to catch up or dropping frames if visual rendering is too slow*

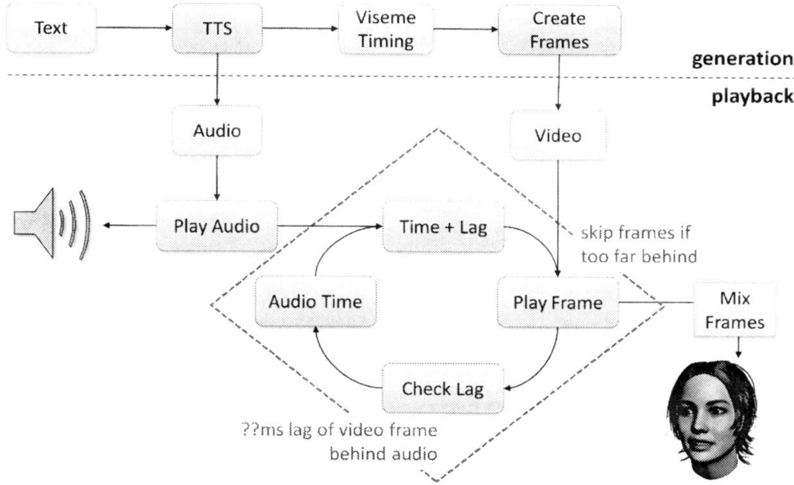

*Figure 4. A screenshot of the conversation module*

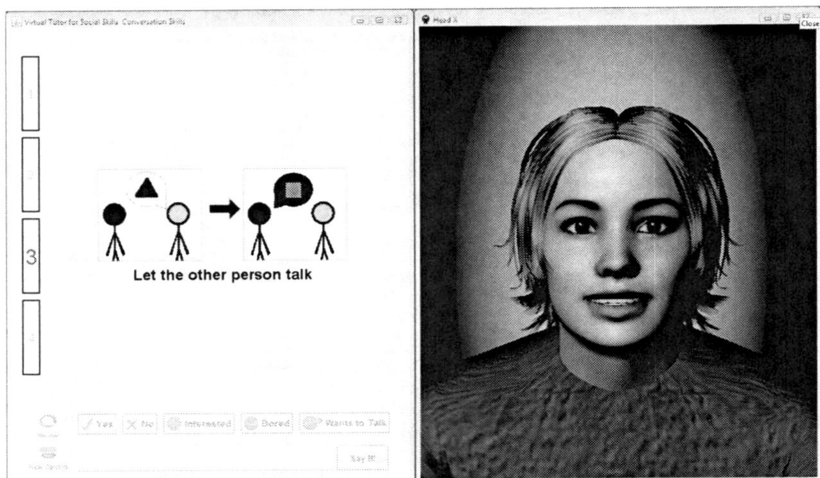


the entire module by clicking icons and could type a response if desired. In the future, incorporating assistive technologies such as speech recognition and touch screens would be desirable.

Due to the communication impairment that is associated with autism, the majority of sufferers tend to be primarily visual learners. Icons with clear meanings rather than text labels are often a good choice, and thus have been used wherever possible in these modules, as can be seen in Figure 4. Timely feedback that explicitly tells the learner how appropriate their response was is essential, as ambiguity can cause anxiety and subtle cues are often missed (Brown et al., 2001; Parsons et al., 2000).

Additionally, any rewards a learner receives must reinforce the task at hand. Davis et al. (2005) found that if this is not the case, learners are likely to rush tasks just to receive the reward at the end. To this end, the virtual tutor praises the student when a correct answer is chosen, and guides them towards the correct answer in a non-judgemental manner if they have difficultly.

Many studies emphasise the importance of self-paced learning and task repetition as it gives individuals with autism a sense of control which reduces anxiety and therefore improves lesson retention (Davis et al., 2005; Brown et al., 2001; Parsons et al., 2000). The structure of the lesson modules follows a predictable pattern and users have the option of having the tutor repeat the last question again, both in an effort to reduce the risk of anxiety.

Our social world is dynamic and very complex, which leads to individuals with autism finding it difficult to learn social skills when they are being bombarded with so much sensory input and so many distractions. Kerr (2002) and Parsons and Mitchell (2002) both emphasise the need for scaffolding, starting with very basic scenarios with lots of prompting and gradually fading the prompts and increasing the complexity and distractions involved.

Figure 5 shows how complex social interactions can be broken down and taught as explicit steps. The strongest advantage of virtual tutors and environments is that the situations can be broken down to the basics and tailored to suit the learner's needs. Parsons and Mitchell (2002) found that with gradual prompt fading, generalisation of social skills to the real world could be achieved.

*Figure 5. Screenshots of the dealing with bullying module showing how complex interactions can be explicitly taught in steps*

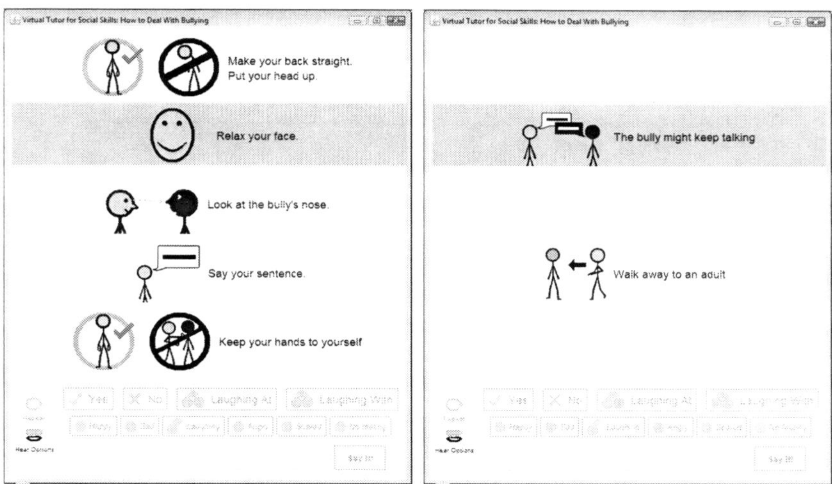


## 6 SYSTEM EVALUATION

There were two evaluations performed in relation to this prototype. The first, an expression evaluation, was performed during the software development stage and the second, the module evaluation, followed completion of the prototype.

The purpose of the expression evaluation was to ensure that the expressions modelled by the virtual tutor, throughout the conversation tutoring module in particular, were sufficiently accurate. This involved evaluating neurotypical adults' perceptions of the expressions used, as if they cannot identify the expressions presented, then we cannot expect children with ASD who suffer from deficits in this area to be able to or to gain any benefit from the use of these expressions.

The primary goal of the second evaluation was to indicate whether it was worthwhile developing a more extensive educational system centred on an autonomous virtual tutor, by evaluating the prototype developed here. There are several aspects to this which were considered, including whether the learners demonstrated an improvement in test scores after using the tutoring software and whether they found the educational experience to be a positive one.

### 6.1 Expression Evaluation

A core aspect of the conversation skills module involves the virtual agent modelling facial expressions for the learner so they can become aware of the nonverbal cues associated with particular emotional-intentional stances, namely boredom, interest and wanting to speak.

The portrayal of expressions associated with feelings of boredom, interest and wanting to speak were informed by combining the work of Grun (1998), Kroes (2007) and Straker (2008). It is unreasonable to expect children with ASD to apply their knowledge of the virtual person's expressions to a real person if neurotypical individuals cannot, and so as part of the developmental stage of the tutoring software, an evaluation was run to assess how realistic neurotypical adults judged the expressions to be.

*Table 1. Multiple choice summary data from the expression evaluation*

| Multiple Choice Question Data | | | |
|---|---|---|---|
| **Target Responses** | **Bored** | **Interested** | **Wants to Talk** |
| **Count** | 25 | 20 | 18 |
| **Percentage** | 100% | 80% | 72% |
| **Significance** *(binomial method)* | $p < 0.0001$ | $p < 0.0001$ | $p < 0.0001$ |

### 6.1.1 Method

Twenty five neurotypical adult participants were involved in the expression evaluation, of which seventeen were male and eight female. Most participants were sourced from various departments within the university, while others were from outside of the university. No participants were involved in the development of the software.

The evaluation was conducted through an automated program developed specifically for this task that presented participants with six non-fiction stories, split into two sections of three stories each. Two Head X instances were launched and controlled by the evaluation program. One with a male identity remained out of sight and read aloud the stories while the other, with a female identity, was visible to participants and displayed expressions in response to the stories. All data was recorded and saved automatically by the purpose-built software.

Three possible emotional-intentional stances to the conversation were investigated, these being boredom, interest and wanting a turn to talk. At the end of each story, participants were prompted to give a response regarding how they perceived the listener throughout the story. For the first three stories, participants were asked *How did she feel while listening? What did she want to do?* and provided with a text box to write their response in. For the last three stories, participants were asked *Which of these best describes her?* and provided with the following six options: bored, interested, wanting to talk, pleased, confused, upset. The open-ended questions were always first and the multiple choice questions were always last, to ensure that the multiple choice options did not influence the responses for the open-ended section. For the multiple choice component, participants scored 1 for each correct answer and 0 for each incorrect answer. For the open-ended questions, participants scored 1 if they used at least one of the expected key words or phrases in their response, and 0 if they did not.

Throughout each story, the listening virtual person would make facial expressions and in some cases use verbal cues that were intended to give an indication of one of three possible emotional-intentional stances to the conversation: boredom, interest or wanting a turn to talk. Six non-verbal cues from the same stance were presented during each story, resulting in two stories dedicated to bored expressions, two dedicated to interested expressions and two dedicated to wanting to talk expressions.

### 6.1.2 Results

Table 1 shows a summary of participants' selections in the multiple choice section. All participants answered correctly in the Bored condition and over 70% answered correctly in both the Interested and Wants to Talk conditions. A binomial test of significance confirmed these findings ($p < 0.0001$ for all conditions).

Table 2 summarises participants' responses in the open-ended section. In all conditions, over 75% of participants used at least one of the target

*Table 2. Open-ended summary data from the expression evaluation*

| Open-Ended Question Data | | | |
|---|---|---|---|
| **Target Responses** | **Bored** | **Interested** | **Wants to Talk** |
| **Keywords and Phrases** | bored / disinterested / uninterested | interested / wanted to hear more / fascinated / intrigued | wanted to talk / interrupt / ask a question |
| **Count** | 24 | 22 | 19 |
| **Percentage** | 96% | 88% | 76% |

words or phrases in their response. These results indicate that participants were able to successfully interpret the presented expressions, even in the open-ended condition where they were not given any cues to guide their decisions.

It is noteworthy that there is a strong correlation between the responses in the multiple choice condition and the responses in the open ended condition ($R = 0.94$ and $R^2 = 0.88$). Given the assumption that the open-ended condition provides at least as many implicit choices as the closed, multiple choice condition and that the percentages in all open-ended cases exceed the lowest percentage response in Table 2, it may also be concluded that these results are significant to $p < 0.0001$ (by binomial test, based on assumption of choice from at least 6 alternatives).

### 6.1.3 Discussion

The data obtained from this experiment indicate that the depiction of boredom presented to participants is sufficiently accurate, as all 25 participants were able to answer correctly in the multiple choice stage ($p < 0.0001$, by binomial method) and in the open-ended section, 24 of the 25 participants used at least one of the key words and phrases of 'bored', 'disinterested' or 'not interested' in their description of the virtual person. Combined, these results indicate that participants were able to successfully interpret the non-verbal cues presented by the virtual person in this condition, and hence suggest that the portrayal of boredom used here was sufficiently accurate for use in the prototype tutoring software.

For the Interested and Wanting to Talk conditions, the results indicate that participants were able to successfully interpret the given expressions the majority of the time, supporting the notion that the depiction of these expressions was sufficient. However, the results also reflect the limitations of the current technology and the challenges inherent in presenting the somewhat similar expressions of interested and wanting to talk effectively.

In the multiple choice section, 20 of 25 participants responded correctly for the Interested condition and 18 of 25 chose the correct response in the Wanting to Talk condition ($p < 0.0001$ for both). Supporting this, over 75% of participants used at least one of the listed key words or phrases in their description of the interested and wanting to talk expressions in the open-ended stage. Incorrect responses for the Interested condition indicated that some participants felt the virtual person was making a routine show of listening but was not truly interested or felt that she was amused, while in the Wanting to Talk condition some felt she was amused or simply being a good listener and encouraging the speaker to continue.

Interestingly, for the Wanting to Talk condition, there was disagreement between participants about whether the motivation for the virtual person wanting to speak was that she was interested and wanted to contribute, disinterested and wanted to change the subject or frustrated at not being given a chance to speak. While there is clearly room for improvement, this outcome indicates that the current expressions for the Interested and Wants to Talk conditions should be adequate for conversation training.

From informal observation and discussion, we noted that many participants felt the virtual person's nodding movements when combined with a leaning forward movement appeared unnatural. This may have had some impact on their perception of the virtual person's feelings and intentions, and as such could be one of the causes of the lower percentage of correct responses in the Wants to Talk condition, where this combination was used.

More importantly, it may be that this expression requires significant refinement to truly be a useful teaching aide to children with autism. If neurotypical individuals perceive it as unnatural, it is unlikely that children with ASD who struggle to generalise concepts will be able to successfully apply their knowledge of the virtual person's modelled body language to a real person. Given the limitations of the technology as it stands, particularly the limited movement of the shoulders in relation to the head, this was the closest representation that could be achieved. However, the technology is research in progress in itself, both by our own researchers and those in the wider community, and as such a more realistic portrayal of these expressions should be achievable in future.

## 6.2 Module Evaluation

Two lesson modules were developed for use with the ECA, one focussing on the identified area of need surrounding conversation skills, and the other teaching a simple strategy to help children with autism deal safely with bullying. The virtual agent used for this evaluation is an autonomous social skills tutor, as participants use the software independently, the software has sufficient decision making capabilities to not require outside input, and the skills it teaches are aimed at improving the learner's skills in human-human social interactions.

### 6.2.1 Conversation Skills Lesson

The aims of the conversation skills lesson were to teach students how to recognise the facial expressions that indicate when their conversation partner is feeling bored, interested or wants a turn to speak, and to encourage children to take notice of these expressions through developing an understanding of the importance of being a good conversation partner. Additionally, the lesson plan aimed to foster an understanding of appropriate actions to take when these expressions are recognised, e.g. changing the topic of conversation when the person listening appears bored or giving them the opportunity to speak when they wish to.

### 6.2.2 Dealing with Bullying Lesson

The dealing with bullying skills lesson is heavily based on work by Carol Gray (2001), which refers to 'social mistakes' to explain inappropriate behaviour between peers, and explains that these mistakes only become bullying when they are repeated over and again, helping learners understand the difference between bullying and a once-off conflict. Additionally, learners were taught about the difference between laughing with and laughing at someone. The strategy for dealing with bullying involves three simple steps; think about a true fact, say one sentence and walk away to an adult. This is concise and explicitly taught, and it is hoped that this will help learners to use good self-control and successfully deal with bullying situations.

### 6.2.3 Method

Fourteen participants were involved in the study, three with high functioning autism, ten with Asperger Syndrome and one with classic autism. The study was advertised in the AutismSA e-newsletter and families contacted the researcher to become involved. Anecdotally, many parents stated that

*Figure 6. A screenshot of the dealing with bullying module*

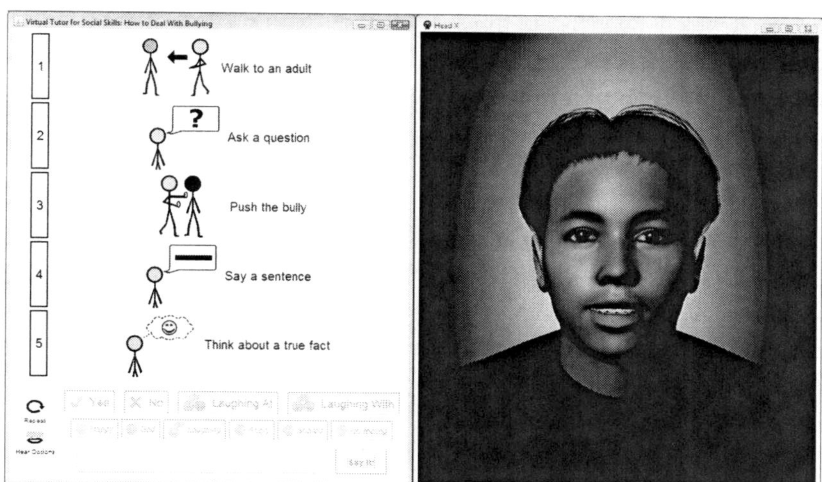


their interest in the study stemmed from their child's interest in computers.

Six of the participants were involved in the evaluation of both tutors, four participated in just the conversation skills tutor and four participated in just the dealing with bullying skills tutor. This resulted in ten children participating in the conversation tutor evaluation (mean age: 10.5, range 6 to 15) and ten participating in the dealing with bullying skills tutor evaluation (mean age: 9.9, range 6 to 15). The evaluation was conducted using a desktop computer for ten of the participants, with the other four participants using a laptop computer. In both cases an external optical mouse and external speakers were used.

Several practical issues had to be considered during the design of the evaluation process, including that the participants are young and as such are likely to get bored quickly. Conversely, we needed to gather enough data to achieve informative results. For this reason, we constructed the evaluation process in such a way that an individual can complete the whole process in roughly an hour. The evaluation process for both the conversation tutor and dealing with bullying skills tutor was identical, each consisting of three rounds of interaction with the virtual tutor. Each round was designed to take approximately fifteen minutes, with a five minute break between each.

Each fifteen minute lesson block was automated by the tutoring software, including pre-testing for each of the three rounds and post-testing for the final round. All lesson content was spoken aloud by the Head X tutor, which was launched and controlled by an application that was custom-built for this experiment. Accompanying icons, words and other interactive features such as streaming video were displayed on this custom-built component, an example of which can be seen in Figure 6.

All data was recorded automatically by the program. At the conclusion of each module, a survey was completed which investigated participants' thoughts about their experience and provided an opportunity to offer ideas for future development. All participants are considered high-functioning and thus are capable of providing reliable responses.

Before starting the software, each participant was shown a printed screen capture of it. The behaviour of all buttons was explained and participants were encouraged to watch and listen to the tutor carefully. This was aimed at reducing anxiety, as participants were given prior warning about what to expect during the program. Parents remained in the room with the child but were not permitted to assist. This was in an effort to minimise any stress that may have been experienced by the participants being in an unfamiliar situation.

Each fifteen minute block started with a set of questions, considered to be pre-test questions in round one and delayed interim post-test questions in rounds two and three. Round three also ended with a set of questions identical to the pre-test questions. This resulted in rounds one and two having tests only at the beginning, and round three having tests at the beginning and end.

Initially, all rounds were going to have tests at the start and end, however due to time constraints, the already repetitive nature of the lessons and a concern that participants would become bored, it was decided that the question blocks described here would be adequate. This avoided participants undergoing testing before and after their five minute break. It was decided that a test after the break would give a better indication of participants' learning, rather than testing before the break when participants may just be remembering facts instead of applying concepts. The pre-test and post-test were designed to test all lesson content, while the interim tests focused on the lesson content of only the preceding fifteen minute block.

In the conversation tutor there were three types of questions. In 'face test' questions, the virtual tutor modelled a facial expression, possibly accompanied by a verbal cue, and participants were asked to appropriately label the modelled expression. In 'action test' questions, the virtual tutor asked a question such as, *If the person you are talking to is bored, which of these is the best thing to do?* and participants were asked to choose the appropriate action from a list of options. In 'combined test' questions, participants were presented with an expression and asked to determine the appropriate action to take from the listed options, in essence combining the previous two question types.

In the dealing with bullying skills tutor, there were four types of questions. In 'strategy steps' questions, participants were asked to identify what they would do first, next and last if confronted with a bullying situation by clicking on options presented on the screen. In 'is friendly' and 'is bullying' questions, participants were asked to identify whether a scenario was a friendly or bullying situation. In 'laughing test' questions, participants were asked to identify whether a presented scenario constituted laughing with or laughing at someone.

All sets of questions were presented in random order to reduce the effect that any particular ordering may have had on the outcome, and the delayed post-test questions were also partially random in that the particular expression tested was randomly chosen from a set of possibilities. Throughout these question blocks no feedback was given and a new question was provided as soon as a response was made to the presented question. At the end of each block, the virtual person thanked the participant for answering their questions and the tutor moved onto the instructional component.

### 6.2.4 Results

Comparison of the pre-test from round one and the post-test from round three revealed that most participants achieved at least a small improvement in their test scores. For the conversation skills tutor, the mean and median improvements were both 1.8 out of a total of nine questions, representing a 32% improvement on average.

Using a Wilcoxon Signed Rank test, this overall improvement was found to be statistically significant ($p < 0.05$) supporting the notion that it was the use of the tutoring software that lead to this outcome. A visual representation of each participant's pre-test to post-test scores can be seen in Figure 7a. On further analysis of the data, significance was reached for the 'face test' question section ($p < 0.05$, Wilcoxon Signed Rank test) but was not reached for the 'action test' or 'combined test' sections, with many participants answering

*Figure 7. Comparison of pre-test and post-test scores for both tutors*

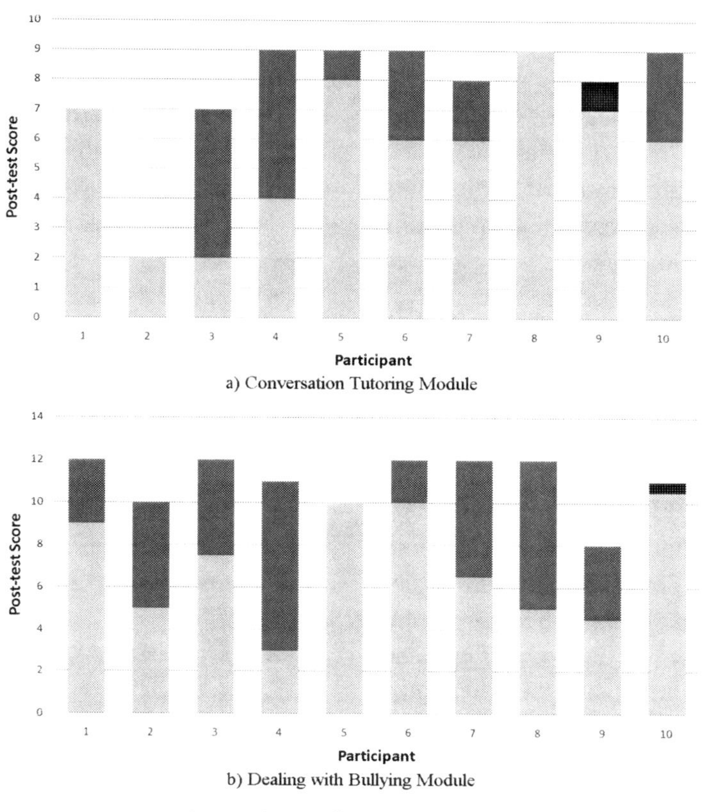


correctly in the pre-test and thus having no room for improvement in the post-test.

The data gathered for the dealing with bullying skills tutor indicates that in all but two cases, participants made at least a small improvement from pre-test to post-test. The mean improvement for the dealing with bullying skills tutor was 3.8 and the median was 4 out of a total of twelve questions. This represents a 54% improvement on average. A summary of participant's pre-test to post-test scores can be seen in Figure 7b. This result was found to be significant through a Wilcoxon Signed Rank test ($p < 0.01$), supporting the notion that, as in the results for the conversation tutor, the improvement here is the result of participants' interaction with the social skills tutoring software.

For both modules, the interim tests were analysed to investigate whether the participants gained any benefit from undertaking the fifteen minute lesson block more than once. In all but one module section, participants made a significant improvement between the pre-test of round one and the pre-test of round two ($p < 0.01$, Wilcoxon Signed Rank test), but no significant improvements after that. The exception was when participants were learning to distinguish between interested and wanting to talk expressions, where a significant improvement between the pre-test of round two and the pre-test of round three was also found ($p < 0.01$, Wilcoxon Signed Rank test), indicating that in this case it was beneficial to undertake two fifteen minute rounds with the tutoring software.

For the conversation tutor, an analysis was done on each of the components of the test. The test results were divided into a 'strategy steps' component and a 'situational reasoning' component. Statistical significance was reached only for the 'strategy steps' section ($p<0.01$, Wilcoxon Signed Rank test). Again, a high number of participants answered the 'situational reasoning' questions correctly in the pre-testing stage, so in these cases there was no scope for increased scores.

The seven-point Likert scale data from the conversation tutor survey was analysed, and it was found that for all conditions the mode was six or higher, indicating a high level of agreement with all statements. For both the mean and median, a response of five or more was obtained for all questions except the 'helped me learn' question, which had a response of over four. A visual depiction of the frequency data can be seen in Figure 8a. From observation it becomes clear that most responses were in agreement with the statements, suggesting that overall participants' experiences with the conversation tutor were positive. Most notable is that all participants in the conversation tutoring evaluation strongly agreed with the statement 'the tutors were friendly'.

For all Likert scale statements in the dealing with bullying skills tutor survey the mode is six or more, with the exception of the 'helped me learn' question which has dual modes of five and seven. The median for all questions is five or more, and the mean is five or more for all questions except the 'helped me learn' condition, in which it is over four. As four is the middle point of the Likert scale, and hence assumed to indicate neither agreement nor disagreement, these results suggest that overall participants had a positive experience with the dealing with bullying skills tutoring software.

Figure 8b provides a visual depiction of the multiple choice survey data for the dealing with bullying tutor. It can be seen that the majority of responses are five or higher, indicating agreement with the statements presented. Once again, all participants gave a rating of six or seven for the statement 'the tutors were friendly'. Some disagreement was obtained for the statements 'it helped me to learn', 'it was fun' and 'it was easy to understand what the tutors said'. These ratings are supported by the results of the open-ended questions, which can be seen in Table 4.

A summary of participants' comments for the open ended survey section for both the conversation tutor and dealing with bullying tutor is given in Tables 3 and 4, respectively. Common issues included the length of the evaluation process and the voice of the tutors, in particular the male tutor. Conversely, common strengths included the variety of interactive content, especially the streaming video, the appearance of the virtual people, the clearly worded questions and content and having the opportunity to repeat tasks.

### 6.2.5 Discussion

On a very positive note, we found that the overall improvements in participants' test results reached significance for both tutors, strongly suggesting that the gains made were due to the use of the tutoring software and not simply due to chance or other external factors. On breaking the pre- and post-tests down into their constituents, it appears that only the 'face test' component in the conversation tutor and the 'strategy steps' component in the dealing with bullying tutor reached significance; however, other sections such as the 'combined test' questions in the conversation tutor were nearing significance also.

In several cases participants answered a high number of questions correctly in the pre-test, leaving little scope for improvement. This suggests that for some participants the lesson content and difficulty level of the given questions was not sufficiently challenging. As the evaluation included six to fifteen year olds, the content had to be simple enough for the younger and lower functioning participants to cope with; consequently, it was not sufficiently challenging for many of the

*Figure 8. Summary of Likert scale survey data for both tutors*

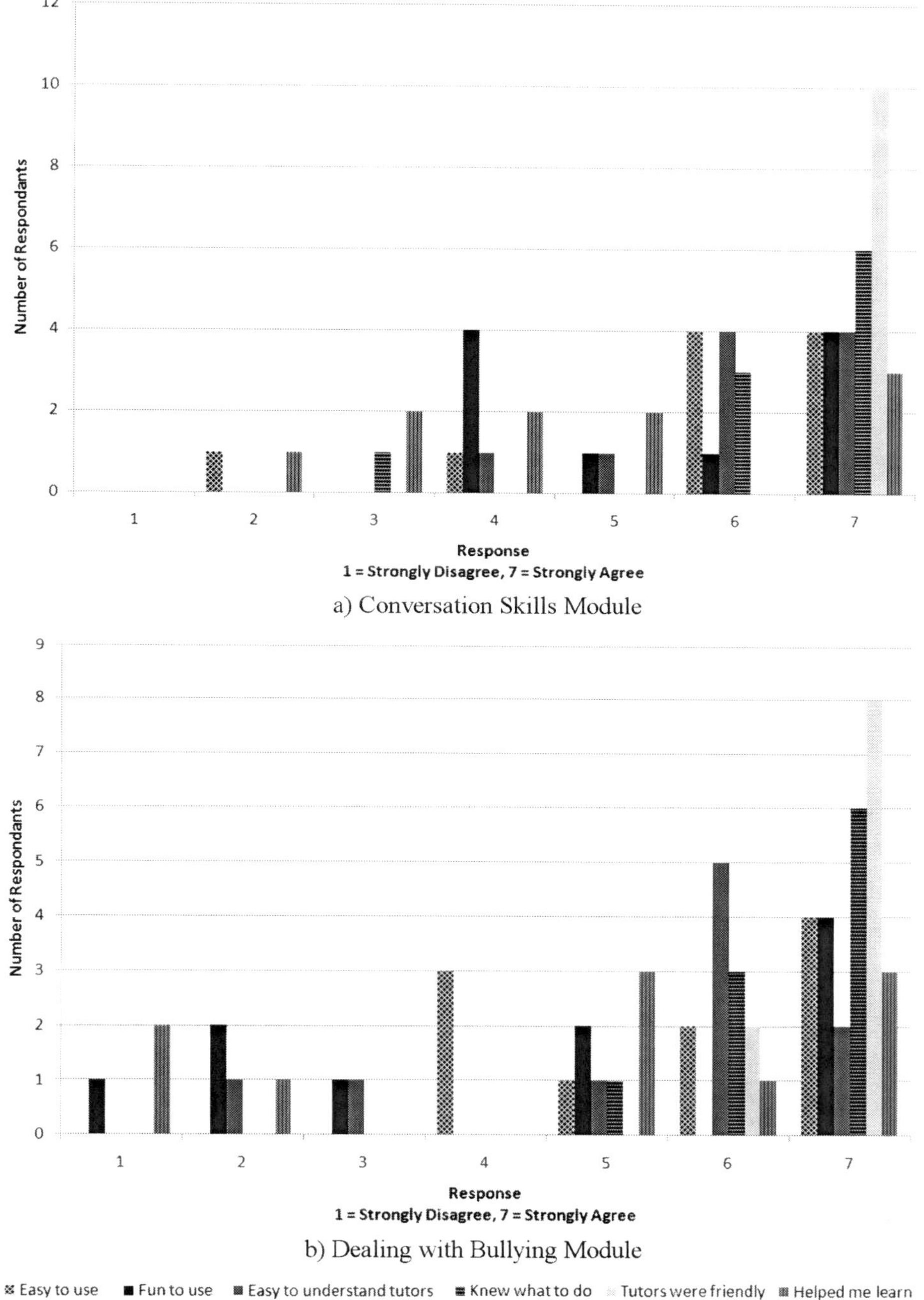


a) Conversation Skills Module

b) Dealing with Bullying Module

older and higher-functioning participants. Ideally, participants should be screened prior to involvement in the study to ensure that only those who the lesson content is appropriate for are included, but project time limitations prevented this from being a viable option.

The lower rating that some participants gave for 'it was fun' may be connected to the comments that

*Table 3. Summary of open-ended responses from the conversation tutor survey*

| Positive Aspects | Negative Aspects |
|---|---|
| The appearance of the tutors (3 participants) | The tutor's voices (3 participants) |
| Taking a photo of myself (3 participants) | Took a long time (2 participants) |
| Questions were easy to understand (2 participants) | The tutor's clothes are outdated |
| Repetitiveness (2 participants) | Repetitiveness |
| Lesson content (2 participants) | Expressions with nodding need to be more explicitly taught |
| Very interactive (2 participants) | Having to wait for people to stop talking |
| The people were friendly | Sometimes hard to understand tutor's meaning |
| Non-stressful learning | Asked me things I already knew |
| Clicking on the pictures | |
| Easy | |
| Fun | |

*Table 4. Summary of open-ended responses from the dealing with bullying tutor survey*

| Positive Aspects | Negative Aspects |
|---|---|
| The people (5 participants) | Took too long (3 participants) |
| Lesson content (5 participants) | Tutor's voice (3 participants) |
| It said my name (2 participants) | Boring (2 participants) |
| It was fun (2 participants) | Repetitive (3 participants) |
| The graphics | Technical difficulties |
| Acting along with scenarios | Need more sentence options for older kids |
| Great learning tool | Had to say my sentence out loud |
| Liked clicking the words | Tutor's clothes are outdated |
| Easy to use | It wasn't a real person |
| | Needed a bigger pool of questions |

the evaluation process took too long, potentially resulting in boredom and disengagement where the initial reaction was quite positive. Anecdotally, most parents commented that their children seemed to enjoy the first round but got bored doing the same type of task for an hour, even with breaks. It may be that the length of the evaluation led to lower concentration, which may have led to lower levels of improvement on test scores than could have been achieved had the evaluation process been spread out across multiple, shorter sessions. There were several participants whose caregivers expressed surprise at their incorrect post-test choices and stated that this must have been because they were experiencing fatigue. Providing the software to homes and schools and spreading the evaluation sessions across multiple days should alleviate this.

Along with the length of the evaluation, the repetitiveness of the lessons in terms of the content across the three sessions and the questions asked within a single session was a concern. However, repetitiveness was also mentioned as a positive by a number of participants. For those who needed lesson content repeated for practice, it was very helpful, and it should be noted that this was our aim in structuring the modules. However, for those who picked the lesson content up quickly or already knew it, it was unnecessary and led to disengagement. Future development would ideally involve a mechanism that continually assesses the learner's level of proficiency and repeats only where necessary or explicitly desired by the learner. Additionally, while the repetitiveness of lessons was an issue for some, the content of the lessons was cited as a positive aspect by several participants, confirming that the choice of lesson topics was appropriate and worthwhile for this learner group, as was hoped.

Overall, the survey results for both tutors were very positive, with all participants strongly agreeing with the statement about the tutors being friendly. One child reported that in the bullying skills tutor, having to say their sentence out loud made them uncomfortable, and from informal observation there were several children who said it very quietly or not at all, presumably for the same reason. Other than this, no-one reported feeling uncomfortable using either module, and one participant specifically reported that they felt it was good for non-stressful learning.

As one of the aims of this project was to provide a non-judgemental learning opportunity, this is a very positive result and suggests that this goal was achieved, further supporting the notion that overall the participants' experiences with the tutoring software were positive. With respect to saying the sentence out loud, it is important that the child be able to fully enact the bully-proof strategy, and if they struggle to say the sentence to the tutor, they are likely to struggle to say it in a real situation. However, there is certainly scope for putting in intermediate steps and options so that the sentence is only practiced out loud when the child is ready to.

A commonly cited issue was the voice of the tutors, especially the male voice. Participants and caregivers noted that they did not always sound natural or exhibit correct intonation, and this caused some confusion in the Interested condition, as the intonation of a verbal utterance such as 'oh' could indicate a variety of things including interest, disappointment or confusion, depending on the tone and context. This was in particular an issue for individuals who reported auditory processing difficulties. While the best voices accessible were used, this is still noteworthy and it is expected that in future as the technology develops, more realistic voices will become available. The tone of voice contributes to the meaning of non-verbal cues, and as such it is important that this be accurately portrayed. This is one factor likely to have influenced the survey ratings for the statement 'it was easy to understand what the tutors said', one of the lower rated statements.

One of the most commonly noted strengths of the tutor, especially by caregivers, was the manner in which the lessons were structured. It was noted that the questions and information were worded clearly, concise sentences were used, and the step by step structure of the lessons was appropriate to this learner group. Another strength of the tutor, in particular the conversation skills tutor, was the interactivity of the content and the program in general.

Most participants particularly enjoyed being able to take a photograph of themselves using the streaming video 'mirror' and others specifically stated that they enjoyed clicking on the buttons to answer questions. Many participants cited that the virtual people, particularly their appearance and movement, were their favourite aspect of the tutoring program. This is a very positive response because, as mentioned previously, some individuals with autism can suffer from sensory tolerance issues. The positive response towards the virtual tutors' faces is motivating, confirming that this has the potential to be a very useful tool for teaching non-verbal social cues.

## 7 FUTURE RESEARCH DIRECTIONS

Evaluation of our prototype has exposed a clear need for improved speech and facial gesture synthesis. Additional controls over voice intonation and the movement of the virtual head and shoulders are being developed to address this issue. In fact, employing ECAs as tutors also offers incentive for advancing a whole range of other, associated ECA technologies.

Of particular interest to us is emotion recognition, as we can thereby automatically monitor learners' interest levels and take action to avoid disengagement with the learning material, which was a major issue in our study. It may also be used to help children investigate their own expressions of emotion, as the virtual tutor can explain how it perceives the expression they are presenting and why.

Such an emotion classification system will have to be customisable and contain individual profiles, as children with autism may have distinct markers of particular emotions that may have very different meanings for others – for example, rocking backwards and forwards may indicate frustration in one individual but excitement in another. Our emotion recognition system will be based on video and audio inputs from conventional webcams, as ultimately the tutoring software is to be deployed in homes and schools.

Emotion recognition combined with continuous in-built assessment of student responses to lesson content would be used to monitor learner progress. Through this and by developing learning materials in the format of short, sequential modules, content that is appropriate to the learner's current needs can be delivered. It is certainly worth investigating whether software that autonomously adapts its lesson content and sequence to the individual learner can improve the quality and enjoyment of the educational experience for learners. Most importantly, however, future research must focus on whether the gains shown here through comparison of pre- and post-testing can be translated into improvements in other contexts, such as interaction ability in real social situations, as generalisation of skills is a major concern in all forms of interventions for children with autism.

Another direction for future research involves a joint literacy and conversation skills program. Children with autism learn best when each step of a task is explicitly taught. Reading comprehension, arguably an important life skill, is an area where this strategy is traditionally somewhat neglected. Speech interaction of this kind could be extended to discussions on lesson content, which is not only useful for assessment, but also to facilitate learning of important conversational skills, such as turn-taking, in a non-judgemental environment.

This approach gives context to the conversation which is advantageous from a technical viewpoint because it will facilitate effective dialogue management, potentially allowing for quite realistic conversation practice that has not yet been achieved. However, further research into the area of speech recognition may be required to support this. Current technology works best when it can predict what likely utterances are, which is particularly difficult in the context of children with ASD, who may not always behave according to social conventions and expectations.

## 8 CONCLUSION

The primary aim of our study was to ascertain whether it is worthwhile expending further time and effort into the development of an extensive social skills tutoring program centred on autonomous virtual peers. While other studies have provided such evidence for autonomous language skills tutors, such as Baldi and Timo (Bosseler and Massaro, 2003) and authorable social skills tutors such as Sam (Tartaro and Cassell, 2008), evidence was lacking for autonomous tutors that teach social skills.

Given the limited public availability and feature set of software suitable for this purpose, a new virtual speaking agent software was developed for the purposes of this and related studies. Uniquely, the software is based on a parametric face model, which offers full customization of the agent's appearance to suit the needs of the audience. In conjunction with a simple but capable developer's interface, we could thus shift our focus to the teaching logic and swiftly build the autonomous tutoring modules.

Comparison of pre and post-test scores in both the conversation skills tutoring module and the dealing with bullying skills module showed significant average gains in scores. This suggests that further research into developing an autonomous social skills tutor is indeed justified. Another important goal of this research was to provide a non-judgemental learning environment for participants. In the surveys for both our tutors, mean scores for all statements fell on the 'agreement' side of the scale, with many in range of strong agreement, indicating that participants typically found the program easy and enjoyable to use.

All participants perceived the virtual people as being friendly, which suggests that our aim of providing a non-judgemental learning environment was successfully met. Thus, further research into developing an autonomous social skills tutor has the potential to result in an effective and enjoyable social skills intervention that will relieve some of the time pressure that carers and educators of children with autism face.

A few challenges were encountered during the study. Several participants answered a high percentage of the pre-test questions successfully, suggesting that for these individuals the presented lesson content was too easy and that many more lessons are required on a wide range of topics if we are to cater to learners' changing needs successfully. Many participants found the length of the sessions too long and became disengaged. While this format was necessitated by the time limitations of the study, it is proposed that in future research the software be deployed in a realistic setting, such as on a home or school computer, allowing participants to interact with the software for a short time each day over an extended period. It is hoped that this will not only reduce boredom, but also increase educational gains.

Technical issues that need to be addressed include that some participants had difficulty understanding the synthesised voices, which raises a need for improved voices or recorded voices accompanied by subtitles. Furthermore, some nonverbal cues appeared awkward and require improvement; nonverbal cue expression could be enhanced by adding the ability to control the virtual tutor's head and shoulders separately.

Participants and their caregivers responded enthusiastically to the notion of the virtual tutor for social skills teaching, caregivers being particularly keen to hear of any future development, as participants in general found it engaging, non-threatening and an overall positive experience. There is much scope for expansion of the social skills tutoring software and related technologies, particularly in the area of a combined reading comprehension and conversation skills program, within the context of which technologies such as mood detection and speech recognition can be further developed, applied, and their usefulness investigated. With further development and the ability to cater to individual learners' needs, the use of the autonomous virtual tutor for teaching social skills may prove highly beneficial for children with autism and other special needs.

## ACKNOWLEDGMENT

This work was supported by the 'Thinking Head' project, a Special Research Initiative of the Australian Research Council (ARC) and the National Health and Medical Research Council (NH&MRC) (Burnham et al., 2006-2011).

## REFERENCES

American Psychiatric Association. (2000). *Diagnostic and statistical manual of mental disorders* (4th ed., text revision). Washington, DC: APA.

Bickmore, T., & Cassell, J. (2005). Social dialogue with embodied conversational agents. In van Kuppevelt, J., Dybkjaer, L., & Bernsen, N. (Eds.), *Advances in natural, multimodal dialogue systems* (pp. 23–54). New York, NY: Kluwer Academic. doi:10.1007/1-4020-3933-6_2

Blanz, V., & Vetter, T. (1999). A morphable model for the synthesis of 3D faces. In *Proceedings of the 26th Annual Conference on Computer Graphics and Interactive Techniques (SIGGRAPH)*, (pp. 187-194). New York, NY: ACM Press.

Bosseler, A., & Massaro, D. (2003). Development and evaluation of a computer-animated tutor for vocabulary and language learning in children with autism. *Journal of Autism and Developmental Disorders*, *33*(6), 653–672. doi:10.1023/B:JADD.0000006002.82367.4f

Brown, D. J., Standen, P. J., Proctor, T., & Sterland, D. (2001). Advanced design methodologies for the production of virtual learning environments for use by people with learning disabilities. *Presence (Cambridge, Mass.)*, *10*(4), 401–415. doi:10.1162/1054746011470253

Burnham, D., et al. (2006-2011). *From talking heads to thinking heads: A research platform for human communication science*. Retrieved from http://thinkinghead.uws.edu.au

Cassell, J. (2001). Embodied conversational agents: Representation and intelligence in user interfaces. *AI Magazine*, *22*(3), 67–83.

Davis, M., Robins, B., Dautenhahn, K., Nehaniv, C., & Powell, S. (2005). A comparison of interactive and robotic systems in therapy and education for children with autism. In Pruski, A., & Knops, H. (Eds.), *Assistive technology: From virtuality to reality*. IOS Press.

Gray, C. (2001). How to respond to a bullying attempt: What to think, say and do. *The Morning News, 13*(2).

Grun, U. (1998). *Visualization of gestures in conversational turn taking situations*. Retrieved 10 July, 2009, from http://coral.lili.uni-bielefeld.de/Classes/Winter97/PhonMM/UlrichGruen/

Gulz, A., & Haakeb, M. (2006). Design of animated pedagogical agents—a look at their look. *International Journal of Human-Computer Studies*, *64*, 322–339. doi:10.1016/j.ijhcs.2005.08.006

Herrera, G., Alcantud, F., Jordan, R., Blanquer, A., Labajo, G., & De Pablo, C. (2008). Development of symbolic play through the use of virtual reality tools in children with autistic spectrum disorders: Two case studies. *Autism*, *12*(2), 143–157. doi:10.1177/1362361307086657

Kerr, S. J. (2002). Scaffolding: Design issues in single & collaborative virtual environments for social skills learning. In *Proceedings of the Workshop on Virtual Environments 2002*. Barcelona, Spain: Eurographics Association.

Kopp, S., Sowa, T., & Wachsmuth, I. (2004). Imitation games with an artificial agent: From mimicking to understanding shape-related iconic gestures. In Braffort, A., Gherbi, R., Gibet, S., Richardson, J., & Teil, D. (Eds.), *Gesture-based communication in Human-Computer Interaction* (pp. 436–447). Berlin, Germany: Springer-Verlag. doi:10.1007/978-3-540-24598-8_40

Kroes, S. (2007). *Detecting boredom in meetings* (pp. 1–5). Enschede, Netherlands: University of Twente.

Massaro, D. (2004). Symbiotic value of an embodied agent in language learning. In R. H. Sprague, Jr. (Ed.), *IEEE Proceedings of 37th Annual Hawaii International Conference on System Sciences*, Computer Society Press.

Massaro, D. W. (2003). A computer-animated tutor for spoken and written language learning. In *Proceedings of the 5th International Conference on Multimodal interfaces (ICMI '03),* Canada, ACM, (pp. 172-175).

Moreno, R., & Flowerday, T. (2006). Students' choice of animated pedagogical agents in science learning: A test of the similarity-attraction hypothesis on gender and ethnicity. *Contemporary Educational Psychology*, *31*, 186–207. doi:10.1016/j.cedpsych.2005.05.002

Oh, I., & Stone, M. (2007). Understanding RUTH: Creating believable behaviors for a virtual human under uncertainty. In Duffy, V. G. (Ed.), *Digital human modeling* (pp. 443–452). Berlin/Heidelberg, Germany: Springer-Verlag. doi:10.1007/978-3-540-73321-8_51

Parsons, S., Beardon, L., Neale, H. R., Reynard, G., Eastgate, R., Wilson, J. R., et al. Hopkins, E. (2000). Development of social skills amongst adults with Asperger's Syndrome using virtual environments: The 'AS Interactive' project. *Proceedings of the 3rd International Conference on Disability, Virtual Reality & Associated Technologies*, (pp. 163-170).

Parsons, S., & Mitchell, P. (2002). The potential of virtual reality in social skills training for people with autistic spectrum disorders. *Journal of Intellectual Disability Research, 46*(5), 430–443. doi:10.1046/j.1365-2788.2002.00425.x

Parsons, S., Mitchell, P., & Leonard, A. (2005). Do adolescents with autistic spectrum disorders adhere to social conventions in virtual environments? *Autism, 9*(1), 95–117. doi:10.1177/1362361305049032

Poggi, I., Pelachaud, C., de Rosis, F., Carofiglio, V., & De Carolis, B. (2005). GRETA: A believable embodied conversational agent. In Stock, O., & Zancarano, M. (Eds.), *Multimodal intelligent information presentation* (pp. 3–25). Netherlands: Springer-Verlag. doi:10.1007/1-4020-3051-7_1

Putnam, C., & Chong, L. (2008). Software and technologies designed for people with autism: What do users want? In *Proceedings of the 10th International ACM SIGACCESS Conference on Computers and Accessibility* (pp. 3-10). Halifax, Canada: ACM Press.

Rapin, I., & Tuchman, R. F. (2008). Autism: Definition, neurobiology, screening, diagnosis. *Pediatric Clinics of North America, 55*(5), 1129–1146. doi:10.1016/j.pcl.2008.07.005

Schröder, M., & Trouvain, J. (2003). The German text-to-speech synthesis system MARY: A tool for research, development and teaching. *International Journal of Speech Technology, 6*, 365–377. doi:10.1023/A:1025708916924

Silver, M., & Oakes, P. (2001). Evaluation of a new computer intervention to teach people with autism or Asperger Syndrome to recognize and predict emotions in others. *Autism, 5*(3), 299–316. doi:10.1177/1362361301005003007

Singular Inversions. (2009). *FaceGen SDK 3.6*. Retrieved from http://www.facegen.com

Straker, D. (2008). Using body language. *Changing Minds*. Retrieved 10 July, 2009, from http://changingminds.org/techniques/body/body_language.htm

Tartaro, A., & Cassell, J. (2006). *Authorable virtual peers for autism spectrum disorders*. Paper presented at the Combined Workshop on Language-Enabled Educational Technology and Development and Evaluation of Robust Spoken Dialogue Systems at the 17th European Conference on Artificial Intelligence (ECAI06), Riva del Garda, Italy.

Tartaro, A., & Cassell, J. (2008). Playing with virtual peers: Bootstrapping contingent discourse in children with autism. *International Conference of the Learning Science*. Utrecht, The Netherlands: ACM Press.

Wang, A., Emmi, M., & Faloutsos, P. (2007). Assembling an expressive facial animation system. In *Proceedings of the ACM SIGGRAPH symposium on Video Games* (pp. 21-26). New York, NY: ACM Press.

## KEY TERMS AND DEFINITIONS

**Authorable Peer:** A virtual agent that takes input from external sources in order to carry out behaviours is said to be authorable. For example, the experimenter may control its actions via a control panel, much like a puppet. (Also known as; human-controlled virtual agent.)

**Autistic Spectrum Disorder (ASD):** A pervasive developmental disorder involving impairment in communication skills, social skills and a tendency towards repetitive patterns of interest and behaviour. Classic or 'low functioning' autism refers to individuals with more severe impairments and often lower IQ. 'High functioning' individuals typically have normal to high IQ. Debate exists about the difference between Asperger Syndrome and high functioning autism however a difference in speech development and motor skill deficits may set the diagnoses apart. (Also known as; autism.)

**Autonomous Peer:** A virtual agent is said to be autonomous when it has the ability to make independent decisions and carry out actions without direct input from external sources. A stand-alone program. (Also known as; autonomous virtual peer, autonomous agent, autonomous virtual agent.)

**Bullying:** A real or perceived power imbalance where the more powerful party repeatedly and intentionally performs negative actions towards a party with less power.

**Conversation Skills:** The ability to interpret verbal and non-verbal signals so as to properly engage and take turns in maintaining a dialogue with another human being. (Also known as; conversation management.)

**Embodied Conversational Agent (ECA):** An animated interface agent (often a virtual human) that engages the user in real-time, multimodal dialogue using speech, gesture, gaze, intonation, and other verbal and nonverbal behaviors.

**Face Synthesis:** The rendering and animation of a human face on a computer screen.

**Social Skills:** The skills required for successful social interaction with others. These skills include but are not limited to nonverbal communication and friendship skills, for example understanding and responding to the nonverbal signals displayed by others and engaging in taking turns.

**Speech Synthesis:** The artificial production of sounds accurately representing another human being speaking. It notably differs from prerecorded speech in that the computer can dynamically compose sentences that have not been spoken before.

**Virtual Tutor:** An animated character that typically acts as a teacher and may exhibit some or all of the capabilities of an ECA. (Also known as; virtual peer.)

# Section 2
# Design of Conversational Agents

# Chapter 3
# Designing ECAs to Improve Robustness of Human–Machine Dialogue

**Beatriz López Mencía**
*Universidad Politécnica de Madrid, Spain*

**David D. Pardo**
*Universidad Politécnica de Madrid, Spain*

**Alvaro Hernández Trapote**
*Universidad Politécnica de Madrid, Spain*

**Luis A. Hernández Gómez**
*Universidad Politécnica de Madrid, Spain*

## ABSTRACT

*One of the major challenges for dialogue systems deployed in commercial applications is to improve robustness when common low-level problems occur that are related with speech recognition. We first discuss this important family of interaction problems, and then we discuss the features of non-verbal, visual, communication that Embodied Conversational Agents (ECAs) bring 'into the picture' and which may be tapped into to improve spoken dialogue robustness and the general smoothness and efficiency of the interaction between the human and the machine. Our approach is centred around the information provided by ECAs. We deal with all stages of the conversation system development process, from scenario description, to gesture design and evaluation with comparative user tests. We conclude that ECAs can help improve the robustness of, as well as the users' subjective experience with, a dialogue system. However, they may also make users more demanding and intensify privacy and security concerns.*

DOI: 10.4018/978-1-60960-617-6.ch003

## INTRODUCTION

Spoken Language Dialogue Systems (SLDSs) are being introduced into the user interfaces of an ever growing range of devices and applications. This is in spite of pervading problems encountered by almost anyone who has had to deal with these systems as users, and which result in low quality, inefficient communication, or even its breakdown altogether.

A widely held view among those interested in improving the users' experience with SLDSs is that Embodied Conversational Agents (ECAs) can be beneficial to the communication process by fostering a more effective, affective and user-friendly interaction (Foster, 2007). Adequate, broadly accepted cognitive and operational models explaining how humans combine speech and gesture have not yet been found (Kopp et al., 2008). Nevertheless, empirical evidence is growing that shows that ECAs provide a supra-linguistic communication channel that, through gestures and other visual cues, may be used to add semantic richness, improve intelligibility by adding redundancy, and display attitudes and moods that open the scope for emotional and empathic dialogue strategies (Buisine et al., 2004; Cassell et al., 2000b; Picard, 2003).

As regards dialogue design, ECAs in research have been approached mainly from linguistic and social interaction perspectives, and from Artificial Intelligence-related fields (a snapshot of efforts containing elements along these lines was offered in the Functional Markup Language workshop at the AAMAS conference in 2008, from which the example references in this paragraph have been taken). The latter approaches (AI) deal with constructing appropriate, "intelligent" responses to users or other agents in a particular context of interaction (as in the ICT virtual human project by Lee et al., 2008); the former are concerned with a variety of elements in a hierarchy of linguistic and, more generally, conversational functions (Heylen & ter Maat, 2008), and they tend to focus primarily on high level aspects such as interpersonal stance (Bickmore, 2008) and social relations (see, e.g., Samtani et al., 2008).

Surprisingly, however, relatively little attention has been given to studying how ECAs can affect dialogue when miscommunication occurs at the lower yet most common levels, and in particular at the speech recognition level. In this chapter we present a relatively simple dialogue system we have built for the purpose of identifying a set of basic dialogue situations that either arise when problems occur (for instance, a no-input or a no-match) or are prone to lead to interaction problems (e.g., turn-taking), and we show the process of designing ECA behaviour for each of these situations.

Our goal is to illustrate how ECAs can help in these low-level interaction problem cases and also to show the overall design, validation and user-centred testing process as a common sense example of the general approach we believe can be applied to interaction problems higher in the hierarchy. As we shall see, some of the strategies will involve an affective element introduced for two reasons: to influence the users' emotions during the interaction so as to obtain a desired result such as success with an error recovery strategy, and, ultimately, to try to improve the users' subjective opinion of the system – even, and especially, when there are problems and recovery strategies don't work well and the task is accomplished inefficiently or fails altogether.

The chapter is structured as follows: we begin with some background on the literature on embodied conversational systems, robustness issues in dialogue systems and how ECAs can help. We then enter the main body of the chapter, which is a case study on ECA behaviour design applied to the improvement of (mostly ASR-related) robustness in SLDSs. First we present a guiding application and interaction scenario and we explain the behavioural strategies devised for the ECAs in the scenario. Next, we describe the user tests we performed to compare interaction performance and the subjective experience of users between a version of the system with ECAs and a version with only speech output, after which we present and discuss a few of the more interesting results we obtained. We then offer a few thoughts on actual and desirable, present and future, research directions. The concluding section summarises and highlights the main points made in the chapter.

## BACKGROUND

### Some Research Trends in Spoken Embodied Conversational Agents

During the past few decades major advancements in various fields, not least in automatic speech recognition and synthesis, have made it possible to develop increasingly complex spoken conversational interfaces. While most dialogue systems to date have been very much task oriented, confined to very specific purposes in information access applications and 'command-and-control' scenarios (Paek & Horvitz, 2000; Rudnicky et al., 1999), we are beginning to see more flexible personal assistants (Bohus & Rudnicky, 2005), interactive tutors (Rickel et al., 2001) and embodied conversational agents – such as Cassell et al.s' (2002) Mack or MIT's FitTrack system (Bickmore & Picard, 2005).

For Justine Cassell, ECAs are representations of 'virtual humans' that are capable of engaging in conversation with humans, understanding what its interlocutors – humans or other ECAs – say and reacting accordingly (and according to its interaction goals) through speech, movement, gesture and facial expression, but also suggesting new paths along which to lead the conversation. Thus, an ECA proper should possess advanced communicative abilities similar to those displayed in face-to-face conversation between humans. This is because, according to Cassell, in order to achieve natural interaction a dialogue system must be designed following human-human communication principles (Cassell et al., 2000b).

ECA technologies have a long way to go yet to produce virtual humans that possess such demanding qualities. Nevertheless, humanlike animated figures that combine and coordinate state-of-the-art spoken dialogue system elements with gestures and facial expressions do exist and are getting ever closer to their ideal.

ECAs can be viewed from a variety of perspectives. They are an object of attention in artificial intelligence and software agent technology, and they can be seen as a piece of (multimedia and multimodal) interface technology. As was mentioned in the introduction, ECAs in dialogue are being studied to explore what they can offer beyond speech, bringing into the scene, as they do, a visual channel for communication which can be very powerful and which open up possibilities in the social and psychological domains.

The potential of ECAs to mediate a more effective, efficient, intuitive and natural interaction with people and to open up a social and emotional dimension is being explored in a wide variety of application areas. Early research efforts already looked into the motivating effects a humanlike presence can have simply by being in an interface (see, e.g., Lester et al., 1997; Van Mulken et al., 1998). Most noteworthy are educational applications for children in which animated agents can be used in different roles such as virtual peers or virtual teachers (Tartaro & Cassell, 2008), to enhance the pupils' motivation through a sense of trust engendered by the ECAs (Atkinson, 2002; Gratch et al., 2007), or as support for learning through imitation by exaggerating both verbal and non-verbal expression (Engwall, 2008; Massaro et al., 2001).

In the Companions Project ECAs are used as a 'humanising' face for a system that inquires about how the user's day has been and then responds empathically giving comfort, encouragement, advice and a sense of companionship through speech and gesture (Companions, 2010). Building long-term 'relationships' is also closely related to the work of Bickmore et al. (2009) with nursing assistance applications. ECAs are also being used as friendly virtual assistants (e.g., Cassell et al.'s (1999) real estate agent REA), guides (e.g., Kopp et al.'s (2005) museum guide), and to help the user conceptualise an intelligent system with ubiquitous qualities (e.g., a home assistant (Amores et al., 2007) or an on-board assistant in a car (Dausend & Ehrlich, 2008)) by providing a physical, corporeal anchor.

ECAs also have their detractors, however, who point out that no interaction benefits have been proved beyond their aesthetic or entertainment value, and warn that they can be confusing, distracting, lead to false expectations and even produce anxiety in the user (Catrambone et al., 2002; Xiao, 2006). These are certainly adverse effects to look out for.

In any case, the role ECAs may play in reducing communication errors and improving the flow of the dialogue has not yet received enough attention (Bell & Gustafson, 2003). In this chapter we will be concerned with Spoken Embodied Conversational Agents understood as spoken dialogue systems with an added human-looking 'presence' that performs gestures in coordination with utterances to help prevent and recover from basic difficulties related to speech recognition (as opposed to the notion of an ECA as an intelligent agent with a physical presence and endowed with cognitive abilities above and beyond those of typical speech-only dialogue systems). These difficulties are described in the following section.

## Robustness in SLDSs

Conceptually, spoken language dialogue systems (SLDSs) involve several elements: speech recognition, natural language understanding, speech synthesis, natural language generation and mechanisms to decide what to say or do at each particular point of the interaction with the user. These decisions are based on considerations such as which information items needed to accomplish specific interaction goals are known, or how well the system understood the utterance from the user.

Miscommunication can arise at different linguistic levels, from the lexical – misinterpreting the meaning of the words in the message – to the discourse and pragmatic levels – misinterpreting the intention with which the message was communicated –, and beyond problems with grounding the content (the referential aspect) it is also worthwhile to consider misalignments of the mutually interpreted emotions (the affective aspect) of the parties engaged in conversation (McTear, 2008).

However, the most common source of errors in spoken human-computer interaction has been found to be the automatic speech recognition (Bohus & Rudnicky, 2008; McTear, 2008). It is, thus, particularly important and challenging to design spoken language dialogue systems that are able to detect and recover from problems related to the quality of speech recognition when these problems occur, and do so staying within a normal, or, might we say, natural flow of the dialogue, without disrupting it. Such ability is said to make dialogue more robust. A major problem, then, with spoken dialogue systems today is their lack of robustness to speech recognition problems (Bohus & Rudnicky, 2008).

Difficulties related to speech recognition include non-understandings, misunderstandings, no-inputs and dealing with low confidence in recognition. These are the types of problems with which we are chiefly concerned in the study we present in this chapter. We now describe each of them briefly:

- Non-understandings occur when the system cannot find a complete and unequivocal interpretation of the output speech recognition module (for instance, if the user says *"the bathroom lights"* but the speech recogniser returns *"the cartoon frights"* which makes no sense in the context of the dialogue task).

- In the case of misunderstandings, the system obtains a response which fits the vocabulary and makes sense in the context of the dialogue task at hand, but it doesn't match what the user actually said (for example, the user says *"living room"* and the system understands *"bathroom"*, which would be a valid response but it happens not to be the correct one).
- No-inputs have to do with speech recognition conceptually, even though technically they usually do not arise in the automatic speech recognition (ASR) module, but a step lower, in the Voice Activity Detection (VAD) module. No-inputs are situations in which no utterance from the user is detected within a reasonable lapse of time. If the reason is that the user didn't say anything, the problem may be one of coordination between the user and the system or misalignment of user's and the system's understanding of the current state of the dialogue, but not one of speech recognition. However, it may happen that the user speaks but the voice detection unit doesn't activate, perhaps because the user spoke too softly or because it was during a system turn in which user interruptions happened to be disabled and VAD or ASR were inactive. Conceptually, we can take this (in a rather unorthodox manner, it has to be said) as a special case of misunderstanding in which the system takes it that the user has not made an utterance when in fact he has.
- Along with the textual transcript of what was recognised as a result of a user utterance, ASR modules usually provide a score that indicates their own degree of confidence in the accuracy of the the recognised message – i.e., it's the system's own estimation of how likely it is that it interpreted the user's utterance correctly. Confidence scores are not always very reliable. Nevertheless, they can be used to define error prevention and recovery strategies (San Segundo et al., 2001; Bohus, 2007). For instance, if the confidence score is low then precautionary measures are usually in order to make sure that a misunderstanding did not occur. Such measures may involve asking more or less overtly for confirmation from the user that what the system understood is in fact correct.

When recognition difficulties are detected it is advisable to initiate a recovery process to find out what the correct communicative intention of the user is. Unfortunately, this may produce frustration in the user (Goldberg et al., 2003). In fact, once an error occurs it is common to enter an error spiral, because as the user becomes increasingly frustrated the system will typically find it more and more difficult to understand her, so further errors are made (Oviatt & VanGent, 1996; Oviatt et al., 1998). A system's robustness will depend on how it deals with all of these situations.

In order to improve the robustness of a spoken dialogue interface is necessary to take into account not only the accuracy and reliability of the speech recognition engine but also the capabilities of the dialog manager and the design of the interaction flow. More specifically, turn-taking and interruption handling provide another family of problems that fit this slightly broader notion of robustness. The classical model of turn-taking describes it as both depending only on the local context, and a predictive phenomenon where turn endings can be anticipated by following combined syntactic, semantic and prosodic signals (Sacks et al., 1974). It feels natural enough in human-to-human conversation (especially face-to-face), but in a two-party spoken dialogue knowing when to speak and when to listen can be rather difficult, especially if one of the parties is a machine.

Some SLDSs allow *barge-in*, essentially enabling the user to interrupt the system at any time. The obvious risk is that the system may take noise, background speech or user attention cues (e.g., filled pauses such as "aha") as barge-in attempts by the user, resulting in confusion and, possibly, the beginning of a frustrating and unfruitful stretch of dialogue.

Another, a common problem in dialogue systems arises when the user isn't sure what the system has understood, what it is doing and whether or not the dialogue process is working normally. In other words, as we anticipated in the previous paragraph, the user may be confused as to the state of the dialogue at a particular point in time (Oviatt, 1994).

To sum up all of the above, the robustness of a conversational system can be seen as the ability to prevent, detect and recover from difficult situations, situations which may lead to inefficiency in reaching, or inability to reach, the interaction goals, to unnaturalness and to the dissatisfaction of the user.

## How Can ECAs Help?

The visual channel provided by the ECA can convey different kinds of information. It can offer redundancy over the spoken message, stressing words or gesturing certain features of the meaning that the words convey; it can also provide information that complements the speech (such as pointing in a certain direction, or winking to show that what was said was meant with humorous irony) (Kopp et al., 2008). Then, also complementing the spoken message is the emotional content conveyed by facial expressions. All of these elements can be explored to improve dialogue robustness. Gaze, gestures, intonation and body posture all play an important role in creating adequate conversational behaviour when initiating and terminating the dialogue, taking and giving turns, handling interruptions, providing feedback and correcting errors (Cassell et al., 2000a).

Hone (2006) has observed that ECAs can help limit user frustration in error recovery processes. Indeed, emotional strategies can be used to greater effect with an animated agent taking the blame, apologising and playing out 'remorse' when it didn't understand an utterance from the user. As a result, the user's motivation and trust in the system can rise while her stress is reduced (Cassell & Tartaro, 2007). Turn-taking and user interruption handling can be made to go more smoothly with appropriate facial and verbal feedback (White et al., 2005), and body language and expressiveness have been used, beyond reinforcing the spoken message, to help regulate the flow of the dialogue (Bickmore & Cassell, 2005).

ECAs have been used, to the greater satisfaction of users, as 'visual fillers' to improve turn management in applications that keep the user on hold for extended lengths of time (Edlund & Nordstrand, 2002). Synchronisation strategies overlapping gesture and speech can be devised to improve user satisfaction with turn-taking mechanisms (ter Maat & Heylen, 2009). Breazeal et al. (2005) underlines the importance of non-verbal communication (in human-robot interaction) to reduce user confusion regarding the state or flow of the dialogue (i.e., where the dialogue is at any particular time and where it is heading), and Marsi & van Rooden (2007) has shown that users prefer visual cues over verbal ones in the face of uncertainty.

Furthering these efforts, we set out to explore the extended and enriched information that can be conveyed through ECAs, and the closer social engagement with the users that they can nurture, focusing on the benefits that may be derived in connection with basic dialogue robustness and user acceptance.

# CASE STUDY: ECA BEHAVIOUR DESIGN AND COMPARATIVE RESEARCH (ECA VS. NO ECA)

As mentioned in the introduction, we put together a dialogue system that would allow us to observe problem situations related to speech recognition, dialogue management and the flow of the dialogue, as well as task failure (i.e., failure to successfully complete the task that motivated the interaction). The goal was to see if we could design specific ECA behaviour for each of these situations that would improve dialogue robustness and provide a more satisfying experience for the users, as compared with the same system without the presence of ECAs in the visual interface. We now describe a scenario as an example of use of the system with the ECAs.

## Description of the Dialogue System

### The Scenario

Our dialogue system allows users to conduct two independent but related tasks in succession. This is the scenario:

Guillermo is away from home, let's say he's attending a conference on human-machine interaction, and suddenly he is struck by the suspicion that, just like poor Passepartout after setting off to travel around the world with Phileas Fogg, he may have forgotten to turn the heating off. With beads of cold sweat starting to form on his forehead, he immediately picks up his mobile phone and calls his home automation system. When the system answers, Isidro, a male ECA, appears on the screen of Guillermo's phone and asks him to provide a voice sample (a sequence of numbers) so that the system may biometrically authenticate his identity using its speaker recognition unit. Guillermo's first attempt is unsuccessful because the sequence of numbers recognised by the system does not match the requested sequence (i.e., there has either been a speech recognition error or Guillermo simply said the wrong numbers), so the ECA politely asks Guillermo to repeat the sequence. His second attempt isn't good enough – in a sense it fails –, this time not because the system recognised an incorrect sequence of numbers but because the system couldn't match the acoustic features extracted from Guillermo's utterance closely enough with those stored as his model at the time of enrolment. That is, the speaker verification module remains undecided as to whether the person speaking is really Guillermo or an impostor. The system then seeks to obtain a further sample of speech from Guillermo in order to have more acoustic material with which to increase its level of certainty either way. So, Isidro asks Guillermo to say another number sequence (i.e., he is given a *second* chance – of a total of three that the biometric access system allows before it declares finally that verification has failed –; the first attempt doesn't count because of the speech recognition error). At this point Guillermo, who is already impatient enough to get through, is getting rather annoyed and frustrated, and this increases the chances of further recognition errors (of both types: speech and speaker). Nevertheless, after Guillermo's third number sequence utterance the system finally does decide it is certain enough that Guillermo is the person who is speaking (i.e., it succeeds in verifying Guillermo's identity), and Isidro grants him access to the remote home automation system. Isabel, a female ECA, welcomes Guillermo and asks him what he would like to know or do. Guillermo then asks Isabel whether he left the heating on. She responds affirmatively, to Guillermo's despair, so he asks her to turn it off. Isabel forwards the request to the heating control unit, checks that the heating has in fact been switched off, and then she informs Guillermo, who breathes a sigh of relief.

The scenario, as we can see, has two phases: the biometric identity verification (speaker recognition) phase and the remote home automation phase. To underline the separation between the two in the mind of the user we employ two different ECAs, one male and the other female. Some authors have suggested that users tend to prefer interacting with a male or female personality depending on the application (McTear, 2008); for instance, a male voice or, by extension, a male ECA tends to be associated with authority (Nass & Brave, 2005 – as noted in McTear, 2008), so we have left the mean business of letting users in or keeping them out to Isidro; while a female voice (or ECA) tends to be perceived as being more sensitive to and demonstrative of emotions (*ibid.*), which partly motivated our decision to let Isabel handle the remote home automation application.

## The Dialogue Phases In Detail

### The Biometric Access Phase

From the point of view of the system, the goal of this phase, to state it once again, is to authenticate the identity of the user (or to reject impostors) through the recognition of distinctive qualities in his (or her) voice in order to grant him (or her) access to the home automation phase. The goal from the point of view of the user is, obviously, to gain access to the next phase.

Applying dialogue systems to speaker recognition is an area of research that has received relatively little attention. Seeking to maximise efficiency, and so as not to tire users, instead of making them provide one long sample of speech most systems ask users to produce a series of shorter voice samples, for example by asking them to read or repeat a short text, until the acoustic parameters collected are sufficient to make a match with a level of confidence that is higher a pre-established threshold, or until a certain number of failed matching attempts have been made, at which point the verification task is declared unsuccessful (Eckert, 2006). Anxiety may creep into the user with every new utterance he (or she) is asked to produce, however. This brings us to our goal, as designers, with this dialogue phase: we would like to see whether an expressive embodied conversational agent that empathises with the user aids a dialogue strategy already designed to try to maximise efficiency, effectiveness and user satisfaction, and so leads to better results than when no ECA is present.

The dialogue in this stage follows a request-answer scheme: in order to collect a sample of the speaker's voice the system (Isidro) asks the user to repeat a short (4-digit) random number sequence. The user then replies, and if the utterance (as understood by the speech recogniser) does not coincide with the requested number sequence he (or she) is asked to repeat it. If it does coincide, the utterance is passed on to the speaker verification unit. Then the dialogue proceeds according to the outcome of the verification attempt. The system does *not* inform the user when it is unable to reach an authentication decision (acceptance or rejection). Instead, a new (different) random sequence of numbers is presented. The reason for not telling the user that authentication result was inconclusive is to limit the user's frustration at the system's 'incompetence' and to try to keep him (or her) in a positive mood. As soon as the acoustic material, accumulated from all of the user's number sequence utterances from the beginning of the interaction up to that instant, is enough for the system to accept or reject the user's claimed identity with a high enough degree of certainty (i.e., the match with his (or her) stored acoustic features is deemed to be close enough), the system informs the user that his identity was successfully authenticated. But after three consecutive inconclusive speaker recognition outcomes, or after the first 'conclusive' rejection – which could be a false rejection –, the authentication task is deemed to have failed.

In the system design that we put together for testing we asked the test users to verify their identity with the system three times, and we explained that each time they would have three attempts to succeed in entering. However, the output of the speaker recognition unit was actually ignored and in its place we substituted a predetermined verification outcome. We did this for two reasons: first, our focus is on speech recognition problems and other closely related dialogue situations; we were not on this occasion particularly interested in looking at speaker recognition rates. Secondly, we wanted all of our users to experience all and the same biometric verification outcomes: success on the first attempt (with one number sequence, but correct recognition of the number sequence itself, as opposed to recognition of the speaker's voice, may require several repetitions by the speaker), success on the second attempt, and failure to verify the user's identity after three attempts (an 'access denied' situation).

So, the system asked users to verify their identities three times in a row, one for each of the predetermined outcomes we have just described. Importantly, as mentioned above, speech recognition was active, and system and user had to resolve whatever miscommunication issues arose (misunderstandings, non-understandings, no-inputs, etc.). Thus, the task is exactly the same for all users as respects the outcome of verification attempts, and the users' opinions of the system will not differ as a result of actual differing success with the biometric access task, although different users might have differing *impressions* of their success with the task and, in fact, observing whether this is indeed the case is an important part of the experiment. As was just mentioned, all of the users were made to 'fail' in one of the three verification tasks they were required to perform, and it is interesting to see whether the presence of an empathetic ECA can exert a positive influence on the users' subjective experience with the system even when they have faced task failure.

### The Remote Home Automation Phase

After the biometric access phase the user enters the remote home automation phase. Here the goal is one of *information retrieval*: the scenario is a service with which users call 'home' using mobile phones (simulated on a computer screen) to check the state of various home appliances. At the beginning of each 'call' the system speaks a welcome message and reminds the user of what the application does: provide information about various home devices – lights, TV, fan, heater, etc. – and/or carry out actions with them – e.g., switch them on or off.

The communicational goal in each call is for the system to collect the three information items that form the user's request: a device, a location (a room) and an action. Once the system is confident it has correctly understood of which device in which room the user wants to do which action, it answers appropriately. For example, a faultless call might go like this:

**USER:** Are the bathroom lights off?
[Here the action is to request information regarding the status (on/off) of a device.]
**SYSTEM:** The lights in the bathroom are switched on.

Misunderstandings and non-understandings may occur at the item (or *slot*) level (i.e., the system might not properly get what device or which room the user inquired about). Recognition confidence – high or low – is also evaluated at the slot level, and it can happen that the system understands part of the information (e.g., the place) with a high degree of confidence and another part (e.g., the device) with low confidence. We will see that dialogue strategies will be different depending on the combination of recognition confidence levels.

## Development of ECA Gestures for the Chosen Situations

We designed a set of ECA behaviours and animation effects to respond to a set of dialogue situations in which robustness (or the lack of it) can be an issue, as we discussed previously.

These ECA behaviours have a verbal component and a gestural component. That is, the ECA says something appropriate to the situation and also moves or performs a gesture. The design and implementation of ECA gestures is a broad field of research. For the purposes of this chapter, however, the following notes will provide sufficient background.

The most commonly used procedures to extract the information necessary to develop a gesture sequence are based on the observation of human-human communication (Cassell et al., 2000b). Indeed, classic literature on human nonverbal behaviour is a widely employed resource to develop ECA gestures (de Rosis et al., 2003). In order to develop more specific gestures, human actors are often used, existing videos analysed (Kipp, 2001) or user tests conducted in specific contexts (Theune et al., 2007).

As regards the implementing the gestural repertoire of ECAs, one approach is to do so automatically. For instance, the BEAT system allows the automatic annotation – in XML – of text with gestures, which are then performed through the action of a gesture execution rule set (Cassell et al., 2001b), and more recently Zoric et al.'s approach of generating gestures from the prosody of the speech signal (Zoric et al., 2009). Another, simpler, route is to tailor gestures for specific situations (with speech and gesture synchronization, therefore, done by hand (Theune et al., 2007).

For our case study, we decided to design situation-specific behaviour based on the literature on nonverbal behaviour. We then performed user test to validate each of the ECA gestures we had designed – in the vein of Hartmann et al. (2005). The gestures worked acceptably well with the test subjects: overall, they were correctly interpreted, regarded as natural, and they did not generate undesirable or unexpected effects (López-Mencía et al., 2007).

We now look at the specific dialogue situations we have focused on and the ECA behaviours we have designed for them. In the following subsections we will see the point of each behaviour for each particular dialogue situation. The general goal is to get the dialogue to move forward as easily and efficiently as possible while trying to keep the user in a positive attitude. The strategies involve managing the communication of information, including complementarity and redundancy provided by gestures, and manipulating affect (e.g., showing empathy with the user). In addition we have added mild visual effects (involving lighting intensity and 'camera' distance to the ECA) to stress turn possession.

In the following subsections we describe selected dialogue situations, we explain the associated ECA behaviour for each of them and we underline the motivation for each behavioural response, as well as the communicative elements the response carries. As was mentioned above, the gestural behaviour can have an affective role and/or convey information that complements, provides redundancy over, or anticipates the verbal message. Our attention to complementarity and redundancy of verbal and non-verbal information is motivated by the discussion in Kopp et al. (2008) and Cassell et al. (2000b).

The gesture repertoire of our ECAs is partially based on relevant gestures described in Cassell et al. (2000b), Bickmore & Cassell (2005) and Pelachaud (2003), as well as on recommendations in Kendon (1990), Cassell et al. (2001a) and San Segundo et al. (2001), to which we have added a few ideas of our own. Specific sources are given, as appropriate, in the corresponding subsections for the dialogue situations. Each section has a figure depicting one or several phases of the ECA's behavioural sequence, which is composed of gestures and some visual effects – the 'gesture line' in the figures – and the verbal output – the 'speech line'. In addition we show at which points the ASR engine is operating. This is important, especially in the turn-taking sequences, as we shall see, due to the fact that our dialogue interface does not allow barge-ins.

## Dialogue Initiation

An ECA tends to 'humanise' the system in the eyes of the user (Oviatt & Adams, 2000), who may, as a result, have higher expectations regarding the communicative capability of the system than he otherwise would. This can lead to disappointment and even to worse dialogue performance if the user has spoken more complex utterances because of the ECA's presence. Furthermore, ECAs can

Figure 1. Behavioural routine for dialogue initiation

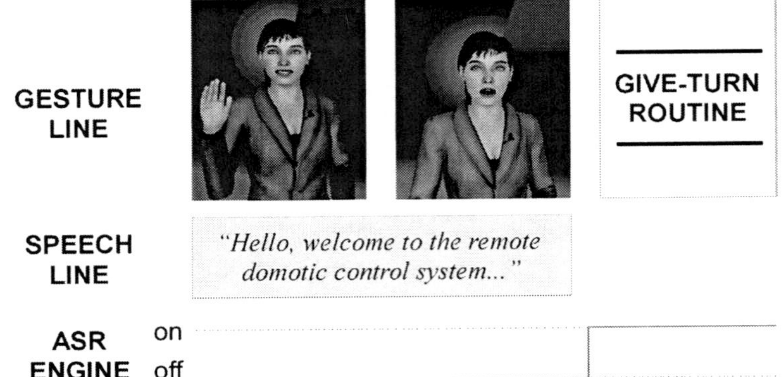


potentially distract users and lead them to pay less attention to what it is saying and to the task at hand (Schaumburg, 2001; Catrambone et al., 2002). Thus, the goal is to present a humanlike interface that is not too distracting upon first contact and which clearly 'sets the rules' of the interaction and conveys to the user the realistic limits of conversation with the system.

With the previous goals in mind, we have designed welcome gestures for our ECAs based on the recommendations in Kendon (1990): a smile and a wave of the hand. We have also played with the 'camera zoom' (the size and the position of the ECA on the screen). Figure 1 shows the gesture for Isabel, our female ECA. It also shows that after speaking the welcome message Isabel performs the turn-giving gesture routine to invite the user to speak. (Note that the give-turn routine itself is not shown here. We will describe it later, in its own dedicated subsection.)

## Speaker Verification Success

If the system was able to verify the user's identity (i.e., the system considers there was a close enough match), Isidro, the male ECA, informs the user, smiles and nods. The object of this simple behaviour is to connect with the user's satisfaction at having succeeded in the verification task and gained access to the next phase (the home automation application), to give the user the impression that the system shares his satisfaction.

From the point of view of communicative value or content, here the ECA conveys an emotion (which complements the message) and, partly by so doing, provides redundancy over the spoken confirmation of task success. The nodding is purely to reinforce this redundancy.

## Speaker Verification Error

As we saw in our scenario description, when the system is unable to verify the identity of the user after one or two valid attempts (i.e., when the recognised utterance corresponds to the number sequence the system requested), Isidro kindly informs the user:

*"I wasn't able to verify your identity."*

Isidro says this with a sad expression on his face to show empathy with the user in order, hopefully, to control his frustration and keep him in a calm mood. Again, our goal is to see whether an empathetic ECA makes for a better subjective experience even in the worst possible situation: task failure.

*Figure 2. Wrong number sequence routine*

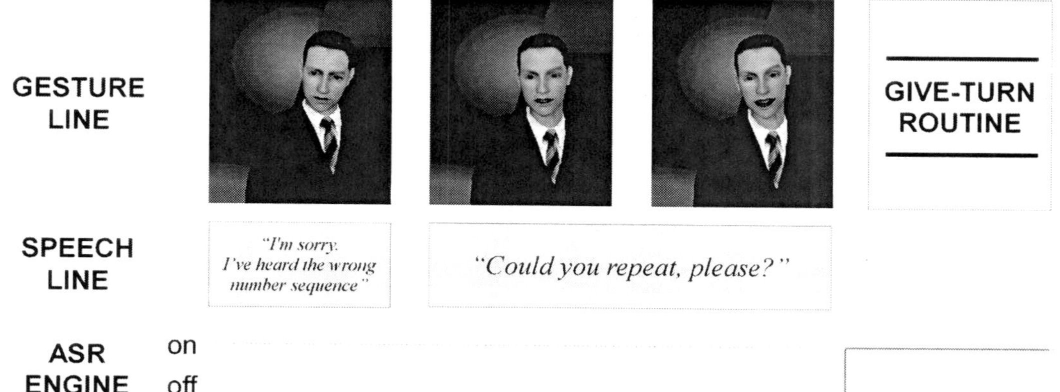


## Wrong Number Sequence

If the speech recognition unit produces an output which does not correspond to the number sequence it had requested, then we can assume that there has been a recognition error (since the utterance the user is asked to provide is a simple, concise sequence of numbers, which would be hard to get wrong if a user is cooperating).

Isidro responds with a two-part behaviour (Figure 2): first he displays a facial expression that involves lowering the head and putting on a 'eyebrow of sadness' – elements that Pelachaud (2003) has associated with remorse – while he says:

*"I'm sorry. I've heard the wrong number sequence."*

Then Isidro lifts his head up, opens his eyes, smiles and says:

*"Could you repeat, please?"*

We have tried to show remorse at having made a mistake followed by an expression of interest. Again, the motivation for this is to show empathy towards the user and let him know that the system is trying its best to understand what he says and remains optimistic that it will succeed, thus, it is hoped, infusing the user with optimism and motivation.

Therefore communicative content of the ECA's non-verbal behaviour provides redundancy of information regarding both the current state of the dialogue – there has either been a speech recognition error or the user has said something different to what he was supposed to – and what the user is expected to do next. Again, it also complements the verbal message by conveying that the system is trying to do its best to understand.

## Non-Understanding

A non-understanding occurs when the system fails to obtain a representation of the user's utterance that is intelligible within the scope of its grammar (Bohus & Rudnicky, 2008). When this happens it is important to make sure that the user realises what has happened, and also to get him to try again. We also want to avoid a build up of anxiety, frustration or disappointment in the user, which would reduce his motivation to continue to engage with the system.

The motivating idea for the ECA behaviour we have designed to respond to non-understandings is that, by engaging more closely with the user, chances are he may feel more encouraged to try to resolve the communication problem. In Figure

*Figure 3. Behavioural routine for non-understandings*

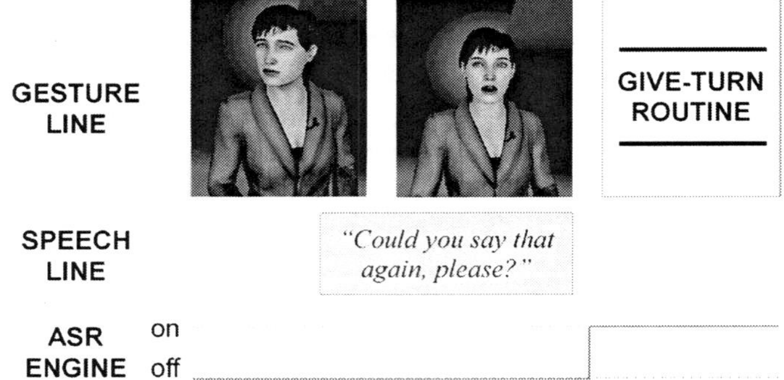


3 we see the gesture sequence: Isabel first stops smiling and brings her head forward very slightly, and turns it to one side while mildly squinting. One thing we are looking to achieve is to enhance the sense of engagement with the user by subtly closing the distance with him, but without making it too obvious, as then the movement could be seen as threatening.

Indeed, it has been suggested that confidence can by manipulated by altering the interpersonal distance (Altman & Vinsel, 1977). We also want to show that the system is making an effort to understand and to recover from the situation – which is taken seriously, hence the losing of the smile –, sending the encouraging message that the system probably expects the problem will be easily solved. Our gesture takes some elements from the *wh-question* intention gesture and the *sorry-for* and *sadness* affective state gestures suggested in Pelachaud (2003).

The verbal response that accompanies the gesture sequence is chosen randomly from one of the following:

a. "*Could you say that again, please?*"
b. "*I didn't catch that. Please tell me what you want again.*"

Notice that (a) and (b) are different recovery strategies. (a) is a typical request for the user to repeat the last utterance (although the user may choose to rephrase). With (b), on the other hand, the system first notifies the user of the non-understanding, and adds a request which reminds the user broadly of what he is expected to do – to query the system or instruct it to do something – without biasing him towards repeating or rephrasing. In neither strategy does the system apologise.

It could seem more polite to do so, and indeed apologising would imply taking the blame for the problem, which is a common psychological strategy in dialogue system design (although some authors tend not to recommend it – see, e.g., Nass & Brave, 2005). However, we have chosen not to include an apology to distinguish this situation from the more blameful and dangerous one of misunderstanding something the user says (i.e., taking the user to have said something different to what he actually said, rather than simply not understanding the utterance). We saw above an example of a misunderstanding recovery strategy with apology for the 'wrong number sequence' situation.

The gestural strategy is the same for messages (a) and (b). It is both an affective and an informative strategy which complements the verbal message by manipulating the interpersonal distance between the system and the user and showing that the system is making an effort to understand. The same gesture also adds redundancy over the verbal component to reinforce the message that the system did not understand the user's utterance.

## Confidence in the Accuracy of Recognition

The system's interpretation of a user utterance is qualified by an estimation of the probability of having made a mistake. If this probability is high – higher than a pre-determined threshold – the system then checks to see if it has all the pieces of information it needs – the action, the device and the location. If it does, it performs the action (e.g., it responds to the user's query). If one or more slots of information are missing it asks the user following a strategy of implicit confirmation of the known piece of information (to give the user an opportunity to correct the information if, against the estimated odds, the system has got it wrong). For instance:

*"Which lights do you want me to turn on?"*

We haven't associated a specific gestural behaviour with this situation, however.

If the system's confidence in having understood the user correctly is low, on the other hand, the recovery strategy is one of explicit confirmation, e.g., *"Did you ask about the bathroom lights?"*. Now, a common problem with explicit confirmation in these cases is that users will often reply with a short utterance like *"yes"* or *"no"* and without putting too much breath into it. Such utterances are hard for the system to detect, and easy to get wrong if it does detect them.

In order to prevent the occurrence of this sort of problem we added a second part to the ECAs behaviour, reiterating that the system needs the user to confirm the accuracy of a certain piece of information (*"Am I correct?"*). Accompanying this utterance is a gesture designed both to show interest and to engage optimistically with the user. Again, as with the non-understanding, the ECA leans forward slightly to catch the user's attention and to enhance the social engagement and enter a space of mutual trust. The gesture combines elements from the *I propose* intention gesture in – "head forward, raised eyebrow, look at [the user]" – and the *hope* affective state gesture – "raised eyebrow, large eye aperture" – suggested in Pelachaud (2003). The object of this optimistic stressing of the utterance is to elevate the user's motivation and induce him to increase the energy, and perhaps also the amount of words, he puts into his response.

The communicative content of this gesture sequence therefore complements the utterance with a display of interest combined with information to the effect that the system believes that it understood correctly. It also engages affectively with the user.

## Taking and Giving Turns

ECA body language and expressiveness may be exploited to help the flow the dialogue (Bickmore & Cassell, 2005). In particular, turn changing can be smoother with facial feedback provided by avatars (White et al., 2005). Turn changing involves two basic actions: taking turn and giving turn. Dialogue fluency improves and fewer errors occur if alternate system and user turns flow in orderly succession with the user knowing when it is his turn to speak.

It is important to stress that we have not allowed barge-in (i.e., the user cannot interrupt the system because the system doesn't listen to the user during its turn as the speech recogniser is then inactive). This makes for a less flexible dialogue than may be generally desirable, but we hope it offers at least two advantages: firstly, in the sort of problem situations we are interested in exploring it may advisable not to allow the user to interrupt while the system is trying to reach stable, mutually understood ground.

Secondly, if users try to speak during the system's turn (our users are not told they cannot interrupt the system) this usually leads to no-inputs (when the system remains waiting for an utterance that the user has already uttered), non-understandings and misunderstandings (because the system only listens to an incomplete utterance). Turn management then becomes more critical, and the consequences of confusion regarding who's turn it is more obvious. Thus, any effect an ECA may have on the mutual understanding of turn possession and turn transitions should be more visible.

The gestural behaviour we have designed for our ECAs is as follows (Figures 4.a and 4.b): When it's the ECA's turn the camera zooms-in slightly and the light becomes brighter. While the ECA approaches it raises a hand into the gesture space to 'announce' that it is going to speak. When it's the user's turn the camera zooms out, lights dim and ECA raises the eyebrow.

The sequence is not symmetric in that when the system initiates the turn-taking routine the ASR is disabled from the beginning (see Figure 4.a). After all, the system took the turn in the first place because it detected that the user had stopped speaking. When the system gives the turn, on the other hand, it allows the user to speak during the turn-giving transition routine, as is shown in Figure 4.b. This seems the more natural way to do it, and we anticipated that users might start speaking in the middle of a transition, as soon as they realized they were being handed the floor.

This strategy is a combination of gesture and other visual effects. It has been shown that users tend to prefer a gestural approach to indicate who has the floor – system or user – over other visual signs such as a light going on and off, a colour code or an hourglass (Edlund & Nordstrand, 2002). Since we only mark turn *transitions* with gestures, we thought that adding information that remained visible throughout an entire turn might help the user distinguish when it is the system's turn and he should not speak from when he is expected to

*Figure 4. (a) Isabel's take-turn routine: visual sequence of turn transition from user to ECA. (b) Isabel's take-turn routine: visual sequence of turn transition from ECA to user.*

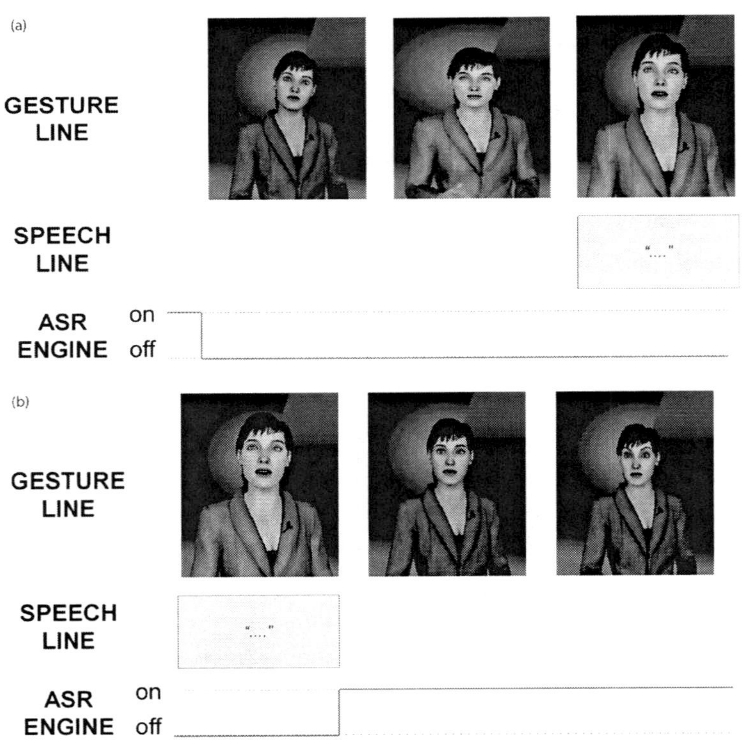

do so. Thus, we have tried combining gestures for the transition and other visual cues that remain in view once a transition has finished. Hopefully the user will learn to associate different gestures, camera shots and levels of light intensity with user turns and system turns.

This gestural and visual strategy complements the verbal cues indicating that the ECA has stopped speaking and, it is hoped, is more socially engaging.

## No Input

A no-input, to reiterate what was said earlier, is a situation in which the system is waiting for the user to say something for a lapse of time long enough to indicate that there may be a problem. The problem may be that the user does not know it is his turn yet, or that he is confused and doesn't know what to do, or maybe he is trying to speak but the VAD module doesn't detect his voice, or perhaps the user spoke before the ASR was enabled and the user doesn't realise it is *still* his turn since the system didn't register his utterance.

The no-input recovery routine is shown in Figure 5. The system decides there is a no-input situation when there has been a timeout. At this point the ECA does nothing. After a second timeout the ECA performs a gesture sequence to show that it is waiting: Isabel (or Isidro) leans back slightly, crosses her arms and brings her left hand to her face, and she shifts her 'weight' slightly onto her left leg. (This gesture sequence is largely our own design, but we drew inspiration from Fagerberg et al. (2003).) If the user still does not react before a third timeout then the ECA takes the turn and says:

*"I haven't heard you say anything yet. You can ask me for help, if you need it."*

This lets the user know that the system was expecting him to say something but heard nothing, and it also suggests a line of action (asking for help) in case the cause of the problem was that the user is unsure of what he is supposed to say.

The gestural strategy in this case *anticipates* the verbal message. The goal is to solve the problem (i.e., get the user to say something) before having to resort to taking the turn from him, which would make the dialogue more inefficient and could cause further problems (e.g., barge-in attempts if the user finally reacts when it is no longer his turn).

# User Tests: Experimental Design

## Test Architecture

The architecture of our test environment is based on web technology, with which we simulate a mobile phone interface. We implemented two different

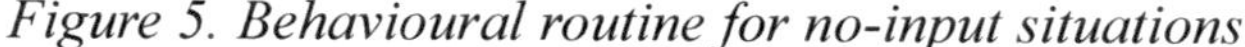

*Figure 5. Behavioural routine for no-input situations*

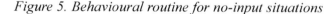

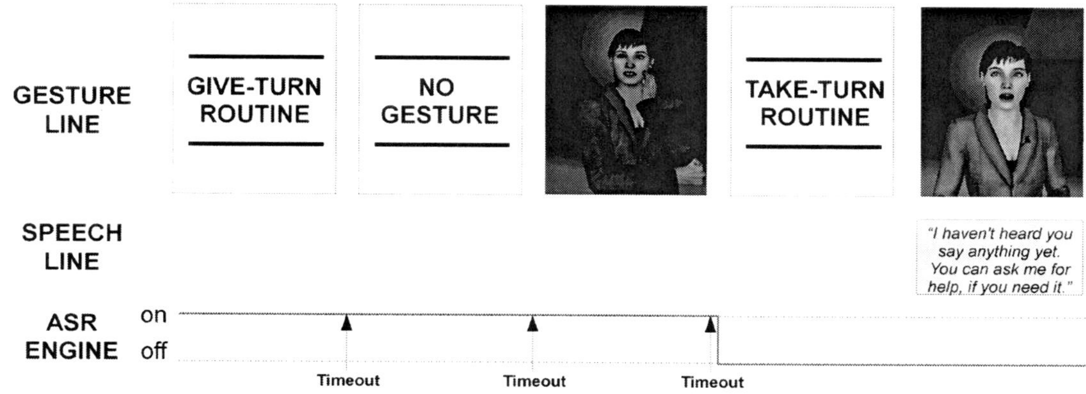

interaction scenarios: one with ECAs (specific dialogue situations for it have been described earlier) and the other without (voice-only output for the dialogue system). The system is implemented on a web page that contains two frames. In the left frame there is a column of labels that show the test user what stage of testing he or she is (not to be confused with the dialogue stage which is not indicated). The main interface is displayed in the right frame and shows a mobile phone running a videotelephony application.

All the technical elements of the evaluation environment are hosted on an Apache Tomcat web server. Throughout the test, users face a series of evaluation questionnaires and dialogue interactions. The questionnaires are implemented using HTML forms, and the information collected on them is transferred to JSP files and then stored in a database. Our test environment uses Nuance Communications' speech recognition technology (www.nuance.com). The ECA character was created by Haptek (www.haptek.com). The dialogues are implemented with Java Applet technology, and they are all packed and signed to guarantee fast download and access to the audio resources. Dialogue dynamics are programmed. Nuance's speech recognition engine provides a useful Java API that allows access to different grammars and adjusting a range of parameters depending on the characteristics of each application. Finally, interaction parameters (such as utterance durations, number of turns, number of recognition errors, etc.) are recorded automatically during the test interactions.

## Description of the Experiment

We tested the system with 40 users divided into two groups, one interacting with the ECA and the other only receiving a speech output from the system. Due to system errors during the interaction, two users (1 from each group) were excluded. Therefore, we obtained results from 38 people (19 users in each group). Users were mainly students (28 out of the 38 – 74%) and under 24 years of age (25 out of the 38 – 69%). 16 were female and 22 male. Regarding their prior experience with virtual agents, about 60% of the users have ever used a system where an agent is included. Finally, a high percentage of users (81.6%) indicated they had previously used traditional spoken dialogue systems. However, only 52.6% of our test users had had some prior use experience with SLDSs that had natural language capabilities. Regarding user satisfaction with SLDS technology, only 13.2% of the users describe their previous interaction experiences as having been 'good'.

Testing was carried out in a small meeting room. Users were seated at the head of a long table in front of a 15" screen. Two different views of the user interacting with the system were video-recorded to provide us with visual data to inspect and annotate the subject's behaviour: a frontal view was taken from the top edge of the user's screen (see Figure 6), and a lateral view was recorded from a wide-angle position to the right of the user. Both views were taken with Logitech Quickcam Pro 4000 webcams. Users spoke to system through headset microphone, and the system prompts were played through two small speakers. All user-system dialogue was in Spanish. The entire test procedure was designed to take roughly 30 to 45 minutes, with minimal intervention on the part of experimenter.

*Figure 6. ECA interface for the speaker verification task*

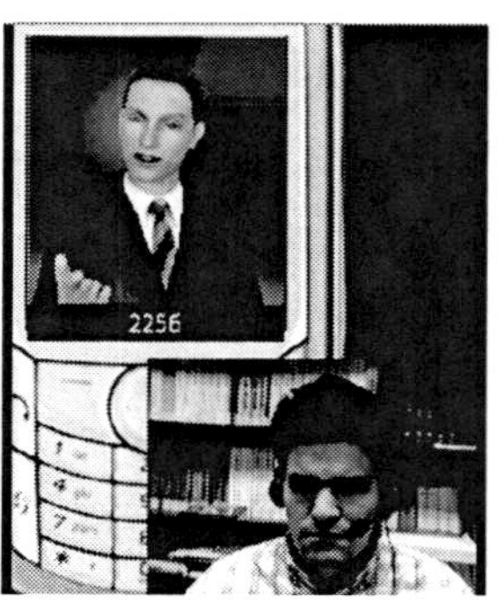

The stages of the evaluation are as follows:

1. *Brief explanation:* The user is told what the general purpose (to "evaluate automatic dialogue systems") and methodology of the evaluation are, as well as the tasks that lie ahead for him/her.
2. *Opening questionnaire* to learn about the user's prior experience and expectations.
3. *Training phase:* The user is asked to enrol in a secure access system, which requires interacting in guided dialogue with an application that registers his/her voice traits (the system asks the user to repeat four four-digit sequences).
4. *Post-enrolment questionnaire* to capture the user's opinions on the form of access and related aspects such as privacy and security.
5. *Verification phase (secure access task):* The user does three successive verification exercises (as was discussed above).
6. *Post-verification questionnaire:* Similar to the post-enrolment questionnaire, to see if users' opinions change after using the biometric access system.
7. *Domotic dialogue phase (query task):* Users are asked to find out the state (on/off) of three household devices ("the bathroom lights", "the fan in the bedroom", and "the living-room television set").
8. *Final questionnaire:* To obtain the user's overall impression of the system, its main elements and the most important aspects of using it. Some questions are the same as in previous questionnaires, so that we may observe how user perceptions evolve throughout the various stages of using the system.

## User Tests: Presentation and Discussion of Results

In this section, we present some of the more interesting results we have obtained from comparing the performance and the users' subjective experience of user-system interaction with ECAs and with a voice-only interface, both scenarios and dialogue systems otherwise being identical, with the exception that some system turns were slightly longer with the ECA to allow full execution of gesture sequences.

Our questionnaires are based on Hone and Graham's (2001) SASSI 'subjective assessment' tool for dialogue systems and on the ITU-T P.851 recommendation on questionnaire design for the evaluation of spoken dialogue systems for general telephone services (ITU-T, 2003), which we expanded to include dimensions (as sets of questions) to evaluate aspects of the users' experience related with biometric access and with the presence and behaviour of an ECA. Our combined performance and user experience approach was inspired initially by the PARADISE method (Walker et al., 1997), and more recently by the work of Möller et al. (2007).

We have obtained the results detailed below by a) comparing performance and questionnaire responses in the ECA group of users with those in the voice-only group; and b) observing how performance and responses to certain questions evolve throughout the test. We used two sample t-tests, Mann-Whitney tests and Spearman correlation coefficients, setting the significance level at 5% ($p=0.05$). Questionnaire responses were collected on Likert-type 5-point response formats. User comments were also collected.

## Interaction Parameters

### Overall Accumulated Data

ITU-T Suppl. 24 to P-Series Recommendation (ITU-T, 2005) lists the most common objective parameters for quantifying quality of interaction with a spoken dialogue system. In Table 1 we summarise the main observations in which we found differences between the ECA and the voice-only interfaces, as regards user-system interaction.

*Table 1. Dialogue performance data for the ECA and voice-only interfaces*[1]

| **Dialogue- and communication-related interaction parameters** | | | |
|---|---|---|---|
| **Abbrev.** | **Description** | **With ECA** | **Voice only** |
| *DD* | Overall dialogue duration (sec.) | 343.15 | 368.45 |
| STD | Average system turn duration (sec.) | 7.17 | 6.57 |
| *UTD* | Average user turn duration (sec.) | 3.57 | 3.87 |
| *# Turns* | Accumulated number of turns throughout all interaction (all users) | 933 | 1055 |
| **Meta-communication-related interaction parameters** | | | |
| **Abbrev.** | **Description** | **With ECA** | **Voice only** |
| *# Time Out* | Number of time-outs | 7 | 15 |
| *# ASR Reject.* | Number of non-understandings | 22 | 32 |
| *# Barge-in* | Number of times users tried to speak when the ASR module was inactive.[2] | 30 | 68 |
| **Task-related interaction parameters** | | | |
| **Abbrev.** | **Description** | **With ECA** | **Voice only** |
| *TS* | Task success rate (%) | 98,25 | 98,25 |
| Speech-input-related interaction parameters | | | |
| Abbrev. | Description | With ECA | Voice-only |
| *%PA:CO* | Percentage of correctly parsed user utterances | 76.29 | 68.38 |
| *%PA:PA* | Percentage of partially parsed user utterances | 5.67 | 5.38 |
| *%PA:IC* | Percentage of failed-to-be-parsed user utterances | 18.04 | 26.23 |

1 Averages or totals for all users in the respective test groups, accumulated from both phases in the test scenario (biometric access and home automation).

2 In our user tests, in addition to the number of barge-in attempts the figures include the number of times users tried to jump the welcome message.

The parameters listed are taken from the above-mentioned ITU-T recommendation. The figures in the table are averages or totals (depending on the parameter) for all users in the respective test groups, and include all of the interactions accumulated from both phases in the test scenario (biometric access and home automation).

We can see that overall dialogue duration was similar for both interaction scenarios, as was average user-turn duration and average number of turns in the dialogue, with figures for the ECA interface being slightly lower. However, system turns were slightly longer with the ECA, which, combined with the fact we just mentioned that average DD and UTD are slightly shorter for the ECA interface, seems to indicate that voice-only interactions were, on average, slightly less efficient.

This is confirmed when we look at the second ('meta-communication') block of parameters. The total number of time-outs (when the system is waiting for the user to say something) for the voice-only interface (15) is twice that of the version with the ECA (7), and the total number of non-understandings is about 50% higher (32 *vs.* 22). We performed Mann-Whitney tests on these two variables, and in the case of the ASR Rejections the difference is statistically significant at the p =.05 level.

Inspired in the smoothness parameter proposed in Weiss et al. (2010), we computed a parameter we called *roughness* derived from several performance parameters related to complications in the interaction. Specifically,

Roughness = #ASR rejection + #PA:PA + #PA:IC + #Time-out

The median value of roughness for the interactions in the ECA group was 5 *vs.* 8 for the voice-only group. A Mann-Whitney test revealed that the difference is statistically significant (U = 110; p (exact, two-tailed) <.05).

We may infer from these general observations that the ECA is helping users interact more efficiently with the system, as a result of their having, generally, fewer problems and recovering more easily from them – i.e., the system is more robust. The reason may be that the information provided by the ECA throughout the interaction reduces user confusion regarding the state of the dialogue at any particular moment.

More specifically, turn changing and no-input behaviour sequences may be helping them understand when they are required to speak. The number of barge-in attempts was roughly the same for both groups of users. The large difference in the number of times the user tried to speak when the ASR module was inactive is due solely to instances in which users of the voice-only version tried to speak before the system uttered the welcome message. These users had received no cue at all from the system at this point, so they lacked a point of reference regarding turn possession. The ECA group, on the other hand, could see the ECA from the beginning and they all waited for it to begin speaking. This is an interesting observation: the presence of the ECA made users understand that they should wait, effectively inducing them to grant initial control to the system.

The number of barge-ins was not much higher for the ECA group thanks to the fact that the ASR was made active for the system-user turn transition behaviour sequence, because on 201 of these transitions (52% of the total) users began speaking before the end of the sequence. However, certain gesture sequences were too effective in conveying information to the user, and led to barge-in attempts and, as a result (since barge-in is not allowed with our system), to interaction problems. Indeed, upon viewing the recorded interaction videos we observed a few instances in which the first phases of a gesture were enough to prompt a user response. Specifically, this sometimes occurred with the non-understanding gestural sequence described previously. The gesture sequence is performed before the ECA speaks, but some users already react to that. In spite of the interaction problems that this gave rise to because of the peculiarities of our system, it shows the communicative power of this particular gesture sequence.

Effectiveness in reaching the interaction goals was identical in both groups: almost all of the tasks with the home automation system (the queries) were completed successfully.

## The Users' Subjective Experience

### Overall Impression and Expectations

The users' overall impression of the home automation system (response categories: 1 = 'very bad ... 5 = 'very good) was similar in both groups, ECA and voice-only, with a median of 4 in both cases. However, looking at the raw data there is an observable difference in the distribution of answers. The number of people giving a positive rating (categories 4 and 5) is similar for both groups (15 in the ECA group *vs.* 12 in the voice-only group), but there are noticeable differences in categories 4 and 5 considered separately. While there were equal numbers of users (6) rating 4 and 5 in the voice-only group, in the ECA group most of the positive ratings were on a 4 (12 ratings *vs.* 3 for category 5). Thus, users in the latter group seemed more likely to avoid the extreme positive rating regarding their overall impression.

Another question addressed whether the system had surprised users negatively or positively (response categories: 1 = 'very negatively' ... 5 = 'very positively'). The responses show that voice-only interface users were very slightly more positively surprised by the system's dialoguing capability than ECA users ($\mu_{ECA}$ = 3.9, $\mu_{voice}$ = 4.3; medians were 4 for both groups). A Mann-Whitney test to compare both groups on this question, however, revealed that differences were not quite statistically significant at the p =.05 level (two-tailed exact p =.073). Still, the observation is interesting; especially in view of the fact that in terms of actual dialogue performance, the interactions of the voice-only group fared objectively worse than those of the ECA group, as we related above.

These findings in relation to the two previously mentioned questions (*overall impression* and *surprise*) suggest that ECAs may generate greater expectations which lead them subsequently to being less impressed with the system's performance compared to voice-only users, even if on average they had fewer interaction problems.

## Efficiency

Users' perception that "*Dialoguing with the system led quickly to solve the task proposed*" (1 - totally disagree... 5 - totally agree) was on average greater in the ECA group ($\mu_{ECA}$ = 4.2) than in the voice-only group ($\mu_{voice}$ = 3.2) (t(12)=3,16; p<0.01). Some of the users in the latter said they had felt confused at certain stages of the dialogue (e.g., *"between tasks there were silences and I didn't know if I was supposed to say anything," "a couple of times I think I spoke too early and that's why the system didn't get what I said," "it would be better if some sort of visual sign told you when the system is ready to listen"*). Thus, comments and scores for user impression of efficiency in their interaction are in accordance with the actual performance data presented above. We must be cautious in our interpretation, however, since the users' subjective impression can be positively influenced merely by the presence of a human-like animated figure – the so-called persona effect (Lester et al., 1997).

## Likeability

ITU-P P.851 factors related with pleasantness and amusement display a significant evolution throughout the tests. The average grade users award to the *amusement* value of spoken dialogue interaction grows significantly in the ECA users from the first questionnaire (2.9) to the last (3.6) (t=-2.39; p<0.05). In contrast, the average *pleasantness* score for the voice-only group falls from the first questionnaire (3.6) to the last (3.3) (t=2.05; p<0.05).

A key element in speaker training and verification dialogues is that users feel comfortable during the interaction. If users are comfortable and relaxed there will generally be fewer interaction problems, as we discussed in a previous section. Therefore, in addition to the direct reading of the previous result, which is an indication that the presence of our gesturing ECAs can positively affect the users' subjective experience, it could be helping dialogue performance and the avoidance of interaction problems. Nevertheless, it is difficult to establish the direction of the causal relationship between objective performance and subjective experience, and likeability factors in particular, since they are surely mutually reinforcing.

## Rejection Factors: Privacy and Security Concerns

A major concern in speaker verification systems is privacy. Therefore, 'personifying' with an ECA a system designed to capture sensitive information, as voice features are, requires special care. These are the findings in our study that bear on this issue:

Responses to the question *"I would feel uncomfortable using the remote control system for home devices because I would feel my privacy was being encroached on"* (1 - totally disagree ... 5 - totally agree) evolved significantly in the ECA group, averaging 2.5 in the first questionnaire and 3.3 in the last (t =-2.05; p<0.05). Similarly, for the question *"I would have security concerns using the system, perhaps because I fear that unauthorized people might manage to remotely control my home devices"* (same scale): replies averaged 2.5 in the first questionnaire and 3.5 in the last ($t=-3.06$; $p<0.01$).

These results are in accordance with previous work in which we studied the effect an ECA could have on users interacting with a biometric authentication application (Hernández-Trapote et al., 2007). We found then that the mere presence of an ECA (without any specifically designed gestures and with little expressiveness) can negatively affect users' perception of loss of privacy. However, our new findings seem clearer, suggesting that a more active ECA has a greater negative impact on the users' perception of security and privacy. This could be either because the user feels observed or because an animated figure makes the system look less serious and therefore less trustworthy.

## Correlations between Objective Performance and Subjective Experience

The ultimate test for any technological application is the satisfaction of users and whether or not they are willing to actually use the system; in other words, user acceptance. It is therefore useful, indeed necessary, to find connections between performance data and the impressions of users regarding their experience of use.

In our tests we found that the users' overall impression regarding the system (both groups of users together) was correlated with the roughness parameter we computed ($r_s = -.33$; $p <.05$). Responses to the question *"Overall, did you have positive or negative feelings?"* (response categories: 1 = 'very negative' ... 5 = 'very positive') were also correlated with roughness ($r_s = -.42$; $p <.01$). This general (albeit weak) trend makes sense: the better the interaction goes we should expect a better overall opinion of a dialogue system.

Interestingly, for the voice-only group the correlations are weaker and not statistically significant (the halving of the sample also contributes to this, of course); however, for the ECA group the correlation between overall impression and roughness was stronger ($r_s = -.58$; $p <.01$).

We saw earlier that interactions were generally smoother in the ECA group than in the voice-only group. These correlation results now show that smoother interaction was only correlated significantly to the overall subjective experience in the ECA group, the group that fared better with the dialogue system. It is early to conclude why this is so, but it is plausible that an ECA, which we have seen tends to help the interaction flow better, also makes users more sensitive to interaction problems when they do occur. This effect could also be connected to the greater expectations users have of dialogue systems with ECAs, which are betrayed when there are errors and problems recovering from them.

## Concluding Discussion of the Results

These results suggest that the ECAs we have designed are complementing the verbal message with their gestural behaviour, adding to the overall meaning, the information content that users are able to process cognitively. To begin with, users are attentive to the presence of the ECA and to what it does, as was evidenced by the initial waiting for the ECA to do something and also the immediate responses to some of the gestures before the ECA had begun to say anything.

There are no differences in task success between the two groups of users – probably because of the relatively straightforward nature of the tasks – but the complementary and redundant information conveyed by the ECA does seem to be helping users have a better grasp of where they are in the dialogue and what they can do or are required to do in each particular situation. In other words, interaction with the ECA turned out, in our experiment, to be slightly more robust than with a voice-only output. We have to be prudent, nonetheless, regarding the generalizability of our results due to the context and situation-specific nature of the observations on which they are based, as well as the relatively small sample size of test users (we must note, however, that our sample size lies within the usual range in this type of user studies in the general literature on human-machine interaction).

It is difficult to assess the role of affect in these results. We have seen that users in the ECA group felt that their interaction with the system was clear and efficient to a greater degree than did users in the voice-only group, and the former also liked and enjoyed interacting with the system slightly more than the latter. However, we must further investigate whether these effects are related to the presence and behaviour of the ECA directly or if, on the other hand, they emanate from the improved performance with the ECA, or perhaps both. The correlations we found between robustness (smoothness) and overall impressions and feelings give weight to the first of these interpretations, but do not preclude the second.

Finally, on the negative side our ECAs may be generating in users expectations regarding the systems communicative skills (and perhaps also its functional abilities) that are too optimistic, which then leads to a degree of disappointment. Privacy and security concerns are also heightened when an ECA is present, although further research is needed to confirm this observation, explain it and shed light on its connections with other elements of the users' experience.

## FUTURE RESEARCH DIRECTIONS

The previous discussion of our results suggests that ECAs could be of service to improve robustness of spoken dialogue systems. Nevertheless, we are just beginning to understand how ECAs affect the perceptions of users, upon which the most appropriate design of the ECA's behaviour ultimately depends. What does seem clear is that the design of the ECAs behaviour must take the context of interaction into account.

In this chapter we have shown that users of ECAs are slightly more sensitive to privacy and security matters. Bearing in mind that our experimental scenario was related with biometric identification and personal services this finding opens an interesting line of research regarding the source of this effect, which seems to be an instance of the 'persona effect'. As yet little research of this sort has been undertaken for biometric applications (Krämer et al., 2009), but it is a promising area of application, and the line of research could also be extended to further scenario variations.

The case study presented above was designed for studying very basic situations which occur in a spoken dialogue system in which the flow of the interaction was guided to a certain extent, and the content domain rather limited. Nevertheless, there are numerous initiatives that are beginning to propose more complex behavioural models and based on the user's feedback (Gratch et al., 2006; Edlund & Beskow, 2007). The capacity to deal with more intelligent, broader and less guided interaction strategies is an important step towards which some efforts are currently being made (for instance, the Companions Project funded by the 7th Framework Programme of the European Commission (Companions, 2010)).

For significant progress to be made in the design of this new family of interaction systems it will be invaluable to develop ECA gesture collections. Typically, researchers design ECA behaviour by copying human behaviour or collecting the information from classic literature on human gesture generation or performance. It would be very useful to have a dynamic and standardized framework that can support fast prototyping.

As regards user centred evaluation, we have had to extend international recommendations for dialogue systems that are spoken only, so that they would cover aspects related to the non-verbal channel of communication introduced with the ECA. An extensive amount of further work will be needed to consolidate appropriate evaluation methods, frameworks and recommendations for the context-independent embodied dialogue systems of the present and near future.

## CONCLUSION

In this chapter we have given an overview of the most common low-level, speech recognition-related interaction problems with spoken dialogue systems and presented insights regarding how embodied conversational agents can help improve a system's robustness to these problems and the general smoothness in the flow of the dialogue. We have used our description of a case study – a dialogue system which we developed to carry out comparative user tests – as a vehicle to compile and present a variety of aspects found in different projects, experiments and theoretical approaches in the literature on ECA development, from defining scenarios and contexts of use, to gesture design, coordination of different behavioural elements, user test design and evaluation of the interaction.

We have threaded the various aspects of our account around reflections regarding the information that is conveyed – and the types of information conveyed – between the system and the user (particularly from the system to the user), as well as the affective and attitudinal (empathetic) aspects of the social engagement between the user and the system. This approach has lent a conceptual clarity which has enabled us to draw, however tentatively, encouraging conclusions along the general lines that ECAs who's behaviour is designed to convey information appropriate for specific contexts and situations can reduce user confusion, help recover from interaction problems and make the dialogue flow more smoothly. Furthermore, these benefits tend also to be reflected in the users' general satisfaction with the interaction experience. On the negative side, we have seen that ECAs may also elevate the users' expectations regarding the system's conversational proficiency and make them more sensitive to (and critical of) interaction problems.

It seems, therefore, that ECAs possess features that provide the opportunity to increase dialogue robustness. This realisation suggests applying the notion of affordance as used by Norman (1999) in the field of design (of "everyday things" (Norman, 2002)) and restated for 'smart technology environments' by Jokinen as a set of relationships between users and systems that allow the latter to "lend themselves to natural use without the users needing to think and reason how the interaction should take place in order to get the task completed" (Jokinen, 2009, p. 125). Regarding the relationship between the user and an ECA interface, the expressive possibilities of ECAs, if properly coupled with the user's communicational ability, provide the possibility (are an affordance) for rich, fluent, natural and robust dialogue between the two.

## ACKNOWLEDGMENT

The activities described in this chapter were funded by the Spanish Ministry of Science and Technology as part of the TEC2009-14719-C02-02 project.

## REFERENCES

Altman, I., & Vinsel, A. (1977). Personal space. An analysis of E. T. Hall's proxemics framework. *Human Behaviour and Environment. Advances in Theory and Research*, *2*, 181–259.

Amores, J., Pérez, G., & Manchón, P. (2007). MIMUS: A multimodal and multilingual dialogue system for the home domain. In *Proceedings of the ACL 2007 Demo and Poster Sessions, vol. 45* (pp. 1-4).

Atkinson, R. (2002). Optimizing learning from examples using animated pedagogical agents. *Journal of Educational Psychology*, *94*(2), 416–427. doi:10.1037/0022-0663.94.2.416

Bell, L., & Gustafson, J. (2003). *Child and adult speaker adaptation during error resolution in a publicly available spoken dialogue system*. In 8th European Conference on Speech Communication and Technology-EUROSPEECH 2003 (pp. 613-616). ISCA.

Bickmore, T. (2008). *Framing and interpersonal stance in relational agents*. Paper presented at Why Conversational Agents do what they do. Functional Representations for Generating Conversational Agent Behavior. AAMAS 2008.

Bickmore, T., & Cassell, J. (2005). Social dialogue with embodied conversational agents. In Jan van Kuppevelt, L. D., & Bernsen, N. O. (Eds.), *Advances in natural multimodal dialogue systems* (*Vol. 30*, pp. 23–54). Springer. doi:10.1007/1-4020-3933-6_2

Bickmore, T., Pfeifer, L., & Jack, B. (2009). Taking the time to care: empowering low health literacy hospital patients with virtual nurse agents. In *Proceedings of the 27th International Conference on Human Factors in Computing Systems* (pp. 1265-1274). ACM.

Bickmore, T. W., & Picard, R. W. (2005). Establishing and maintaining long-term human-computer relationships. [TOCHI]. *ACM Transactions on Computer-Human Interaction*, *12*(2), 293–327. doi:10.1145/1067860.1067867

Bohus, D. (2007). *Error awareness and recovery in conversational spoken language interfaces. Unpublished doctoral disseration*. Carnegie Mellon University.

Bohus, D., & Rudnicky, A. (2005). LARRI: A language-based maintenance and repair assistant. In *Spoken multimodal human-computer dialogue in mobile environments, vol. 28* (pp. 203-218). Springer Netherlands.

Bohus, D., & Rudnicky, A. I. (2008). Sorry, I didn't catch that! An investigation of non-understanding errors and recovery strategies. In Dybkjær, L., & Minker, W. (Eds.), *Recent trends in discourse and dialogue* (*Vol. 39*, pp. 123–154). Springer Netherlands. doi:10.1007/978-1-4020-6821-8_6

Breazeal, C., Kidd, C., Thomaz, A., Hoffman, G., & Berlin, M. (2005). Effects of nonverbal communication on efficiency and robustness in human-robot teamwork. In *Proceedings of IEEE/RSJ International Conference on Intelligent Robots and Systems (IROS)* (pp. 708-713).

Buisine, S., Abrilian, S., & Martin, J. (2004). Evaluation of multimodal behaviour of embodied agents. In Ruttkay, Z., & Pelachaud, C. (Eds.), *From brows to trust: Evaluating embodied conversational agents* (pp. 217–238). Springer.

Cassell, J., Bickmore, T., Billinghurst, M., Campbell, L., Chang, K., Vilhjalmsson, H., & Yan, H. (1999). Embodiment in conversational interfaces: Rea. In *Proceedings of the SIGCHI conference on Human factors in computing systems: the CHI is the limit* (pp. 520-527). ACM Press.

Cassell, J., Bickmore, T., Campbell, L., Vilhjálmsson, H., & Yan, H. (2000b). Human conversation as a system framework: Designing embodied conversational agents. In S. P. Justine Cassell, Joseph Sullivan & E. F. Churchill (Eds.), *Embodied conversational agents* (pp. 29-63). MIT Press.

Cassell, J., Nakano, Y., Bickmore, T., Sidner, C., & Rich, C. (2001a). Non-verbal cues for discourse structure. In *Proceedings of the 39th Annual Meeting on Association for Computational Linguistics* (pp. 114-123). Morgan Kaufmann Publishers.

Cassell, J., Stocky, T., Bickmore, T., Gao, Y., Nakano, Y., Ryokai, K., et al. Vilhjálmsson, H. (2002, January). *MACK: Media lab Autonomous Conversational Kiosk*. In IMAGINA'02, vol. 2 (pp. 12-15). Monte Carlo, Monaco.

Cassell, J., Sullivan, J. S. P., & Churchill, E. F. (Eds.). (2000a). *Embodied conversational agents*. MIT Press.

Cassell, J., & Tartaro, A. (2007). Intersubjectivity in humanagent interaction. *Interaction Studies: Social Behaviour and Communication in Biological and Artificial Systems*, *8*(3), 391–410.

Cassell, J., Vilhjálmsson, H., & Bickmore, T. (2001b). BEAT: The behavior expression animation toolkit. In *Proceedings of the 28th annual conference on Computer graphics and interactive techniques* (pp. 477-486). Association for Computational Linguistics.

Catrambone, R., Stasko, J., & Xiao, J. (2002). Anthropomorphic agents as a user interface paradigm: Experimental findings and a framework for research. In W. D. Gray & C. Schunn (Eds.), *Proceedings of the 24th Annual Conference of the Cognitive Science Society* (pp. 166-171). Cognitive Science Society.

*Companions Project*. (2010). Retrieved April 26, 2010, from http://www.companions-project.org

Dausend, M., & Ehrlich, U. (2008). A prototype for future spoken dialog systems using an embodied conversational agent. In *Perception in multimodal dialogue systems* (*Vol. 5078*, pp. 268–271). Springer. doi:10.1007/978-3-540-69369-7_30

de Rosis, F., Pelachaud, C., Poggi, I., Carofiglio, V., & Carolis, B. (2003). From Greta's mind to her face: Modelling the dynamics of affective states in a conversational embodied agent. *International Journal of Human-Computer Studies*, *59*(1-2), 81–118. doi:10.1016/S1071-5819(03)00020-X

Eckert, M. (2006). *Speaker identification and verification applications. (Internal Working Draft)*. VoiceXML Forum Speaker Biometrics Committee.

Edlund, J., & Beskow, J. (2007). Pushy versus meek using avatars to influence turn-taking behaviour. In *Proceedings of Interspeech 2007 ICSLP*. Atwerp.

Edlund, J., & Nordstrand, M. (2002). Turn-taking gestures and hourglasses in a multi-modal dialogue system. In *Proceedings of ISCA Workshop Multi-Modal Dialogue in Mobile Environments*. ISCA.

Engwall, O. (2008). Can audio-visual instructions help learners improve their articulation? An ultrasound study of short term changes. In [ISCA.]. *Proceedings of Interspeech*, *2008*, 2631–2634.

Fagerberg, P., Stahl, A., & Höök, K. (2003). Designing gestures for affective input: an analysis of shape, effort and valence. In Ollila, M., & Rantzer, M. (Eds.), *Proceedings of mobile ubiquitous and multimedia, MUM 2003*. Linköping University Electronic Press.

Foster, M. (2007). Enhancing human-computer interaction with embodied conversational agents. *Universal Access in Human-Computer Interaction. Ambient Interaction*, *4555*, 828–837.

Goldberg, J., Ostendorf, M., & Kirchhoff, K. (2003). *The impact of response wording in error correction subdialogs*. In ISCA Tutorial and Research Workshop on Error Handling in Spoken Dialogue Systems (pp. 101-106). ISCA.

Gratch, J., Okhmatovskaia, A., Lamothe, F., Marsella, S., Morales, M., van der Werf, R. J., & Morency, L. P. (2006). Virtual rapport. In *Proceedings of the 6th International Conference on Intelligent Virtual Agents* (pp. 14-27).

Gratch, J., Wang, N., Okhmatovskaia, A., Lamothe, F., Morales, M., van der Werf, R., & Morency, L. (2007). Can virtual humans be more engaging than real ones? *Lecture Notes in Computer Science*, *4552*, 286. doi:10.1007/978-3-540-73110-8_30

Hartmann, B., Mancini, M., Buisine, S., & Pelachaud, C. (2005). Design and evaluation of expressive gesture synthesis for embodied conversational agents. In *Proceedings of the 4th International Joint Conference on Autonomous Agents and Multiagent Systems* (pp. 1095-1096). Association for Computational Linguistics.

Hernández-Trapote, A., López-Mencía, B., Díaz-Pardo, D., Fernández-Pozo, R., Hernández-Gómez, L., & Caminero, J. (2007). A person in the interface: Effects on user perceptions of multibiometrics. In *Proceedings of the ACL 2007 Workshop on Embodied Language Processing*. Association for Computational Linguistics.

Heylen, D., & ter Maat, M. (2008). *A linguistic view on functional markup languages*. Paper presented at Why Conversational Agents do what they do. Functional Representations for Generating Conversational Agent Behavior. AAMAS 2008. Estoril, Portugal.

Hone, K. (2006). Empathic agents to reduce user frustration: The effects of varying agent characteristics. *Interacting with Computers*, *18*(2), 227–245. doi:10.1016/j.intcom.2005.05.003

Hone, K. S., & Graham, R. (2001). Towards a tool for the subjective assessment of speech system interfaces (SASSI). *Natural Language Engineering*, *6*(3-4), 287–303.

Jokinen, K. (2009). *Constructive dialogue modelling: Speech interaction and rational agents*. John Wiley & Sons.

Kendon, A. (1990). *Conducting interaction: Patterns of behavior in focused encounters*. Cambridge University Press.

Kipp, M. (2001). From human gesture to synthetic action. In *Proceedings of the Workshop on" Multimodal Communication and Context in Embodied Agents held in conjunction with the Fifth International Conference on Autonomous Agents (AGENTS)* (pp. 9-14).

Kopp, S., Allwood, J., Grammer, K., Ahlsen, E., & Stocksmeier, T. (2008). Modeling embodied feedback with virtual humans. *Modeling Communication with Robots and Virtual Humans*, *4930*, 18–37. doi:10.1007/978-3-540-79037-2_2

Kopp, S., Gesellensetter, L., Krämer, N., & Wachsmuth, I. (2005). A conversational agent as museum guide-design and evaluation of a real-world application. In *Intelligent virtual agents* (*Vol. 3661*, pp. 329–343). Springer. doi:10.1007/11550617_28

Krämer, N., Bente, G., Eschenburg, F., & Troitzsch, H. (2009). Embodied conversational agents: Research prospects for social psychology and an exemplary study. *Social Psychology*, *40*(1), 26–36. doi:10.1027/1864-9335.40.1.26

Lee, J., DeVault, D., Marsella, S., & Traum, D. (2008, May). *Thoughts on FML: Behavior generation in the virtual human communication architecture*. Paper presented at Why Conversational Agents do what they do. Functional Representations for Generating Conversational Agent Behavior. AAMAS 2008, Estoril, Portugal.

Lester, J. C., Converse, S. A., Kahler, S. E., Barlow, S. T., Stone, B. A., & Bhogal, R. S. (1997). The persona effect: Affective impact of animated pedagogical agents. In S. Pemberton (Ed.), *Proceedings of the SIGCHI conference on Human factors in computing systems* (pp. 359-366).

López-Mencía, B., Hernández-Trapote, A., Díaz-Pardo, D., Fernández-Pozo, R., Hernández-Gómez, L., & Torre Toledano, D. (2007). Design and validation of ECA gestures to improve dialogue system robustness. In *Proceedings of the ACL 2007 Workshop on Embodied Language Processing* (pp. 67-74). Association for Computational Linguistics.

Marsi, E., & van Rooden, F. (2007). Expressing uncertainty with a talking head in a multimodal question-answering system. In E. R. E. K. I. van der Sluis, & M. Theune (Eds.), *Workshop on Multimodal Output Generation (MOG)* (pp. 105-116). University of Aberdeen, United Kingdom.

Massaro, D. W., Cohen, M. M., Daniel, S., & Cole, R. A. (2001). Developing and evaluating conversational agents. In Hancock, P. A. (Ed.), *Human performance and ergonomics* (pp. 173–194). Academic Press.

McTear, M. (2008). Handling miscommunication: Why bother? In Dybkjær, L., & Minker, W. (Eds.), *Recent trends in discourse and dialogue* (pp. 101–122). Springer Netherlands. doi:10.1007/978-1-4020-6821-8_5

Möller, S., Smeele, P., Boland, H., & Krebber, J. (2007). Evaluating spoken dialogue systems according to de-facto standards: A case study. *Computer Speech & Language, 21*(1), 26–53. doi:10.1016/j.csl.2005.11.003

Nass, C., & Brave, S. (2005). *Wired for speech: How voice activates and advances the human-computer relationship.* MIT Press. Norman, D. A. (1999). Affordance, conventions, and design. *Interaction, 6*(3), 38–43.

Norman, D. (2002). *The design of everyday things.* New York, NY: Basic Books.

Oviatt, S. (1994). Interface techniques for minimizing disfluent input to spoken language systems. In B. Adelson, S. Dumais & J. Olson (Eds.), *Proceedings of the SIGCHI conference on Human factors in computing systems: celebrating interdependence* (pp. 205-210). Association for Computational Linguistics.

Oviatt, S., & Adams, B. (2000). Designing and evaluating conversational interfaces with animated characters. In S. P. Justine Cassell, Joseph Sullivan & E. F. Churchill (Eds.), *Embodied conversational agents* (pp. 319-345). MIT Press.

Oviatt, S., MacEachern, M., & Levow, G. (1998). Predicting hyperarticulate speech during human-computer error resolution. *Speech Communication, 24*(2), 87–110. doi:10.1016/S0167-6393(98)00005-3

Oviatt, S., & VanGent, R. (1996). Error resolution during multimodal human-computer interaction. In *Proceedings of the Fourth International Conference on Spoken Language Processing, vol. 1* (pp. 204-207). Institute of Electrical & Electronics Engineers.

Paek, T., & Horvitz, E. (2000). Conversation as action under uncertainty. In C. Boutilier & M. Goldszmidt (Eds.), *16th Conference on Uncertainty in Artificial Intelligence* (pp. 455-464).

Pelachaud, C. (2003). *Overview of representation languages for ECAs (Project Reports). Paris VIII.* IUT Montreuil.

Picard, R. (2003). What does it mean for a computer to have emotions? In Trappl, P. P. R., & Payr, S. (Eds.), *Emotions in humans and artifacts.* Citeseer.

Rec, I. T. U.-T. (2003). *Subjective quality evaluation of telephone services based on spoken dialogue systems (International Recommendation)* (p. 851). International Telecommunication Union.

Rickel, J., Lesh, N., Rich, C., Sidner, C., & Gertner, A. (2001). *Building a bridge between intelligent tutoring and collaborative dialogue systems.* Paper presented at Tenth International Conference on AI in Education (pp. 592-594), San Antonio, Texas.

Rudnicky, A. I., Thayer, E., Constantinides, P., Tchou, C., Shern, R., Lenzo, K., et al. Oh, A. (1999). *Creating natural dialogs in the Carnegie Mellon Communicator System.* EUROSPEECH'99, Sixth European Conference on Speech Communication and Technology (pp. 1531-1534). ISCA.

Sacks, H., Schegloff, E. A., & Jefferson, G. (1974). A simplest systematics for the organization of turn-taking for conversation. *Language, 50*(4), 696–735. doi:10.2307/412243

Samtani, P., Valente, A., & Johnson, W. (2008). *Applying the SAIBA framework to the tactical language and culture training system*. Paper presented at Why Conversational Agents do what they do. Functional Representations for Generating Conversational Agent Behavior. AAMAS 2008.

San Segundo, R., Montero, J., Ferreiros, J., Córdoba, R., & Pardo, J. (2001). Designing confirmation mechanisms and error recover techniques in a railway information system for spanish. In *Proceedings of the Second SIGdial Workshop on Discourse and Dialogue, vol. 16* (pp. 136-139). Association for Computational Linguistics.

Schaumburg, H. (2001). Computers as tools or as social actors? The users' perspective on anthropomorphic agents. *International Journal of Cooperative Information Systems, 10*(1-2), 217–234. doi:10.1142/S0218843001000321

ITU-T Suppl. 24 to P-Series Rec. (2005). *Parameters describing the interaction with spoken dialogue systems* (International Recommendation). International Telecommunication Union.

Tartaro, A., & Cassell, J. (2008). Playing with virtual peers: Bootstrapping contingent discourse in children with autism. In *Proceedings of International Conference of the Learning Sciences, vol. 2*. International Society of the Learning Sciences.

ter Maat, M., & Heylen, D. (2009). Turn management or impression management? In *Proceedings of 9th International Conference on Intelligent Virtual Agents, IVA 2009* (pp. 467-473). Berlin/Heidelberg, Germany: Springer.

Theune, M., Hofs, D., & Van Kessel, M. (2007). The virtual guide: A direction giving embodied conversational agent. In *Proceedings of the 8th Annual Conference of the International Speech Communication Association (Interspeech 2007)* (pp. 2197-2200). International Speech Communication Association (ISCA).

Van Mulken, S., André, E., & Müller, J. (1998). The persona effect: How substantial is it? In L. N. H. Johnson & C. Roast (Eds.), *People and Computers, Proceedings of HCI-98* (pp. 53-66).

Walker, M. A., Litman, D. J., Kamm, C. A., & Abella, A. (1997). PARADISE: A framework for evaluating spoken dialogue agents. In *Proceedings of the 35th Annual Meeting of the Association for Computational Linguistics (ACL-97)* (pp. 271-280). Association for Computational Linguistics.

Weiss, B., Kühnel, C., Wechsung, I., Fagel, S., & Möller, S. (2010). Quality of talking heads in different interaction and media contexts. *Speech Communication, 52*(6), 481–492. doi:10.1016/j.specom.2010.02.011

White, M., Foster, M., Oberlander, J., & Brown, A. (2005). Using facial feedback to enhance turn-taking in a multimodal dialogue system. In *Proceedings of HCI International, vol. 2*. Lawrence Erlbaum Associates, Inc.

Xiao, J. (2006). *Empirical studies on embodied conversational agents. Unpublished doctoral disseration*. Georgia Institute of Technology.

Zoric, G., Smid, K., & Pandzic, I. (2009). Towards facial gestures generation by speech signal analysis using HUGE architecture. In *Multimodal signals: Cognitive and algorithmic issues* (*Vol. 5398*, pp. 112–120). Berlin / Heidelberg, Germany: Springer. doi:10.1007/978-3-642-00525-1_11

## KEY TERMS AND DEFINITIONS

**Automatic Speech Recognition (ASR):** A technology that allows a programmable device to identify the words that a person speaks into a microphone. The ideal goal with this technology is for it to recognize in real-time and with 100% accuracy all of the words that are intelligibly spoken by any person. However, many factors (such as vocabulary size, noise, speaker characteristics and accent, and channel conditions) can hinder the performance of ASR.

**Embodied Conversational Agent (ECA):** A representation of a virtual human capable of engaging in conversation with humans by both understanding and producing speech, hand gestures and facial expressions.

**Interaction Parameters:** A set of variables that quantify the flow of the interaction, the behaviour of the user and the system, and the performance of the speech technology devices involved in the interaction.

**Nonverbal Communication:** The act of giving or exchanging the part of a message that is not contained in the words spoken (if any).

**Robustness:** Communicative competence of Natural Language Dialogue systems that includes the ability to detect and recover from problems related to the quality of speech recognition and to do so without disrupting the natural flow of the dialogue.

**Speaker Verification:** The process of authenticating a user's identity by comparing acoustic features extracted from live voice samples captured with an input device (microphone) with the reference biometric template obtained during enrolment.

**Voice Enrolment:** The process of obtaining an initial biometric template of acoustic features that characterise the voice of the user of a speaker verification system. The template is typically obtained by processing a number of biometric samples (voice samples) from an appropriate input device (a microphone). As soon as the user has enrolled, he/she can use the system to authenticate his/her identity.

# Chapter 4
# Dialogue Act Classification Exploiting Lexical Semantics

**Nicole Novielli**
*Università degli Studi di Bari, Italy*

**Carlo Strapparava**
*FBK-irst, Istituto per la Ricerca Scientifica e Tecnologica, Italy*

## ABSTRACT

*In this chapter we present our experience with automatic dialogue act recognition using empirical methods for exploiting lexical semantics in an unsupervised framework. Moreover, we show how automatic dialogue act annotation of human-ECA (Embodied Conversational Agent) interactions may be used as a preliminary step in conversational analysis for modeling the users' attitudes. Experiments are presented, by exploiting corpora of English and Italian natural dialogues. In both cases the approaches employed have been conceived as general and domain-independent and may be relevant to a wide range of both human-computer and human-human interaction application domains.*

## 1. INTRODUCTION

In recent years, the research on intelligent interfaces has focused with great enthusiasm on developing intelligent embodied conversationalists, which are better known as Embodied Conversational Agents (ECAs). An ECA is a 'virtual agent that interacts with a User or another Agent through multimodal communicative behavior' (Poggi et al., 2005). It represents the system as a person and the information is conveyed to human users through multimodal behavior, using speech and hand gestures; the internal representation is modality independent and both propositional and nonpropositional (Cassell, 2001). ECAs offer to people the possibility to relate with computer media at a social level (Reeves & Nass, 2003) and, therefore, to make the interaction more natural and enjoyable.

DOI: 10.4018/978-1-60960-617-6.ch004

To be successful an ECA has to be believable and should be perceived as intelligent. To this aim, it has to engage humans in face-to-face natural language interaction by properly adopting the conversation behavior governing human-human dialogues. In natural conversations people can ask for information, agree with their partner, state some facts and express opinions. They proceed in their conversations through a series of dialogue acts to yield some particular communicative intentions. Moreover, humans proved to coordinate themselves in conversations by matching their nonverbal behavior and word use (Niederhoffer & Pennebaker, 2002), and they demonstrate the ability of properly using interactional skills, i.e. knowing when to interrupt, when to give/wait for feedback, which conversational style to adopt, introducing small talk in the dialogue, understanding who is holding the floor in the conversation, etc. (Bickmore & Cassell, 2005). A natural language intelligent interface should be able to emulate these abilities and should give the user the feeling of cooperating with a virtual companion rather than just using a system.

ECAs are one of the forms in which this intelligent kind of interaction promises to be effective. According to Cassell (2001), two kinds of intelligence should be integrated into the reasoning ability of a virtual conversational character: propositional intelligence, regulating the propositional functions (domain-oriented intelligence, ability to retrieve the information that the user needs, internal representation of the knowledge in the domain etc.) and interactional intelligence, regulating interactional functions.

In addition, ongoing research on intelligent interfaces is now focusing on the role played by affective factors during the interaction and aims at developing adaptive conversational systems that can both adjust to individual differences among users and track and adapt to changes in key features of affective states that users experience during the conversation (see Section 2.2 for a review). The more a virtual character succeeds in its goal of appearing intelligent, the more the users are expected to attach anthropomorphic features to the agent and to react also affectively to their virtual interlocutor. ECAs definitely represent a great potential in this sense and should be equipped to show some forms of socio-emotional intelligence in their turn (Mazzotta et al., 2007; De Carolis et al., 2010).

In this perspective, developing a virtual conversationalist able to believably interact with humans means to develop a character endowed with the ability of:

- providing domain and task-oriented support to the user, by managing appropriately its domain knowledge,
- managing the interaction in a way that successfully matches the user expectation and,
- adapting the interaction style to both the affective and cognitive factors of the user state of mind.

Designing an architecture for such an ECA requires, first of all, to deal with the understanding of the conversational structure and dynamic evolution of the interaction: at every step of the interaction the agent should be able to understand who is telling what to whom (i.e. understanding the illocutionary force (Austin, 1962) of the communicative actions of the user). While not constituting *per se* a deep understanding of the dialogue (Cohen & Levesque, 1990), automatic dialogue act tagging is a task that certainly plays a fundamental role in this sense.

Dialogue Acts (DAs), in fact, constitute the basis of everyday conversations and are object of study since long time (Austin, 1962; Searle, 1969; Core & Allen, 1997; Traum, 2000). In this chapter, we describe our experience in investigating the lexical semantics of dialogue moves with the final goal of defining a method for automatic labeling natural dialogues with the proper speech acts (Novielli & Strapparava, 2010a). Moreover, we describe some experiments in recognizing the user attitudes by exploiting conversational analysis techniques for modeling dialogues with embodied agents (Martalò et al., 2008; Novielli, 2010).

The chapter is structured as follows: in Section 2 we provide an overview on the role of Dialogue Acts and affective states in human-ECA interaction; then, in Section 3 we describe the data sets employed for the purpose of the studies reported in this chapter; Sections 4 and 5 report about our experience in, respectively, defining a method for automatic DA annotation and applying conversational analysis for modeling user attitudes toward an ECA; we finally conclude in Section 6.

## 2. BACKGROUND

ECAs have been successfully employed in the role of counselors (Marsella et al., 2003), personal trainers (Bickmore, 2003), healthy living advisors (de Rosis et al., 2004) and in other domains where it is important to settle a long-term relation with the user (Bickmore & Picard, 2005). Regardless of the application domain, agent believability is regarded as probably the most important issue to deal with when designing an ECA.

Building a believable agent, though, is a complex task that requires an architecture conceived so as to combine several modules (De Carolis et al., 2010). According to Cassell (2001), an embodied interface should provide not only 'something pretty and entertaining to look at' (p. 78). On the contrary, it should be equipped so as to demonstrate propositional and interactional intelligence through multi-modality. To Poggi et al. (2005), a key requirement for a believable agent is the ability to express emotions, to behave according to a given personality, culture and style, to demonstrate context-awareness and user sensitivity, that is, at each step of the interaction the agent should be equipped to reason on the combination of these aspects to determine its next contribution to the dialogue.

To achieve believable natural language conversations, ECA systems require the combination of several modules. First of all, the interpretation module should analyze the user input in order to provide to the system the formal representation of what the user said (and of 'how' he said it). Dialogue act annotation of natural language interaction constitutes a preliminary and necessary step towards this goal. In the following subsections we provide an overview on the role of Dialogue Acts in the development of computer conversationalists as well as an overview on the role of affective states in human-ECA interaction.

### 2.1 The Role of Dialogue Act in Natural Interaction with an ECA

Dialogue Acts (DAs) have been well studied in linguistics (Austin, 1962; Searle, 1969) and computational linguistics research for a long time (Core & Allen, 1997; Traum, 2000). Traditionally, speech acts have been analyzed in the action view initiated by Austin (1962): like actions influence the state of affairs in the physical world, speech acts affect the cognitive state of the participants to the dialogue. For some researchers (e.g. (Searle, 1969)) the speech act represents the minimal and primitive unit of linguistic communication; others (Cohen & Levesque, 1995) refer to dialogue acts as more complex events involving interaction between the mental states of the participants to a dialogue.

Our interests in DAs is justified by the fact that they constitute the basis of verbal communication, either in human-human or human-ECA interaction scenarios, as also demonstrated by the following overview on studies about the design of natural dialogues with conversational agents. Dialogue Act modeling can be regarded as both a preliminary step towards the interpretation of the user input and a useful formalism for representing the communicative intention of both the user and the agent.

According to De Carolis et al. (2010), the architecture of an ECA should be designed in order to allow the interpretation of the multimodal input generated by the user, reason on the information it intends to convey, trigger the corresponding communicative goal and achieve these goals by applying a set of communicative plans. In their system, the user moves are treated using a keyword-based approach. The system response is then generated according to the communicative goal triggered by the agent's reasoning module. The ECA architecture is based on the separation between the 'mind' and the 'body' of the agent: the mind module manages the selection of the meaning to express ('what to say') while the body has to convey this meaning according to the agent communicative capabilities ('how to say') that include communicative functions typically used in human-human dialogs such as syntactic, dialogic, meta-cognitive, performative, affective, deictic, adjectival and belief relation functions (Poggi et al., 2000).

In Cassell's REA (Cassell, 2001; Cassell et al., 1999), the input manager collects the multi-modal user input and decides whether it requires instant reaction or deliberate discourse planning. On the other hand, the agent is capable to combine speech and gesture in order to express the propositional content of its move according to the selected communicative goal (i.e. the speech act the agent intends to realize). The approach employed in REA is based on the distinction between propositional and interactional functions: propositional intelligent contributes to determine the content of the conversation, including speech and gesture devices; interactional intelligence guides the appropriate management of conversational processes and actually 'shapes' the conversation by mean of appropriate nonverbal behavior.

In (King et al., 2003), an existing dialogue manager for written text is integrated into the architecture of Kare, a talking head that engages users in either English or Maori dialogues for information-seeking or knowledge-authoring tasks. In this study, the input analyzer processes the user input in order to extract the dialogue act (e.g. assertion, yes/no question, wh-question, clarification-question, acknowledge, yes/no answer, etc.). Analogously, the dialogue manager employs the formalism of dialogue acts to represent the communicative goal of its reply. The surface generation of utterances was originally conceived for written texts and has been extended to support the use of nonverbal behavior according to the language used and, therefore, to culture-specific knowledge.

In (van Deemter et al., 2008) the NECA approach is presented for the generation of dialogues with ECAs. The interaction is represented as a sequence of acts that can be both verbal and non-verbal. Each dialogue act is a complex linguistic object characterized by a set of features describing its communicative function, semantic content and the main emotion to express when performing it.

Finally, in (Dohsaka et al., 2009) conversational agents are employed to foster human communication during a quiz. The scenario described in the study involves two agents and two humans, whose contributions to the conversation are described in terms of domain related dialogue acts (e.g. Present-hint, Give-ans, Show-difficulty, Evaluate-ans, Complete-quiz- with-success, and so on). When a user utterance is input, the system analyzes and converts it into dialogue acts using ad-hoc grammars and the dialogue history is updated. The agent reaction is planned according to preconditions in turn-taking rules defined for each dialogue act.

Recently, the problem of DA recognition has been addressed with promising results and has been often modeled as a text-classification task. In particular, in DA classification the units of learning are the annotated utterances in the dialogues while each class correspond to a label of dialogue act. Supervised frameworks have been widely investigated: Samuel et al. (1998) propose an approach that employs transformation-based learning reporting one of the best performance in literature on a 18 DA classification task. The learnt model consists in a set of rules that are developed starting from the annotated corpus in several experimental settings. The best performance of the system (75.12%) is obtained by employing a combination of dialogue act cues and other features, including contextual information (i.e. features describing the change of speaker and the previous dialogue act). Stolcke et al. (2000) achieve an accuracy of around 70% and 65% respectively on transcribed and recognized words by combining a discourse grammar, formalized in terms of Hidden Markov Models, with evidences about lexicon and prosody. Reithinger and Klesen's (1997) employ a Bayesian approach with uni- and bi-grams, achieving 74.7% of correctly classified labels. A partially supervised framework by Venkataraman et al. (2005) has also been explored, using five broad classes of DA and obtaining an accuracy of about 79%.

Though, it is not always easy to have large training material at disposal, partly because of manual labeling effort and moreover because often it is not possible to find it. Hence, rather than improving the performance of supervised frameworks, we aim at exploring the use of an unsupervised methodology. The method is described in Section 4.

## 2.2 Affective Interaction with an ECA

ECAs have the great potential of improving interaction by engaging users at a social level (Bickmore & Cassell, 2005; Bickmore & Picard, 2005). They foster the natural tendency of people to manifest several forms of anthropomorphic behavior towards technologies (Cassell, 2001; Reeves & Nass, 2003) and, therefore, they should be equipped to appropriately recognize and react to the user cognitive and affective state.

In recent years, we have assisted to the flourishing of research about affective responses of users to ECAs. Studies conducted at the DFKI (André et al., 2000) aim at combining personality traits and emotions to enhance the agent believability in different application domains. Another relevant experience in this sense is the study described in (De Carolis et al., 2001) about the design of a Reflexive Agent in which some forms of emotional intelligence are embedded. The agent is conceived to be able to manifest its emotion by establishing what verbal or nonverbal signals to employ in its communication and how to combine and synchronize them. The reasoning of the agent relies on a representation of both emotion triggering and emotion regulation factors that are employed, respectively, to trigger an emotion and decide when it is appropriate to display it according to the context (i.e. the agent personality, the interlocutor's feature, the relationship between them and their social role, and so on).

Since the concept of 'socially intelligent agents' has been introduced (Dautenhahn, 1999) various terms have been used to denote the user affective and anthropomorphic behavior towards technologies; one of the difficulties in examining the accumulating literature about human-ECA relation is in the plethora of definitions used. Affective states, in fact, vary in their degree of stability, ranging from long-standing features (personality traits) to more transient ones (emotions). Among the huge variety of affective states, in this chapter we report about our research experience in modeling 'interpersonal stances', which are in a middle of this scale.

To Roesch et al. (2005) an interpersonal stance is 'characteristic of an affective style that spontaneously develops or is strategically employed in the interaction with a person or a group of persons, coloring the interpersonal exchange in this situation (e.g. being polite, distant, cold, warm, supportive, contemptuous)' (p. 28). This general concept was named differently in recent research projects, each considering one of its aspects. Some authors denote with empathy the emotional reaction due to perceiving that another person is experiencing or about to experience an emotion (Paiva, 2004); others (Hoorn and Konijn, 2003) talk about engagement, involvement, sympathy and their contrary, distance.

In their research about human-robot conversations, Sidner and Lee (2003) define engagement as 'the process by which two (or more) participants establish, maintain and end their perceived connection during interactions they jointly undertake. Engagement is supported by the use of conversation (that is, spoken linguistic behavior), ability to collaborate on a task (that is, collaborative behavior) and gestural behavior that convey connection between the participants.' (p. 2). Another popular term among e-learning researchers is 'social presence' (or co-presence), which received several definitions, from the general one 'the extent to which the communicator is perceived as real' (Polhemus et al, 2001) to the more ECA-specific one 'the extent to which individuals treat embodied agents as if they were other real human beings' (Blascovich, 2002). Quite interestingly, Bailenson et al (2005) clarify the difference between the two definitions by distinguishing existing research in the domain into studies that focus on people's perception of ECAs and studies that focus on people social response to embodied agents. Blascovich's definition refers to the latter one, which had the main initiators in the Stanford University researchers.

In (Novielli et al., 2010) the 'social attitude' towards a virtual therapist is studied, as well as the factors affecting it. The verbal behavior of subjects is observed during the interaction with an ECA in a Wizard of Oz simulation study. Authors refer to Andersen and Guerrero's definition of interpersonal warmth (1998) to define the concept of warm and cold 'social attitude' towards the agent. A method that combine linguistic and acoustic analysis to recognize this attitude has been proposed in (de Rosis et al., 2007).

Bickmore and Cassell (2005) describe their experience in designing social dialogues with embodied conversational agents. REA, a virtual character playing the role of a realtor agent, is able to use 'small talk', that is sub-dialogues (e.g. talking about the weather) that do not directly relate with the main task of the dialogue. Authors base their study on the use that humans do of small talk in everyday conversations: it is usually employed for building trust, gathering information about the interlocutor, building a common ground on which to base the interaction, increase the sense of intimacy. The study reports interesting results about the use of social dialogue in the interaction: users seem to prefer an interaction style involving small talk, in no time pressure condition. When interacting with REA, users showed a more human-human like behavior rather than a human-computer like one. These findings highlight the need for carefully design the social behavior of agents in order to match the user preferences and expectations.

Another very interesting issue that has been investigated is whether virtual characters really enhance the persuasive power of human-computer interaction, the engagement of users and their sense of social presence. In (Berry et al., 2005),which text-based, voice-based and character-based persuasive messages were compared, and a partially positive answer was given to this question, by concluding that a realistic evaluation of ECAs should consider dialogic interaction rather than single, relatively short messages.

In this chapter (see Section 5) we describe our experience in modeling the attitudes of users towards ECA, by exploiting conversational analysis techniques. Detecting long lasting features of users, such as their level of engagement or their overall attitude (e.g. polemic vs. benevolent, warm vs. cold, cooperative vs. competitive) is a fundamental step towards long-term adaptation of the agent behavior and its dialogue strategy. The described study is based on the assumption that long-term attitudes affect the overall dialogue pattern and the conversational behavior of users. Our assumption is also supported by the use that researchers do of ad hoc measures for conversational analysis. Conversational turn-taking, in fact, is one of the aspects of human behavior that can be relevant for modeling social signaling (see, for example (Core et al., 2003) and (Pentland, 2005)). Therefore, we decided to model categories of users, by looking at differences in the dialogue pattern (Martalò et al., 2008; Novielli, 2010). In particular we argue in favor of the suitability of Hidden Markov Models (HMMs) as formalism for dialogue pattern description. The complete dialogue pattern is modeled according to the goal of predicting the user overall final attitude towards the ECA and towards the task of the dialogue. HMMs modeling enable us to represent differences in the whole structure of the dialogues among subjects showing different attitudes during the interaction.

## 3. DATA SETS

In the present chapter we report about two studies at the intersection of Human-Computer Interaction (with particular focus on advice-giving dialogues with an ECA) and Natural Language Processing (with particular focus on defining a domain and language independent approach for automatic dialogue act annotation). In our research we exploit two different corpora: the Switchboard corpus (Godfrey et al., 1992), which is a collection of transcriptions of spoken English telephone conversations about general interest topics, and an Italian corpus of dialogues in the healthy-eating domain (Clarizio et al., 2006).

The Italian corpus had been collected in the scope of some previous research about Human-ECA interaction: to collect these data a Wizard of Oz tool was employed. This corpus contains overall 60 dialogues, 1448 user utterances and 15,500 words. Sixty graduate students (age 21–28) were involved in the study, in two interaction mode conditions: thirty of them interacted with the system in a written-input setting, using keyboard and mouse; the remaining thirty dialogues were collected with users interacting with the ECA in a spoken-input condition: the agent was displayed on a touch screen and subjects used a microphone to talk to it as well as a touch-screen to send other commands.

In the studies performed for the collection of these dialogues, the ECA was a quite realistic agent named Valentina, with a young woman's appearance. During the interaction, Valentina played the role of an artificial therapist and the users were free to interact with it in natural language, without any particular constraint. They could either simply answer the question of the agent or taking the initiative and start asking questions; users could also make comments about the agent behavior or competence in the domain or even argument in favor or against a system suggestion or persuasion attempts. The Wizard, on his behalf, had to choose among a set of about 80 predefined possible move. More details about the WoZ study and its design can be found in (Novielli et al., 2010; Clarizio et al., 2006).

The annotation of the Italian advice-giving dialogues has been performed in the scope of a study about detecting the user engagement during the interaction with an ECA (see (Novielli, 2010) and Section 5 for more details). The corpus was labeled so we could capture the communicative intention of each dialogue move, according to our final goal of modeling the user attitude during the dialogue. Both system and user moves were classified into appropriate categories of communicative acts. Table 1 reports the markup label employed: system moves (Wizard), though, are already known so they are out of the scope of interest of our study about dialogue act labeling and are kept out from the data set used for the automatic DA annotation experiments described in Section 4 (see Table 2 for an example of annotated dialogue). The 11 labels are a revision of those proposed in SWBDL-DAMSL (Jurafsky et al., 1997) and are defined according to (i) the DAMSL classification rationale, (ii) the frequencies with which they had been employed in the corpus and (iii) the intended use in the user attitude detection task (i.e. their potential descriptive power of the user intention with respect to the engagement modeling task).

The Switchboard corpus is a collection of English human-human telephone conversations (Godfrey et al., 1992). Each conversation involved a couple of randomly selected strangers: they were asked to select one general interest topic and to

*Table 1. Categories of wizard and user moves*

| Dialogue Act | Description |
|---|---|
| ***Wizard*** | |
| OPENING | initial self-introduction by the ECA |
| QUESTION | question about the user eating habits or information interests |
| OFFER-GIVE-INFO | generic offer of help or specific information |
| PERSUASION-SUGGEST | persuasion attempt about dieting |
| ENCOURAGE | statement aimed at enhancing the user motivation |
| ANSWER | provision of generic information after a user request |
| TALK-ABOUT-SELF | statement describing own abilities, role and skills |
| CLOSING | statement of dialogue conclusion |
| ***User*** | |
| OPENING | initial self-introduction by the user |
| REQ-INFO | information request |
| FOLLOW-UP-MORE-DETAILS | further information or justification request |
| OBJECTION | objection about an ECA assertion or suggestion |
| SOLICITATION | request of clarification or generic request of attention |
| STAT-ABOUT-SELF | generic assertion or statement about own diet, beliefs, desires and behaviors |
| STAT-PREFERENCES | assertion about food liking or disliking |
| GENERIC-ANSWER | provision of generic information after an ECA question or statement |
| AGREE | acknowledgment or appreciation of the ECA advice |
| KIND-ATTITUDE-SYSTEM | statement displaying kind attitude towards the system, in the form of joke, polite sentence, comment or question about the system |
| CLOSING | statement of dialogue conclusion |

talk informally about it. The Linguistic Data Consortium distributes full transcripts of these dialogues. A part of this corpus is annotated with DA labels (overall 1155 conversations, for a total of 205,000 utterances and 1.4 million words)[1]. In particular, the Switchboard annotation has been performed by employing a revision of the DAMSL framework (Jurafsky et al., 1997): it modifies the original version of DAMSL by further specifying some categories or by adding extra features (mainly prosodic), which were not originally included in the scheme.

The main difference between the two corpora (besides the spoken language) is that the Switchboard domain itself is essentially task-free while the Italian one is highly constrained and every dialogue strictly reflects the task the interaction is designed to implement, that is the advice-giving process. The two corpora significantly differ also in size, interaction modality and scenario. As already said, the choice of two corpora presenting different characteristics is motivated in the perspective of defining a method for dialogue act annotation which is independent not only from the language but also from the size, the interaction scenario and the domain in which the interaction takes part.

## 4. UNSUPERVISED DIALOGUE ACT RECOGNITION

In this section, we describe our research experience in studying the task of automatic labeling dialogues with the proper speech acts in an unsu-

*Table 2. An annotated excerpt of a transcript from the Italian corpus, using the advice-giving study annotation scheme. The dialogue has been translated from Italian.*

| Label | Speaker | Utterance |
|---|---|---|
| OPENING | User | Ok! Hi, my name is Imma and I'm here, waiting for your suggestions. |
| QUESTION | S | Do you like eating? |
| SOLICIT-REQ-CLARIF | U | Yes, a lot. And I eat everything. Hey, you take a lot of time to answer! So? |
| QUESTION | S | Do you eat a lot? |
| GENERIC-ANSWER | U | well... yes. |
| QUESTION | S | Are you attracted by sweets? |
| STAT-PREFERENCES | U | Of course, I always eat sweets after lunch, with coffee. |
| QUESTION | S | What did you have for dinner? |
| STAT-ABOUT-SELF | U | For dinner? I had... Ah.. sausages with mayonnaise, great! But I don't usually eat this way. Last night, for example, I had a steak and a salad. |
| OFFER-GIVE-INFO | S | I can give you suggestion on how to improve your diet, if you want. |
| AGREE | U | Ok! |
| QUESTION | S | Try to think about what you eat during the day: do you think you have a balanced diet? |
| STAT-ABOUT-SELF | U | I think so: I usually have fruit, vegetables... I like salads a lot. |
| QUESTION | S | What do you think about fried food? |
| STAT-PREFERENCES | U | I like it very much, expecially fried fish. |
| | [...] | |
| PERSUASION-SUGGEST | S | In a balanced diet, at least the 50% of the total amount of calories should come from carbohydrates. |
| FOLLOW-UP-MORE-DET | U | Why? |
| | [...] | |
| ENCOURAGE-SORRY | S | I see that, overall, you pay attention to your diet, congratulation! |
| KIND-ATTITUDE-SYS | U | Thanks! |
| CLOSING | S | It's been nice to interact with you. Feel free to come back and have a chat whenever you like. |
| CLOSING | U | Ok, bye! |
| CLOSING | S | Thanks, see you! |

pervised framework. We define a method for DA recognition by relying on empirical methods that simply exploit lexical semantics of the sentences. Even if prosody and intonation surely play a role (e.g. Stolcke et al., (2000); Warnke et al., (1997)), nonetheless language and words are what the speaker uses to convey the communicative message. Some experiments in both a supervised and unsupervised framework are presented, on both the English and the Italian corpus described in Section 3. In particular we consider the classification of dialogue acts with and without taking into account dialogue contextual features. The use of corpora that differ in the content and in the used language is consistent with our goal of developing a recognition methodology as much general as possible.

## 4.1 Labeling

Dialogue acts mark important characteristics of utterances, indicate the role or communicative

*Table 3. The set of labels employed for dialogue act, with description, examples and distribution in the two data sets*

| Label | Description and Examples | Italian | English |
|---|---|---|---|
| INFO-RE-QUEST | Utterances that are pragmatically, semantically, and syntactically questions - *'What did you do when your kids were growing up?'* | 34% | 7% |
| STATE-MENT | Descriptive, narrative, personal statements - *'I usually eat a lot of fruit'* | 37% | 57% |
| S-OPINION | Directed opinion statements - *'I think he deserves it.'* | 6% | 20% |
| AGREE-AC-CEPT | Acceptance of a proposal, plan or opinion - *'That's right'* | 5% | 9% |
| REJECT | Disagreement with a proposal, plan, or opinion - *'I'm sorry no'* | 7% | .3% |
| OPENING | Dialogue opening or self-introduction - *'Hello, my name is Imma'* | 2% | .2% |
| CLOSING | Dialogue closing (e.g. farewell and wishes) - *'It's been nice talking to you.'* | 2% | 2% |
| KIND-ATT | Kind attitude (e.g. thanking and apology) - *'Thank you.'* | 9% | .1% |
| GEN-ANS | Generic answers to an Info-Request - *'Yes', 'No', 'I don't know'* | 4% | 4% |
| total cases | | 1448 | 131,265 |

intention that the utterances conveys, that is they represent utterances' strength at the level of illocutionary force (Austin, 1962). To address these dimensions of analysis, the NLP community has employed DA definitions with the drawback of being often domain or application oriented. Moreover, in defining dialogue act taxonomies researchers have been trying to solve the trade-off between the need for formal semantics and the need for computational feasibility (see Traum, (2000) for an exhaustive overview).

In the study described in this section (Novielli & Strapparava, 2010a) we refer to a domain-independent framework for DA annotation, the DAMSL architecture (Dialogue Act Markup in Several Layers) by Core and Allen (1997). The two corpora are annotated in order to capture the main communicative intention of each dialogue move. Defining a DA markup language is out of the scope of the present study; hence we employed the original annotation of the two corpora (Novielli, 2010; Jurafsky et al., 1997), which is consistent, in both cases, with the DAMSL scheme. In particular the Switchboard corpus employs the SWBD-DAMSL revision.

Table 3 shows the set of labels employed for the purpose of this study, with definitions, examples, distribution and total number of cases (utterances): it maintains the DAMSL main characteristic of being domain-independent and it is also consistent with the original semantics of the SWBD-DAMSL markup language employed in the Switchboard annotation. The SWBD-DAMSL had been automatically converted into the categories included in our markup language without considering the utterances formed only by non-verbal material (e.g. laughter). Table 4 reports an annotated excerpt from the Switchboard corpus.

## 4.2 Data Preprocessing

To reduce the data sparseness, we used a POS-tagger and morphological analyzer (Pianta et al., 2008) for preprocessing the corpora and we used lemmata instead of tokens. No feature selection was performed, keeping also stopwords. In addition, we augmented the features of each sentence with a set of linguistic markers, defined according to the semantics of the DA categories: we hypothesized these features could play an important role in defining the linguistic profile

*Table 4. An annotated excerpt from the switchboard corpus*

| Speaker | Dialogue Act | Utterance |
|---|---|---|
| A | OPENING | *Hello Ann.* |
| B | OPENING | Hello Chuck. |
| A | STATE-MENT | *Uh, the other day, I attended a conference here at Utah State University on recycling* |
| A | STATE-MENT | *and, uh, I was kind of interested to hear cause they had some people from the EPA and lots of different places, and, uh, there is going to be a real problem on solid waste.* |
| B | OPINION | Uh, I didn't think that was a new revelation. |
| A | AGREE-AC-CEPT | *Well, it's not too new.* |
| B | INFO-RE-QUEST | So what is the EPA recommending now? |

of each DA. The addition of these markers was performed automatically, by just exploiting the output of the POS-tagger and of the morphological analyzer, according to the following rules:

- **WH-QTN**, used whenever an interrogative determiner is found, according to the output of the POS-tagger (e.g. 'when' does not play an interrogative role when tagged as conjunction);
- **ASK-IF**, used whenever an utterance presents some cues of the pattern 'Yes/No' question. ASK-IF and WH-QTN markers are supposed to be relevant for the recognition of the INFO-REQUEST category;
- **I-PERS**, used for all declarative utterances whenever a verb is in the first person form, singular or plural (relevant for the STATEMENT);
- **COND**, used when a conditional form is detected.
- **SUPER**, used for superlative adjectives;
- **AGR-EX**, used whenever an agreement expression (e.g. 'You are right', 'I agree') is detected (relevant for AGREE-ACCEPT);
- **NAME**, used whenever a proper name follows a self-introduction expression (e.g. 'My name is') (relevant for the OPENING);
- **OR-CLAUSE**, used when the utterance is an or-clause, i.e. it starts with the conjunction 'or' (should be helpful for the characterization of the INFO-REQUEST);
- **VB**, used only for the Italian, it is when a dialectal form of agreement is detected.

## 4.3 The Method

Rather than going into deep processing of the meaning of the sentences which compose an utterance, we focus on capturing the dialogue act it conveys, by assuming that if some linguistic communication device/convention exists for meaning, in terms of sense and reference (Searle, 1969), then they should exist also for conveying the illocutionary force of utterances. Language, in fact, plays a fundamental role in determining the illocutionary force of an utterance, as demonstrated by the success of the natural language processing techniques for automatic dialogue act annotation using textual features (see section 2.1).

Acoustic features surely are fundamental in understanding the communicative intention of our interlocutors (see, for example the studies reported in (Stolcke et al., 2000; Warnke et al., 1997; Wright, 1998). Still the language and, in particular, lexical features often act as a primary device in conveying communicative intentions and indicating the discourse structure (Jurafsky et al., 1998; Grosz and Sidner, 1986; Hirschberg and Litman, 1993; Hinkelman and Allen, 1989).

*Table 5. Some example of set of seeds*

| Label | Seeds |
|---|---|
| S-OPINION | Verbs which directly express opinion or evaluation (guess, think, suppose, affect) |
| AGREE-ACC | yep, yeah, absolutely, correct |
| OPENING | Expressions of greetings (hi, hello), words and markers related to self-introduction formula |
| KIND-ATT | Lexicon which directly expresses wishes (wish), apologies (apologize), thanking (thank) and sorry-for (sorry, excuse) |

Moreover, rules of conversational coherence have been shown to govern the use of surface linguistic phenomena, such as cue phrases and choice of reference, in many models of discourse (Litman and Allen, 1990).

Therefore, we decided to focus on the analysis of the lexical semantics of utterances. Schematically, our unsupervised methodology consists of the following steps:

1. Building a semantic similarity space in which words, set of words, text fragments can be represented homogeneously,
2. Finding seeds that properly represent dialogue acts and considering their representations in the similarity space, and
3. Checking the similarity of the utterances.

To get a similarity space with the required characteristics, we used Latent Semantic Analysis (LSA), a corpus-based measure of semantic similarity proposed by Landauer et al. (1998). In LSA, term co-occurrences in a corpus are captured by means of a dimensionality reduction operated by a singular value decomposition (SVD) on the term-by-document matrix T representing the corpus. In LSA, similarity is computed in a vector space in which second-order relations among terms and texts are exploited using cosine. LSA presents the advantage of yielding a vector space model that allows for a homogeneous representation (and hence comparison) of words, sentences, and texts.

For representing a word set or a sentence in the LSA space we use the *pseudo-document* representation technique (Berry, 1992): each text segment is represented in the LSA space by summing up the normalized LSA vectors of all the constituent words, using also a *tf.idf* weighting scheme (Gliozzo & Strapparava, 2005).

The methodology is unsupervised as we do not exploit any 'labeled' training material. For the experiments reported in this chapter, we run the SVD using 400 dimensions (i.e. $k'$) respectively on the English and Italian corpus, without any DA label information. Starting from a set of seeds (words) representing the communicative acts, we build the corresponding vectors in the LSA space and then we compare the utterances to find the communicative act with the highest similarity.

Table 5 shows some example of set of seeds with the corresponding DAs. The seeds are the same for both languages, which is coherent with our goal of defining a language-independent method. We defined seeds by only considering the communicative goal and the specific semantics of every single DA, just avoiding the overlapping between seed groups as much as possible.

An upper-bound performance is provided by running experiment with Support Vector Machines (Vapnik, 1995), which are regarded as the state-of-the-art in supervised learning. To allow comparison, the performance is measured on the same test set partition for both the unsupervised and supervised experiments.

## 4.4 Experimental Results and Discussion

We evaluated the performance of our method in terms of precision, recall and F1-measure

*Table 6. Evaluation of the supervised and unsupervised methods on the two corpora*

| | Italian | | | | | | English | | | | | |
|---|---|---|---|---|---|---|---|---|---|---|---|---|
| | SVM | | | LSA | | | SVM | | | LSA | | |
| **Label** | **prec** | **rec** | **F1** | **prec** | **rec** | **F1** | **prec** | **rec** | **F1** | **prec** | **rec** | **F1** |
| INFO-REQ | .92 | .99 | .95 | .96 | .88 | .92 | .92 | .84 | .88 | .93 | .70 | .80 |
| STATEMENT | .85 | .68 | .69 | .76 | .66 | .71 | .79 | .92 | .85 | .70 | .95 | .81 |
| S-OPINION | .28 | .42 | .33 | .24 | .42 | .30 | .66 | .44 | .53 | .41 | .07 | .12 |
| AGREE-ACC | .50 | .80 | .62 | .56 | .50 | .53 | .69 | .74 | .71 | .68 | .63 | .65 |
| REJECT | - | - | - | .09 | .25 | .13 | - | - | - | .01 | .01 | .01 |
| OPENING | .60 | 1.00 | .75 | .55 | 1.00 | .71 | .96 | .55 | .70 | .20 | .43 | .27 |
| CLOSING | .67 | .40 | .50 | .25 | .40 | .31 | .83 | .59 | .69 | .76 | .34 | .47 |
| KIND-ATT | .82 | .53 | .64 | .43 | .18 | .25 | .85 | .34 | .49 | .09 | .47 | .15 |
| GEN-ANS | .20 | .63 | .30 | .27 | .38 | .32 | .56 | .25 | .35 | .54 | .33 | .41 |
| micro | .71 | .71 | .71 | .66 | .66 | .66 | .77 | .77 | .77 | .68 | .68 | .68 |

(see Table 6) according to the DA labels given by annotators in the datasets. As baselines we can consider (i) most-frequent label assignment (respectively 37% for Italian, 57% for English) for the supervised setting, and (ii) random DA selection (11%) for the unsupervised one.

We got.71 and.77 of F1 respectively for the Italian and the English corpus in the supervised condition, and.66 and.68 respectively in the unsupervised one. The performance is quite satisfying and is comparable to the state of the art in the domain. In particular, the unsupervised technique is significantly above the baseline, for both the Italian and the English corpus experiments. We note that the methodology is independent from the language and the domain: the Italian corpus is a collection of dialogue about a very restricted domain (advice-giving dialogue about healthy-eating) while in the Switchboard corpus the conversations revolve around general topics chosen by the two interlocutors. Moreover, in the unsupervised setting we use the same seed definitions. Secondly, it is independent on the differences in the linguistic style due to the specific interaction scenario and input modality. Finally, the performance is not affected by the difference in size of the two data sets.

*Error analysis.* After conducting an error analysis, we noted that many utterances are misclassified as STATEMENT. One possible reason is that statements usually are quite long and there is a high chance that some linguistic markers that characterize other dialogue acts are present in those sentences too. On the other hand, looking at the corpora we observed that many utterances that appear to be linguistically consistent with the typical structure of statements have been annotated differently, according to the actual communicative role they play. The following is an example of a statement-like utterance (by speaker B) that has been annotated differently because of its context (speaker A's move):

A: 'In fact, it's easier for me to say, uh, the types of music that I don't like are opera and, uh, screaming heavy metal.' STATEMENT

B: 'The opera, yeah, it's right on track.' AGREE-ACCEPT

For similar reasons, we observed some misclassification of S-OPINION as STATEMENT. The only significative difference between the two labels seems to be the wider usage of 'slanted' and affectively loaded lexicon when conveying an

*Table 7. Enriching the data set with contextual features*

| natural language input: | | |
|---|---|---|
| (a1) | STATEMENT | 'I don't feel comfortable about leaving my kids in a big day care center' |
| (b1) | INFO-REQ | 'Worried that they're not going to get enough attention?' |
| (a2) | GEN-ANS | 'Yeah' |
| **correspondent dataset item for the utterance a2:** | | |
| BoW | STATEMENT:1 INFO-REQUEST:1 yeah:1 | |
| Bigram | STATEMENT-INFO-REQUEST:1 yeah:1 | |

opinion (Novielli & Strapparava, 2010b). Another source of confounding is the misclassification of the OPENING as INFO-REQUEST. The reason is not clear yet, since the misclassified openings are not question-like. Eventually, there is some confusion among the backchannel labels (GEN-ANS, AGREE-ACC and REJECT) due to the inherent ambiguity of common words like 'yes', 'no', 'yeah', 'ok'.

Consistently with Levinson's theory of conversational analysis (Levinson, 1983), these findings highlight the role played by the context and suggested us to exploit the dialogue history to improve the DA classification performance, as described in the following section.

## 4.5 Exploiting Contextual Features

Several approaches have been proposed in literature to exploit the dialogue history in DA classification tasks. Stolcke et al. (2000) combine HMM discourse modeling with consideration of linguistic and acoustic features extracted from the dialogue turn. Poesio and Mikheev (1998) exploit the hierarchical structure of discourse, described in terms of game structure, to improve DA classification in spoken interaction. Reithinger and Klesen (1997) employ a Bayesian approach to build a probabilistic dialogue act classifier based on textual input.

In our approach, each utterance is enriched with contextual information (i.e. the preceding DA labels) in form of either 'bag of words' or 'n-grams'. We explore the supervised learning framework, using SVM, under five different experimental settings. Then, we propose a bootstrap approach for the unsupervised setting. To allow comparison, we refer, for both languages, to the same train/test partitions employed in the experiments in Section 4.3

*Supervised.* We have tested the role played by the context in DA recognition, experimenting with:

a. the number of turn (one vs. two turns) considered in extracting contextual features (i.e. the DA labels) based on the dialogue history of a given turn and
b. the approach used for representing the knowledge about the context, i.e. Bag of Words style (BoW) vs. n-grams.

Data preprocessing involves enriching both the train and test sets with contextual information, as shown in Table 7. When building the context for a given utterance we only consider the label included in our DA annotation language (see Table 3). In fact, our markup language does not allow mapping of SWBD-DAMSL labels such as 'non verbal turn' or 'abandoned turn'. According to our goal of defining a method, which simply exploits textual information, we consider all cases originally annotated with such labels as a lack of knowledge about the context.

Table 8 (a) shows the results in terms of precision, recall and F1-measure. As comparison, we also report the global performance when no con-

*Table 8. Overall performance of the different approaches for exploiting contextual information in the supervised setting (a) and bootstrap on the unsupervised method (b)*

| English | | | |
|---|---|---|---|
| Experimental Setting | Prec | Rec | F1 |
| *no context* | *.77* | *.77* | *.77* |
| 1 turn of context | .49 | .49 | .49 |
| BoW (2 turns) | .76 | .76 | .76 |
| Bigrams (2 turns) | .83 | .83 | .83 |
| BoW + Bigrams (2 turns) | .83 | .83 | .83 |
| **Italian** | | | |
| *no context* | *.71* | *.71* | *.71* |
| Bigrams (2 turns) | .82 | .82 | .82 |

(a)

| English | | | |
|---|---|---|---|
| Experimental Setting | Prec | Rec | F1 |
| *no context* | *.68* | *.68* | *.68* |
| Bigrams (2 turns) | .70 | .70 | .70 |
| **Italian** | | | |
| *no context* | *.66* | *.66* | *.66* |
| Bigrams (2 turns) | .72 | .72 | .72 |

(b)

text features are used in the supervised setting. For both the Italian and English corpora, bigrams seem to best capture the dialogue structure. In particular, using a BoW style seems to even lower the performance with respect to the setting in which no information about the context is exploited. Neither combining bigrams with Bag of Words nor using higher-order n-gram improves the performance.

*Unsupervised.* According to the results in the previous section, we decided to investigate the use of bigrams in the unsupervised learning condition using a bootstrap approach. Our bootstrap procedure is composed by the following steps:

1. Annotating the English and Italian corpora using the unsupervised approach described in Section 4.3;
2. Using the result of this unsupervised annotation for extracting knowledge about contextual information for each utterance: each item in the data sets is then enriched with the appropriate bigram, as shown in Table 7;
3. Training an SVM classifier on the bootstrap data enriched with bigrams.

Then performance is evaluated on the test sets (see Table 8 (b)) according to the actual label given by human annotators.

## 5 ATTITUDE DISPLAY IN DIALOGUE PATTERNS

In this section, we describe our experience with the investigation on how affective factors influence dialogue patterns and whether this effect may be described and recognized by Hidden Markov Models (HMM) (Martalò et al., 2008). In particular we present a study about engagement recognition of users interacting with an Embodied Conversational Agent playing the role of an artificial therapist in an advice-giving task about healthy-eating (Novielli, 2010).

This study was performed in the scope of a research project whose main goal is to build an Embodied Conversational Agent (ECA) that is able to inform, persuade and engage a human interlocutor in a conversation about healthy dieting (Mazzotta et al., 2007). In the referred scenario the ECA plays the role of an artificial therapist and employs natural argumentation techniques to persuade the user.

A fundamental requirement for such an agent is the ability to observe the verbal and non verbal behavior of users during the interaction, to infer the cognitive and affective ingredients of their state of mind and to adapt both the dialogue strategy and interaction style accordingly. This is particularly true for advice-giving dialogues in which knowledge of the user characteristics is of primary importance in building an effective persuasion strategy.

## 5.1 Dialogue Representation

The study described in this section is based on the assumption that long-term affective phenomena influence the overall behavior of users during the interaction. As a consequence, such states also impact the overall dialogue dynamics (Sidner & Lee, 2003). This is particularly true for attitudes and social stances, which smoothly evolve during the dialogue.

After becoming a very popular approach for language modeling tasks (Rabiner, 1990; Charniak, 1993), HMMs began to attract the interest of researchers working in the field of conversational analysis. Levin et al. (1998) were among the first to use this formalism for modeling Human-Computer interaction: in their representation, states are associate to system moves while user moves are employed to label transitions. The models are employed to evaluate the cost of different dialogue strategies in terms of distance to the achievement of the application goal. In (Twitchell et al., 2004), HMMs are used to classifying conversations, with no specific application reported.

Finally, the study with which the approach described in this section has more in common is the one proposed in (Soller, 2004) for classifying effective knowledge-sharing episodes in online collaborative learning: aggregates of students' communicative acts are associate to each one of the five state of the HMM model learnt from a corpus of manually labeled 'knowledge sharing' or 'breakdowns' episodes.

In our study (Novielli 2010), interactions are coded as sequences of dialogue acts, according to the mark-up language reported in Table 2, so as to capture the main communicative intention of each dialogue move. Then, dialogue act sequences are represented using HMMs. Formally (Rabiner, 1990; Charniak, 1993), an HMM can be defined as a tuple: $< S, W, \pi, A, B>$, where

- $S = \{s_1,\ldots s_n\}$ is the set of states in the model,
- $W = \{w_1,\ldots w_m\}$ is the set of observations or output symbols,
- $\pi$ are a-priori-likelihoods, that is the initial state distributions: $\pi = \{\pi_i\}$, $i \in S$;
- $A = \{a_{ij}\}$, $i, j \in S$, is a matrix describing the state transition probability distribution: $a_{ij} = P(X_{t+1} = s_j \mid X_t = s_i)$;
- $B = \{b_{ijk}\}$, $i, j \in S$, $w_k \in W$, is a matrix describing the observation symbol probability distribution: $b_{ijk} = P(O_t = w_k \mid X_t = s_i, X_{t+1} = s_j)$.

In our models states represent aggregates of either system or user moves, each with a probability to occur in that specific phase of the dialogue while the transitions represent the possible dialogue sequences. Ideally, transitions start from a system move and end to a user move type and vice versa, each with a probability to occur, although in principle, user-user move or system-system move transitions may occur. HMMs are learnt from the Italian corpus by representing every input dialogue as a sequence of coded dialogue moves. For example, the following dialogue excerpt:

T(S,1)= Hi, my name is Valentina. I'm here to suggest you how to improve your diet. Do you like eating?
T(U,1)=Yes
T(S,2)= What did you eat at breakfast?
T(U,2)=Coffee and nothing else.
T(S,3)=Do you frequently eat this way?
T(U,3)=Yes

T(S,4)= Are you attracted by sweets?
T(U,4)= Not much. I don't eat much of them.
T(S,5)= Do you believe your diet is correct or would you like changing your eating habits?
T(U,5)= I don't believe it's correct: I tend to jump lunch, for instance.

is coded as follows: (OPENING, GENERIC-ANSWER, QUESTION, STAT-ABOUT-SELF, QUESTION, GENERIC-ANSWER, QUESTION, STAT-ABOUT-PREFERENCES, QUESTION, STAT-ABOUT-SELF).

## 5.2 Testing the Descriptive Power of the Model

In order to verify how good such a model is in capturing the main differences in the dialogue pattern due to different attitudes of the users, we first tested the descriptive power of the HMMs (Martalò et al., 2008) by classifying users according to an objective feature about some knowledge that had been acquired in a previous study. The relationship between the 'social attitude' of users towards the ECA and their background was analyzed: people with background in Humanities (HUM) tended to display a 'warmer' social attitude towards the agent with respect to people with background in Computer Science (CS), that is they used more familiar language, asked personal question to the agent, talked more about self (indicating self-disclosure and intention to establishing a common ground), made more positive/negative comments after the agent suggestion (probably denoting an higher perceived 'social presence' and their more prominent attitude to attach humanness-related features to the ECA rather than simply considering it as a 'tool' to be used for gathering information about diet) (de Rosis et al., 2007).

The transcripts of the interactions belonging to the Italian corpus of advice-giving dialogues were therefore classified according to the background of the subjects involved (CS vs. HUM). An HMM model was learnt for each subset of dialogues, using the Baum-Welch algorithm (Rabiner, 1990), which adjusts the model parameters $\mu = (A, B, \pi)$ to maximize the likelihood of the given input observations, that is $P(O|\mu)$.

Figures 1 (a) and (b) show, respectively, the best 8-states[2] HMMs for CS and HUM subjects. States Si correspond to aggregates of system moves: in 1a, an OPENING is associated with S1 with probability 1; a QUESTION to S2 with probability.88; a PERSUASION (p=.57), and OFFER-INFO (p=.20) or an ENCOURAGE (p=.14) with S3, etc. Interpretation of states Uj, to which user moves are associated, can be observed in the figure. Transitions between states in models 1a and 1b have a common core pattern, although with different probabilities: the path (S1, U1, S2, U2, S3, U3), the way back (U3, S2) and the direct link (S1, U3). Other transitions differ. Dissimilarities can be found also in the probability distributions of communicative acts associated with the phases of dialogue opening (S1, U1), question answering (S2, U2), system persuasion (S3, U3) and of a warm phase (S4,U4), in which the user displays a kind attitude towards the system in various forms. The following are the main differences between the models, in these phases:

- *Question-answering* (S2,U2): the only difference, in this case, is that HUM subjects tend to be more specific and eloquent than CS ones, by producing more statements about' self, 'statements about preferences' and less 'generic answers'.
- *Persuasion* (S3, U3): in CS models, users may respond to persuasion attempts with information requests or declarations of consensus. They may enter, as well, in the warm phase (S3, U4 link). In the HUM model, after a persuasion attempt by S, U may stay in the persuasion phase (U3) by making further information requests, objections, solicitations or statements about self. In both models, question answering

*Figure 1. HMM for CS (a) and HUM (b) users*

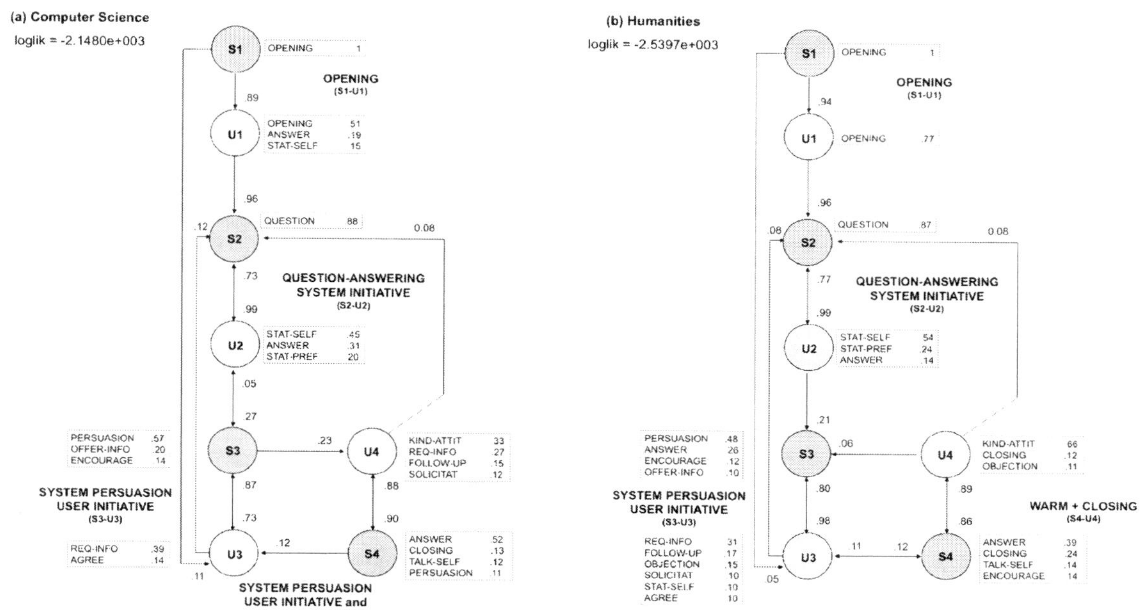


and persuasion may alternate (link U3, S2) in a more varied dialogue.

- *Warm phase* (S4, U4): although this phase exists in both models, communicative acts employed by U, once again differ: the objection move of HUM is substituted by a solicitation in CS model. In this model, the state S4 may contain persuasion moves as well: hence, the whole phase may be called system persuasion-user initiative and warm attitude. The likelihood to produce a kind attitude move (in U4) is, in the HUM model, twice than in the CS model. These differences in the subjects' behavior confirm the findings of our previous studies, by describing them in terms of dialogue structure rather than of individual moves' content.

To test the ability of the learnt model to classify new users, a leave-one-out validation was performed (Martalò et al., 2008). By applying HMM analysis to users background, we aimed at verifying whether any difference between the two categories of users could be found, as well, in the dialogue patterns. Information about this feature was collected with a questionnaire during the WoZ study. Here, it was taken as the external reference in the testing phase. Table 9 shows the results of this analysis: a CS dialogue is recognized correctly in 77% of cases, while a HUM dialogue is recognized correctly in 57% of cases. This is probably due to the higher variability of behavior in HUM users. Also, HUM dialogues tend to be misclassified as CS ones more frequently than the inverse.

## 5.3 Recognizing the User Engagement

We applied the methodology described in the previous section to the recognition of the user engagement in the task of the conversation (i.e. advice-giving in the diet domain) (Novielli, 2010).

*Table 9. Confusion matrix for CS and HUM users*

| | CS | HUM | Precision | Recall | F1 |
|---|---|---|---|---|---|
| CS | .77 | .23 | .64 | .77 | .70 |
| HUM | .43 | .57 | .71 | .57 | .63 |
| micro | | | .67 | .67 | .67 |

Researchers have employed different definitions of engagement according to the domain and task requirements: some studies aim at implementing intelligent media switching (see for example, Yu et al., (2004); Woodruff & Aoki, (2004)) while others (Core et al., 2003) aim at tailoring the interaction to the user needs. The study described in this Section fits in the scope of a long-term research project whose goal was to design an agent capable to engage and persuade users in the healthy eating domain (de Rosis et al., 2006; Mazzotta et al., 2007), hence we refer to a concept of engagement defined accordingly to this goal.

In advice-giving dialogues two tasks are integrated: the provision of domain specific information and the persuasion to abandon a wrong behavior. By analyzing the Italian corpus of dialogues, we found that some users typically adopt an attitude aimed at the extraction of information and the testing of the reliability of this information. We therefore named 'Information-Seeking' (IS) the users asking several questions, either for requesting information or challenging the application, sometimes even right after the system self introduction.

In another category of users (AG, from 'Advice-Giving'), subjects seem to be more involved in the persuasion goal of advice-giving: they show a more cooperative attitude towards the system, by providing extra-information to the agent so as to build a shared ground of knowledge about their habits, desires, beliefs etc., they react to the agent suggestions and/or attempts of persuasion by providing a constructive feedback in terms of objections, comments (either positive or negative) and follow-up questions.

Finally, we have a third category of Not-engaged (N) users who do not show any interest in any of the two mentioned tasks. They rather give a passive contribution to the interaction and demonstrate to be barely reactive by mainly answering the systems questions, usually with general answers (e.g. 'yes' or 'no'); their dialogues are usually shorter than the others and tend to be driven by the system (that sometimes seems to struggle to protract the interaction).

Distinguishing among the three levels of engagement is relevant for adaptation: IS users might be either supported in their information seeking goal or leaded by the system to get involved also in the advice giving task; AG users might perceive an increased satisfaction about the interaction if the agent is believable in playing its role; N users represent a real challenge for the system since the reasons for their attitude are actually unknown (e.g. either a lack of interest in the domain or a lack of trust in the agent ability to manage the dialogue).

The complete corpus of Italian dialogues has been annotated according to the provided definition of engagement: each dialogue received one of the three labels (AG, IS, N) with respect to the overall attitude shown by the user during the interaction as described in (Martalò et al., 2008; Novielli, 2010). The corpus is not equally distributed (N = 28%, IS = 44%, AG = 28%), which is an undesirable circumstance when the available set of data is not particularly wide, as in our case.

An HMM model has been trained for each subset of dialogues identifying a class of users: figures 2(a), (b) and (c) show, respectively, the best 8-state HMMs for N, IS and AG subjects. The results of training reflect the differences in

*Figure 2. HMM for neutral (a), information seeking (b) and advice-giving (c) dialogues*

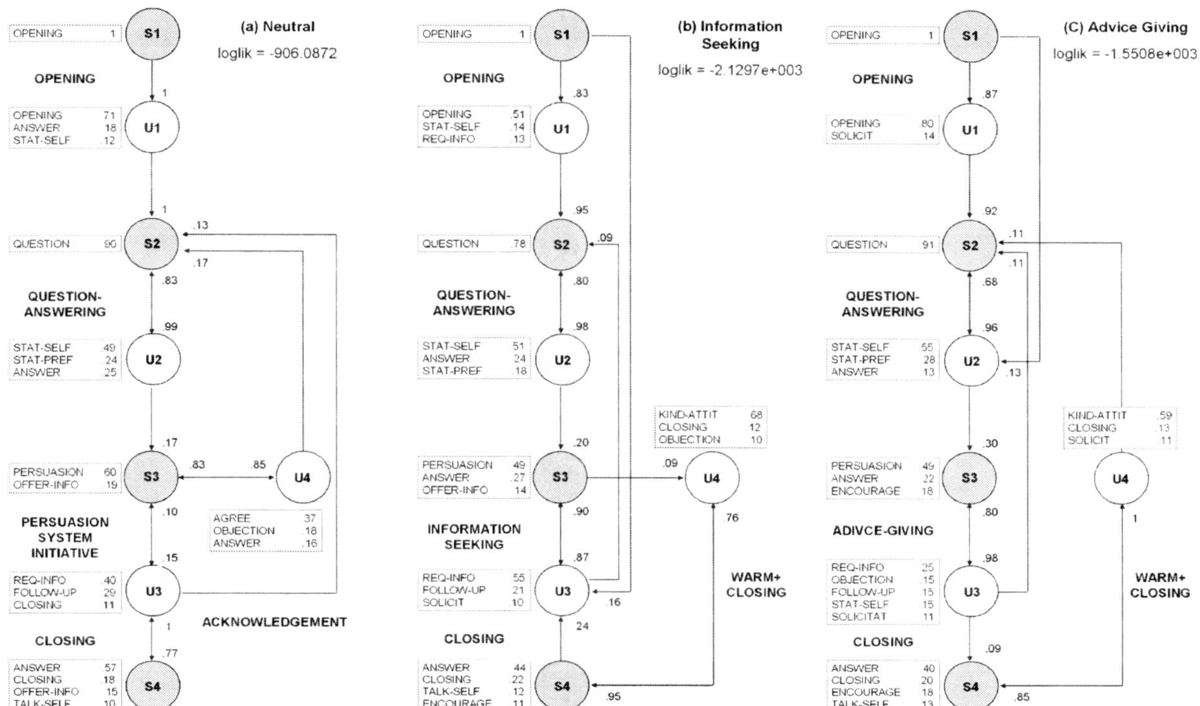


the users' behavior that led us to the definition of the three class of engagement. In particular, the main differences are in the Persuasion phase (S3, U3), which is named in each model according to the differences in the observable user categories of moves. In the N model, the users may respond to persuasion attempts with information requests, follow-up questions and even with a closing move: so we named this phase persuasion with system initiative.

IS users have the highest probability of performing a request of information and do not provide any kind of personal information (information seeking phase). In the AG models, users are clearly involved in an advice-giving phase: the probability of information requests is lower and the variety of reactions to system suggestions is wider, according to the user goal of either enhancing the construction of a shared ground of knowledge about healthy eating, or giving a positive feedback to the ECA. Also, for this model we observe a higher likelihood of entering the persuasion phase, core of the advice-giving process, after the initial assessment of the user situation performed by the ECA through the question-answering (S2, U2). Moreover, the duration of the persuasion phase for N users is usually very short, as described by the low transition probabilities between S3 and U3. On the contrary, a long phase of either information seeking or advice-giving can be observed for, respectively, IS and AG users.

To test the ability of the models in recognizing the user overall engagement, once again leave-one-out cross-validation has been performed. Results are quite satisfying (see Table 10) and are comparable to the state of the art in the domain (Soller, 2004). Though, in spite of the high inter-rater agreement (Kappa=.90) and of the good descriptive power of the HMMs, the analysis

*Table 10. Confusion matrix for N, IS and AG users*

| | N | IS | AG | Precision | Recall | F1 |
|---|---|---|---|---|---|---|
| N | .76 | .24 | 0 | .76 | .81 | .78 |
| IS | .04 | .85 | .12 | .85 | .73 | .79 |
| AG | .12 | .24 | .65 | .65 | .69 | .67 |
| micro | | | | .77 | .77 | .77 |

shows a lack of robustness for AG models, due to the unequal distribution of the data set, the restricted amount of available data and the higher variability of behavior observed in AG users. A detailed discussion and further investigation about dynamic recognition of engagement during the dialogue may be found in (Novielli, 2010).

## 6. CONCLUSION AND FUTURE WORK

In this chapter, we have briefly reported on our research experience with natural dialogues. We have described two studies lying at the intersection of two main research area that is Natural Language Processing and Human-Computer Interaction, with particular attention to natural dialogues with an ECA. In particular, we have shown how we exploit empirical methods to define a domain and task independent approach for automatic labeling natural conversations with the proper Dialogue Acts (DAs). Then, we have proposed a method that exploits conversational analysis techniques for recognizing the user attitude during a dialogue with an embodied agent.

As far as automatic DA annotation is concerned, we have described our method based on exploiting the lexical semantics of utterance in dialogues: we have defined linguistic profiles for DAs through a similarity study in latent semantic spaces automatically acquired from dialogue corpora. To ensure the independence of our DA profiles from the language used, the application domain and other important features such as the interaction mode, we focused our experiments on two different corpora of natural dialogues, both annotated with DA labels and presenting different languages, tasks, application domain, interaction modality and size. Some experiments in both a supervised and unsupervised framework have been performed, on both the English and the Italian corpus, with and without taking into account dialogue contextual features, obtaining good performance. The results of our experiments confirm the hypothesis about lexical knowledge playing a fundamental role in characterizing DA labels. Language and domain independence is also demonstrated: the results in both the supervised and the unsupervised case showed that the performance is not affected by the difference in the language used, the size and the domain of the conversations belonging to the two corpora exploited. The approach employed can be easily extended to other languages by simply redefining the seeds (lexical cues) used in the definition of the DA profiles and by using a POS-tagger and a morphological analyzer trained on the target language.

Then we have shown how automatic DA annotation of natural language interaction may be exploited in modeling the user attitudes during a dialogue with an ECA. In particular, we described studies about user attitude modeling in the domain of persuasion dialogues with an ECA playing the role of an artificial advisor, in which we achieved satisfying results. In our research we have provided experimental results regarding the validation of this approach on advice-giving dialogues in the healthy-eating domain. Though, the method is based on domain independent conversational analysis techniques and uses a domain-independent framework for dialogue act annotation. Therefore, it can be easily generalized according to different attitude-detection needs, also in different domains or interaction scenarios. This is one of the direction we intend to follow in our future research.

To conclude, the methods employed in the experiments described in this chapter are not necessarily restricted to the field of natural interaction with ECAs. On the contrary, they may be relevant for a wide range of applications about human-human and human-machine interaction, such as forum and chat log analysis for opinion mining, automatic meeting summarization and so on. With the advent of the Web, a large amount of material about natural language interaction has become available, raising the attractiveness of empirical methods of analysis on this field. Manual labeling of such a huge amount of data is an error-prone and time-consuming activity. Automatic DA recognition based on unsupervised approaches is of great potential interest along this perspective.

## REFERENCES

Andersen, P. A., & Guerrero, L. K. (1998). *Handbook of communication and emotions. Research, theory, applications and contexts*. New York, NY: Academic Press.

André, E., Klesen, M., Gebhard, P., Allen, S., & Rist, T. (2000). Integrating models of personality and emotions into lifelike characters. In Paiva, A. (Ed.), *Affective interactions: Towards a new generation of computer interfaces, Lecture Notes In Computer Science* (*Vol. 1814*, pp. 150–165). New York, NY: Springer-Verlag.

Austin, J. (1962). *How to do things with words*. New York, NY: Oxford University Press.

Bailenson, J. N., Swinth, K. R., & Hoyt, C. L., Persky, Susan, D. A., & Blascovich, J. (2005). The independent and interactive effects of embodied agents appearance and behavior on self-report, cognitive and behavioral markers of copresence in Immersive Virtual Environments. *Presence (Cambridge, Mass.)*, *14*(4), 379–393. doi:10.1162/105474605774785235

Berry, D. C., Butler, L. T., & de Rosis, F. (2005). Evaluating a realistic agent in an advice-giving task. *International Journal of Human-Computer Studies*, *63*, 304–327. doi:10.1016/j.ijhcs.2005.03.006

Berry, M. W. (1992). Large-scale sparse singular value computations. *The International Journal of Supercomputer Applications*, *6*(1), 13–49.

Bickmore, T. (2003). *Relational agents: Effecting change through human-computer relationships*, Ph.D. thesis, media arts & sciences, Massachusetts Institute of Technology.

Bickmore, T., & Cassell, J. (2005). Social dialogue with embodied conversational agents. In van Kuppevelt, J., Dybkjaer, L., & Bernsen, N. O. (Eds.), *Advances in natural multimodal dialogue systems* (pp. 23–54). Springer. doi:10.1007/1-4020-3933-6_2

Bickmore, T. W., & Picard, R. W. (2005). Establishing and maintaining long-term human-computer relationships. *ACM Transactions on Computer-Human Interaction*, *12*, 293–327. doi:10.1145/1067860.1067867

Blascovich, J. (2002). Social influences within immersive virtual environments. In Schroeder, R. (Ed.), *The social life of avatars* (pp. 127–145). London, UK: Springer-Verlag.

Cassell, J. (2001). Embodied conversational agents: Representation and intelligence in user interfaces. *AI Magazine*, *22*, 67–83.

Cassell, J., Bickmore, T., Billinghurst, M., Campbell, L., Chang, K., Vilhjalmsoon, H., & Yan, H. (1999). Embodiement in conversational interfaces: Rea. In *Proceedings of the CHI'99 Conference* (pp. 520–527).

Charniak, E. (1993). *Statistical language learning*. The MIT Press.

Clarizio, G., Mazzotta, I., Novielli, N., & de Rosis, F. (2006). Social attitude towards a conversational character. In *Proceedings of the 15th IEEE International Symposium on Robot and Human Interactive Communication*, (pp. 2–7), Hatfield, UK.

Cohen, P. R., & Levesque, H. J. (1990). Rational interaction as the basis for communication. In Cohen, P. R., Morgan, J., & Pollack, M. E. (Eds.), *Intentions in communication* (pp. 221–256). MIT Press.

Cohen, P. R., & Levesque, H. J. (1995). Communicative actions for artificial agents. In *Proceedings of the First International Conference on Multi-Agent Systems* (pp. 65–72). AAAI Press.

Core, M., & Allen, J. (1997). Coding dialogs with the DAMSL annotation scheme. In *Working Notes of the AAAI Fall Symposium on Communicative Action in Humans and Machines* (pp. 28-35). Cambridge, MA.

Core, M. G., Moore, J. D., & Zinn, C. (2003). The role of initiative in tutorial dialogue. In *Proceedings of the ITS Workshop on Empirical Methods for Tutorial Dialogue Systems*, (pp. 67–74).

Dautenhahn, K. (1999). Socially situated life-like agents: If it makes you happy then it can't be that bad?! In *Proceedings VWSIM'99, Virtual Worlds and Simulation Conference*. Retrieved from http://homepages.feis.herts.ac.uk/~comqkd/papers.html

De Carolis, B., Mazzotta, I., & Novielli, N. (2010). Enhancing conversational access to information through a social intelligent agent. In G. Armano, M. de Gemmis, G. Semeraro and E. Vargiu (Eds): *Intelligent Information Access, Studies in Computational Intelligence*, 2010, Volume 301/2010 (pp. pages 1-20), Springer Berlin / Heidelberg.

De Carolis, B., Pelachaud, C., Poggi, I., & de Rosis, F. (2001). Behavior planning for a reflexive agent. In *IJCAI'01: Proceedings of the 17th international Joint Conference on Artificial intelligence,* San Francisco, CA, USA, (pp. 1059–1064). Morgan Kaufmann Publishers Inc.

de Rosis, F., Batliner, A., Novielli, N., & Steidl, S. (2007). You are sooo cool, Valentina! Recognizing social attitude in speech-based dialogues with an ECA. In Paiva, A., Prada, R., & Picard, R. W. (Eds.), *Affective computing and intelligent interaction. Lecture Notes in Computer Science* (*Vol. 4738*, pp. 179–190). Berlin/Heidelberg, Germany: Springer-Verlag. doi:10.1007/978-3-540-74889-2_17

de Rosis, F., Carolis, B. D., Carofiglio, V., & Pizzutilo, S. (2004). Shallow and inner forms of emotional intelligence in advisory dialog simulation. In Prendinger, H., & Ishizuka, M. (Eds.), *Life-like characters: Tools, affective functions, and applications (Cognitive Technologies)* (pp. 271–294). Springer Verlag.

de Rosis, F., Novielli, N., Carofiglio, V., Cavalluzzi, A., & De Carolis, B. (2006). User modeling and adaptation in health promotion dialogs with an animated character. *Journal of Biomedical Informatics*, *39*, 514–531. doi:10.1016/j.jbi.2006.01.001

Dohsaka, K., Asai, R., Higashinaka, R., Minami, Y., & Maeda, E. (2009). Effects of conversational agents on human communication in thought-evoking multi-party dialogues. In *SIGDIAL '09: Proceedings of the SIGDIAL 2009 Conference,* Morristown, NJ, USA (pp. 217–224). Association for Computational Linguistics.

Gliozzo, A., & Strapparava, C. (2005). Domains kernels for text categorization. In *Proceedings of the Ninth Conference on Computational Natural Language Learning (CoNLL-2005)* (pp. 56–63), University of Michigan, Ann Arbor.

Godfrey, J., Holliman, E., & McDaniel, J. (1992). SWITCHBOARD: Telephone speech corpus for re-search and development. In *Proceedings of the IEEE International Conference on Acoustics, Speech and Signal Processing (ICASSP),* San Francisco, CA, (pp. 517–520). IEEE.

Grosz, B. J., & Sidner, C. L. (1986). Attention, intentions, and the structure of discourse. *Computational Linguistics, 12*, 175–204.

Hinkelman, E. A., & Allen, J. F. (1989). Two constraints on speech act ambiguity. In *Proceedings of the 27th Annual Meeting on Association for Computational Linguistics* (pp. 212-219). Vancouver, British Columbia, Canada.

Hirschberg, J., & Litman, D. (1993). Empirical studies on the disambiguation of cue phrases. *Computational Linguistics, 19*, 501–530.

Hoorn, J. F., & Konijn, E. A. (2003). Perceiving and experiencing fictional characters: An integrative account. *The Japanese Psychological Research, 45*(4), 221–239. doi:10.1111/1468-5884.00225

Jurafsky, D., Shriberg, E., & Biasca, D. (1997). *Switchboard SWBD-DAMSL shallow-discourse-function annotation coders manual*, draft 13. Technical Report 97-01, University of Colorado Institute of Cognitive Science.

Jurafsky, D., Shriberg, E., Fox, B., & Curl, T. (1998). Lexical, prosodic, and syntactic cues for dialog acts. In *Proceedings of ACL/COLING-98 Workshop on Discourse Relations and Discourse Markers* (pp. 114–120). Montreal, Canada.

King, S. A., Knott, A., & McCane, B. (2003). Language-driven nonverbal communication in a bilingual conversational agent. *In CASA '03: Proceedings of the 16th International Conference on Computer Animation and Social Agents (CASA 2003)* (p. 17). Washington, DC: IEEE Computer Society.

Landauer, T. K., Foltz, P., & Laham, D. (1998). Introduction to latent semantic analysis. *Discourse Processes, 25*, 259–284. doi:10.1080/01638539809545028

Levin, E., Pieraccini, R., & Eckert, W. (1998). Using Markov decision process for learning dialogue strategies. In *Proceedings of the IEEE International Conference on Acoustic, speech and signal processing* (pp. 201–204).

Levinson, S. C. (1983). *Pragmatics*. Cambridge, UK & New York, NY: Cambridge University Press.

Litman, D. J., & Allen, J. F. (1990). Discourse processing and commonsense plans. In Cohen, P. R., Morgan, J. L., & Pollack, M. E. (Eds.), *Intentions in communications* (pp. 365–388). The MIT Press.

Marsella, S. C., Johnson, W. L., & Labore, C. M. (2003). *Interactive pedagogical drama for health interventions*. In AIED 2003, 11th International Conference on Artificial Intelligence in Education, Australia, (pp. 341–348). IOS Press

Martalò, A., Novielli, N., & de Rosis, F. (2008). Attitude display in dialogue patterns. In *Proceedings of AISB 2008 Convention on Communication, Interaction and Social Intelligence*. Retrieved from http://www.aisb.org.uk/convention/aisb08/proc/proceedings/02%20Affective%20Language/01.pdf

Mazzotta, I., Novielli, N., Silvestri, V., & de Rosis, F. (2007). O Francesca, ma che sei grulla? Emotions and irony in persuasion dialogues. In R. Basili & M. T. Pazienza (Eds.), *Proceedings of the 10th Congress of the Italian Association For Artificial intelligence on AI*IA 2007: Artificial intelligence and Human-Oriented Computing, Lecture Notes In Artificial Intelligence, vol. 4733*, (pp. 602-613). Berlin/ Heidelberg, Germany: Springer-Verlag.

Niederhoffer, K. G., & Pennebaker, J. W. (2002). Linguistic style matching in social interaction. *Journal of Language and Social Psychology, 21*, 337–360. doi:10.1177/026192702237953

Novielli, N. (2010). HMM modeling of user engagement in advice-giving dialogues. *Journal on Multimodal User Interfaces, 3*(1-2), 131–140. doi:10.1007/s12193-009-0026-4

Novielli, N., de Rosis, F., & Mazzotta, I. (2010). User attitude towards an embodied conversational agent: Effects of the interaction mode. [Elsevier Science.]. *Journal of Pragmatics, 42*(9), 2385–2397. doi:10.1016/j.pragma.2009.12.016

Novielli, N., & Strapparava, C. (2010a). Exploring the lexical semantics of dialogue acts. *Journal of Computational Linguistics and Applications, 1*, 9–26.

Novielli, N., & Strapparava, C. (2010b). Studying the lexicon of dialogue acts. In N. Calzolari, K. Choukri, B. Maegaard, J. Mariani, J. Odijk, S. Piperidis, M. Rosner & D. Tapias (Eds.), *Proceedings of the Seventh Conference on International Language Resources and Evaluation (LREC'10)*. Retrieved from http://www.lrec-conf.org/proceedings/lrec2010/index.html

Paiva, A. (Ed.). (2004). *Empathic agents*. Workshop in conjunction with AAMAS'04.

Pentland, A. S. (2005). Socially aware computation and communication. *Computer, 38*, 33–40. doi:10.1109/MC.2005.104

Pianta, E., Girardi, C., & Zanoli, R. (2008). The TextPro tool suite. In N. Calzolari, K. Choukri, B. Maegaard, J. Mariani, J. Odjik, S. Piperidis & D. Tapias (Eds.) *Proceedings of the Sixth International Language Resources and Evaluation (LREC'08)*. Retrieved from http://www.lrec-conf.org/proceedings/lrec2008/.

Poesio, M., & Mikheev, A. (1998). The predictive power of game structure in dialogue act recognition: Experimental results using maximum entropy estimation. In *Proceedings of ICSLP-98*, Sydney.

Poggi, I., Pelachaud, C., & De Rosis, F. (2000). Eye communication in a conversational 3d synthetic agent. *AI Communications, 13*, 169–181.

Poggi, I., Pelachaud, C., de Rosis, F., Carofiglio, V., & De Carolis, B. (2005). GRETA: A believable embodied conversational agent. In Stock, O., & Zancanaro, M. (Eds.), *Multimodal intelligent information presentation* (pp. 1–23). New York, NY: Kluwer. doi:10.1007/1-4020-3051-7_1

Polhemus, L., Shih, L.-F., & Swan, K. (2001). *Virtual interactivity: The representation of social presence in an online discussion*. Annual Meeting of the American Educational Research Association.

Rabiner, L. (1990). A tutorial on hidden Markov models and selected applications in speech recognition. In Waibel, A., & Lee, K. (Eds.), *Readings in speech recognition* (pp. 267–296). San Francisco, CA: Morgan Kaufmann Publishers.

Reeves, B., & Nass, C. (2003). *The media equation: How people treat computers, television, and new media like real people and places (CSLI Lecture Notes)*. Center for the Study of Language and Inf.

Reithinger, N., & Klesen, M. (1997). Dialogue act classification using language models. In. *Proceedings of EuroSpeech, 97*, 2235–2238.

Roesch, E. B., Banziger, T., & Scherer, K. R. (2005). *D3e – proposal for exemplars and work towards it: Theories and models*. (HUMAINE, Human-Machine Interaction Network on Emotions, IST-FP6 Contract No 507422). Retrieved from http://emotion-research.net/projects/humaine/deliverables/D3e%20final.pdf

Samuel, K., Carberry, S., & Vijay-Shanker, K. (1998). Dialogue act tagging with transformation-based learning. In *Proceedings of the 17th International Conference on Computational Linguistics*, Morristown, NJ, USA, (pp. 1150–1156). Association for Computational Linguistics.

Searle, J. (1969). *Speech acts: An essay in the philosophy of language*. Cambridge/London, UK: Cambridge University Press.

Sidner, C. L., & Lee, C. (2003). *An architecture for engagement in collaborative conversations between a robot and humans*. (MERL Technical Report, TR2003-12), June 2003.

Soller, A. (2004). Computational modeling and analysis of knowledge sharing in collaborative distance learning. *User Modeling and User-Adapted Interaction*, *14*, 351–381. doi:10.1023/B:USER.0000043436.49168.3b

Stolcke, A., Coccaro, N., Bates, R., Taylor, P., Ess-Dykema, C. V., Ries, K., & Meteer, M. (2000). Dialogue act modeling for automatic tagging and recognition of conversational speech. *Computational Linguistics*, *26*, 339–373. doi:10.1162/089120100561737

Traum, D. (2000). 20 questions for dialogue act taxonomies. *Journal of Semantics*, *17*, 7–30. doi:10.1093/jos/17.1.7

Twitchell, D. P., Adkins, M., Nunamaker, J. F., & Burgoon, J. K. (2004). *Proceedings of the 9th International Working Conference on the Language-Action perspective on Communication Modelling* (pp. 121-130).

van Deemter, K., Krenn, B., Piwek, P., Klesen, M., Schröder, M., & Baumann, S. (2008). Fully generated scripted dialogue for embodied agents. *Artificial Intelligence*, *172*(10), 1219–1244. doi:10.1016/j.artint.2008.02.002

Vapnik, V. (1995). *The nature of statistical learning theory*. Springer-Verlag.

Venkataraman, A., Liu, Y., Shriberg, E., & Stolcke, A. (2005). Does active learning help automatic dialog act tagging in meeting data? In *Proceedings of EUROSPEECH-05*, Lisbon, Portugal.

Warnke, V., Kompe, R., Niemann, H., & Noth, E. (1997). Integrated dialog act segmentation and classification using prosodic features and language models. In *Proceedings of 5th European Conference on Speech Communication and Technology, vol. 1,* Rhodes, Greece (pp. 207–210).

Woodruff, A., & Aoki, P. (2004). Conversation analysis and the user experience. *Digital Creativity*, *4*, 232–238. doi:10.1080/1462626048520184

Wright, H. (1998). Automatic utterance type detection using suprasegmental features. In *Proceedings of the International Conference on Spoken Language Processing (ICSLP-98)* (pp. 1403-1406). Sydney, Australia.

Yu, C., Aoki, P. M., & Woodruff, A. (2004). Detecting user engagement in everyday conversations. In *Proceedings of the 8th International Conference on Spoken Language Processing (ICSLP '04)* (pp. 1–6).

## KEY TERMS AND DEFINITIONS

**Affective Computing:** Research field that studies how to develop systems able to recognize, simulate and adapt their behavior to affective states of users, such as emotions, moods, attitudes or other emotion-related states.

**Automatic Dialogue Act Annotation:** Is the task of assigning a Dialogue Act label to an utterance or a dialogue turn in natural language. In literature, it has been recently treated as a task of text-classification. Many NLP tasks, in fact, can be modeled as a classification problem, that is the problem of assigning a category label to a linguistic object (i.e. assigning a DA label to the utterance in input).

**Dialogue Acts (DAs):** DAs constitute the basis of communication. In Austin's view (1962), a DA can be identified with the communicative goal of a given utterance. Researchers use different labels and definitions to address similar concepts. For example, Searle (1969) talks about *speech act* while Cohen and Levesque (1995) focus more on the role speech acts play in interagent communication. In this chapter we refer to the domain-independent Dialogue Act taxonomy defined by Core and Allen (1997).

**Hidden Markov Models (HMM):** Is a statistical model (Rabiner, 1990; Charniak, 2003) in which the Markov property holds (the past has no impact on the future given the present). The phenomenon modeled is assumed to be a Markov process with unobserved states. In the study presented in this chapter, interactions are coded as sequences of dialogue acts. Then, dialogue act sequences are represented using HMMs in which states are aggregates of either system or user moves, while the transitions describe the possible dialogue sequences.

**Human-Computer Interaction (HCI):** Research field that investigates issues related to the interaction with technological devices (e.g. usability, interaction design, user modeling, evaluation of the user satisfaction).

**Latent Semantic Analysis (LSA):** LSA is a corpus-based measure of semantic similarity (Landauer et al., 1998) in which term co-occurrences in a corpus are captured by means of a dimensionality reduction operated by a singular value decomposition (SVD) on the term-by-document matrix representing the corpus.

**Lexical Semantics:** It is the study of how and what the words of a language denote. In particular if focuses on what individual lexical items mean, why they mean what they do, how we can represent all of this, and where the combined interpretation for an utterance comes from.

**Natural Language Processing (NLP):** Research field that studies how to automatically process written or spoken texts in natural language.

**Part of Speech (POS) Tagging:** Is the NLP task of marking up the words in a text with the corresponding part of speech.

**Stopwords:** Words that, due to their high frequency in a given language (e.g. articles, prepositions or conjunctions) are usually considered of poor importance in tasks such as determining the semantics a text or defining the query for a search engine and so on.

## ENDNOTES

1. ftp.ldc.upenn.edu/pub/ldc/public_data/swb1_dialogact_annot.tar.gz
2. To establish the number of states to include in our models, three alternatives were tested: 6, 8 and 10 states. The robustness analysis led us to choose the 8-state HMM model and is described in more details in (Martalò et al., 2008).

# Chapter 5
# A Cognitive Dialogue Manager for Education Purposes

**Roberto Pirrone**
*University of Palermo, Italy*

**Vincenzo Cannella**
*University of Palermo, Italy*

**Giuseppe Russo**
*University of Palermo, Italy*

**Arianna Pipitone**
*University of Palermo, Italy*

## ABSTRACT

*A conversational agent is a software system that is able to interact with users in a natural way, and often uses natural language capabilities. In this chapter, an evolution of a conversational agent is presented according to the definition of dialogue management techniques for the conversational agents. The presented conversational agent is intended to act as a part of an educational system. The chapter outlines the state-of-the-art systems and techniques for dialogue management in cognitive educational systems, and the underlying psychological and social aspects. We present our framework for a dialogue manager aimed to reduce the uncertainty in users' sentences during the assessment of his/her requests. The domain is the development of a new generation of Intelligent Tutoring Systems (ITS) enabled with meta-cognitive abilities to make the learning process more effective. The architecture of the developed systems is explained in detail, along with some experimental results, and a possible vision for the future of these systems is presented.*

## INTRODUCTION

A conversational agent is a software system that is able to interact with users in a natural way, and often uses natural language capabilities. Many aspects have to be considered when defining the architecture of a conversational agent. At first, one has to design a natural interaction process able to trigger the user's interest.

DOI: 10.4018/978-1-60960-617-6.ch005

Many conversional agents are employed as artificial tutors to improve the user knowledge in a particular field. We focus our researches in the field of artificial tutors. A system acting as a tutor has to reproduce some of the dynamics used in the learning processes. The design and the development of an intelligent interface involve many advanced topics in human-computer interaction.

One of the major aspects we investigate is related to the definition of intelligent user interfaces able to adapt the presentation of contents and the flow of the conversation according to the particular task that has to be performed. To be more effective, a system should be able to interact with the user both in natural language and graphically. Moreover, it should be able to adapt itself to the context of the interaction and the user's needs. This adaptability is often limited to the front-end of the interface.

The task is probably hardier if a similar ability referred to the back-end of the interface is expected. A system able to either modify or update also the contents it manages is able to adapt what it says, and not only its actions. To this purpose we propose a methodology able to increase the knowledge of the system based on the interaction with users. The focus of our work is on a conversational agent acting as an intelligent tutoring system in a particular field of interests.

Intelligent tutoring systems (ITSs) can have learning agents embodied in an interactive system. They have to improve effectively the student's skills using different learning modalities to achieve major learning objectives such as knowledge acquisition, comprehension, application, analysis, synthesis, and evaluation. The effectiveness increases if the student has a good perception of the gaps she is bridging and a clear explanation of how the learning strategies are performed.

Another important aspect is related to the student's capabilities to mix the efforts useful to increase her knowledge. We refer to self regulated learning as a way to increase both students' skills and system knowledge in a push-pull process. According to (Pintrich, 2000) a self regulated learning is a process with tree main directions in the strategies' definition:

- Cognitive learning strategies
- Meta-cognitive and regulation strategies
- Resource management strategies

We are developing strategies in all the three mentioned fields to define a complex system able to reply to students' needs in a natural and intuitive way. In particular, in this work, we present Graphbot (Pirrone, Cannella, & Russo, 2008) and WikiArt (Pirrone et al., 2009) where the latter system is an improvement and extension of the first one. The design of Graphbot addressed the problems related to the natural language interaction, the graphical interaction, and the integration of these two distinct modalities. Graphbot has been adopted in a more complex system devoted to the specific domain of Arts, which is WikiArt. The design of this new version of the system has added to the focus aspects related to the automatic enrichment of the system's knowledge. Both of them have been developed as conversational agents.

Many conversational agents can be programmed in Artificial Intelligence Markup Language (AIML) an XML dialect used to define the procedural knowledge of the chatbots. This language can be used to describe atomic interactions, called *categories* and composed by a stimulus produced by the user (<pattern>) and a corresponding reply of the system (<template>). The <category> element can be referred to a specific context through the optional <that> element. In the simplest case, the chatbot replies directly with the content of the <template> element. In other cases, the reply of the system is obtained combining the content of many categories together. The <topic> element is used to group similar categories.

The chatbot replies with the corresponding template when the input of the user matches with one pattern of the categories. <that> elements can be used to distinguish between many different behaviors for a same input in different contexts.

A.L.I.C.E. (A.L.I.C.E., 2008) is the most famous chatbot programmable with AIML code. Our work started from this very basic system. It represents the core of Graphbot. All the innovations presented in this work have been developed as new modules of this system. AIML has been extended too. As explained in subsequent sections, both of them grew together. The result is very different from the starting point. The new system is able to merge linguistic and graphical interaction modes.

Moreover, the control of the conversation flow has been modified. WikiArt is able to plan the conversation on the basis of a probabilistic reasoning. It is a probabilistic agent. Other new modules add the ability to manage ontological knowledge, and to interact with WordNet. The AIML language has been extended with new terms referred to the graphical interaction modality, and to the interaction with all new developed modules. The name of the new version of the language is Graphical AIML (GAIML) (Pirrone, Cannella, & Russo, 2008).

WikiArt includes all the new functionalities we developed. It is a specialized wiki system able to supply an advanced service to users interested in Arts. It is not a simple wiki. It is an ontology-based information retrieval system, which is able to interact either in linguistic and graphical manner.

The development of WikiArt started up with collecting a huge corpus of documents treating subjects as artists, works of art, artistic movements, and so on. The documents contain data about more then 15000 artworks and more than 4000 artists, besides artistic movements, and specific techniques employed by artists. The documental corpus represents the information level of the system.

All these documents have been organized semantically, on the basis of a knowledge base about Arts managed by the system. Each document is related to one or more concepts in the ontology. This ontology represents the knowledge level of the system. Ontology browsing corresponds to documents browsing. This solution differs from the one adopted in a common semantic wiki, where the semantic relations involve documents directly, and are inserted in them.

The system is able not only to supply contents from a tag composition query, as in a common wiki. It can plan an entire browsing path on the basis of the relationships between the concepts in the ontology. Paths are built starting from a collection of exploration patterns.

Finally, the system has a huge database, storing all the main data regarding Arts (data about artists, artworks, etc...). This database represents the data level of the system. The schema of the database has been designed according to the specific characteristics of the domain. This approach is very different from normal wikis where documents and data are stored in a database with a standard schema.

The definition of ontology instances and concepts directly associated to a wiki page has leaded to the definition of the so-called Semantic Wikis (Volkel et al., 2006; Kawamoto, Kitamura, and Tijerino, 2006; Quan, Yuying, and Jing, 2008). In this way, wiki links and annotations are related to concepts, while pages are related with each other. The navigation of the ontology and the definition of rules allow obtaining more accurate matching and better retrieval of pages.

The subsequent sections of this chapter are organized as follows. The next section describes the state of the art of the many different research fields involved for the design of WikiArt. The third section offers a brief overview of the architecture of WikiArt, while sub-sections detail each component. The fourth section describes the modules of the system devoted to the natural language interaction. It is focused on two distinct and complementary aspects: understanding the users' sentences, and planning the conversation flow. The fifth section explains the graphical interaction with the system, and how it is combined with the linguistic one. The sixth section describes how the system manages, and enriches its own knowledge that is coded symbolically in the ontology. Finally, the last section presents conclusions and future works.

## STATE OF THE ART

### Intelligent Tutoring Systems

According to Bloom, learning activity in whatever domain has three main objectives (cognitive, affective, and psychomotor) that are subdivided in classes such as knowledge, comprehension, application, analysis, synthesis, and evaluation. An agent enabled with strong interaction capabilities designed to support learning, has a primary goal to improve effectively the student's skills with different modalities. Software systems able to improve the knowledge of a student in a particular field are known as Intelligent Tutoring Systems (ITSs).

The architecture of an ITS is arranged as a series of modules working in cooperation (Wolff et al., 1998; Rickel, 1989). The main modules are: the expert model, the student model, the instructional model, and the learning environment (Piramuthu, 2005). The student model defines the student's individual needs. The expert model is able to track student knowledge and to perform corrections and hints. The instructional model is used to present knowledge in a way oriented to student's skills acquisition. Many theoretical models have been proposed to build an ITS, while the most used ones are Model-Tracing Tutors (MTTs) (Gertner and VanLehn, 2000) and Constraint-Based Model Tutors (CBMTs) (Mitrovic, Martin, and Suraweera, 2006; Mayo, Mitrovic, and McKenzie, 2000; Gonzalez, Burguillo, and Llamas, 2007).

Besides the previous approaches, the literature reports the Bayesian one (Butz, Hua, and Maguire, 2006) while another important effort is towards the definition of cognitive architectures (Goh and Quek, 2007; Samsonovich et al., 2008). A cognitive architecture is software architecture willing to reply some of the mechanisms belonging to humans. It can be defined according to the modules and the functionalities used to achieve a particular goal.

The Human Information Processor Model (HIPM) is one of the main models developed to describe human cognitive processes. It has inspired the Model Human Processor (MHP). According to this model, a cognitive architecture is composed by a series of modules. Each module performs a specific function involved in the cognitive processes. Modules can belong to three main categories: perceptual module, cognitive module, and sensory motor module. The sensor/motor modules are the most basic set of modules able to interact with the environment. The information provided by sensors modules is filtered by the perceptual modules that are used to better understand the nature of the external stimuli. The cognitive modules are used to put together different perceptions in order to perform reasoning and memorization of complex information.

EPIC (Executive Process-Interactive Control) is a cognitive architecture inspired to MHP focusing both on the human cognition and on the performance (Kieras, Wood, and Meyer, 1997). The production-rule cognitive processor generates a proper action in response to a certain stimulus. The main perceptual processors are the visual and the auditory ones.

ACT-R (Anderson et al., 2004; Newell, 1994) is a hybrid system based on chunking. The ACT-R architecture consists of a module aimed to retrieve information from a declarative memory, a procedural memory, a goal stack to manage the current goal, and a visual module to identify objects. The declarative memory containing the chunks, and the procedural memory containing rules are symbolic structures. They are accessed by a neural activation mechanism. Access to declarative chunks is determined by an activation representing the probability the chunk has to be retrieved. In this way ACT-R is defined as a goal-oriented system.

## Interface Definition and Management

When dealing with highly interactive agents in support of the learning process, interface definition is a crucial topic. In the past, many formal interface description languages have been proposed. Some of them allow defining very sophisticated multimodal interfaces. Whereas complex interfaces were used for stand-alone applications, nowadays many of the most recent web applications provide as much functionality as the desktop ones.

Moreover, web applications show remote capability and platform/device independency. For these reasons, many interface description languages are used to define web interfaces. Most of them are markup languages. An example is XForms. It allows minimizing the use of scripts, adopting a declarative approach for the definition of data and event management. It can be embedded into code in other languages, and interpreted by the client.

Such languages have been used to program chatbots too. For example, The Multimodal Presentation Markup Language (MPML) is an XML dialect used to program the verbal and nonverbal behavior of a 2D character. It supports multimodal presentations, including graphics, music, and video, which are combined with natural language synthetic expositions. Facial displays, hand gestures, head movements, and body posture of the character can be controlled too. The group, which developed MPML, has defined also the Dynamic Web Markup Language that is used to build WIMP web interface. This language is no more supported.

Another possible approach to interface design is task-based. TRIDENT (Bodart et al., 1995) generates an interface from the activity flow of the task. The task is decomposed into a series of subtasks described through an *abstract interaction model* (AIO). An AIO can correspond to *concrete interaction objects* (CIO), which implement the interface components. XIML is a system able to generate a Java Swing interface through an XSLT transformation of data expressed in XML (Puerta and Eisenstein, 2001).

XML can be used to generate concrete interfaces implemented in a particular programming language, such as Java Swing, HTML, VoiceXML, and so on. In some cases, the generation is guided by the explicit knowledge of the system as in UIDE (Foley, Gibbs, & Kovacevic, 1988). Its knowledge base is arranged in taxonomies of frames and describes the interface components, the interface actions, the parameters, and the pre- and post- conditions of the tasks to be executed. The project MECANO (Puerta, 1996) developed a similar knowledge base useful to generate interfaces described in a specific formal language. Finally, the Extended Set description Language (ESDL) proposed by Ardizzone et al. (2004) allows to define interfaces that can be generated thorough first order logic rules, which are expressed in Prolog and are inspired to the Model-View-Control paradigm.

## Knowledge Base Development

Another crucial aspect in the development of an ITS is the definition of the knowledge base. The system must be targeted for a specific subject. The implementation of a new instance needs a huge effort in developing a new ontology of the domain and a new semantic space of document treating the new subject.

Moreover, these instances need to be frequently updated. This is a typical problem in ITS literature. In particular, new documents treating the subjects of the domain could be published, and need to be included into the semantic space. These limitations are due mainly to the systems inability to learn from experiences. The knowledge is static, and can change only thank the manual intervention of the developer. A common way to express the knowledge domain is related to the definition of an ontology.

An ontology typically provides a formal explicit representation of a domain of interest

*Figure 1. The architecture of the system: the memory module and the Chatbot engine with the main components*

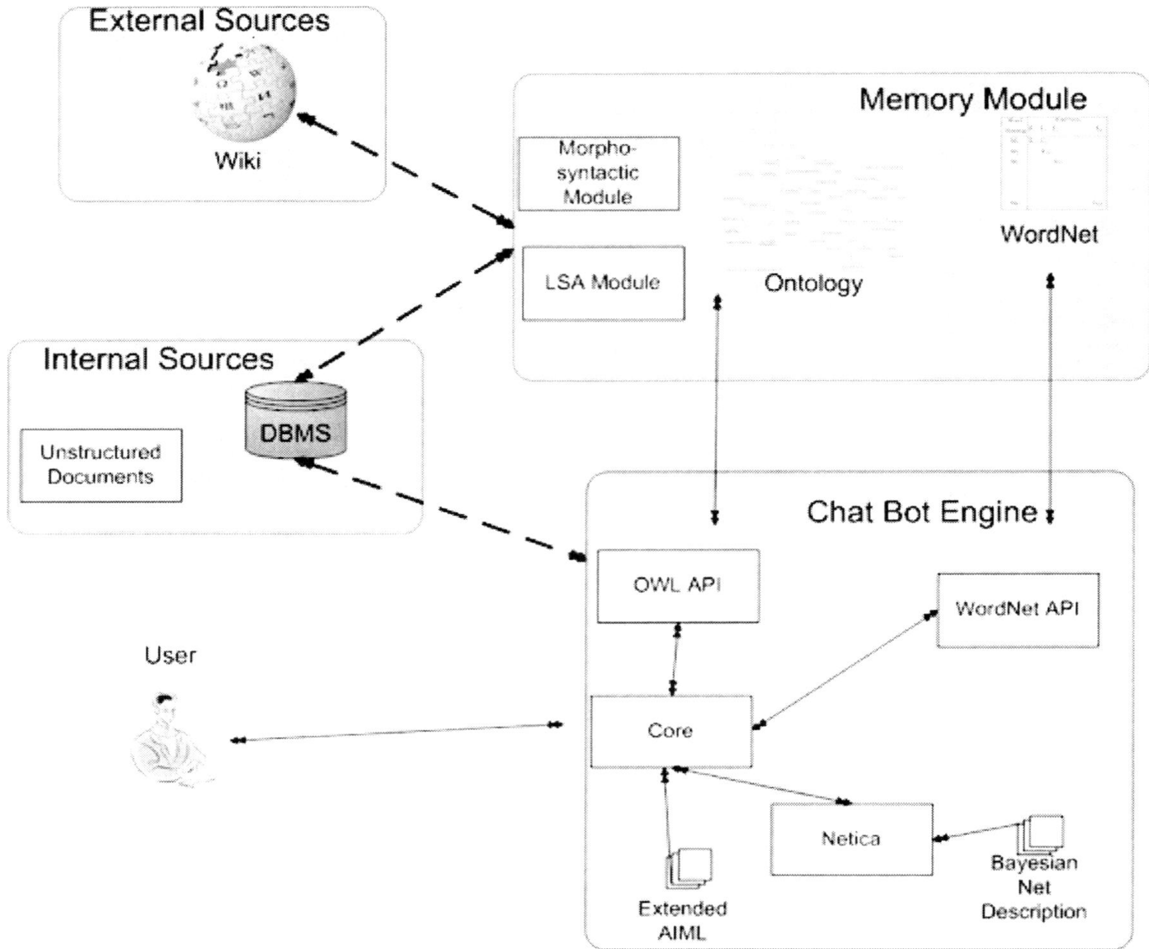


(a space of knowledge identified by a name), in terms of specification of relevant concepts of the domain and in terms of identification of the relations between them. Ontologies cover several data or conceptual models, like database schema, classifications, thesauri, and so on.

Each concept in the domain is modeled in a class of the ontology: a class has a set of properties describing various features and attribute of the concept, called slots or roles, and restrictions on slots (facets, sometimes called role restriction).

## ARCHITECTURE OF WIKIART

The architecture of WikiArt has been designed according to the HIPM paradigm, so WikiArt implements the Model Human Processor (MHP) (see Figure 1).

Memory modules in WikiArt manage both symbolic and sub-symbolic information. Symbolic information is managed in the ontology module where the domain is represented, the WordNet module that is used to disambiguate English terms, and in the procedural memory describing the behavior rules of the chatbot during the interaction. Rules are expressed in GAIML.

Sub-symbolic information is stored in the LSA module and in the morpho-syntactic one. The first one uses Latent Semantic Analysis (Landauer, Foltz, & Laham, 1998) to create a semantic space that is shared by documents and concepts in the ontology. Points close in that space represents elements with similar meanings. At the same manner, a sub-symbolic memory is represented by the semantic space produced through the morpho-syntactic analysis of documents. LSA and morpho-syntactic module are part of the linguistic module, which is devoted to the analysis of the user's sentences and to dialogue planning. As further explained, dialogue planning can be either deterministic or probabilistic.

All the listed memories are long-term memories. The short-term memory (or working memory), that records stimuli from the environment and executed actions, is embedded in the chatbot engine. Sensor-motor modules perform both natural language and graphical interaction with the environment. The chatbot engine is the core of the whole system. It coordinates other modules. It manages the interaction on the basis of the GAIML rules stored in the procedural memory. To this aim, it has to interact with the ontology module to control the flow of topics in the conversation, and with the linguistic one to understand the sentences in the conversation.

## The Linguistic Module

As previously explained, this module is in charge of managing natural language interaction as a whole. This implies performing many complex tasks together. For this reason, the module has been designed as built by different components and each is devoted to a specific aspect of the interaction.

The conversation involves many aspects and can be analyzed at different levels of granularity. At first, every single sentence in a conversation must be understood. On the other hand, the whole conversation has a main goal and needs to be planned in some way.

The problem of language understanding is very far from being fully solved. The proposed solution tries to combine hints from the analysis of different aspects of a sentence: lexicon, structure, and semantics. The WordNet and LSA modules carry out respectively lexicon analysis and extraction of rough semantics from the content of a phrase, while the morpho-syntactic module analyzes structure. All these data are used to compare a user's sentence with a huge collection of sentences describing the domain. The interpretation is guided by the result of lexical, semantic, and structural matching.

As regards conversation planning, one can notice that whole conversation is guided by a global goal but each dialogue move (i.e. an interaction step) has a specific goal. As a consequence, a two levels planning has been developed.

Next, two sub-sections explain in detail respectively the joint work of LSA and WordNet modules, and the structure analysis in the morpho-syntactic one. LSA-based techniques cannot understand what a sentence says, but there are information retrieval methods in order to assess the topic covered by a certain phrase. The LSA module works jointly with the WordNet module that is used to disambiguate the terms in a sentence.

All the components of the linguistic module interact with the chatbot engine using a collection of new AIML tags whose processors have been developed suitably to manage the whole linguistic interaction. All modifications maintain the compatibility with the original A.L.I.C.E. system.

## The LSA and WordNet Modules

The task of the LSA module is rough semantic analysis of the sentence of the user by means of Latent Semantic Analysis. This is a technique very used in natural language processing. In this framework, a textual document is transformed into a numerical vector from the frequency of its terms. The measure used in this analysis is TF-IDF (term frequency – inverse document frequency).

The gained vector space is called a "semantic space". Two vectors near in the space (according to the cosine distance) are related to documents whose topics are either similar in a semantic sense or highly correlated as regards the most frequent terms. LSA is a bag-of-word technique, i.e. it ignores the mutual positions of the words in a sentence. In this way, it is not able to fully understand the meaning of a sentence. It can be used to understand only the topic of a sentence. This module is very useful at the beginning of the conversation, when the system needs to understand what the user wants to speak about. Its usefulness is reduced as the dialogue goes on and LSA allows only tracing the evolution of the topic of the conversation. The LSA module is activated by a proper AIML tag.

As already said, language understanding suffers from many limitations as regards correct interpretation of sentences. One source of uncertainty is the ambiguity of terms in natural language. The chatbot has been extended with a new module for WordNet interaction to face this problem. A set of suitable tags allow the agent to make queries to the thesaurus, and to browse the relations between words, such as synonymy, hypernymy, and hyponymy. In this way, the chatbot can control the degree of specificity of lexicon used in the conversation.

For instance, synonymous or antonymous words can be used to enlarge the range of the conversation, including new topics not considered by the user. The new tags translate the WordNet API enriched with some formatting functions to put data returned by WordNet into the conversation.

## The Morpho-Syntactic Module

LSA technique suffers from many limitations. The main drawback is due to the nature of LSA as a bag-of-word approach for modeling documents. In a bag-of-word model the structure of sentences is not preserved and information about the context is lost. Moreover, the same word can be used with very different even conflicting meanings. As a consequence LSA technique has a very good performance when trying to discover the topics covered in a sentence. On the contrary, it is not useful to understand the actual meaning of a sentence.

As already stated, the space created using LSA is called a "semantic space". Lowe (2001) defines semantic space as a quadruple *{W, L, S, R}*. Here *W* is the set of basis elements that define the vocabulary. Many possible examples of *W* can be used: a set of uncorrelated words, a set of tagged words, or a set of words syntactically related in some order. *L* is the lexical function applied to the elements of *W*. The most used *L* function is the identity function that counts raw frequencies of the basis elements in the corpora. *S* is a similarity measure computing the similarity of two samples in the space. *R* is a transformation aimed to reduce the dimensionality of the space.

We extended the previous definition to cope with the problem of understanding a sentence. A new semantic space based on the tree representation of phrases has been defined. The new semantic space has been created by a new definition of *W*, *L*, and *S*. No attention has been devoted to *R*, preferring consolidated techniques, as Single Value Decomposition (SVD). The *W* set is the result of a multi-step process. At first, the system retrieves a documents corpus. Part of these documents is pre-loaded by the programmer, while the rest is downloaded from web sites such as Wikipedia.

Some pages in wiki resources contain useless information and have been discarded. This is the case of disambiguation pages, which contain links to the different meanings retrieved for the same term. In general, links are a very interesting source of information because they actually carry the relationships between two topics. For this reason, links are used during the conversation planning. On the contrary, disambiguation pages would connect terms that should not be related.

Documents are grouped according to their subject after retrieval to reduce the computational load. Each group is related to a single topic. When the dialogue is focused on a particular subject the system can discard all the documents grouped in other topics. Representative words for each topic are compiled manually. Next, documents are stemmed and they are transformed into words' TF-IDF vectors that are clustered by a Self-Organizing Map (SOM). A document may deal with multiple topics. As a consequence, clustering is refined inside each primary group and all the pages that are linked by a page belonging to a certain cluster are added to that cluster.

Content analysis is performed on the main text sections of the page. Parts like references, related pages, forms, and images are discarded. Selected sections are decomposed into sentences after being preprocessed using text chunking, abbreviations replacement, and tokenization. Sentences are grouped on the basis of their constituting words to reduce the computational load. Each phrase is associated to the set of relevant words. The database storing the sentences is arranged according to a multilevel phrase clustering. Level $n$ contains the clusters of phrases with exactly $n$ words. All the layers constitute the $W$ set.

The lexical function $L$ is built by representing sentences in a topological tree space. Each sentence is parsed by both the Stanford parser (Klein & Manning, 2003) and the FreeLing (Atserias et al., 2006) software. The corresponding parse tree with POS (Part-Of-Speech) and morpho-syntactic information is obtained and represented in XML using the Penn TreeBank notation (Marcus et al., 1994). Trees are stored in a eXist DB, a native XML database. Tree generation represents the $L$ function of the semantic space.

The similarity measure $S$ defines a metric distance between two sentences projected onto $W$. In particular, $S$ is a suitable topological distance between two parse trees. Trees are projected into a mathematical structure, defined in (Billera, Holmes, & Vogtmann, 2001). Each point of this space is related to a rooted semi-labeled tree with $n$ leaves and positive branch lengths on all interior edges. Many n-leaves trees are possible. Trees are grouped on the basis of their structures. Trees with similar structures can differ only for the lengths of their branches. Each tree corresponds to a vector belonging to a positive open orthant whose elements are the ordered lengths of its branches.

A degenerative tree can be defined, which has zero weighted edges. Such a tree belongs to all the sets of trees with similar structures except for that edge, so it belongs to more than one orthant. As a consequence, each orthant has a not null intersection with the other ones.

In case two trees share a common structure, they correspond to two points in a same orthant their distance can be defined as the Euclidean distance. On the contrary, two trees with different structures are projected into two points not belonging to the same orthant. If their respective orthants are intersecting, a path crossing their intersection points joins them. More complex paths can be traced through many orthants when two points do not belong to intersecting orthants. In both cases, the distance of the two points is the length of the path.

We adopted the distance described in (Owen and Provan, 2010). Each possible node of a parse tree is associated to a positive value. Each edge is weighted using the value of the child node. Values do not reflect a real meaning. They only allow distinguishing nodes in the tree. Moreover, this distance computation reflects all the structure differences between two trees. For these reason, the systems lists all the matches above some specified threshold for a given input sentence and performs further point-to-point comparisons to find the best matching. The global distance between an input sentence and the corresponding best match is measured as the weighted sum of the LSA and the tree distance, to take into account both semantics and structure.

## PLANNING THE CONVERSATION

As previously mentioned, the flow of the conversation is guided by a series of temporary goals for single conversational acts, while a global goal guides the whole conversation. Local goals are due to the motivation of a particular conversational act. A speaker makes a question because s/he needs to know its reply, or s/he affirms something to communicate it. As a matter of fact, the whole conversation has its own motivations. This mechanism allows facing the problem of conversation management as a hierarchical planning problem.

### Short-Time Planning

In the original AIML, the programmer can specify the reply of the system to each possible input. Obviously, the choices of the programmer are due to her intentions. S/he wants the system to provide a certain reply to reach a specific goal. Any way, the goal is not explicitly stated in the code. The new version of the language (i.e. GAIML) allows defining an action's goal explicitly. In this way, it is possible to join all the different reactions of the system to the same input according to their goals.

GAIML provides the <type> and <goal> tags to this purpose. Both of them are used inside categories. The latter assigns a goal to an AIML category. Similar inputs can match the same pattern with different templates. The <goal> tag allows distinguishing between such templates and classifying different replies to the same stimulus on the basis of the different goals the chatbot tries to reach in different contexts. Actions of the chatbot can be grouped on the basis of their goal. Moreover, goals can be organized logically into hierarchies. This is a very simple way to model pragmatics inside the chatbot. While the chatbot is a general framework, many possible models for pragmatics can be proposed.

The <type> tag is more general than the <goal> one even if they behave similarly. Types have been defined to fit the programmer's specific needs. Many categories can share a common pattern and they can be distinguished on the basis of their type. This is the case when the agent has to exhibit different interaction modes, or when the programmer wants to characterize its mood.

It should be noted that these two tags do not modify the agent model of the chatbot. It remains a simple reflex agent, which reacts to external stimuli in a pre-programmed manner. Goals and types add new parameters to make the control of the chatbot behavior more flexible. Such tags define only local goals and the way to reach them by a single dialogue move. The whole conversation is planned using a global probabilistic technique.

### A Probabilistic Approach to Conversation Planning

The basic behavior of the chatbot as described so far is strictly deterministic. The agent's reaction to the environmental stimuli is fixed by the rules defined in the categories. We assume the system has exact perceptions and its reactions are predefined. As a matter of fact, natural language interaction is prone to many possible mistakes. Natural language understanding techniques are not able to gain always complete and sure results. As an example LSA techniques suffers from the bag of words limitations: the words in a phrase are not discriminated according the role (subject, verb, adjective,...). The conversation planning process can be affected by the deterministic behavior of the system too. Ideally, an action is chosen by the system because it should affect the user in a certain way. Obviously, the effect is not guaranteed.

To face all these problems, a probabilistic approach has been followed and the chatbot has been extended with two new probabilistic modules. Each module can be used to program the chatbot as a probabilistic agent.

The first module implements Bayesian reasoning with a tool called Netica. A set of new tags in the language have been defined for the interaction with this new module. These tags allow programming the chatbot as a Bayesian system. The choice of the reaction to a specific stimulus is made using probabilistic reasoning, while the chatbot only executes actions. At the beginning, the chatbot loads the Bayesian network by the <loadBN> tag. The network can be used to estimate the state of the environment.

When the chatbot perceives a stimulus from the world, it asserts or denies a fact using the <enterState> and <enterStateNot>) tag respectively. The <getBelief> tag is used to evaluate the probability of some event on the basis of the asserted facts. Finally, the net can be reset and deleted using the <retractFindings> and <delBN> tag respectively.

The net can be used to plan the actions too. The <getExpectedUtils> tag returns the rewards of all possible actions and the <getBestDecision> tag returns the best action. The second probabilistic module has been focused mainly on the problem of planning the entire conversation. It implements a Partially Observable Markov Decision Process (POMDP) (Porta et al., 2006).

A POMDP is defined as a tuple $\{S, A, O, T, R, Z\}$ where:

- $S$ represents a finite set of states
- $A$ represents a finite set of actions
- represents a set of observations
- $T$: $S \times A \times S \rightarrow \Pi(S)$ is the state transition function where $T(s' \mid s, a)$ is the conditional probability of passing state $s'$ when the action $a$ has been executed in the state $s$
- $R$: $S \times A \rightarrow \mathbf{R}$ is the reward function and $R(s, a)$ is the expected reward for taking an action $a$ when the agent is in the state s
- Z: $O \times S \times A \rightarrow \Pi(S)$ is the observing function and $Z(o \mid s, a)$ is the conditional probability function of observing $o$ when the agent is in the state $s$ after performing the action $a$.

The POMDP has been used because it models all the working conditions of the agent. The chatbot has no direct access to the state of the world, so the environmental conditions are estimated as a set of probabilistic evaluations from a set of perceptions. The system can only select the action it presumes to be the best one on the basis of this indirect analysis. Moreover, it has to cope with the uncertain effects of its actions. A long list of new AIML tags has been developed to manage the POMDP when planning the interaction with the user step by step.

## GRAPHICAL INTERACTION

The original ALICE interface is rather poor. It is a simple WIMP (Window, Icon, Menu, Pointing device) interface with a reduced number of widgets like a text field where the user and the system can write their sentences, and a button. On the contrary, recent chatbots own more sophisticated interfaces such as avatars acting in virtual worlds.

Chatbots interact with user in a pretty linguistic fashion using text and/or speech. This can result in too long annoying statements in case the conversation is focused on a complex domain were structured data have to be accessed by the user. Here WIMP GUIs can help the interaction to be quick with no misunderstandings. We designed a new model were pure linguistic interaction is mixed with dynamic instances of GUI widgets depending on the context devised in the conversation.

To reach this aim, we have enriched AIML with tags containing information about GUI building. We called the new language GAIML, that is, Graphical AIML. Interface generation code is implemented using both XHTML and JavaScript. Interface patterns are described through XML schemata to be transformed into GUI instances. Finally, GAIML allows writing rules to generate interfaces for data not matching any known pattern. In both cases, the interface generation is guided by data structures managed throughout the conversation.

We extended the original ALICE chatbot to merge natural language and graphical interaction modes by GAIML programming. The new agent is called Graphbot and it is able to provide the user with a graphical reply using a GUI. Three different cases have been defined. Interfaces can be either defined explicitly or they are generated automatically starting from predefined patterns or they result from a composition process.

The interface generation is based on the data model, described through the "interaction step patterns" (ISPs). An ISP describes a data structure and it is joined to the corresponding "interface pattern" (IP) an interface template implemented in XHTML and JavaScript. An XSLT transformation maps ISPs to IPs.

GraphBot is able to generate new IPs for unknown ISPs. To this aim, it compares the input ISP to known ISPs, and creates a new IP as composition of the known IPs corresponding to the most similar ISPs. ISPs (and IPs) are structured as trees, and a comparison between two ISPs (or two IPs) corresponds to measure the distance between their corresponding trees.

We adopted the tree edit distance, which gives a similarity degree for two trees and supplies the sequence of changes (insertions, deletions, and renaming of nodes) allowing to transform the first tree into the second one. When combining two IPs, a rename operation consists of changing a graphical element with another one inside a pattern. The delete operation removes a component from the interface, while the insert operation adds a component.

New IP generation for unknown ISP is governed by a set of rules, which are applied to already known patterns on the basis of a priority level. The main rules are stated in the following:

- Maximum pattern covering: such rules try to cover the major portion of unknown pattern.
- Minimum composition weight: the patterns to be changed are expressed in a way that the composition weight (described with a proper cost function) tends to be minimum.
- Preference for insert and delete operations: preferred operations on the IPs are insertion and deletion.

A side effect of using rules is that the application contexts can also be inherited. This is an important feature because the context definition provides the constraints on the interface usage and on involved data types. The programmer can define new rules to bind a pattern to another one.

## DOMAIN REPRESENTATION AND KNOWLEDGE ACQUISITION

In our framework, we use the Web Ontology Language (OWL) (Euzenat & Shvaiko, 2007) to represent knowledge. OWL is a World Wide Web Consortium (W3C) standard language, which is aimed to write ontological statements. It has been developed as the follow-on to RDF and RDF Schema (RDFS). OWL is meant to be a language for the World Wide Web and all its elements (classes, properties and individuals) are defined as RDF resources, and are identified by URIs.

Using OWL, one can represent a domain in a way suited for applications that need to process the information content instead of just presenting information to humans. OWL has three increasingly-expressive sublanguages: OWL Lite, OWL DL, and OWL Full.

OWL usually defines the kinds of entities in a domain by specifics constructs. In particular, the classes of the domain are introduced in OWL by the OWL:Class notation, while the individuals are defined by the OWL:Thing construct.

Relations between classes are introduced in OWL by the OWL:ObjectProperty construct. A knowledge domain may have some parts whose values are not individuals, while having a specific type like string, integer number and so on. This is the case of a concept's attributes, which define its features. These parts of the domain could be defined using relations: in the case of the attributes, a class is linked with the values of its attributes. These relations are called "data type relations" whose OWL definition is the OWL:DatatypeProperty construct.

In OWL a new concept can be created as the intersection of two distinct classes, by OWL:intersectionOf. Similarly, a concept could be defined as the union of two distinct classes, using OWL:unionOf. Moreover, an OWL concept can be simply a restriction of a relation. For example, the class Author can be interpreted as the set of individuals that have created at least one artwork, like in the following example:

```
<OWL:Restriction>
<OWL:onProperty rdf:resource="hasCrea
tedArtWork"/>
<OWL:minCardinality rdf:datatyp
e="&xsd:nonNegativeInteger">1</
OWL:minCardinality>
</OWL:Restriction>
```

A knowledge base can own different types of relations: i.e. the instantiation links a class with its instances. It is expressed in OWL by rdf:type. The specialization defines the inclusion relation between two concepts or two properties, and it is defined in OWL by rdfs:subClassOf for concepts and rdfs:subPropertyOf for properties.

Conversely, if two classes or two properties have nothing in common, they could be declared to be mutually exclusive, and an exclusion relation links them. In OWL, the construct for this kind of relation is OWL:disjointWith.

## The Wikiart Ontology

The Wikiart ontology has been modeled from the Arts domain, which includes concepts and relations aimed to describe artists, their artworks, their biographies, and their cultural relations as being exponents of the same artistic movement.

The domain addressed by WikiArt is also represented in a database, as it is a wiki system. We modified the standard wiki entity-relation diagram (ERD) to address specific issues of the Arts domain. As a consequence, modeling the WikiArt ontology requires the WikiArt database must to be mapped in OWL ontology, following a suitable procedure. OWL representation overcomes plain ERD because it integrates the organization of the domain with semantics aspects, allowing reasoning engines to expand the information contained in the knowledge base, and to integrate existent data with new knowledge retrieved from Web sources.

The rules to transform an ERD diagram into OWL ontology are defined by Fahad (2008). Each entity in the ERD is mapped into a class of the ontology (for example, the table *Person* in the database is the class Person in the ontology). Entities can have simple, composite, and multi-valued attributes that can be defined as primary keys too.

A different OWL Mapping has been devised for each attribute type: simple attributes are mapped in OWL:DatatypeProperty elements (for example, the attribute "age" of a *Person* entity is an integer OWL:DatatypeProperty for the class Person). Composite attributes are mapped in elements, which reflect the nesting of the composite attributes. For example, the attribute "address" of a *Person* entity is composed by different sub-attributes, including for example "city" and "nation": this attribute is mapped into a OWL:DatatypeProperty including other similar elements to code each sub-attribute.

Multi-valued attribute can be defined using multi-valued OWL:DatatypeProperty elements, which has different types (i.e. the union of integer or string values); a primary key attribute is simply a functional OWL:DatatypeProperty that can have only a unique value.

Relations between entities are mapped into OWL ontology by an object property linking the classes used to map entities. Cardinality can also be defined for the relations, using restrictions. Mapping rules have been implemented by a proper XML DTD. A concept is related to a set of tables; each table has a set of attributes, which define the

*Figure 2. A fragment of the WikiArt ontology*

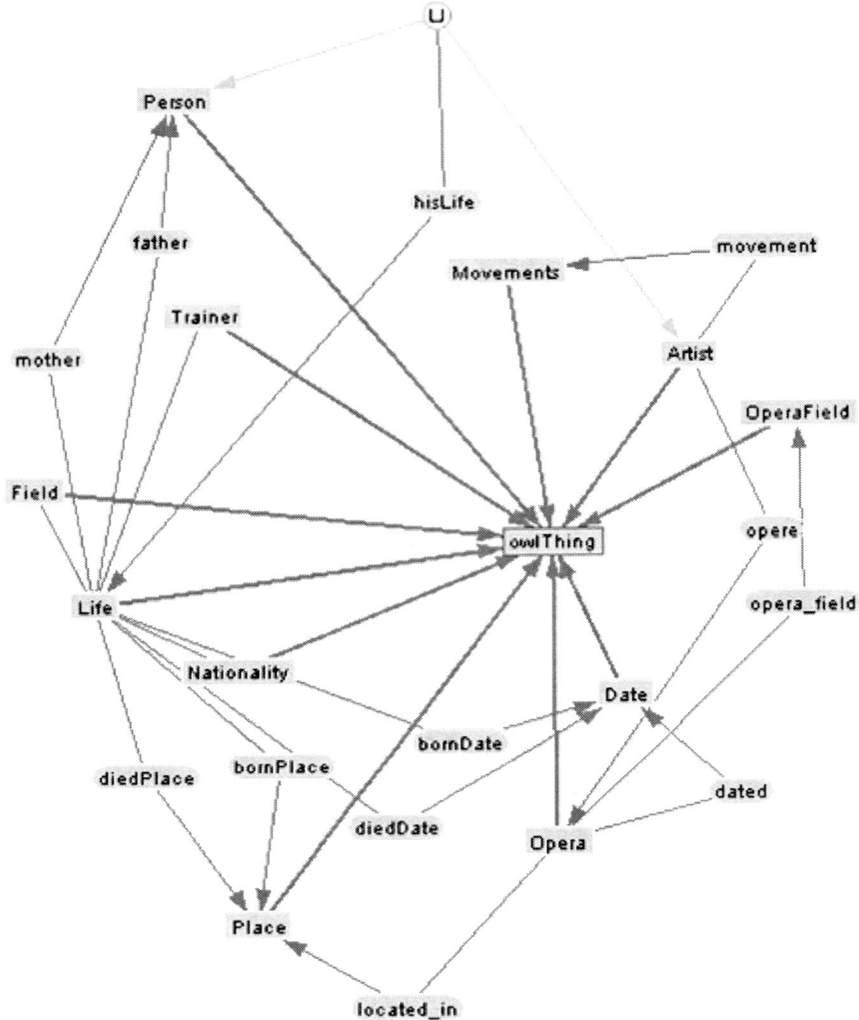


features of the entity represented in the table, the values for attributes and how they have to be used (attributes can be related with the OR, AND, and NOT logical connectives).

The level of granularity that can be reached is very precise. Furthermore, the definition of the instances on the database is obtained simply querying the tables that are mapped to the concept. For a more accurate definition of the methodology the reader is referred to a previous work of some authors (Russo et al. 2009).

The OntoWikiArt.OWL ontology is compliant to the OWL-DL profile. The next figure shows a fragment of the WikiArt ontology.

## Acquisition of New Knowledge from External Sources

WikiArt can have three types of users: authors, administrators and visitors/students. Authors contribute to the growth of the system's knowledge by inserting new topics or integrating existent arguments, and they have to be authenticated before writing. Contributions are allowed in many languages: Italian, English, German, French, Spanish, Chinese, Portuguese, Russian, Arabian, and Albanian.

Administrators have all privileges: they can admit new authors. Finally, visitors/students consult the wiki to learn about a topic with no need of authentication or registration. In this case, it may happen that an argument is not present in the knowledge base, or it is incomplete and does not satisfy the needs of the user. Acquisition of new information to expand the knowledge base is an important aspect of the system: to this aim, it is necessary to retrieve new data (texts, video or images about the topic of interest) from external information sources like the Web. New contents must be structured according to the ontological formalism based on OWL representation to merge it into the knowledge base. Ontology matching integrates the process of acquisition of new information. This topic will be cleared in the next paragraph.

Information sources may be structured or un-structured. Structured sources organize the information in semantic way, using a tagging system to provide data with semantics. As an example, words in a textual sentence are instances of generic concepts and could be tagged with the name of the class. In the sentence "Rome hosted the 1960 Olympic Games", the word "Rome" could be tagged with <city> because "Rome" is an instance of the concept "City". Accordingly, "1960" could be tagged with <date>.

In the same way, a portion of image or video could be tagged with the name of generic concept it represents or with the name of the subject (i.e. the individual) shown in the shot or in the image. An example of structured source is the semantic wiki (Semantic MediaWiki). This is a kind of wiki whose words in the text of the pages are tagged according to several possible dictionaries. It is possible to extract contents from structured sources using reasoning engines that know the semantic organization of the information, and arrange them in the OWL formalism. However, these kinds of sources have some limits. They require the set of tags to be shared by the users community and each tagger (automatic or not) has to refer to it. Expert systems used to extract knowledge should be based on these tags: no standard tags dictionary has been defined until now.

Most information sources are unstructured, and the retrieval of data requires direct extraction of semantics from contents. The most popular unstructured source is Wikipedia, that since 2001 is the "free encyclopedia that anyone can edit" and has over 10 millions of articles written in many languages. Wikipedia has a high degree of reliability as it is demonstrated by a study performed by (Giles, 2005) and its accuracy is comparable to Britannica. It organizes its contents in categories, which represent all possible arguments. Our approach to semantic sense extraction from Wikipedia pages is based on the page's table of contents. The table specifics the sections of the page, and it is possible represented it by a tree, where the category of the page is the root and sections are nested in the tree like nodes.

It is possible to infer the semantic sense of each section and sub-section by matching the tree of the table with a domain ontology corresponding to the category of the page. Once the topic of each section has been devised, it is possible to define the most frequent natural language sentences referring to it. We model in advance several statement patterns regarding different topics in the knowledge base, then pattern matching is applied throughout the section to retrieve the linguistic structures related to its topic.

In the case of a biography, sentences like "born in", "he is from" are often used to refer where and when the subject of the biography is born. When we find these sentences in the text of the section Biography of an artist like Michelangelo, we can know where and when the artist is born, and we can instantiate these new pieces of information in the knowledge base of the system. New inferred contents are stored in the database; the procedure is used to annotate unstructured contents in the web using inferred semantic sense.

## Application Example

An application example is presented to better show the implications of the proposed methodology. The key idea is related to keep track of the interaction process between students and the system in order to add new and previously unknown concepts to the knowledge base. The two main drivers are related to a self-regulated model of the student able to intercept his/her needs. The procedure is executed iteratively until the student feedback becomes positive so the focus of conversation is moved to another concept.

The macro-steps of the procedure are the following:

1. User requests are inferred from the dialogue performed through the chatbot interface.
2. On-line services are used to retrieve knowledge about a topic with low Feeling of Knowing (FOK). The FOK is a measure of the degree of accuracy for recognizing or knowing a task or answer.
3. New knowledge is mapped into the domain ontology.
4. Results are shown to the user.

Here follows the main parameters involved in the process:

- $D$: the domain ontology (represented as an OWL file).
- $N$: the number of concepts in $D$ (number of classes).
- $f$: the first level concept of $D$ (a direct subclass of OWL:Thing that is the ontology root).
- $x$: a generic concept.
- $O$: a generic object property
- $G$: a sub-graph of $D$.
- $S$: the service that exports a document page of a semantic wiki in OWL-DL format.
- $D_{xy}$: the distance between concept x and y measured according to a similarity measure.
- $T$: the threshold for similarity measure. $x$ and $y$ are assumed to be similar if $D_{xy} < T$.
- $V_c$: the selected concepts vector whose components are interesting concepts selected indirectly by the user.
- $M$: the dimension of $V_c$.
- $V_u$: the URL vector, its components are the ontology URLs of the wiki documents exported by $S$.
- $M_d$: the $N{\times}M$ distance matrix that is used when concepts belonging to $V_c$ have to be retrieved in $D$. $M_d(i,j) = D_{ij}$: $i \in D$, $j \in V_c$.

The chatbot module manages the dialogue with the student, and copes also with uncertainty in the conversation as already explained. It is able to assess the user, and to put in $V_c$ interesting concepts that are extracted from his/her most relevant sentences. Each component of this vector corresponds to a candidate document. Then the procedure calls $S$ and evaluates the existence, in an external wiki, of a document that is related to each component $c$ in $V_c$. If the document exists, an ad-hoc service function of $S$ is used to retrieve new documents in OWL format to extend $D$. If the documents do not exist in the wiki, $D$ cannot be extended and information must be retrieved in $D$ about the topic. This is obtained through the computation of the similarity distance $D_{xy}$ between whatever concepts $x$ and $c$.

## CONCLUSION

The chapter presented a conversational agent able to interact with user in a mixed way. The most important aspect is the definition of a cognitive architecture to develop the agent's behaviors based on the Self Regulated Learning Theory and the acquisition of new knowledge from external sources as the results of a continuous push-pull with users. The main components of the architecture have been presented. The system has to deal with many real problems according to the definition of a new generation of conversational agents able to interact with user in a very intuitive way.

One of the major issues in the presented agent is that the conversation has not to be necessarily guided on the basis of some predefined topics, but it has to address the self-regulated behaviours of the student. To solve this problem, we have enlarged the flow control model of the chatbot that is able to treat the relations between topics in the knowledge domain and the behavioural type of actions that the agent has to implement. The major challenges in the proposed approach are related to model the self-regulated processes for the users as a key to enhance a better comprehension of the user's knowledge state.

Finally, another important challenge is related to the definition of the system's behaviours according to the lack of information in a particular field. During the interaction, deficiencies can be discovered not only in the student, but in the system too. The student could make questions about topics that the system does not know. A particular module of the system is devoted to enriching automatically the knowledge of the system. New knowledge can be added through a process made up by the following steps: finding new information sources, retrieving information, interpreting retrieved information, and storing it into a repository.

## FUTURE RESEARCH DIRECTIONS

An Intelligent Tutoring System has to be able to support a student during a training session, supplying learning material customized to her needs, skills, and goals. To reach this goal, many different approaches focusing on different aspects of the learning process have been adopted. Recently, a growing interest has been devoted to adopt cognitive and meta-cognitive strategies in guiding the interaction with the system, and the learning process. The goal of these strategies is the promotion of comprehension and retention of new knowledge by the user. Such a goal can be attained by stimulating self-regulation in students while they are learning.

Resorting self-regulation needs the ability to understand the cognitive state of the student. On the other hand, self-regulation has to be developed in the student, improving his/her self-evaluation and self-management. Self-evaluation can be exercised engaging the student into an interaction intended to assess the level of training of the student. This interaction can get the student to focus on his/her knowledge about a specific topic. The interaction has been designed to contextualize each topic in a wider domain. In this way, the student can place the topic in his/her own interior conceptual map.

At the same time, the student's assessment allows to plan a learning strategy that is suitable to the student's knowledge state, referring to his/her previous knowledge, and taking advantage of it.

## REFERENCES

A.L.I.C.E. (2008). *A.L.I.C.E. homepage*. Retrieved from http://alice.sunlitsurf.com/alice/about.html

Anderson, J. R., Bothell, D., Byrne, M., Douglass, S., Lebiere, C., & Qin, Y. (2004). Integrated theory of the mind. *Psychological Review*, *111*, 1036–1060. doi:10.1037/0033-295X.111.4.1036

Ardizzone, E., Cannella, V., Peri, D., & Pirrone, R. (2004). *Automatic generation of user interfaces using the set description language*. In the 12th International Conference in Central Europe on Computer Graphics, Visualization and Computer Vision (pp. 209-212). UNION Agency - Science Press.

Atserias, J., Casas, B., Comelles, E., González, M., & Padru., M. (2006). *Freeling 1.3: Syntactic and semantic services in an open-source NLP library*. In the 5th International Conference on Language Resources and Evaluation (LREC 2006), ELRA.

Billera, L. J., Holmes, S. P., & Vogtmann, K. (2001). Geometry of the space of phylogenetic trees. *Advances in Applied Mathematics*, *27*(4), 733–767. doi:10.1006/aama.2001.0759

Bodart, F., Hennebert, A., Leheureux, J., Provot, I., Sacre, B., & Vanderdonckt, V. J. (1995). Towards a systematic building of software architecture: The trident methodological guide. In *Interactive systems: Design, specification and verification* (pp. 77–94). Springer.

Butz, C. J., Hua, S., & Maguire, R. B. (2006). A Web-based Bayesian intelligent tutoring system for computer programming. *Web Intelligent and Agent Systems*, *4*(1), 77–97.

Euzenat, J., & Shvaiko, P. (2007). *Ontology matching*. Berlin, Germany: Springer Verlag.

Fahad, M. (2008). ER2OWL: Generating OWL ontology from ER diagram. [Springer.]. *Intelligent Information Processing*, *288*(4), 28–37.

Foley, J., Gibbs, C., & Kovacevic, S. (1988). A knOWLedge based user interface management system. In CHI '88: *Proceedings of the SIGCHI conference on Human factors in computing systems*, (pp. 67–72). New York, NY: ACM.

Gertner, A., & VanLehn, K. (2000). Andes: A coached problem solving environment for physics. [Springer.]. *Lecture Notes in Computer Science*, *1839*, 133–142. doi:10.1007/3-540-45108-0_17

Giles, J. (2005). Internet encyclopaedias go head to head. *Nature*, *438*, 900–901. doi:10.1038/438900a

Goh, G. M., & Quek, C. (2007). EpiList: An intelligent tutoring system shell for implicit development of generic cognitive skills that support bottom-up KnOWLedge construction. *IEEE Transactions on Systems, Man, and Cybernetics*, *37*(1), 58–71. doi:10.1109/TSMCA.2006.886340

González, C., Burguillo, J. C., & Llamas, M. (2007). *Integrating intelligent tutoring systems and health Information Systems*. In 18th International Workshop on Database and Expert Systems Applications, (pp. 633–637), IEEE CS.

Kawamoto, K., Kitamura, Y., & Tijerino, Y. (2006). *Kawawiki: A semantic wiki based on RDF templates*. In Web Intelligence and Intelligent Agent Technology Workshops, (pp. 425–432). WI-IAT.

Kieras, D. E., Wood, S. D., & Meyer, D. E. (1997). Predictive engineering models based on the epic architecture for a multimodal high-performance human-computer interaction task. *ACM Transactions on Computer-Human Interaction*, *4*(3), 230–275. doi:10.1145/264645.264658

Klein, D., & Manning, C. D. (2003). Fast exact inference with a factored model for natural language parsing. *Advances in Neural Information Processing Systems*, *15*, 3–10.

Landauer, T., Foltz, P., & Laham, D. (1998). An introduction to latent semantic analysis. *Discourse Processes*, *25*, 259–284. doi:10.1080/01638539809545028

Lowe, W. (2001). *Toward a theory of semantic space*. In the 22nd Annual Conference of the Cognitive Science Society, 1, (pp. 675–680).

Marcus, M., Kim, G., Marcinkiewicz, M. A., Macintyre, R., Bies, A., Ferguson, M., et al. Schasberger, B. (1994). *The Penn treebank: Annotating predicate argument structure*. In ARPA Human Language Technology Workshop, Morgan Kaufmann.

Mayo, M., Mitrovic, A., & McKenzie, J. (2000). *APIT: An intelligent tutoring system for capitalization and punctuation.* International Workshop on Advanced Learning Technologies, (pp. 151–154).

Mitrovic, A., Martin, B., & Suraweera, P. (2006). Intelligent tutors for all: The constraint-based approach. *IEEE Intelligent Systems*, *22*(4), 38–45. doi:10.1109/MIS.2007.74

Newell, A. (1994). *Unified theories of cognition.* Cambridge, MA: Harvard University Press.

Owen, M., & Provan, J. S. (2010). *A fast algorithm for computing geodesic distances in tree space. IEEE/ACM Transactions on Computational Biology and Bioinformatics*. PrePrints.

OWL. (2004). *W3C Semantic Web, Web Ontology Language (OWL).* Retrieved from http://www.w3.org/2004/OWL/

Pintrich, P. R. (2000). The role of goal orientation in self regulated learning. In Boekaerts, M., Pintrich, P. R., & Zeinder, M. (Eds.), *Handbook of self-regulation* (pp. 451–502). San Diego, CA: Academic Press. doi:10.1016/B978-012109890-2/50043-3

Piramuthu, S. (2005). Knowledge-based Web-enabled agents and intelligent tutoring systems. *IEEE Transactions on Education*, *48*(4), 750–757. doi:10.1109/TE.2005.854574

Pirrone, R., Cannella, V., Gambino, O., Pipitone, A., & Russo, G. (2009). *Wikiart: An ontology-based information retrieval system for arts.* Intelligent Systems Design and Applications Conference,(pp. 913–918).

Pirrone, R., Cannella, V., & Russo, G. (2008). *GAIML: A new language for verbal and graphical interaction in Chatbots.* In Complex, Intelligent and Software Intensive Systems Conference, (pp. 715–720).

Porta, J. M., Vlassis, N., Spaan, M. T. J., & Poupart, P. (2006). Point-based value iteration for continuous POMDPS. *Journal of Machine Learning Research*, *7*, 2329–2367.

Puerta, A. (1996). The Mecano project: Comprehensive and integrated support for model-based interface development. In *Computer-aided design of user interfaces* (pp. 5–7). Namur University Press.

Puerta, A., & Eisenstein, A. (2001). XIML: A common representation for interaction data. In *Proceedings Intelligent User Interfaces Conference*, (pp. 214–215). ACM.

Quan, L., Yu-ying, J., & Jing, C. (2008). Uimwiki: An enhanced semantic wiki for user information management. In *IT in medicine and education*, (pp. 930–934). IEEE.

Rickel, J. W. (1989). Intelligent computer-aided instruction: A survey organized around system components. *IEEE Transactions on Systems, Man, and Cybernetics*, *19*(1), 40–57. doi:10.1109/21.24530

Russo, G., Gentile, A., Pirrone, R., & Cannella, V. (2009). *XML-based knOWLedge discovery for the linguistic atlas of Sicily (ALS) project.* In Complex, Intelligent and Software Intensive Systems, International Conference, (pp. 98–104).

Samsonovich, A. V., Kitsantas, K. D. J., Peters, E. E., Dabbagh, N., & Kalbfleisch, M. (2008). Cognitive constructor: An intelligent tutoring system based on a biologically inspired cognitive architecture (BICA). Artificial General Intelligence 2008: Proceedings of the First AGI Conference. *Frontiers in Artificial Intelligence and Applications, 171*(1), 311–325.

Semantic Media. (n.d.). *Wiki*. Retrieved from http://semanticweb.org/wiki/SemanticMediaWiki

Volkel, M., Krotzsch, M., Vrandecic, D., Haller, H., & Studer, R. (2006). Semantic Wikipedia. In *WWW '06: Proceedings of the 15th International conference on World Wide Web*, (pp. 585–594). New York, NY: ACM.

Wolff, A. S., Bloom, C. P., Shahidi, A., Shahidi, K., & Rehder, R. E. (1998). Using quasi-experimentation to gather design information for intelligent tutoring systems. In *Facilitating the development and use of interactive learning environments*, (pp. 21-51).

## ADDITIONAL READING

Banko, M., M. J. Cafarella, S. Soderland, M. Broadhead & O. Etzioni. (2007). Open information extraction from the Web, *IJCAI*, 2670-2676.

Chakrabarti, S. (2003). *Mining the web*. Morgan. Kaufmann Publishers.

Copestake, A., Flickinger, D., Sag, I., & Pollard, C. (2005). Minimal Recursion Semantics: an introduction. *Journal of Research on Language and Computation*, *3*(2-3), 281–332. doi:10.1007/s11168-006-6327-9

Fellbaum, C. (Ed.). (1998). *WordNet: An Electronic Lexical Database*. Cambridge, Massachusetts: The MIT Press.

Nakayama, K., Hara, T., & Nishio, S. (2008): *Wikipedia Link Structure and Text Mining for Semantic Relation Extraction, Towards a Huge Scale Global Web Ontology*. SemSearch 2008, CEUR Workshop.

Ponzetto, S.P. & Strube, M. (2007). Deriving a large scale taxonomy from Wikipedia. *AAAI*, 1440-1445.

Suchanek, F. M., Kasneci, G., & Weikum, G. (2007). YAGO: A core of semantic knowledge. *WWW*, 697-706.

Völkel, M., Krötzsch, M., & Vrandecic, D. (2005). *Wikipedia and the Semantic Web – the missing link.* 1st Int Wikimedia Conf, Wikimania.

Wu, F., & Weld, D. (2008). *Automatically Refining the Wikipedia Infobox Ontology.* WWW 2008/ Refereed Track: Semantic/Data Web - Semantic Web 3.

## KEY TERMS AND DEFINITIONS

**Chatbot (or Chatterbot):** Is a computer program able to have a conversation in an intelligent manner with one or more users.

**Latent Semantic Analysis (LSA):** Technique in natural language processing, used to analyze relationship between a set of documents and the terms they contain by producing a set of concepts related to the documents and terms. It starts from the term-document matrix, describing the occurrences of terms in documents. LSA finds a low-rank approximation of this matrix, with the aims of identifying synonymies between terms, similarity in contents between documents, and relations between terms and documents.

**Ontology Mapping:** Alignment of two different ontologies by pairing defined concepts.

**Ontology:** Formal representation for a knowledge domain by defining relevant terms (concepts), their properties and relations between them.

**Orthant:** In geometry, an orthant is the analogue in n-dimensional Euclidean space of a quadrant in the plane or an octant in three dimensions. In general, an orthant in n-dimensions can be considered the intersection on n mutually orthogonal half-spaces.

**OWL:** Language for authoring ontologies endorsed by W3C (World Wide Web Consortium).

**Partially Observable Markov Decision Process (POMDP):** A generalization of a Markov Decision Process. A POMDP is a model of a decision process. The system is assumed to be determined by an MDP, but the state can not be observed directly by the agent. For this reason, it must maintain a probability distribution over the possible states, based on observations and corresponding observation probabilities, and the underlying MDP.

**Part-of-Speech (POS) Tagging:** POS tagging is the process of marking up the words (or fragment texts) in a documental corpora as corresponding to a specific part of speech. The process can be based on the definition of the part of speech, or on the context. Once performed by hand, POS tagging is now done automatically through means developed in the computational linguistics field, on the basis of algorithms.

**Semantic Space:** A quadruple W{*W, L, S, R*}. *W* is the set of basis elements that define the vocabulary. *L* is the lexical function applied to the elements of *W*. The most used *L* function is the identity function that counts raw frequencies of the basis elements in the corpora. *S* (0..1) is a similarity measure computing the similarity of two samples in the space. *R* is a transformation to reduce the dimensionality of the obtained space.

# Chapter 6
# Building a Social Conversational Pedagogical Agent:
## Design Challenges and Methodological approaches

**Agneta Gulz**
*Linkoping University, Sweden & Lund University, Sweden*

**Magnus Haake**
*Lund University, Sweden*

**Annika Silvervarg**
*Linkoping University, Sweden*

**Björn Sjödén**
*Lund University, Sweden*

**George Veletsianos**
*University of Texas at Austin, USA*

## ABSTRACT

*This chapter discusses design challenges encountered when developing a conversational pedagogical agent. By tracing the historical roots of pedagogical agents in Intelligent Tutoring Systems (ITS), we discern central developments in creating an agent that is both knowledgeable and fosters a social relationship with the learner. Main challenges faced when attempting to develop a pedagogical agent of this kind relate to: i) learners' expectations on the agent's knowledge and social profile, ii) dealing with learners' engagement in off-task conversation and iii) managing potential abuse of the agent. We discuss these challenges and possible ways to address them, with reference to an ongoing Research & Development project, and with a focus on the design of a pedagogical agent's visual embodiment and its conversational capabilities.*

DOI: 10.4018/978-1-60960-617-6.ch006

# 1. INTRODUCTION

## 1.1 Conversational Pedagogical Agents

In this chapter a "pedagogical agent" refers to a computer-generated character employed in an educational setting in order to fulfill pedagogical purposes. Such agents (or characters) can serve numerous pedagogical roles (Chou, Chan, & Lin, 2003; Baylor & Kim, 2005; Haake & Gulz, 2009). For instance, they have been presented and studied as instructors, coaches, tutors, and learning companions.

The concept of an "agent" denotes an entity with some degree of "intelligence" and capacity for autonomous action. Agents, or intelligent agents as used within the computer science discipline, refer to a *computer programs* that can "act" on their own (i.e. autonomously). When referring to "pedagogical agents" in today's educational contexts, it is also assumed that the agent has a corresponding *visual representation*. *Conversational* pedagogical agents refer to a subgroup of pedagogical agents, namely those that can engage in a conversation with a learner, through dialogue, and, often through elaborate body language movements including gestures, facial expressions, etc.

In this chapter, we focus on conversation via natural language, and limit our treatment to text-based interaction (typed conversation via the keyboard). Thus, we do not discuss the challenges and potentials surrounding speech recognition and production. We also exclude complex non-verbal interaction (often explored in Embodied Conversational Agents research (e.g., Cassell, Sullivan, Prevost, & Churchill, 2000; Ruttkay & Pelachaud, 2004), where the agent's body is used for demonstrating, showing, pointing, and for giving feedback via gestural and emotional expressions. We discuss *animated pedagogical agents* where the visual animations are less complex, mainly aimed at making the agent appear more life-like and appealing.

## 1.2 Chapter Outline

We begin our discussion by tracing the historical roots of pedagogical agents in the *Intelligent Tutoring Systems* (ITS) paradigm, and discussing two central lines of development that have transformed agents from the nonsocial and impersonal characters of the past to the tangible, social and personal pedagogical agents of today: i) development of their visualization and embodiment and ii) development of their conversational capacities. These developments, we argue, carry with them important potential, as well as challenges, for research and development within the field.

In section 3, we present an ongoing Research & Development (R&D) project within the pedagogical agent domain – a web-based game focusing on mathematics learning for children – which serves to illustrate and contextualize our discussion.

In Section 4, we present the guiding framework that we use for designing and researching the project: *the Enhancing Agent-Learner Interaction framework* (*EnALI*) (Veletsianos, Miller, & Doering, 2009).

In section 5, we discuss central challenges that we hold as being common in pedagogical agent design and development endeavors:

1. how to deal with students' (often heightened) expectations regarding pedagogical agents' knowledge and social competencies (including the problem of setting proper constraints),
2. how to deal with students' varying degree of engagement in social interaction with the pedagogical agent, and
3. how to deal with the risk of verbal abuse known to arise when students interact with conversationally-capable pedagogical agents.

We illustrate these challenges and possible ways to address them, with reference to our ongoing project and with reference to the EnALI framework. The list of challenges above is of course not exhaustive or applicable to *all* pedagogical conversational agent projects. Still, we consider them as representative of main issues that are likely to occur when developing pedagogical conversational agents. Numerous design decisions and challenges are involved in the design of agent-based educational software such as the one we will discuss. A complete list of all these design decisions would hardly be useful for readers. What *is* useful however, is the example of how one can reason about dealing with the complexity of decisions within design frameworks and still make progress towards a small number of well-defined, educational goals.

Our hope is that our discussion will inspire and benefit researchers and designers within the field who face similar issues. Our overall goal is to demonstrate how the field of conversational pedagogical agents represents a unique combination of theory and research intertwined with practice.

## 2. BACKGROUND

### 2.1. Intelligent Tutoring Systems

The development of pedagogical agents within digital learning environments finds its historical origins in *Intelligent Tutoring Systems* (ITS), which can be traced back to the early 1970's (Laurillard, 1993; Wenger, 1987). A crucial step towards the development of ITS is often credited to a landmark paper by Carbonell (1970) where the concept of (human) *intelligence* was ascribed to an artificial system assisting a learner in an educational context. This system, called *SCHOLAR*, tutored students on South American geography by posing or answering questions via natural language in text format (*ibid.*).

An intelligent tutoring system exhibits certain characteristics and skills recognized in a *human tutor* such as being able to survey a student's learning progress and provide feedback to relevant actions, including contextual advice and support for problem solving within the learning environment (Laurillard, 1993). Furthermore, as frequently held forth through its history, an ITS allows for *individualization*: it adapts to individual students though various actions, such as offering help on request or recognizing the kinds of mistakes that a learner frequently makes in order to provide personalized feedback (*ibid.*). Individualization in this sense is, however, strictly performance-based and not aimed at establishing a social relationship with the student. *Personal interaction* is absent, and therefore, students do not develop personal relationships with virtual tutors. The *classic* ITS is an impersonal, non-social and abstract pedagogical agent whose sole purpose is to tutor.

In the 1990's this scene changed radically. A new generation of pedagogical agents entered the arena. This development can be ascribed to significant technological developments within two domains: the *visual embodiment area* and the *dialogue systems area*. These agents have been characterized as personal and relational artifacts. Next, we will describe how visual embodiment and dialogue systems have developed and what these developments mean for today's pedagogical agents.

### 2.2. From ITS to Present-Day Pedagogical Agents

#### 2.2.1. Visualization and Embodiment

Imaging and video techniques progressed rapidly during the late 1980's and the early 1990's. Present day pedagogical agents are – in contrast to classical tutoring systems – *visually embodied*, and often animated. They have a face and often a body or torso and are usually humanlike in their appearance.

This makes a modern pedagogical agent more tangible and less abstract than a classical ITS, which in turn increases the likelihood of learners approaching agents as *social entities* and as *personas* (Lester et al., 1997). The visual dimension of pedagogical agents is a powerful means for engendering affordances for social interaction, since it contributes strongly to the experience of a *character with a personality* (Isbister, 2006; Gulz & Haake, 2006) rather than simply a computer artifact. Such effects have recently come in the forefront of the pedagogical agent field. For instance, researchers have investigated the extent to which learners stereotype pedagogical agents and the degree to which such behavior impacts learning (Veletsianos, 2010).

The visual dimension is also a powerful tool for exploiting pedagogically central phenomena such as social models and identification. A social model, or role model, can influence attitudes and motivation as well as learner behaviors (Schunk, 1981; Bandura, 1986). A large set of studies show that pedagogical agents can function as (virtual) social models and similarly influence attitudes, motivation and learner behavior (Baylor, Rosenberg-Kima, & Plant, 2006; Kim, Wei Xu, Ko, & Llieva, 2007; Baylor, 2009; Gulz & Haake, 2010).

A particularly effective social model is either (a) one that is similar to the observer in significant aspects – so that the observer can identify herself with the model – or (b) one representing someone whom the observer aspires to be like. One key factor in this discussion is the visual appearance of the social model (Bandura, 1986), since appearance carries important and immediate information regarding an individual's gender, age, status, ethnicity, style, etc. This applies to human beings as well as to anthropomorphic agents. Another visual factor that matters for the potential effectiveness of a social model is visual attractiveness. For a discussion of this, we refer to Baylor (2009) and Gulz & Haake (2010).

In other words, the visual design of a pedagogical agent is far from a cosmetic or surface aspect (Veletsianos, 2007). The choice of visual design of an agent can have considerable pedagogical consequences as a result of its potential function as a social model. A well-chosen visual design can positively impact learners' attitudes towards and interests in a subject (Baylor et al., 2006; Kim et. al, 2007; Plant, Baylor, Doerr & Rosenberg-Kima, 2009; Gulz & Haake, 2010).

It can also significantly impact learners' *self-efficacy beliefs*. These are beliefs in ones' capacity to accomplish certain tasks in a certain domain, which in turn are a predictor for actual success (Bandura, 2000). A number of studies within the domains of mathematics and technology, show the importance of the visual design of a pedagogical agent (most notably in terms of gender, ethnicity, age, and "coolness") for positively influencing learners' self-efficacy beliefs (Baylor, 2009; Kim, Baylor, & Shen, 2007; Baylor & Plant, 2005).

Overall there is growing evidence that the visual design of virtual characters effects actual accomplishments within a subject domain (Yee & Bailenson, 2007; Yee, Bailenson, & Duchenaut, 2009). For a recent overview of the importance of visual design in pedagogical agents see Baylor (2009). In her review Baylor underlines that the *presence of a visual character* in a computational system as well as the character's *specific visual appearance* are two critical features for the design of an effective pedagogical agent – regardless of its underlying level of computational functionality.

Pedagogical agent visual design is not without challenges however: lack of analysis of visual design decisions can lead to pitfalls such as activating misleading expectations (Haake & Gulz, 2008) and unintentionally reproducing social stereotypes (Baylor, 2005).

### 2.2.2. Developing Conversational Capacities

The first well-known conversational agent is *ELIZA*, which simulated a Rogerian psychotherapist (Weizenbaum, 1966). ELIZA is an example of what is today usually referred to as chatbot, a system with the goal to appear humanlike and engage in social conversation regarding a wide range of issues within an unrestricted domain. Many attempts to build conversational agents followed but the area subsided in the beginning of the 1980s due to the complexity of natural language processing, the problem of representing world knowledge, and the lack of research on connected dialogue and discourse.

The late 1980's and 1990's saw breakthroughs in these areas (cf. Grosz & Sidner, 1986; Smith, 1992; Jönsson, 1997), which in turn led to development of new kinds of dialogue systems which were more task-oriented and dealt with restricted domains, such as *Galaxy* (Goddeau et al., 1994; Seneff et al., 1998) *RailTel* (Bennacef et al., 1996) *TRAINS* (Allen et al., 1995) and *Verbmobil* (Alexandersson, Maier & Reithinger, 1994). These systems were considerably more powerful in the way they could efficiently and smoothly assist a person in solving a task. Furthermore, these systems (a) relied on reasoning mechanisms dealing with knowledge of the domain, the task, the user and the dialogue (Flycht-Eriksson, 2003), and (b) often used complex strategies for dialogue management to achieve fluid interactions and mixed initiative between user and system.

A special type of these task-oriented dialogue systems are tutoring/tutorial dialogue systems that combine the pedagogical functions of intelligent tutoring systems with natural language conversations. In this type of system, natural language conversation is used mainly for a tutor to ask questions, ask a student to elaborate on his/her examples, elaborate on answers, provide further information, summarize answers, correct misconceptions, or provide hints and directions. For examples of research in this area see Graesser, Wiemer-Hastings, Wiemer-Hastings, Kreuz & the Tutoring Research Group (1999), Graesser, Chipman, Haynes & Olney (2005), and VanLehn et al. (2007).

More recently, there has been a revival of *chatbots* developed for various purposes and deployed on the Internet, most frequently developed using the AIML architecture (http://www.alicebot.org/aiml.html). A common use is their deployment as information-providing agents on websites, but these have also been used in education, automatic telephone help desks, business and e-commerce.

Chatbot systems usually have shallow or no understanding of the dialogue, but work by processing the surface text using keyword spotting, pattern matching and information retrieval techniques. They also have no knowledge representations about the world, but can "talk" about a multitude of topics in a dialogue that usually consists of question and answer turns. Connected discourse is limited and the initiative usually belongs either to the user or to the system. However, with improved methods for data mining and machine learning, and the availability of corpora and robust linguistic annotations standards like XML, development and application of chatbot systems are becoming more practical (Shawar & Atwell, 2007).

In between chatbots and task-oriented dialogue systems, a new system category emerged, termed Virtual humans (Traum, Swartout, Gratch, & Marsella, 2008). The main differences between these three systems are presented in Figure 1.

Virtual Humans are agents that *have a goal of both being humanlike and being able to complete tasks in an efficient manner.* From a pedagogical perspective, this development introduces unique new potentials and challenges. Connected and mixed-initiative dialogue, along with the possibility to keep track of a dialogue history, enables educators to develop learning scenarios that capitalize on humanlike interaction (e.g. by enabling learners to discuss issues of historical significance with historical agents). They also offer possibilities to combine elements from task-oriented dialogues in restricted domains with elements from broader, but shallower, dialogues of the kind used in chatbots. At the same time, the knowledge representations and processing of the dialogue can be less extensive and simpler than in traditional task-oriented dialogues.

A central point to make here is that *Virtual Humans* offer enhanced possibilities for simulating human conversation due to the possibility of shift-

*Figure 1. Characteristics in chatbots, virtual humans, and task-oriented dialogue systems*

| | Chatbots | Virtual Humans | Task Oriented |
|---|---|---|---|
| **Domain** | unrestricted | somewhat restricted | restricted |
| **Goal** | be human-like | be human-like and complete task | complete task efficiently |
| **Understanding** | shallow or no understanding of progression of dialogue needed | shallow understanding of dialogue progression needed | deep understanding of dialogue progression needed |
| **Operating level** | surface text | surface text or dialogue-act | dialogue-act |
| **Method** | keyword-spotting, pattern matching, corpus based retrieval | information-state based or corpus based retrieval | information-state based, form based |

ing between task- and domain-oriented conversations, on the one hand, and a broader and more socially oriented conversation, on the other hand. An important implication of this combination of task- and domain-oriented conversation with social conversation is that it opens up the possibility for a student and a pedagogical agent to engage in what Bickmore (2003) calls "relation-oriented conversation". To some extent this development parallels the development of visual embodiment of pedagogical agents. Both these developments amplify the affordances of a pedagogical agent as someone to have a *personal relationship with.*

## 2.3. Intentional Relation Building

The basis for relation building between student and agent presumably lies in the media equation, formulated by Reeves & Nass (1996) who discovered that humans tend to respond to media, including computer artifacts, in manners that are surprisingly similar to how humans respond to other humans. With present-day development of pedagogical conversational agents – visually embodied in a humanlike shape and entertaining a humanlike conversation – the human disposition to respond socially to media is *intentionally* exploited as, in education "the establishing of personal relationships is absolutely crucial" (Bickmore, 2002, p. 1) Pedagogical conversational agents also enable individuals to introduce crucial elements of social context and personal relations, regarded as primary conditions for cognitive and social development (John-Steiner & Mahn, 2003), into a digital learning environment (Baylor & Kim, 2005; Gulz, 2005; Hall et al., 2004; Johnson, Kole, Shaw, & Pain, 2003; Paiva et al., 2004, Wang et al., 2008).

It is within this context that we introduce an ongoing R&D project in the next section. The project focuses on the design and development of an educational math game that includes a pedagogical agent. The agent shares similarities to a traditional ITS, in that it is abstract (minimally embodied) and strictly domain- and task-oriented in its interactions with the learners. The project sets out to develop a present day pedagogical conversational agent, by means of *visual embodiment* and *conversational capacities*. The goal is to enable effective interaction and purposeful learning, within the context of an agent architecture that fosters agent-learner relationships.

# 3. THE ILLUSTRATIVE R&D PROJECT

## 3.1. The Original Game: An Educational Math Game with a Teachable Agent

The math game on which the present R&D project is based, has been developed by Pareto and Schwartz (Pareto, 2004; Pareto, Schwartz, & Svensson, 2009). The educational content of the game is basic arithmetic with a particular focus on base-10 concepts. The math game contains several different 2-player board games that intertwine game play with learning content.

The *pedagogical agent* in the game is a *Teachable Agent* (TA) (Biswas, Katzlberger, Brandford, Schwartz, & TAG-V, 2001). This is a class of pedagogical agents that build upon the pedagogy of *learning by teaching* (Bargh & Schul, 1980) – a pedagogy that has proven to be beneficial for learning in an educational game context (Chase, Chin, Oppezzo, & Schwartz, 2009).

In this game students teach their agents to play the math games, and depending on the quality of the student's teaching, the TA constructs a mathematical model by means of artificial intelligence (AI) algorithms. Thereafter, the TA's mathematical knowledge is continuously reflected in its skill to play the different board games. The game includes two modes. In the first mode, the student demonstrates to the agent how to play the game, and in the second mode "tries to play" by proposing cards that the student can either affirm or replace with another card. In both modes, the agent poses multiple-choice questions to the student that relate to game happenings. Proper (or improper) answers impact corresponding skills in the teachable agent via the AI algorithms. We will refer to the multiple-choice questions module as "on-task conversation," acknowledging that this is a limited and rudimentary form of "conversation,"

As seen in Figure 2 (where two agents play against each other in the "Try and play" mode), the original game includes a very basic visual embodiment of the agent in the form of a simple iconic static image.

The present R&D project involves development of visual embodiment and capacities for conversation (Figure 3). Note that the two areas being added to the original agent of the game are those that were presented in Sections 2.2. and 2.3. With these developments we strengthen the agent's affordances as "a persona" and "a social entity". It should be noted, however, that the media equation (Reeves & Nass, 1996) predicts that the agent in the original game will be approached as a social entity, even though it does not allow any sophisticated interaction and is visually rudimentary.

According to the media equation, minimal social cues from a computer artifact, such as a pair of eyes, a face, linguistic output of some kind, leads users to spontaneously respond and make attributions to the artifact *as if* the artifact is a social entity. For example, students who played the original game made the following remarks about the teachable agents, indicating that they applied human attributes to them (Lindström, Haake, Sjödén & Gulz, in press).

- "What is she doing? Is she *nuts*?!"
- "My agent is pretty smart, but he is not in the lead now"
- "The most important thing is not the outcome, the most important thing is that the agents are having fun!"

## 3.2. Visual Embodiment of the Teachable Agent and a Novel Conversational Module

In the system under development, the original agent image (to the left in Figure 4) has been replaced, via iterative development and testing, with more elaborated visual figures. A first set can be seen to the right in Figure 4, and a second iteration of some of them in Figure 5. Figure 6 provides

*Figure 2. On-task conversation in the original game. See David's agent in the upper left.*

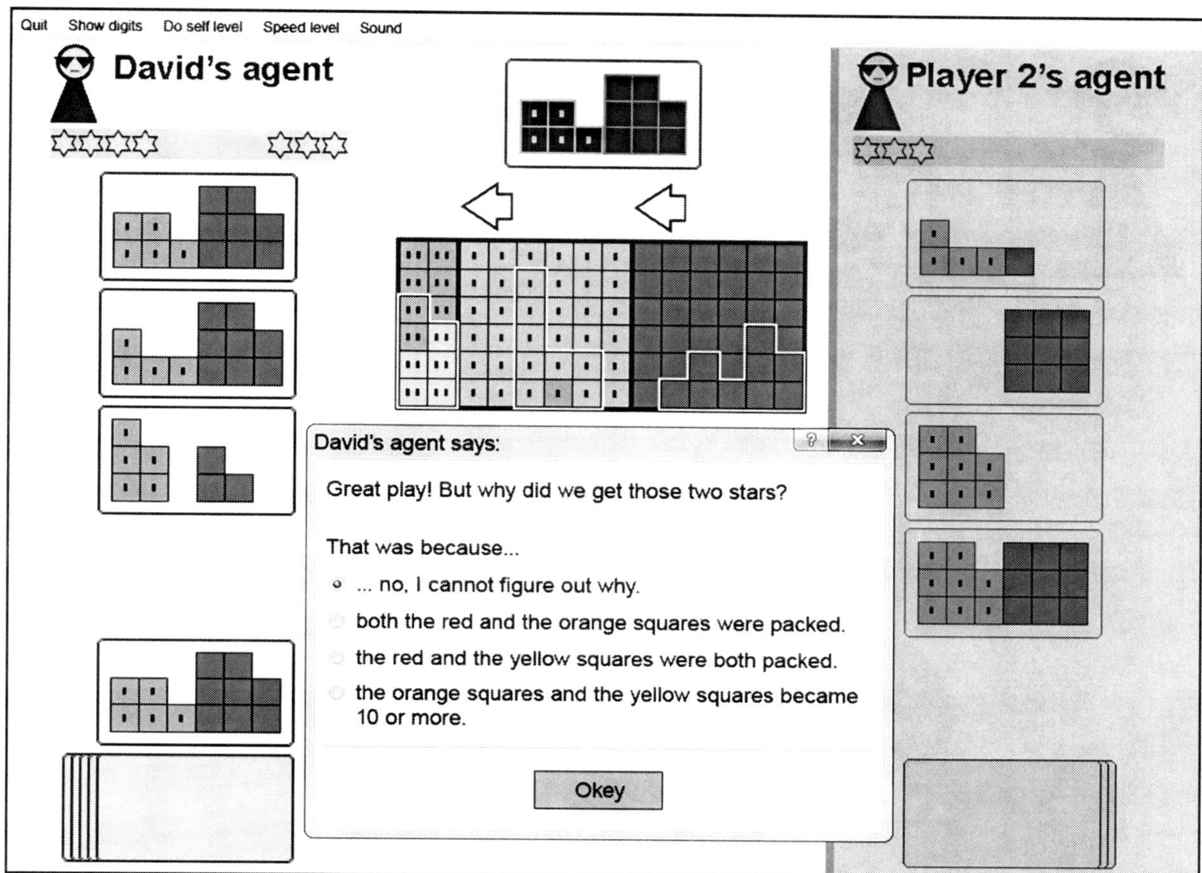


*Figure 3. Enhancements to the original math game: visual embodiment and conversational capacity*

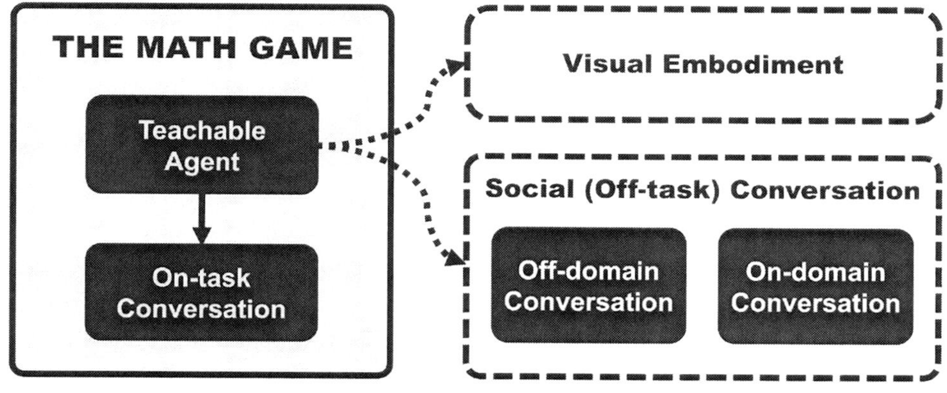

*Figure 4. The embodiment of the pedagogical agent in the original math game to the left with some of the novel visual characters to the right*

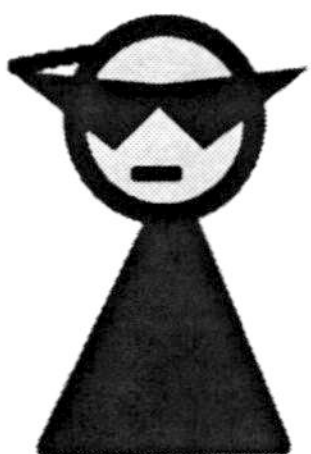
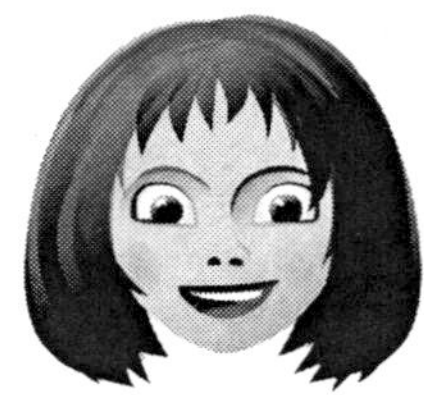
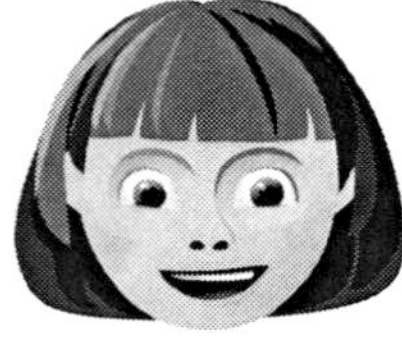
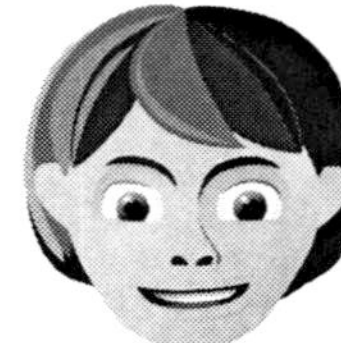
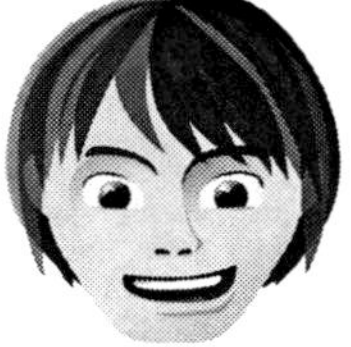

*Figure 5. Second iteration of agents for the math game*

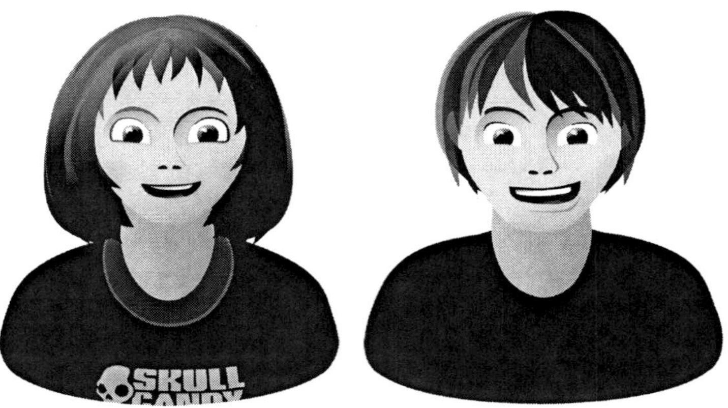


a view of an agent when a student is playing the math game against the computer.

Thorough user testing with the target group in question is essential in these iterative processes, given the importance of visual features for establishing affinity and for role-modeling and identification as described in section 2.2.1.

Note that we explicitly avoid a naturalist or even semi-naturalist style for the pedagogical agent representation. The main reason is that we want to downplay expectations that students may have relating to the agent behaving and conversing *just like* a human being: a conflict between the abilities of an agent and the learners' perception of these abilities, has been shown to cause frustration in a learner.

Dowling (2000), with reference to Masterton (1998), claims that many users "express a higher tolerance of the limitations of a 'character' that is represented in less detail, for instance through cartoon-like graphics." (*ibid.*, p. 30). Likewise, Dehn and van Mulken (2000) review studies that indicate that agents with a more naturalistic visual appearance can indeed hamper learning by misleading the learner to believe that the agent resembles human beings in other cognitive and emotional aspects as well. They may, for instance, expect empathy from the agent or expect conversational capacities, that the agent does not live up to, leading to disappointment and frustration (Veletsianos, Scharber, & Doering, 2008).

The second main development – the focus of this chapter – consists of a module that allows the student to engage in free-form conversation with the agent between game sessions (vis a-vis a conversation that is steered by multiple-choice options, see Figure 3).

*Figure 6. Novel embodiment of the agent in its game context. Note: The word "Dator" under the upper right icon is Swedish for "Computer".*

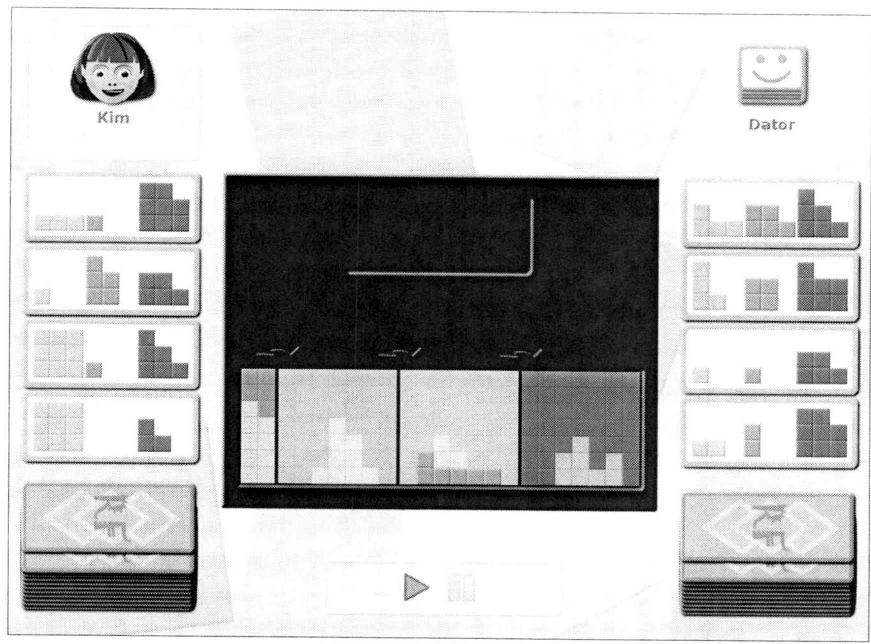


Whereas we refer to the multiple-choice format conversation while playing a particular board game as *on-task* conversation – we refer to the module for freer conversation with the agent in the form of a chat window as *off-task* conversation. In turn, we distinguish two off-task conversation categories with respect to the topic or content[1].

- *Off-task/on-domain* conversation is free conversation relating to the math game, mathematics in general, and school. Conversations that focus on how fun or boring certain board games were or about whether one thinks mathematics is difficult or not, would classify as off-task/on-domain conversation.
- *Off-task/off-domain* conversation can be about any topic other than the ones above. For instance conversations about music, being tired, sports, and food are classified as off-task/off-domain conversations.

The underlying dialogue architecture for a pedagogical agent that will handle such off-task conversation, together with topics that relate to the specific math games being played, has to be a combination of a chatbot-like system and a task-oriented ITS-like system (compare Figure 1).

In our system we are implementing the agent's ability to engage in off-task conversation as a mixed-initiative dialogue strategy in order to allow both the agent and the user to direct the dialogue (e.g. by introducing new topics and posing questions). The agent keeps a history of the utterances in the dialogue, both in the current and previous sessions. This gives us a possible tool for obtaining a balance between on-domain and off-domain topics in the off-task conversation. For instance, the pedagogical agent may attempt to bring the learner back to the task by (re)introducing particular topics of conversation: if the student has persisted in discussing music, the agent can ask about school-related music lessons with the aim to guide the subject back to school-related topics.

Next, we expand on the underlying *reasons* for introducing off-task conversation in a pedagogical agent system by discussing potential pedagogical benefits. We start by looking at human-to-human teaching and the combination of on-task and off-task conversation in that context.

## 3.4. Potential Educational Benefits of Off-Task Conversation

In traditional teaching situations such as lessons, lectures, tutorials, etc., there is always a mixture of *on-task* conversation that strictly pertains to the subject content and tasks of the lesson, and some *off-task* conversation. Instructors regularly digress from the content they are teaching: they may bring up a matter of general interest, comment on their own personal relation to the subject of the lesson, share a joke, and so on. In fact, it is unusual to find a teacher who is completely focused and does not at all deviate from the task and topic of a lesson.

A number of pedagogical motives exist for including opportunities for off-task conversations in a digital learning environment.

Off-task conversations may encourage emotional engagement and create additional possibilities for remembering content. This is supported by findings that brain processes of memory coding and storage are stimulated by emotional engagement (Hamann, 2001). Nevertheless, this is not to say that all off-task interactions are equally engaging. For instance, "small talk" can promote trust and rapport-building, and at the same time bring in task-related information (Bickmore & Cassell, 1999; Bickmore & Cassell, 2000). An example from a real classroom would be a chemistry teacher who engages her students in discussion about school and relates an anecdote about the time she caused a fire during a laboratory lesson as a student. Kumar, Gweon, Joshi, Cui & Rosé (2007) conducted an experiment along this line of thought with a dialogue agent within the mathematics domain, where the agent accompanied student pairs in collaborative learning via a chat. The agents came in two versions: one with cognitive support agents only, and one with both cognitive support agents and social dialogue agents. The latter were designed to show personal interest in the students by asking them to reveal their personal preferences about extra-curricular domains. The student preferences were then used as input when the math problems were constructed. If one student answered that she would prefer a long car ride to a long flight, and the other student in the pair responded that books are more amusing than movies, the math activities presented to these students would include a car ride and books. The intention was that the social dialogue should give students the impression that the agent takes personal interest in them. Results showed that the addition of the social dialogue agents had a strong positive effect on the attitude that students displayed towards agents as well as a slight positive effect at learning outcomes. The authors argued that "social prompts are not just extraneous entertainment, but can affect student's attitudes and behavior."

Off-task conversation can make a learner feel more comfortable, relaxed and at ease with a learning task or topic. It can even help to release mental blockages that beset some students with regard to certain educational material, for example mathematics or technical subjects (van Mulken, André, & Müller, 1998). Math anxiety for instance, is a feeling of tension, apprehension, or fear that interferes with math performance and is a well-documented phenomenon (Hembree, 1990). The potential exists to use an agent's off-task conversation to encourage a more relaxed atmosphere when learning mathematics. An agent can also act as role model for ways to cope with difficulties (cf. Schunk, Hanson & Cox, 1987).

Finally, it has often been suggested that off-task conversation of a social and relational kind, can result in increased motivation or engagement with the task and domain in question. For instance, Ryu & Baylor (2005) hold forth "the '*Engaging* factor' or 'the *positive social presence* of the agent' as it is 'there' for the learners and motivating them" (p. 26). In turn, such motivating effects – gained from the social dimensions of interacting with a pedagogical agent – may affect learning outcomes in terms of improved understanding, memory, problem solving, etc. (e.g. Lester *et al.*, 2000; Moundridou & Virvou, 2002; Johnson *et al.*, 2003). According to André and Rist (2000), a person possibly learns more about a subject matter if he/she is willing *to spend more time* with a system. Moreno, Mayer, Spires, and Lester (2001) suggest that a *social* agency environment built around a conversational pedagogical agent will encourage learners to *make a stronger effort* to understand material.

In sum, by adding an off-task conversation module to the original game and pedagogical agent, we simulate a natural part of traditional educational settings, hoping that this will have positive effects on the motivational qualities of the game. In addition we set out to explore whether the conversational module can be the basis of pedagogical interventions to affect students' math self-efficacy and attitudes towards math as a school subject.

## 4. GUIDING FRAMEWORKS

### 4.1 The Enhancing Agent-Learner Interaction (EnALI) Framework

Researchers have long called for a refined approach to the design of virtual agents (Dehn & van Mulken, 2000), and during the last few years pedagogical agent researchers have proposed a number of frameworks to enhance pedagogical agent implementations (e.g., Kim & Baylor, 2008; Woo, 2009).

In this chapter, we use the *Enhancing Agent-Learner Interaction* (EnALI) framework (Veletsianos et al., 2009) to guide our work. The EnALI framework, consists of practical guidelines for the effective design of pedagogical agents that are in close alignment with design inquiry and practice, taking an encompassing view of design that addresses social, conversational, and pedagogical issues. These guidelines focus on enhancing agent-learner interaction, agent message, and agent characteristics and are presented in Table 1. We will return to these in the sections that follow.

It is important to observe that these guidelines may overlap and influence one another. For instance, one guideline suggests that agents "maintain an appropriate balance between on- and off-task communications" and another suggests that agents "establish [their] credibility and trustworthiness." Notably, both on-task and off-task interactions can establish or shatter credibility or trustworthiness: correct on-task responses to learner questions and off-task remarks (e.g. remembering a learner's name after an initial interaction) may establish rapport, while incorrect on-task responses to learner questions and off-task remarks at inappropriate times (e.g. when the learner is requesting assistance with an especially challenging aspect of a learning activity) may ruin the agent's credibility.

### 4.2 Design Based Research

The methodology that we use to enhance pedagogical agent deployments is termed Design based research (DBR) and is a relatively new research methodology that aims to assist in understanding learning in context (Brown, 1992; Collins, 1992). Wang and Hannafin (2006, p.6) describe DBR as "a systematic but flexible methodology aimed to improve educational practices through iterative analysis, design, development, and implementation, based on collaboration among researchers and practitioners in real-world settings, and leading to contextually-sensitive design principles and theories."

DBR attempts to understand the "how" while valuing ecological validity and exploration in messy educational contexts. For instance, we

*Table 1. The enhancing agent learner interactions (EnALI) framework (from Veletsianos, Miller, & Doering, 2009)*

| | Design focus | Guidelines |
|---|---|---|
| 1 | User interaction | *Agents should be attentive and sensitive to the learner's needs and wants by:*<br>• Being responsive and reactive to requests for additional and/or expanded information.<br>• Being redundant.<br>• Asking for formative and summative feedback.<br>• Maintaining an appropriate balance between on- and off-task communications. |
| 2 | Message | *Agents should consider intricacies of the message by:*<br>• Making the message appropriate to the receiver's abilities, experiences, and frame of reference.<br>• Using congruent verbal and nonverbal messages.<br>• Clearly owning the message.<br>• Making messages complete and specific.<br>• Using descriptive, non-evaluative comments.<br>• Describing feelings by name, action, or figure of speech. |
| 3 | Agent characteristics | *Agents should display socially appropriate demeanor, posture, and representation by:*<br>• Establishing credibility and trustworthiness.<br>• Establishing role and relationship to user/task.<br>• Being polite and positive (e.g., encouraging, motivating).<br>• Being expressive (e.g. exhibiting verbal cues in speech).<br>• Using a visual representation appropriate to content. |

ask, (a) how does pedagogical agent appearance influence the way agents and learners interact, (b) how do iterative modifications enhance learning, (c) and how does knowledge from this exercise inform theory and practice? More formally, DBR is a multi-step methodological approach aimed at enhancing learning and teaching processes by means of theory development, research in authentic and naturalistic environments, and the sharing of knowledge amongst practitioners and researchers (The Design-Based Research Collective, 2003). Phenomena are studied in their "messy contexts," outside of experimental labs (Brown, 1992) because any insights gained from investigations undertaken in out-of-context environments have limited applicability in the classroom.

## 5. DESIGN CHALLENGES AND POSSIBLE WAYS TO APPROACH THEM

We identify four main design challenges that we confronted in the development process of the pedagogical conversational agent in the math game. The challenges in question all arise from the decision to develop the original agent into a social and personal kind of agent – by means of *visual embodiment* and an *extension of its conversational capacities*. These challenges are therefore likely to be faced by others who aim to develop the kind of pedagogical agent previously categorized as a "virtual human":

1. **The challenge of student expectations regarding the pedagogical agent's knowledge:** how to handle students' expectations on the knowledge and *knowledge profile* of the pedagogical agent.
2. **The challenge of student expectations regarding the pedagogical agent's social abilities:** how to manage students' expectations on the *social profile* of the pedagogical agent.
3. **The challenges of students' engagement in off-task conversation:**
    a. how to manage students' possible over-engagement in off-task conversation with the pedagogical agent,
    b. how to manage students' possible under-engagement in off-task conversation with the pedagogical agent.

4. **The challenge of abusive student comments**: how to manage the pedagogical agent's responses to inappropriate or abusive user language without ending the conversation.

## 5.1. The Challenge of Student Expectations Regarding the Pedagogical Agent's Knowledge Profile

Students need to experience a pedagogical agent as *useful* for information purposes and for their learning task at hand (Veletsianos, 2010). A corresponding design challenge is to create a pedagogical agent that lives up to this task. However, this challenge applies to all pedagogical agents, including classical ITS systems.

According to the EnALI framework, a pedagogical agent should be able to promptly provide complete and specific information that is appropriate to the student's abilities, experiences and frame of reference. Again the corresponding design challenge is not unique to present day conversational agents but applies to classical tutoring systems too. However, when we introduce a pedagogical agent whose conversation capacities expands from the ability to engage in a limited, domain-specific and task-oriented conversation to also being able to engage in broader, humanlike conversation, the challenge of creating an *appropriate knowledge profile* becomes considerably more complex.

As soon as the pedagogical agent appears on the screen, and throughout the conversation, the student will develop expectations regarding the *agent's conversational abilities*. Can the agent discuss strategies of the math game? Can it tell whether it finds mathematics a boring subject? Can it discuss music? Can it give an answer to whether it has a best friend or not?

In our example system we need to handle students' expectations of the agent's conversational capacity as pertaining both to *on-domain* and *off-domain* content. Selecting its particular off-task knowledge areas – what it should be capable to talk about and not with the 12-14 year olds in the target group – is a non-trivial and challenging task in itself. Importantly, the R&D team (with a mean age of around 45) needed input from the target audience. This task especially important for off-task/off-domain areas, where the main purpose is to increase student engagement with the game and system (and hopefully have a spill-over towards the mathematical content of the game, attitudes to math, etc.) In order to decide which domains the agent should have knowledge on and be interested in, we collected information from the student target group in an iterative design-redesign process. In concrete terms, focus group interviews provide the input for a Wizard-of-oz role-play (where two students are engaged in a computer mediated, text based chat – one of them taking the role of the pedagogical agent). The collected data in iterations is subject to a dialogue corpus analysis, to provide input for the iterative prototyping of our conversational system. The dialogue logs are then analyzed together with the material from surveys and other focus group interviews.

Our first round of iterative studies and development was completed as follows: for the focus group sessions, twenty 13-14 year-old students played the game for 30 minutes. In these sessions, the agent was present and posed on-task questions. The students were thereafter split into four focus groups that discussed the agent's personality and interests, the agent's visual appearance and any additional information that they wanted to provide about the agent.

Regarding the latter we found it valuable to compare the outcome with the topics that the R&D group had suggested beforehand as probable desired topics for off-task conversation. The students discussed some of these topics (for example, off-task conversations about friends and school). We also discovered that the students did not discuss various topics that we originally thought they would discuss (e.g., film and traveling). In addition, students consistently proposed topics that the

R&D group had not previously considered (e.g. sports, music, and computer games).

On the basis of the material from the focus groups, we developed a sketch of the agent's persona as a basis for a role-play activity, in which students simulated off-task conversations in the game (Wizard-of-Oz study). Agent players were asked to act in accordance with the persona, and if dialogue topics occurred outside of the persona's knowledge scope, they were asked to improvise. The resulting 12 dialogues were analyzed, and again novel topics emerged.

Thereafter a system prototype was developed that was tested by another 38 representatives from the target group. After a short introduction to the system the students played the game for 10 minutes, chatted with the agent for 5 minutes, played the game for another 5 minutes, and chatted with the agent for 5 additional minutes. This was repeated with a revised prototype with the same group of students[2]. These two cycles of iteration led to a refinement and extension of the off-task conversational module. In sum, the user studies described allowed us to expand, revise, and refine the off-task/off-domain topics that we, as researchers and designers, had devised. The target group, acting as designers, helped refine the topics, language, and content used.

For the off-task/on-domain topics the situation is different. We have pedagogical motives for incorporating conversational topics that relate to the domain of mathematics: attitudes towards math, math self-efficacy, etc. However, the conversational architecture must be designed so that conversations on these topics are not perceived as strained in the conversations as a whole. Part of our approach to deal with this comes from our view on on-task conversation and off-task conversation as *interrelated.* The interconnecting factor is represented by the *agent,* which integrates selected on-domain knowledge with (limited) off-domain knowledge (i.e. the agent is an 11-year old student that goes to school and is learning to play the math game, but also has interests like music and sports that it pursues in its spare time). Even when the free conversation is primarily oriented towards off-task/off-domain topics, the agent can also comment on the *game play* (i.e. on-task/on-domain topics), as well as introduce off-task/on-domain topics related to school, math, the math game, etc.

We also introduced a dedicated use of anecdotes and narrative storytelling. As evidenced by the work of Bickmore and Cassell (1999; 2000), anecdotes and small-talk have a social and trust-building function even when the interlocutor is a virtual character. At the same time, the content of small talk can be designed to convey something *relevant about the subject domain*. For our agent we plan to include anecdotal material relating to school and mathematics (e.g., the agent telling a story about "my friend, who turned the math book upside down and found the homework to be very difficult"; or about "the other day in school when we had math and the teacher was explaining on the whiteboard but made a mistake and could not get the right answer, but I saw the mistake and could show him").

One issues that we faced relates to the large number of human cultural domains that humans know at least something about – but that the agent will know nothing about, especially contemporary news. The challenge is to position an agent so as to minimize the friction between "pretty good knowledge on some cultural domains" (for instance TV-shows, computer games, being friends, sports, etc.) and "very limited or no knowledge on others" (for instance cooking, dancing, playing chess). Part of such positioning can be achieved by an appropriate visual embodiment. Using an embodiment that is devoid of naturalism serves to downplay expectations regarding the agent acting and responding *like* a human being. Appropriate dialogue strategies are another important means for addressing this challenge. One needs to handle different classes of the cases where the agent will not understand the student's input. That is, we needed to build a dialogue architecture that can use varied and appropriate responses, such as for instance, in the following cases: asking for clarification, indicate misunderstanding, move on with the conversation, etc. (Artstein et al., 2009; Traum, Swartout, Gratch, & Marsella, 2008).

There is yet another sub-challenge that relates to the idea of combining on-task conversation, strictly targeted at a task, and off-task conversation of a broader and socially oriented kind: if a student finds the *social conversation* with an agent satisfying and engaging, a failure of the same agent to be of use to the student on on-task activities will also cause disappointment.

Finally, one may observe that the challenges of constructing an adequate knowledge profile need further refinement in the case of *teachable* agents. A TA is unusually straightforward as to what it appears to know about its assigned subject. It is the student's task to train it and the agent will explicitly convey *not knowing anything at all* about the learning domain. A TA is not an expert, nor does it belong to any other kind of authoritative pedagogical agents (Haake & Gulz, 2009), and thus there is no risk for student disappointment because the agent discloses that it "knows too little." But when – like in our project – the TA is engaged in task-oriented conversations *and* socially-oriented interactions, there may be a clash between student expectations on the pedagogical agent's knowledge as to the math game (not knowing much at all) and its knowledge of general subjects.

The present section has dealt with student expectations on *what* the agent can/will talk to the student about. We have discussed our approach of iteratively collecting data relating to our target population, and in the next section we discuss student expectations on *how* the agent can/will talk to the student.

## 5.2. The Challenge of Student Expectations Regarding the Pedagogical Agent's Social Profile

From the very first time a student enters the learning environment, s/he will have expectations as to what kind of character the pedagogical agent will be. In comparison to the agent's knowledge profile, we refer to the agent's *social profile* as the manner in which its knowledge is being communicated. Not only does a student have expectations on *what* the agent can talk about to his/her but also on *how* it can and will talk to him/her.

These expectations are also linked to how the student perceives the agent's general personal features, for example in terms of it being a kind or a mean character, extrovert or introvert, humorous or serious, happy or sad, etc. In addition, for any interaction, humans seem to expect some degree of *consistency* with respect to such characteristics. They will not expect – and not appreciate – changes in a pedagogical agent's exhibited attitudes or moods that are random and inconsistent (Isbister & Nass, 2000).

Now, what kind of social profile of a pedagogical agent will be appropriate for a given setting can be hard to predict beforehand. Nevertheless it is an important challenge to address, since a good match between student expectations of an agent's social profile is likely to enhance the pedagogical objective of making the conversation engaging, encouraging and motivating.

Already in the beginning of the design process with our present system, we have an illustrative example of how the EnALI framework can be fruitfully combined with a design-based research strategy for contextualizing, and exemplifying, some of the EnALI guidelines. In the case to be presented we started out from the "Agent Characteristics" guidelines (see Table 1) that suggest that the agent should be credible and trustworthy, establish a role to the user and be polite and positive. Inspired by Wang et al. (2008), who argue specifically for the so-called "politeness effect", our focus for this example is on the politeness aspect. The design process in question can be described as follows: (1) making a raw sketch of the agent character, (2) using this sketch as a basis for preliminary design decisions by the research team, (3) refining the design decisions through focus group interviews with actual students and (4) discussing design implications of the outcome based on the focus group results:

- *Step 1:* Starting from the EnALI guidelines, we made a raw sketch of an "Agent character". A very first set of preliminary design decisions were taken, directed by our knowledge and experience from other pedagogical agent systems as well as from our experience as teachers and considerations about the technical feasibility. Notably, we conceived of the pedagogical agent as being "overall positive, nice and polite" in its conversation, in line with previous suggestions.
- *Step 2:* The first sketch became subject of much discussion, which highlighted the complexity of the student-agent relationship in relation to our various research goals. We are interested in the pedagogical agent's potential to influence students' attitudes towards math, with respect to math self-efficacy as well as to the general attitude towards math as a school subject. At the same time, these are factors we want to be able to manipulate in order to make empirically-based decisions, for example comparing an agent which exhibits low math self-efficacy to one with high math self-efficacy. Results from previous studies proved too ambiguous to serve as an empirical basis for definitive design decisions in these respects, which is why we turned to focus groups to gather input from students.
- *Step 3:* We conducted focus group interviews with four groups of 4-5 teenagers each (13-14 years old), who had the opportunity to play the math game, look at agent images (Figure 4) and listen to material about the game. In these discussions the students reinforced some of our preliminary design decisions regarding the agent's personal qualities, such that it should be friendly, curious, eager to learn, and like school. However, students insisted that the agent should not be too polite, but express some "attitude". Interestingly, it could be inferred from the interviews that a "too soft, nice and polite" character seemed to elicit skepticism among the students, rendering the agent untrustworthy (for the age group in question). This is an example of how a particular user group may give input that diverges from general design guidelines (Veletsianos, Miller & Doering, 2009; Wang et al., 2008) which thus highlights the importance of involving target user groups in design.
- *Step 4:* We turned to possible interpretations, and design implications, of the result regarding the agent being "polite" versus "having some attitude". One interpretation is that the preference for a somewhat "plucky" agent with a bit of an attitude simply is an expression of students wanting to have fun. On the one hand this could be a positive design feature because it may introduce some playful conflict between agents and students. But, on the other hand, an agent having an attitude could be quickly marked as confrontational and conversations could quickly escalate to abuse (cf. Veletsianos, Scharber, & Doering, 2008). Another interpretation is that by stating things like "She/he should be positive, yes, but not over-positive, she/he should have some attitude" or "She/he should be nice

but also have some attitude", the students are searching for an agent that does not return scripted, robot-like responses. The agent should not reply or react in the same way whenever the student types the same comment. This does not prevent the agent from exhibiting an overall positive attitude, but its behavior as well as its mood should vary. In the social conversations, the agent can vary its utterances. In short, given that there are multiple interpretations of the result we see a need to continue exploration of this topic with input from the target group. In particular we need to capture in more detail what "expressing some attitude" means for the target group, and to what extent it relates to unpredictability, interesting personality, sarcasm, humor, and so on.

In conclusion, our considerations about the pedagogical agent's social abilities illustrate that a successful design depends a lot on informative input from actual students on which to make further iterations and implementations of the system. This is also what contemporary design-based approaches to educational technology enhancements suggest.

## 5.3 The Challenges of Off-Task Engagement

A third challenge relates to students' level of engagement in *off-task conversation* with conversational pedagogical agents. There are actually two sub-challenges that are the opposites of one another. On the one hand: an off-task conversation can become *so engaging* that the student completely deviates from the learning task. On the other hand: a student can find off-task conversation completely uninteresting and therefore not (want to) engage in it at all.

### 5.3.1 The Appeal of Off-Task Conversation

There are examples of students becoming so strongly immersed in conversation with a pedagogical agent that they forego the learning task, as demonstrated by Veletsianos and Miller (2008). This appears as a possible drawback of deploying a module "too elaborated" for social conversation, as students come to focus more on the social interaction than the present learning goal. Relating back to the EnALI framework, there is surely a fine line between students being engaged and being immersed to the point of losing focus on the task. As stated in the EnALI guidelines (Table 1), it is important to maintain an appropriate balance between on- and off-task activities.

Our way to address this in the system under development is by dedicatedly bridging the gap between what is *clearly task-oriented* (playing the math game and having a conversation on this) and what is *completely unrelated to the task* (discussing the music style of a rock singer or saying one wants to go and buy an ice-cream) with the *in between* category. *Off-task/on-domain conversation* is social and free conversation *but on the math game, on math, on school*, etc.

By combining a basic chatbot system architecture based on AIML with dialogue management and dialogue history techniques used in dialogue systems, the agent can handle a mixed initiative dialogue and by taking the initiative also steer away from long off-domain conversations and reintroduce the learning task. The pedagogical agent can in this way (re)introduce particular subjects of conversation, drawing from its knowledge database. For example, if the student comments on something in "school", the pedagogical agent can relate the fact that mathematics is a school subject and select between associated responses, such as for instance "I had a pretty good day at school, but it was a very long one. I was tired during the last lesson of the day (math). Did you have math today too?" This provides a tool to work on a balancing between on-task and off-task conversations between agent and student.

### 5.3.2 The Non-Appeal of Off-Task Conversation

On the other hand, some students show very *little* interest in engaging in off-task conversation (Gulz, 2005; Veletsianos, 2009), and may experience off-task conversation as unnecessary and meaningless, taking time from the task. In a study with ninety 12-15-year-old school children from a Swedish secondary school (Gulz, 2005), 37 out of 90 said that they would prefer a pedagogical agent that was strictly task-oriented in its conversation rather than also engage in socially oriented off-task conversation. The arguments fell into four categories: i) off-task conversation with the agent would be *trying, tiresome and a nuisance,* ii) there is a risk of *getting distracted* by off-task conversation, iii) off-task conversation would involve doing *unnecessary or meaningless things instead of focusing* on what is important, and iv) minimal interest in developing a socially oriented relationship with a computer. Similar results of *diverging* attitudes towards agents' off-task conversation have been presented by Bickmore (2003) and by Hall et al. (2004). In other words, the notion that social dimensions of virtual characters increase learners' motivation and engagement may be less straightforward than is sometimes hypothesized (Gulz, 2005).

We tackle this challenge through various approaches. First, we constructed our system in such a way that it can detect a student's lack of engagement in off-task conversation (which is relatively easy to determine from simply the amount of typed text and certain indicative comments or questions). The agent can then take the initiative to finish a conversation and return to the game: "Let's play again", "Do you want to play another game?" Another approach is to enable the learner to end the social conversation by adding a button to 'return to game' by which a student can chose to terminate an off-task conversation before the chat-time (pause-time) has passed.

### 5.3.3 Finding the Balance and Allowing Flexibility for Individuals

Some students are considerably more attracted to an agent that engages in off-task conversation than others. Simply placing preference for pedagogical agent engaging in off-task conversation against preference for a pedagogical agent not doing so is an oversimplification. The *amount* of off-task conversation in relation to task-oriented conversation and the *kind* of off-task conversation are important parameters that can influence preferences. These parameters affect a learner's judgment of the value and worth of off-task interactions.

In fact, there is evidence that a pedagogical agents' engaging in off-task conversation can lead to a stronger focus on the task by the part of the students. In a study by Ai and colleagues (Ai, Kumar, Nguyen, Nagasunder & Rosé, 2010) student pairs interacted with one another within a collaborative software, where a conversational agent in the role of a tutor participated with the students in a chat. The conversational agent was presented in three different versions that differed in the amount of social behaviors and attitudes exhibited by the agent in the conversation. The non-social tutor agent was strictly task-oriented in its conversation, whereas the Low social and the High social agents differed in the frequency of bringing in socially oriented utterances in the conversation. Results showed that the students who interacted with the social agents focused more on the task rather than engaging in off-task conversations with each another.

The system that we develop includes off-task conversations that relate to the task at hand – these aspects we call off-task/on-domain. The agent can use this aspect of off-task conversation to boost the students' accomplishments– for instance the agent could say: "It would not have been easy to learn this without your help", or "I never thought that math could be this fun, thanks to you". The R&D project will explore how this can be used as a way to influence students' self-efficacy beliefs in math (cf. section 2.2.1 above).

In the off-task/off-domain conversation, very different kinds of topics can be discussed. It is expected that students are likely to have different opinions on the usefulness of this type of conversation and be differently willing to engage in it. As discussed above we will opt for design solutions that allow flexibility and choice in order to meet this challenge. Our rationale for this choice comes from the study mentioned above (Gulz, 2005), where students responded that the ideal, as they saw it, would be to be able to choose which agent they wanted to interact with: "Sometimes one would feel like talking more and chatting, but sometimes one would prefer an agent that is quiet and sticks to the task.' [....]; 'It depends, sometimes I would like one that is talkative and social, but sometimes I cannot stand that and want to be spared from it' (ibid. p. 413)."

## 5.4 The Challenge of Abusive Student Comments

A fourth challenge relates to avoiding conversations in which students abuse the pedagogical agent (Branham & De Angeli, 2008; De Angeli & Branham, 2008). The EnALI framework suggests several guidelines for addressing this challenge. Relating to the agent characteristics, for example, the agent should display socially appropriate demeanor and representation and use a visual representation appropriate to the content.

Previously this challenge has been addressed by making the agent give very neutral responses to as student's verbal abuse. Veletsianos, Scharber, and Doering (2008) allowed the pedagogical agent respond to abuses by informing the user that foul language is inappropriate. This response however, resulted in continued abuse. Our current approach involves the pedagogical agent noting that it is not interested in certain topics and not wanting to comment on them. Another strategy being evaluated involves refraining from provocative responses while at the same time refraining from avoiding the presence of abusive language.

Additionally, visual appearance can play an important role in guiding expectations and managing such interactions. In a related study (Gulz & Haake, 2010) a female pedagogical agent in the role of coach for a technology domain was given two different embodiments, one more feminine-looking and one more neutral-looking. The more feminine-looking character was more frequently commented upon in derogative terms, whereas the more neutral-looking was discussed in more positive terms. We will continue to explore what influence manipulations of visual gender can have.

For the early versions of our systems and the visual characters as in Figure 5, the results so far indicate that the amount of agent abuse is considerably smaller and takes milder forms than in the study from Veletsianos et al. (2008). The comparison should, however, be taken with caution, since there are differences not only in the visualization of agents but also in the educational systems used, the period of time for use, age of students as well as the cultural context.

# 6. FUTURE TRENDS AND RESEARCH DIRECTIONS

While this chapter has described challenges, design thinking, and possible solutions to common problems when implementing pedagogical agents, it is important to highlight the ways future research can support the extension of this way of thinking.

To the extent that off-task conversation fulfills the purpose of establishing a social relationship with the learner, there is a potential for pedagogical interventions that deserve further attention – such as pedagogical interventions based on identification and role-modeling. To the best of our knowledge, this project represents the very first implementation of off-task interaction in educational software intentionally designed to serve a set of pedagogical interventions.

An important area that needs to be explored further, in relation to the above, and in relation to other issues is *long-term studies*. What can be accomplished when a pedagogical agent based educational system is used for a longer period of time? The need for such research has been pointed out for quite some time and by several researchers (e.g. Dehn & van Mulken, 2000; Gulz, 2004; Bickmore & Picard 2004). With more mature agent-based educational systems, the time has come where such studies can actually be carried out. For example, it is known that a well-designed conversational pedagogical agent during short-term use can positively influence self-efficacy beliefs in students (Baylor, 2009; Kim, Baylor, & Shen, 2007; Baylor & Plant, 2005) but little is known about long term effects. Regarding the role of visual appearance of pedagogical agents on self-efficacy beliefs and other pedagogical measurements, again most studies have dealt with short-time use. The field stands before the exciting task of also examining the role of appearance when a human-agent social relationship persists over time (cf. Baylor, 2009).

An important and much-needed trend in the field is that studies on conversational pedagogical agents have become considerably more fine-grained than they used to be a decade ago. It is no longer discussed whether educational systems are better with or without conversational pedagogical agents. Instead studies are concerned with what kinds of agent can affect what aspects of performance or attitudes in which learners. Another example of studies becoming more fine-grained is how studies of agent gender do not stop at comparing male and female agent characters, but involve different aspects of femininity and masculinity in appearance (Gulz & Haake, 2010).

In addition to research trends and research areas that necessitate our attention, we see a need to rethink the methodological approach we take to pedagogical agent research. Specifically, Design-Based Research (DBR) methodologies allow researchers and practitioners to fully understand pedagogical agent implementations, challenges, solutions, and theories, and we suggest employing such methodologies for future interventions.

Edelson (2002) suggests that three types of theories can be generated from DBR studies. We see our work as informing two of these three theories. Specifically:

- Domain theories: the implementations and iterations described in this chapter enhance our understanding of interactions between learners and agents within digital learning environments.
- Design Frameworks: the design, implementation, evaluation, and redesign of the pedagogical agents described herein inform and improve the design guidelines proposed by the EnALI framework (Veletsianos, Doering & Miller, 2009).

In sum, DBR affords researchers with the opportunity to experiment with interventions in authentic environments to explore what happens in the "real world". Future work in the pedagogical agent domain can fine-tune and enhance situated practice while also enhancing theory on agent-learner interactions if we employ a DBR approach to pedagogical agent research. In line with DBR methodologies, this chapter describes our thinking and initial design decisions for the project described herein. We will be revisiting the ideas presented here and will be revising the intervention continuously based on data from the field, feedback from teachers and students, assessment results, and evaluations of the learning experience.

## 7. CONCLUSION

This chapter has provided examples of how one can reason about dealing with the complexity of decisions within one coherent framework (the EnALI guidelines) and still make progress towards a small number of well-defined, educational goals. Unlike traditional, experimental research which provides a "yes" or "no" answer to a given research question, or the rejection or acceptance of a hypothesis, a design-based approach to development maintains the focus on the "how" in an on-going enhancement process as to *what actually works in a virtual learning environment* and the socio-cultural environment in which it is being used. The results we obtain in terms of what manipulations yield a positive or negative effect, for example, might be more or less limited to the implementation context. Yet, of greater benefit is the generalizability and applicability of the lines of reasoning, data collection procedures, and strategies for dealing with enacted interventions at different stages of development, which are likely to inform similar endeavors of enhancing interactions in real-world learning environments.

In our case, we have aimed to demonstrate how the field of conversational pedagogical agents represents a unique combination of theory and research intertwined with practice. This chapter has highlighted the fact that design and research knowledge are important in developing effective, efficient, and engaging pedagogical agents that not only capitalize on technological advancements, but are also sensitive to cognitive, emotional, and social considerations as they relate to educational issues. Taking a design-based approach lends promise to enhancing design practices of conversational agents not as pedagogical tools in isolation, but to improving and understanding the dynamics of the actual learning environment as a whole, with respect to particular measures and treatments as well as to theories and interpretations that lead to usable knowledge.

## REFERENCES


Ai, H., Kumar, R., Nguyen, D., Nagasunder, A., & Rosé, C. (2010). Exploring the effectiveness of social capabilities and goal alignment in computer supported collaborative learning . In Aleven, V., Kay, J., & Mostow, J. (Eds.), *ITS 2010, part II, LNCS 6095* (pp. 134–143). Berlin/Heidelberg, Germany: Springer-Verlag.

Alexandersson, J., Maier, E., & Reithinger, N. (1994). *A robust and efficient three-layered dialogue component for speech-to-speech translation system.* Technical Report~50, DFKI GmbH. Retrieved April 29, 2001, from http://www.dfki.uni-sb.de/cgi-bin/verbmobil/htbin/doc-access.cgi

Allen, J., Schubert, L., Ferguson, G., Heeman, P., Hwang, C.-H., & Kato, T. (1995). The TRAINS project: A case study in building a conversational planning agent. *Journal of Experimental & Theoretical Artificial Intelligence, 7*, 7–48. doi:10.1080/09528139508953799

André, E., & Rist, T. (2000). *Presenting through performing: On the use of multiple kifelike characters in knowledge-nased presentation systems. IUI 2000* (pp. 1–8). New Orleans, LA, USA: ACM Press.

Artstein, R., Gandhe, S., Gerten, J., Leuski, A., & Traum, D. (2009). Semi-formal evaluation of conversational characters . In Grumberg, O., Kaminski, M., Katz, S., & Wintner, S. (Eds.), *Languages: From formal to natural. Essays dedicated to Nissim Francez on the occasion of His 65th Birthday (Lecture Notes in Computer Science 5533)* (pp. 22–35). Heidelberg, Germany: Springer.

Bandura, A. (1986). *Social foundations of thought and action: A social cognitive theory*. Englewood Cliffs, NJ: Prentice-Hall.

Bandura, A. (2000). *Self-efficacy: The foundation of agency*. Mahwah, NJ: Lawrence Erlbaum.

Bargh, J. A., & Schul, Y. (1980). On the cognitive benefits of teaching. *Journal of Educational Psychology*, *72*, 593–604. doi:10.1037/0022-0663.72.5.593

Baylor, A. (2005). The impact of pedagogical agent image on affective outcomes. In *Proceedings on the Workshop on Affective Interactions: Computers in the Affective Loop, the 2005 International Conference on Intelligent User Interfaces* (San Diego, CA).

Baylor, A. (2009). Promoting motivation with virtual agents and avatars: role of visual presence and appearance. *Philosophical Transactions of the Royal Society of London. Series B, Biological Sciences*, *364*(1535), 3559–3566. doi:10.1098/rstb.2009.0148

Baylor, A., & Kim, Y. (2005). Simulating instructional roles through pedagogical agents. *International Journal of Artificial Intelligence in Education*, *15*(1), 95–115.

Baylor, A., & Plant, E. (2005). Pedagogical agents as social models for engineering: The influence of appearance on female choice . In Looi, C. K., McCalla, G., Bredeweg, B., & Breuker, J. (Eds.), *Artificial intelligence in education: Supporting learning through intelligent and socially informed technology, 125* (pp. 65–72). Amsterdam, Holland: IOS Press.

Baylor, A., Rosenberg-Kima, R., & Plant, E. (2006). Interface agents as social models: The impact of appearance on females' attitude toward engineering. In *CHI'06 Extended Abstracts on Human Factors in Computing Systems* (Montréal, Québec, Canada, 2006), (pp. 526-531). New York, NY: ACM.

Bennacef, S., Devillers, L., Rosset, S., & Lamel, L. (1996). Dialog in the RAILTEL telephone-based system. In *Proceedings of International Conference on Spoken Language Processing* (pp. 550-553). ICSLP'96, 1, Philadelphia, USA, October 1996.

Bickmore, T. (2003). *Relational agents: Effecting change through human-computer relationships*. PhD Thesis, Media Arts & Sciences, Massachusetts Institute of Technology.

Bickmore, T., & Cassell, J. (1999). Small talk and conversational storytelling in embodied interface agents. *Proceedings of the AAAI Fall Symposium on Narrative Intelligence* (pp. 87-92). November 5-7, Cape Cod, MA.

Bickmore, T., & Cassell, J. (2000). How about this weather: Social dialog with embodied conversational agents. *Proceedings of the American Association for Artificial Intelligence (AAAI) Fall Symposium on Narrative Intelligence*, (pp. 4-8). November 3-5, Cape Cod, MA.

Biswas, G., Katzlberger, T., Brandford, J., Schwartz D., & TAG-V. (2001). Extending intelligent learning environments with teachable agents to enhance learning. In J. D. Moore, C. L. Redfield, & W. L. Johnson (Eds.) *Artificial intelligence in education* (pp. 389–397). Amsterdam, The Netherlands: IOS Press.

Branham, S., & De Angeli, A. (2008). Special issue on the abuse and misuse of social agents. *Interacting with Computers*, *20*(3), 287–291. doi:10.1016/j.intcom.2008.02.001

Brown, A. (1992). Design experiments: Theoretical and methodological challenges in creating complex interventions in classroom settings. *Journal of the Learning Sciences*, *2*(2), 141–178. doi:10.1207/s15327809jls0202_2

Carbonell, J. R. (1970). AI in CAI: Artificial intelligence approach to computer assisted instruction. *IEEE Transactions on Man-Machine Systems*, *11*(4), 190–202. doi:10.1109/TMMS.1970.299942

Cassell, J., Sullivan, J., Prevost, S., & Churchill, E. (Eds.). (2000). *Embodied conversational agents*. Cambridge, MA: MIT.

Chase, C. C., Chin, D. B., Oppezzo, M. A., & Schwartz, D. L. (2009). Teachable agents and the protégé effect: Increasing the effort towards learning. *Journal of Science Education and Technology*, *18*(4), 334–352. doi:10.1007/s10956-009-9180-4

Chou, C. Y., Chan, T. W., & Lin, C. J. (2003). Redefining the learning companion: The past, present, and future of educational agents. *Computers & Education*, *40*, 255–269. doi:10.1016/S0360-1315(02)00130-6

Collins, A. (1992). Towards a design science of education . In Scanlon, E., & O'Shea, T. (Eds.), *New directions in educational technology* (pp. 15–22). Berlin, Germany: Springer.

De Angeli, A., & Brahnam, S. (2008). I hate you! Disinhibition with virtual partners. *Interacting with Computers*, *20*(3), 302–310. doi:10.1016/j.intcom.2008.02.004

Dehn, D., & van Mulken, S. (2000). The impact of animated interface agents: A review of empirical research. *International Journal of Human-Computer Studies*, *52*(1), 1–22. doi:10.1006/ijhc.1999.0325

Dowling, C. (2000). Intelligent agents: Some ethical issues and dilemmas. In . *Proceedings of, AICE2000*, 28–32.

Edelson, D. C. (2002). Design research: What we learn when we engage in design. *Journal of the Learning Sciences*, *11*(1), 105–121. doi:10.1207/S15327809JLS1101_4

Flycht-Eriksson, A. (2003). Representing knowledge of dialogue, domain, task and user in dialogue systems - how and why? *Electronic Transactions on Artificial Intelligence*, *3*(2), 5–32.

Goddeau, D., Brill, E., Glass, J., Pao, C., Philips, M., & Polifroni, J. … Zue, V. (1994). GALAXY: A human-language interface to on-line travel information. In *Proceedings of International Conference on Spoken Language Processing*, ICSLP'94, Yokohama, Japan, September 1994 (pp. 707-710).

Graesser, A., Chipman, P., Haynes, B., & Olney, A. (2005). AutoTutor: An intelligent tutoring system with mixed-initiative dialogue. *IEEE Transactions on Education*, *48*, 612–618. doi:10.1109/TE.2005.856149

Graesser, A., Wiemer-Hastings, K., Wiemer-Hastings, P., & Kreuz, R. Tutoring Research Group. (1999). AutoTutor: A simulation of a human tutor. *Journal of Cognitive Systems Research*, *1*, 35–51. doi:10.1016/S1389-0417(99)00005-4

Grosz, B., & Sidner, C. (1986). Attention, intentions, and the structure of discourse. *Computational Linguistics*, *12*(3), 175–204.

Gulz, A. (2004). Benefits of virtual characters in computer based learning environments: Claims and evidence. *International Journal of Artificial Intelligence in Education*, *14*, 313–334.

Gulz, A. (2005). Social enrichment by virtual characters - differential benefits. *Journal of Computer Assisted Learning*, *21*(6), 405–418. doi:10.1111/j.1365-2729.2005.00147.x

Gulz, A., & Haake, M. (2006). Pedagogical agents – design guidelines regarding visual appearance and pedagogical roles. In *Proceedings of the IV International Conference on Multimedia and ICT in Education (m-ICTE 2006)*, Sevilla, Spain.

Gulz, A., & Haake, M. (2010). Challenging gender stereotypes using virtual pedagogical characters . In Goodman, S., Booth, S., & Kirkup, G. (Eds.), *Gender issues in learning and working with Information Technology: Social constructs and cultural contexts*. Hershey, PA: IGI Global. doi:10.4018/978-1-61520-813-5.ch007

Haake, M., & Gulz, A. (2009). A look at the roles of look & roles in embodied pedagogical agents – a user preference perspective. *International Journal of Artificial Intelligence in Education*, *19*(1), 39–71.

Hall, L., Woods, S., Dautenhahn, K., Sobral, D., Paiva, A., Wolke, D., & Newall, L. (2004). Designing emphatic agents: Adults versus kids . In Lester, J., Vicari, R. M., & Paraguacu, F. (Eds.), *Intelligent tutoring systems* (pp. 604–613). Berlin/Heidelberg, Germany: Springer. doi:10.1007/978-3-540-30139-4_57

Hamann, S. (2001). Cognitive and neural mechanisms of emotional memory. *Trends in Cognitive Sciences*, *5*(9), 394–400. doi:10.1016/S1364-6613(00)01707-1

Hembree, R. (1990). The nature, effects, and relief of mathematics anxiety. *Journal for Research in Mathematics Education*, *21*(1), 33–46. doi:10.2307/749455

Isbister, K. (2006). *Better game characters by design: A psychological approach*. San Francisco, CA: Morgan Kaufmann.

Isbister, K., & Nass, C. (2000). Consistency of personality in interactive characters: Verbal cues, non-verbal cues, and user characteristics. *International Journal of Human-Computer Studies*, *53*(2), 251–267. doi:10.1006/ijhc.2000.0368

John-Steiner, V., & Mahn, H. (2003). Sociocultural contexts for teaching and learning . In Reynolds, A., William, M., & Miller, G. (Eds.), *Handbook of psychology: Educational psychology* (*Vol. 7*, pp. 125–151). New York, NY: John Wiley and Sons.

Johnson, W. L., Kole, S., Shaw, E., & Pain, H. (2003). *Socially intelligent learner-agent interaction tactics*. AI-ED 2003. Retrieved May 19, 2004, from www.cs.usyd.edu.au/~aied/papers_short.html

Jönsson, A. (1997). A model for habitable and efficient dialogue management for natural language interaction. *Natural Language Engineering*, *3*(2/3), 103–122. doi:10.1017/S1351324997001733

Kim, C., & Baylor, A. L. (2008). A virtual change agent: Motivating pre-service teachers to integrate technology in their future classrooms. *Journal of Educational Technology & Society*, *11*(2), 309–321.

Kim, Y., Baylor, A. L., & Shen, E. (2007). Pedagogical agents as learning companions: The impact of agent emotion and gender. *Journal of Computer Assisted Learning*, *23*(3), 220–234. doi:10.1111/j.1365-2729.2006.00210.x

Kim, Y., Wei, Q., Xu, B., Ko, Y., & Ilieva, V. (2007). *MathGirls: Increasing girls' positive attitudes and self-efficacy through pedagogical agents*. Paper presented at 13th International Conference on Artificial Intelligence in Education (AIED 2007): Los Angeles, CA.

Kumar, R., Gweon, G., Joshi, M., Cui, Y., & Rose, C. P. (2007). Supporting students working together on math with social dialogue. In *SLaTE-2007 (Speech and Language Technology in Education) Proceedings*, (pp. 96-99).

Laurillard, D. (1993). *Rethinking university teaching: A framework for the effective use of educational technology*. London, UK: Routledge.

Lester, J., Towns, S., Callaway, C., Voerman, J., & Fitzgerald, P. (2000). Deictic and emotive communication in animated pedagogical agents . In Cassell, J., Sullivan, J., Prevost, S., & Churchill, E. (Eds.), *Embodied conversational agents* (pp. 123–154). Cambridge, MA: MIT Press.

Lester, J. C., Converse, S. A., Kahler, S. E., Barlow, S. T., Stone, B. A., & Bhogal, R. S. (1997). The persona effect: Affective impact of animated pedagogical agents. In *Proceedings of CHI '97*, (pp. 359-366). ACM Press.

Lindström, P., Gulz, A., Haake, M., & Sjödén, B. (in press). Matching and mismatching between the pedagogical design principles of a maths game and the actual practices of play. *Journal of Computer Assisted Learning*.

Masterton, S. (1998). Computer support for learners using intelligent educational agents: The way forward. In . *Proceedings of ICCE, 98*, 211–219.

Moreno, R., Mayer, R., Spires, H., & Lester, J. (2001). The case for social agency in computer-based teaching: Do students learn more deeply when they interact with animated pedagogical agents? *Cognition and Instruction, 19*, 177–213. doi:10.1207/S1532690XCI1902_02

Moundridou, M., & Virvou, M. (2002). Evaluating the persona effect of an interface agent in a tutoring system. *Journal of Computer Assisted Learning, 18*, 253–261. doi:10.1046/j.0266-4909.2001.00237.x

Paiva, A., Dias, J., Sobral, D., Aylett, R., Sobreperez, P., Woods, S., et al. (2004). Caring for agents and agents that care: Building empathic relations with synthetic agents. In *Proceedings of the Third International Joint Conference on Autonomous Agents 2004*, (pp. 194-201).

Pareto, L. (2004). The Squares Family: A game and story based microworld for understanding arithmetic concepts designed to attract girls. In L. Cantoni, & C. McLoughlin (Eds.), *Proceedings of World Conference on Educational Multimedia, Hypermedia and Telecommunications 2004* (pp. 1567-1574). Chesapeake, VA: AACE.

Pareto, L., Schwartz, D. L., & Svensson, L. (2009). Learning by guiding a teachable agent to play an educational game. In *Proceedings of the International Conference on Artificial Intelligence in Education*, July 6-10, 2009.

Plant, E. A., Baylor, A. L., Doerr, C., & Rosenberg-Kima, R. (2009). Changing middle-school students' attitudes and performance regarding engineering with computer-based social models. *Computers & Education, 53*, 209–215. doi:10.1016/j.compedu.2009.01.013

Reeves, B., & Nass, C. (1996). *The media equation: How people treat computers, television, and new media like real people and places*. New York, NY: Cambridge University Press.

Ruttkay, Z., & Pelachaud, C. (Eds.). (2004). *From brows to trust: Evaluating embodied conversational agents*. Dordrecht, The Netherlands & London, UK: Kluwer.

Ryu, J., & Baylor, A. L. (2005). The psychometric structure of pedagogical agent persona. *Technology, Instruction . Cognition & Learning, 2*(4), 291–319.

Schunk, D. H. (1981). Modeling and attributional effects on children's achievement: A self-efficacy analysis. *Journal of Educational Psychology, 73*, 93–105. doi:10.1037/0022-0663.73.1.93

Schunk, D. H., Hanson, A. R., & Cox, P. D. (1987). Peer model attributes and children's achievement behaviours. *Journal of Educational Psychology, 79*, 54–61. doi:10.1037/0022-0663.79.1.54

Seneff, S., Hurley, E., Lau, R., Pao, C., Schmid, P., & Zue, V. (1998). GALAXYII: A reference architecture for conversational system development. In *Proceedings of International Conference on Spoken Language Processing*, ICSLP'98, 3, Sydney, Australia, December 1998 (pp. 931-934).

Shawar, B. A., & Atwell, E. S. (2007). Chatbots: Are they really useful? *LDV-Forum, 22*, 31–50.

Smith, R. W. (1992). Integration of domain problem solving with natural language dialog: The missing axiom theory . In *Proceedings of Applications of AI X* (pp. 270–278). Knowledge-Based Systems.

The Design-Based Research Collective. (2003). Design-based research: An emerging paradigm for educational inquiry. *Educational Researcher, 32*(1), 5–8. doi:10.3102/0013189X032001005

Traum, D. R., Swartout, W., Gratch, J., & Marsella, S. (2008). A virtual human dialogue model for non-team interaction . In Dybkjaer, L., & Minker, W. (Eds.), *Recent trends in discourse and dialogue* (pp. 45–67). New York, NY: Springer. doi:10.1007/978-1-4020-6821-8_3

Van Mulken, S., André, E., & Müller, J. (1998). The persona effect: How substantial is it? In H. Johnson, L. Nigay, & C. Roast (Eds.), *People and Computers XIII: Proceedings of HCI'98* (pp. 53-66). Berlin, Germany: Springer.

VanLehn, K., Graesser, A., Jackson, G. T., Jordan, P., Olney, A., & Rosé, C. P. (2007). Natural language tutoring: A comparison of human tutors, computer tutors, and text. *Cognitive Science, 31*(1), 3–52. doi:10.1080/03640210709336984

Veletsianos, G. (2007). Cognitive and affective benefits of an animated pedagogical agent: Considering contextual relevance and aesthetics. *Journal of Educational Computing Research, 36*(4), 373–377. doi:10.2190/T543-742X-033L-9877

Veletsianos, G. (2009). The impact and implications of virtual character expressiveness on learning and agent-learner interactions. *Journal of Computer Assisted Learning, 25*(4), 345–357. doi:10.1111/j.1365-2729.2009.00317.x

Veletsianos, G. (2010). Contextually relevant pedagogical agents: Visual appearance, stereotypes, and first impressions and their impact on learning. *Computers & Education, 55*(2), 576–585. doi:10.1016/j.compedu.2010.02.019

Veletsianos, G., & Miller, C. (2008). Conversing with pedagogical agents: A phenomenological exploration of interacting with digital entities. *British Journal of Educational Technology, 39*(6), 969–986. doi:10.1111/j.1467-8535.2007.00797.x

Veletsianos, G., Miller, C., & Doering, A. (2009). EnALI: A research and design framework for virtual characters and pedagogical agents. *Journal of Educational Computing Research, 41*(2), 171–194. doi:10.2190/EC.41.2.c

Veletsianos, G., Scharber, C., & Doering, A. (2008). When sex, drugs, and violence enter the classroom: Conversations between adolescent social studies students and a female pedagogical agent. *Interacting with Computers, 20*(3), 292–302. doi:10.1016/j.intcom.2008.02.007

Wang, F., & Hannafin, M. J. (2005). Design-based research and technology-enhanced learning environments. *Educational Technology Research and Development, 53*(4), 5–23. doi:10.1007/BF02504682

Wang, N., Johnson, W. L., Mayer, R. E., Rizzo, P., Shaw, E., & Collins, H. (2008). The politeness effect: Pedagogical agents and learning outcomes. *International Journal of Human-Computer Studies, 66*, 96–112. doi:10.1016/j.ijhcs.2007.09.003

Weizenbaum, J. (1966). ELIZA - a computer program for the study of natural language communication between man and machine. *Communications of the ACM, 9*, 36–45. doi:10.1145/365153.365168

Wenger, E. (1987). *Artificial intelligence and tutoring systems: Computational and cognitive approaches to the communication of knowledge*. Los Altos, CA: Morgan Kaufmann.

Woo, H. L. (2009). Designing multimedia learning environments using animated pedagogical agents: Factors and issues. *Journal of Computer Assisted Learning, 25*(3), 203–218. doi:10.1111/j.1365-2729.2008.00299.x

Yee, N., & Bailenson, J. N. (2007). The Proteus effect: The effect of transformed self-representation on behavior. *Human Communication Research, 33*, 271–290. doi:10.1111/j.1468-2958.2007.00299.x

Yee, N., Bailenson, J. N., & Ducheneaut, N. (2009). The Proteus effect implications of transformed digital self-representation on online and offline behavior. *Communication Research, 36*, 285–312. doi:10.1177/0093650208330254

## KEY TERMS AND DEFINITIONS

**Conversational Pedagogical Agent:** A pedagogical agent that is able to engage in a (textual or spoken) conversation with a learner.

**Design Based Research:** Design Based Research (DBR) is defined by Wang and Hannafin (2006, p.6) as, "a systematic but flexible methodology aimed to improve educational practices through iterative analysis, design, development, and implementation, based on collaboration among researchers and practitioners in real-world settings, and leading to contextually-sensitive design principles and theories."

**Dialogue System:** A computer system that interacts with a user using spoken or written language, and possibly other modalities, in a connected dialogue consisting of several turns.

**Embodiment:** The case where a virtual character is presented as a bodied character. Minimal embodiment refers to the agent being represented as a static feature, while advanced embodiment refers to the agent's ability to use his/her body (e.g., engage in gaze, movement, gesture, etc).

**Enhancing Agent-Learner Interaction (EnALI):** It refers to the framework proposed by (Veletsianos, Miller, & Doering (2009) to guide pedagogical agent design. The framework consists of practical guidelines for the effective design of pedagogical agents that are in close alignment with design inquiry and practice. These guidelines focus on enhancing agent-learner interaction, agent message, and agent characteristics.

**Intelligent Tutoring Systems (ITS):** Systems that provide learners with instructions and feedback that adapt based on learner characteristics, preferences, and objectives.

**On-Task and Off-Task Conversation:** On-task conversation refers to conversation between learners and pedagogical agents that is strictly focused on a lesson's and the processes required to complete the lesson. Off-task conversation is any conversation between learners and agents that is unrelated to the lesson.

**Pedagogical Agent:** Computer generated characters in a pedagogical role. Examples include virtual instructors, mentors, coaches or learning companions. Such characters appear in numerous educational settings including formal education (e.g., pre-school and university settings) and informal education (e.g., video games).

**Social Agent:** A pedagogical agent that is able to relate socially with a learner, and engage in social-oriented dialogue as well as task-based dialogue.

**Teachable Agent:** A type of pedagogical agent that is taught by learners. Such agents are grounded on the notion that learners learn best when they teach others. In this instance, learners learn by teaching computer-generated characters.

**Web-Based Education:** Education that is enhanced with the use of the World Wide Web.

## ENDNOTES

1. These distinctions are important when it comes to evaluating the pedagogical function of off-task conversations and optimizing their potential for promoting actual learning.
2. For both prototypes two questionnaires were filled in by the students, one regarding the experience of using the learning environment and one regarding the experienced personality of the agent.

# Chapter 7
# Design and Implementation Issues for Convincing Conversational Agents

**Markus Löckelt**
*German Research Center for Artificial Intelligence, Germany*

## ABSTRACT

*This chapter describes a selection of experiences from designing and implementing virtual conversational characters for multimodal dialogue systems. It uses examples from the large interactive narrative VirtualHuman and some related systems of the task-oriented variety. The idea is not to give a comprehensive overview of any one system, but rather to identify and describe some issues that might also be relevant for the designer of a new system, to show how they can be addressed, and what problems still remain unresolved for future work. Besides giving an overview of how characters for interactive narrative systems can be built in the implementation level, the focus is on what should be in the knowledge base for virtual characters, and how it should be organized to be able to provide a convincing interaction with one or multiple characters.*

## 1. INTRODUCTION

The design and implementation of a non-trivial system where the user can interact with virtual characters via natural language or other modalities is still a creative challenge besides being an engineering task. This chapter aims to explain some issues that were encountered when designing and implementing dialogue systems for narrative purposes, especially the *VirtualHuman* system. *VirtualHuman* as a whole is quite large, as dialogue research projects go: about 25 people worked on it for its duration of four years. Not surprisingly, the number of issues and lessons learned is big and cannot be covered entirely. Therefore, we decided to limit the scope, and to talk about only a selected subset of issues that could – in our opinion – provide relevant and helpful cues for the reader who wants to work on the creation of future systems in that area. Also, during the course of discussion, some of the still numerous shortfalls will be described that still need to be addressed.

DOI: 10.4018/978-1-60960-617-6.ch007

After a general overview of related work in the area, the basic setup of *VirtualHuman* will be explained. The main matter of the chapter describes several important issues regarding the representation of the knowledge base for character design and control, and how they are addressed in the system to create an immersive and convincing interaction. The ideas and techniques presented here are not in any way meant to constitute definite or complete solutions. They should instead be taken as examples of how the issues they relate to can be approached and as food for thought to nudge towards further improvements.

## 2. BACKGROUND AND RELATED WORK

Most implementations in dialogue research are task-oriented systems intended to solve a clearly-defined problem, or to examine a given research topic. However, the less straightforward genre of virtual narratives is gaining importance and attention in the scientific community, and improved storytelling is also increasingly used in commercial software. Some design principles, including the basic modular approach for the *VirtualHuman* system, are derived from a line of task-oriented research systems, most prominently the *Verbmobil* and *SmartKom* systems.

One reason for the dominance of task-oriented systems, in addition to their applicability in many practical areas, might be that such interactions tend to be reasonably focused and predictable *practical dialogues* that are less complex than general dialogue (Jönsson, 1993). The domain – the task – can also usually be defined by formal means such as task completion criteria and limited sets of actions with pre-conditions and post-conditions that can achieve the goals of the interaction.

Task-oriented frameworks require rational agents that ideally help the user to get to the goal quickly and/or effectively. On the other hand, interactive narratives are more complicated and multifaceted. Good narratives will certainly require more elaborate language than purely task-focused prose. Also, a character acting in a narrative setting does not have to be rational; in a story, the main goal is to entertain users, and this above all requires that the interaction is *interesting* and the actors are *believable*. A character in a play can very well act in a decidedly irrational manner, as long as the audience can understand its motivations.

Following the increased interest, there is currently substantial research in the area of interactive narrative systems. Notable research systems include the *Mission Rehearsal Exercise*, a military emergency simulator (Swartout et al., 2006); the *FearNot* system, intended to train children to cope with bullying situations (Hall et al, 2006); and *Façade*, an enacting of a couple's breakup (Mateas & Stern, 2003). Commercial applications mainly fall into two categories, edutainment / instructional software and, of course, games.

A well-known example is the series *The Sims* that models the motivations of its simulated characters very similarly to the *BDI* (belief-desire-intention) paradigm originating from academic research (Rao & Georgeff, 1991). For current games, there is also a growing trend towards more serious and mature stories like the 2010 title *Heavy Rain*, which is a rather gloomy experience that emphasizes narrative depth and moral choices rather than striving for player satisfaction. However, commercial producers are not inclined to publish details about the inner workings of their software.

The perspective of the designer of the dialogue and the application content is often neglected in dialogue systems research. There are not many frameworks available that are ready to use for authors who are not specialists in the fields of linguistics or computer science. This has much to do with the fact that in research, system and content design is frequently done by members of the same team or even by the same person, usually being computer scientists or linguists rather than professional creative writers. Consequently, the available frameworks tend to not be very accessible for non-technical authors, because they require the use of unfamiliar specification methods, like state diagrams or expressions in predicate logic.

In the area of storytelling, some systems have emerged to address this shortcoming. One example is the *Erasmatron* system (Crawford, 1999) and the successor *Storytron*, designed for writers with non-technical background. The stories created by *Erasmatron* are emergent narratives without goal-based guidance. Also, built-in editors of games like *Quake* or *The Sims* can be employed to create animated stories with game engines (so-called "Machinima" movies). However, the plot of these stories is fixed in advance and allows few (if any) interactions from the user that could significantly affect the outcome of the story.

Some variation can be added by employing story generators such as the *SceneMaker* tool (Gebhard et al., 2003) that script stories by representing them as scenes connected by conditional transitions in scene graphs. A more integrated approach was used by the *Inscape* project that developed editors that allow designing story content and the environment in a graphical fashion (Göbel, Becker & Feix, 2005). These approaches generally do not implement a separation between the overall story structure and the interaction of the story participants.

## 3. THE EXAMPLE SYSTEM

### 3.1. Basic Setup of the VirtualHuman Scenario

*VirtualHuman* is a dialogue system that features up to three virtual characters interacting with two users. The setting is an "interactive narrative", which means that it is a kind of story that unfolds from the interaction between the human and virtual participants. In the first phase, two human users compete as contestants against each other in a live quiz about soccer. (see Figure 1)

To make things more interesting, the virtual characters take on different roles in the quiz and are not always interested to cooperate with each other. One character – the "moderator" – impersonates the quiz host and is responsible for guiding the interaction, the other two represent soccer experts with different background knowledge that have the task to assist the users in their guesses by giving them tips and advice. The experts do not like each other and both also have the intention to demonstrate that they are more knowledgeable than their counterpart. These three agents can be called the "actors" in the play and can pursue short-term goals and tasks. The unfolding of the story as a whole is overseen by a fourth (invisible) character, the so-called "director". The director is in control of the overall sequence of scenes and can at any stage of the play give sub-goal instructions to the actors to ensure that the purpose of the narrative is met. He can dynamically change the sequence of scenes or schedule new sub-interactions, for example, triggering an additional runoff question if the contestants are in a draw.

In the second phase, the winner of the quiz interacts with the moderator and one of the experts to compile an "ideal" lineup for the national soccer team against a given opponent. The user manipulates via speech and gesture the player positions on a virtual representation of a soccer field. The virtual characters comment on the decisions of the user, who can also ask the expert for advice. Each virtual character has an independent knowledge base: the soccer experts have individual (and different) opinions about, e.g., which soccer player is suitable for which position, while the moderator has no knowledge about soccer, but only the rules of the quiz.

On the technical side, the system comprises a set of modules that are dedicated to the separate tasks necessary for a multimodal dialogue system. They are loosely coupled by a blackboard archi-

*Figure 1. The VirtualHuman scenario: phase 1 (left) and phase 2 (right)*

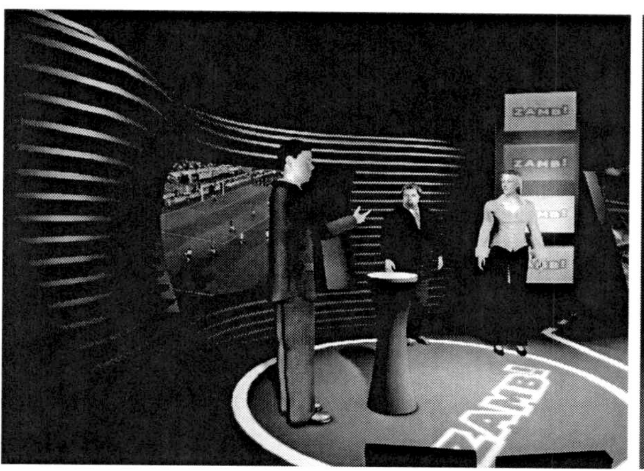

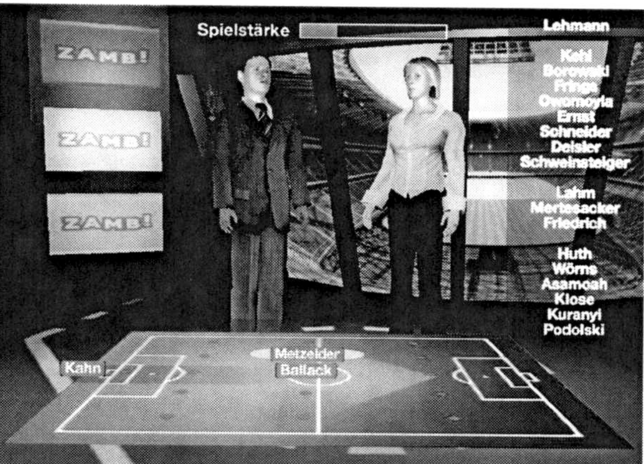


tecture that offers a publish/subscribe mechanism to distribute messages asynchronously.

The main processing, however, follows a pipeline succession that goes as follows: a set of multimodal recognizers gather user input in a parallel fashion. A module called FADE ("Fusion and Discourse Engine") manages the discourse context and uses it to "fuse" inputs in different modalities together to produce a modality-agnostic representation of a communicative act (Pfleger, 2007). It can also resolve references this way. Then, the conversation manager is a multi-agent system of so-called conversational dialogue engines (CDEs). Each CDE represents one of the characters with individual knowledge base and goals. Multimodal output from the conversation manager passes through a scheduler module that calls a TTS module to generate speech output and determines the precise relative timings of the contributions of the characters (speech, gestures, gaze, and posture data). Finally, a 3D presentation module renders the behavior of the characters. Besides the main pipeline, there is also a module called affect engine, which uses a model of the individual traits of the characters and the current interaction situation to compute the affective state of the characters in real-time.

The system was presented to the public on a number of occasions, e.g., as an exhibit at the CeBIT 2006 fair. Unfortunately, the *VirtualHuman* project did not include a formal evaluation to acquire recorded dialogues with a larger number of users to measure the quality of the realized interactions and user satisfaction.

## 3.2. The Designer's Perspective

The most important question that has to be examined when designing a conversational agent for a planned system is what the system will be used for, and what the role of the agent will be. The initial assessment of the designer, especially concerning the second part, will also probably be re-examined several times during the realization, and especially during the test phase.

If the designer is not self-honest in this regard, or the system design is too inflexible, it can lead to suboptimal results and dissatisfied users. It is not difficult to think of instances of conversational agents that failed. One of the most well-known examples is *Clippy*, a cartoon character that was created to provide personalized assistance in *Microsoft Office 97* products. *Clippy* received many strongly adverse reactions from users that

*Figure 2. The interaction triangle*

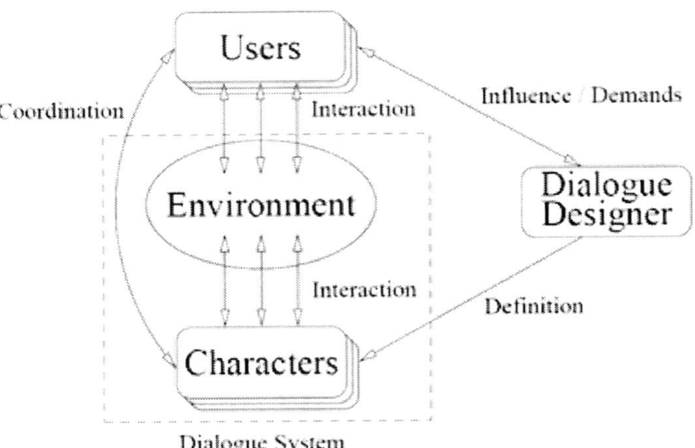


perceived it as annoying, interruptive, and generally unhelpful (Swartz, 2003).

Ideally, the quality of an agent concept should be assessed together with all elements that contribute to the interface of the system as a whole. The depiction in Figure 2 illustrates this overall context in an "Interaction Triangle". The system itself comprises the virtual characters together with the environment they are situated in. This does not necessarily require that the characters are in a 3D environment or even embodied. The environment could also be an interactive web page or maybe just a command line.

It is not confined to the screen, but comprises all available channels of communication, including speech via loudspeakers and microphones and possibly other modalities, such as mouse input. The main point is that the interactions between users and characters go *via* some shared environment that the interacting parties can observe. The communication effects that the actions of users and characters can be coordinated to arrive at the goals of the interaction. The job of the dialogue designer is to cater to the demands of the users by defining the parameters of the system. The relation goes the other way, too, since the actual setup of the system also influences the expectations and possibilities of the user in return.

A useful technique to gather user expectations and to evaluate their opinion about the system as early as in the design stage is to conduct so-called *Wizard-of-Oz Experiments*: a mockup of the (not yet implemented) system as planned is created that is controlled by a (hidden) human operator. Test users – who may or may not be aware of the simulated nature of the system – conduct an interaction with the mockup, and the operator uses a "script sheet" that maps expected user inputs to system reactions, to simulate the system (including the behavior of the conversational agent). The results of such an experiment that was conducted for the *SmartKom* system are described in (Schiel & Türk, 2006).

Beyond the imperative "do not annoy the user", there are some guidelines that the designer can use, depending on the domain. The subject matter of the following sections covers three fields located in the lower half of the Interaction Triangle: modeling the knowledge base (the "definition" arc), action planning with building blocks and expectations (how the characters operate), and realizing a convincing interaction with one or multiple characters including perception filtering (the "interaction" arc between the characters and the environment).

Figure 3. Knowledge types for virtual characters

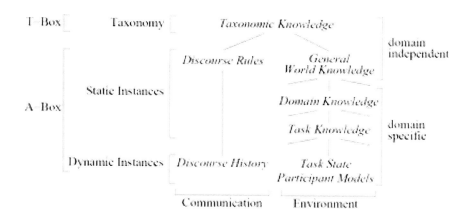


## 4. REPRESENTING AND USING KNOWLEDGE

### 4.1. The Knowledge Base

The knowledge base of the system has to be represented in some formal way. In the past, it was common practice to design custom representations tailored to the concrete system at hand. In the wake of the Semantic Web, it becomes increasingly attractive to employ an ontological representation. While the basic effort might seem greater, besides the inferential power this has the advantage of being able to rely on standardized representation languages, such as RDF(S) and OWL, and upper model ontologies that may already provide a set of pre-defined basic concepts that can be reused.

A dialogue designer needs to deal with several kinds of knowledge in order to encode the character definitions and their contributions. In most cases, the knowledge modeling and management task is made easier by the possibility to separate resources along module boundaries: speech interpretation rules should not have much influence in the dialog manager, and a presentation module should not need to know the planned dialogue structure. For the design of virtual characters, four types of knowledge are central: character (or more generally, participant) models, interaction elements, world and domain knowledge and task knowledge.

Knowledge types can be organized in a hierarchy (see Figure 3). Parts of the hierarchy can be realized independently of the domain (and therefore re-used across systems), for example, dialogue act types such as *Question* or *Answer* are near-universal. As can be seen in the figure, there also is a distinction between static and dynamic instances of information items. Static instances constitute the background knowledge and thus define the system setup. Dynamic instances are created depending on the interaction, while the system is running, and represent the so-called *information state* of the system.

The information state is a store of items with semantic content that describe the state of the world in general and the dialogue in particular from the point of view of the system. As the interaction progresses, new information becomes available (e.g., the utterances made by the participants and their content), and the system adds it to the information state by an "update" operation (Traum & Larsson, 2003). Several approaches for update are in use: simple overwriting fails at preserving old information, and unification does not deal gracefully with conflicts between new and old information.

For many cases, a better solution is using *overlay*, an operation similar to default unification (Alexandersson & Becker, 2001). This operation allows merging new information while preserving pre-existing background information that does not conflict. A model that represents an individual character will usually consist of static as well as dynamic parts to capture both rigid personality traits that are stable across interactions, and aspects that can be changed via the information state update, such as affective state and information the character gathers from the dialogue.

Discourse rules define which types of interaction are possible, and what their effects are. On the most basic level, this comprises a set of atomic actions characters (or the users) can do. The units used to represent dialogue actions on this level are generally called *dialogue acts*, but when the focus is on multimodal interaction, this can be extended to include acts in other modalities such as gestures, facial expressions, and so on, resulting in a set of *communicative acts*.

The dialogue act set is an open set, and what exact information should be encoded in an act is also an open research question in the field of dialogue act theory (cf. Traum, 2000). In practice, for a given system the available dialogue (and communicative) acts and their content are often defined *ad hoc* with regard to the interactions the system is intended to exhibit. Examples of "typical" dialogue acts are *Inform* (giving information to another participant, stating a fact encoded in the content) and *Question* (requesting information about something encoded in the content).

Some communicative acts can easily be realized in a non-linguistic modality (or several modalities combined), for example a *Greeting* or an *Apology*. In *VirtualHuman*, the modality distinction was abandoned altogether for dialogue management, resulting in modality-agnostic processing in this module. However, other parts of the system, such as discourse modeling and presentation, can sometimes make use of the modality information (e.g., the presentation module may prefer to use the same modality in an output utterance that was used in the input).

The boundaries between world and task knowledge is not as clear-cut. The world knowledge of a character, in the concrete example of the soccer quiz, includes personal information about soccer players, their preferred playing positions, strengths and weaknesses etc. together with some trivia that are used to enable the expert characters to make more colorful comments. The task knowledge is more on the procedural side and defines how the different stages of the virtual narrative should proceed. An example for this is a rule "there will be two quiz turns to determine a winner, followed by a decision round if there is a draw."

In systems with multiple computer-controlled characters, it is sensible to let each character have a separate, individual knowledge base to reflect different beliefs and opinions. However, the basic concepts and their taxonomic order must be compatible for all characters to enable mutual understanding (however, in a narrative context, an author could deliberately make use of differing world views to produce, e.g., an "emergent comedy of errors" or other intentional misunderstanding effect).

## 4.2. Modeling Character Personality Traits

For a satisfying experience with virtual characters, it is not enough to get their "dialogue lines" right. Beyond recital, the job of a human actor is to tailor their entire behavior to match the requirements of their role, including posture, prosody, gestures, and many other means of expression. Apart from the situational context of a particular scene, this behavior is on the most basic level parameterized by the personality structure of the character, which an actor is supposed to emulate.

To achieve good results with a virtual actor, there has therefore to be a model of the personality traits of the character it is to play, a way to influence it depending on the situation, and means to express relevant aspects for the audience. A relatively straightforward way to avoid much of the modeling is to directly specify the desired expressions beforehand; but this approach is not very flexible and can be difficult to manage. For example, in the role-playing game *Oblivion*, characters use dialogues that were pre-recorded by voice actors that did their best to use appropriate prosody. However, the overall number of speech snippets is quite large and presumably ones appearing in the same scene were not always recorded in one session.

As a result, it may happen during the course of one interaction that a character's prosody switches from, e.g., a relaxed conversation tone to a rather angry one and back for no apparent reason, which hurts the experience of the player. Given the proper tools, a more flexible approach is to maintain a dynamically updated model of the character's state, and to use it to parameterize its behavior. Such tools are available for a number of modalities, including speech prosody, facial expression, body posture and dynamically generated gestures.

Especially for characters that are meant to possess and express some depth, such as the roles in a virtual performance, the modeling of personality traits can influence strongly how they are perceived by the user, provided that the character also has the means to show them via the interaction or other behavior. In *VirtualHuman*, the characters can exhibit affective state such as anger, anxiety, and joy (see Figure 4).

The kind and the intensity of affect change as a reaction to events happening in the interaction is parameterized using an approach following the so-called *OCEAN* model from psychology: five numerical factors expressing values for openness, conscientiousness, extroversion, agreeableness, and neuroticism define the "affect personality" of the character, and position its "neutral mood" in a space spanned by those five dimensions. An event that occurs in the interaction can be interpreted as exerting a force given by a combination of *OCEAN* values, changing the mood of the character temporarily (e.g., making it angry); however, after some time the mood will drift back to the "neutral position". An elaborate description on affect modeling using this scheme can be found in (Gebhard, 2007).

## 5. THE CHARACTERS IN INTERACTION

### 5.1. Action Planning and Story Control

Action planning means the procedure that decides on the actions of the characters and triggers their execution in a coordinated fashion. Each character has a repertoire of action types it can perform. According to the current goals, actions need to be instantiated with parameters and performed in a meaningful order, respecting constraints if there are any. A main distinction here is the structure of the action plans, and how they are generated and selected.

- *Direct mapping*: this is a basic approach that is only suitable for very simple domains with little structure and dependence on context.
- A *state-based* action planner represents the domain in a graph of states with connecting transition edges. Edges can be traversed, leading to another state, given that their associated conditions are fulfilled. Such conditions can come in different forms from literal user input to logical assertions. The main context in this case is the state the system is currently in.
- *Plan-based*: this approach describes the task in logical terms and gives operators with preconditions and postconditions that change the state of the virtual world when applied. For a given task represented by a logical goal description, a planner can be used to devise an action plan consisting of

*Figure 4. On the left: Expert Kaiser in self-confident vs. docile posture; on the right: Expert Lebacher with friendly vs. angry facial expression*

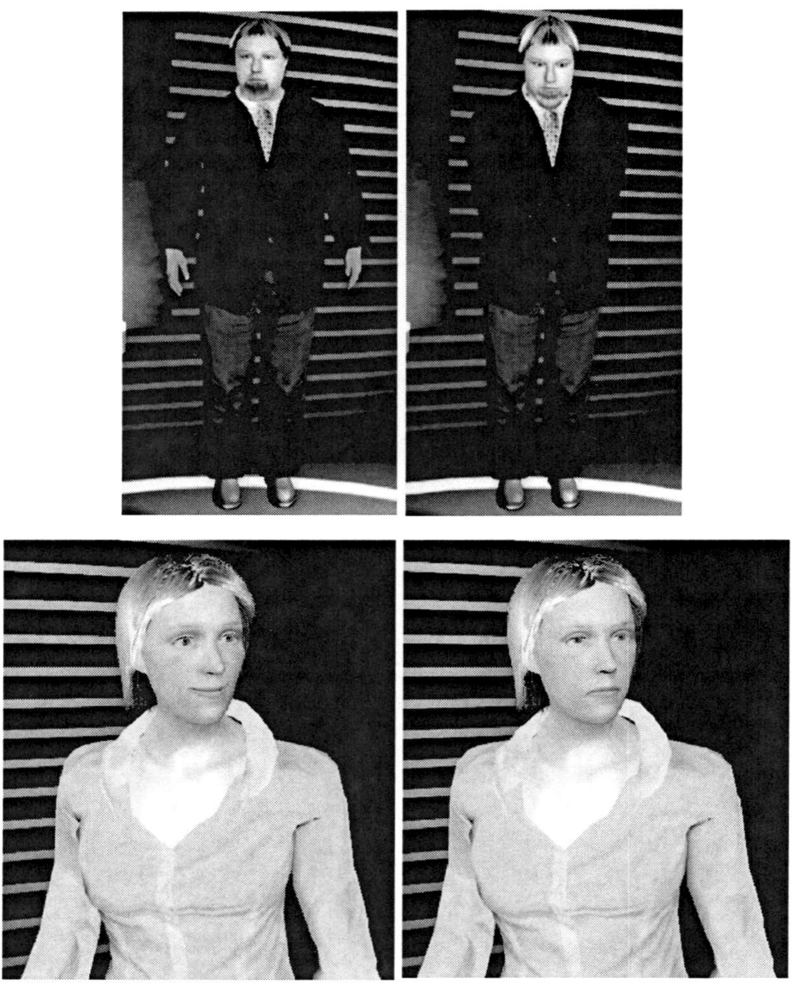

a sequence of operators that leads to the goal.

- *Recipe-based*: this is similar to the plan-based approach, with the exception that the action plans are not computed dynamically. Instead, the system has a library of pre-made plans, called "recipes" that can be applied depending on the situation.

Depending on the complexity of the task, different action planning methods are suitable, and the dialogue designer needs to be aware of their respective capabilities and shortcomings. For example, state-based approaches are very common for interactive narratives. The downside is that more complex stories can comprise many states, and if they are strongly connected, the number of transitions can grow very large (exponentially), leading to a representation that is difficult to understand and manage.

In some cases, it can be a good idea to combine several approaches for different aspects of the system to exploit their relative strengths in different areas. *VirtualHuman* uses such a hybrid approach.

Character deliberations on the highest level (the activity level) are done via planning. The atomic operators used by the planner are *dialogue games*, which themselves are a kind of recipe-based formalism (Hulstijn, 2000) to determine a sequence of dialogue acts. That way, it is not necessary to execute (computationally expensive) full planning all the way; instead, the dialogue game recipes can be used as larger building blocks. For simple reactions that need to happen quickly, such as gazing at another participant in response to being talked at, the characters use a direct mapping approach. The action planning approach in *VirtualHuman* is described in (Löckelt, 2005) and in more detail in (Löckelt, 2008).

During the character design process, some thought should be given to the matter of what the atomic building blocks of action on several levels of interaction for the characters should be. The larger the building blocks are, the less work must be done during execution for assembling and scheduling the course of action. The building blocks should also be parameterizable to allow versatile reuse. For example, proper reusable building blocks for James Bond stories should include the *Evil Villain Confrontation* activity (parameterized by villain, planned execution method for Bond, means of escape) which triggers (among others) the subordinate dialogue game *Evil Speech* (parameters: evil plan, James Bond's witty response) which in turn triggers (among others) a sequence of *Statement* dialogue acts used by the villain to explain the evil plan to James Bond.

It is important to ensure that the characters can achieve the story goals, even if the user actively works against them (which will be quite often the case). Task-oriented dialogue systems can afford to have a more straightforward approach to interaction control. If the goal of the interaction is to solve a particular, well-defined task in cooperation with the user, usually there exists a single best-suited subtask to address at each point in the interaction. This also lends itself to one-sided initiative: either the user states at each point what s/he wants to do next, or the system directs the interaction because it knows "what has to come next".

In addition, it is in the best interest of users in such a context to act cooperatively. Interactive narratives, by their nature, allow more freedom and action alternatives almost by definition. The audience wants to participate and influence how the story goes; otherwise the "interactive" part would not make much sense after all. To summarize, while task-oriented interaction aims to arrive at previously defined goals – as fast and efficient as possible – and interactive narratives are more about managing the (voluntary) branching in the storyline. Ensuring that the story comes to a sensible end necessitates preventing that the user jeopardizes the story goals. One option to achieve this is to prevent story-breaking actions by the user, or changing their outcome. Some techniques for this are described in (Riedl & Stern, 2006).

In the *VirtualHuman* system, an approach was adopted that divides the task of story control between the individual characters and a "supervisor", also known as the director. The goals of the narrative are placed into three categories: one or more main goals (e.g., finish a quiz phase), intermediate goals (e.g., moderate a quiz turn with several participants) and small sub-goals (e.g., get an answer from one participant). The director observes the state of the interaction and sets main goals in order to ensure that the storyline proceeds as planned, and that the high-level intermediate goals of the interaction can be met. The characters receive goals on the intermediate level from the director to that end and devise their own subordinate plans for the sub-goals individually.

In this approach, the characters can act with local knowledge and motivation and it is not necessary to burden them with knowledge about dramatic necessities. Technically, the director is realized as just another character: it gives its directions by exchanging communicative acts with the other characters – in this case, it orders to adopt goals and feedback about success or failure to accomplish goals. The main difference is that the user can not perceive the director, since it has no virtual body and its contributions are not rendered in the environment.

The logic for the director's actions can be implemented in a number of ways. In the main *VirtualHuman* system, the director module is based on a state machine where different states represent different dramatic situations (scenes), and transitions between states are dependent on conditions (such as "user has answered all the questions"). This is similar to the *SceneMaker* approach (cf. Gebhard et al. (2003)). In the student-created spin-off system *Clue*, the story is represented by plan operators, and the director uses the JSHOP planner to decide the next scene (Gholamsaghaee, 2006).

## 5.2. Realizing a Convincing Interaction

The acceptance of a system is strongly dependent on coherent behavior. Especially if virtual characters are involved, or the system purports to have a "personality", it must act believably. This does not necessarily have to mean that a character's actions have to be logically consistent, or human-like. The main requirement is that the character's behavior be plausible given the information (or mental image) the user has about its inner life. This can lead to situations where a character that is less humanlike is actually more believable when exhibiting a certain behavior, namely in the case of *asymmetric interaction*.

It is frustrating to encounter a dialogue system that uses elaborate "canned" text, which leads to the expectation that it actually can engage in free conversation, only to earn repeated misunderstandings when it turns out that the understanding is not up to par with generation. As a rule, a sensible user today does *not* really assume to be interacting with an agent that is intelligent on a human level. It is important, however, that a mental model can be constructed to enable the user to have some idea of what can reasonably be expected from the agent.

To support believability in a narrative context, it is crucial to be able to *express* actions and emotions in addition to the task of *selecting* them. To recall an observation from the background section: for behavior to be suitable for a narrative character, it must be *consistent* and *interesting* instead of *effective* (Doyle, 2002). An additional issue contributing to believability is the variety of utterances a character is able to produce. Like what was said about interaction asymmetry, it can be acceptable to use a uniform utterance schema across cases that are similar. This is especially true for task-oriented systems. It can even be beneficial in this case to strive for a simplified, predictable, and unambiguous interaction, since the user can concentrate on the task and is not distracted. On the other hand, in systems that are predominantly meant to entertain, poor variation and overly plain language harms the atmosphere and believability. The emphasis with such systems is not on conveying information in the most efficient and reliable way.

Depending on the purpose of a system, user immersion has varying degrees of importance from crucial for acceptance to irrelevant. Part of the requirements for immersion is that the user experiences a sense of agency, that is, the actions of the user have a manifest effect on the environment. Narrative systems with life-like virtual characters also rely to some degree on the *Eliza Effect*, i.e., that the user implicitly assumes their actions to be guided by motives and thinking processes similar to a human's. The contributions of the dialogue partner(s) must be adequate (in the sense of the *maxims* proposed by (Grice, 1975) in the conversation, i.e., exhibit the right degree of informativeness, be relevant and clear, and be founded on an understanding by the system.

Narrative systems that try to produce adequate feedback solely for atmospheric purposes, even on user input that was not understood properly, are in danger of failing miserably, like in the following example of an interaction with the *Eliza* system gone awry:

**USER:** Like I said earlier, I hate the rain.
**ELIZA:** Why do you like you said earlier, you hate the rain?
**USER:** What do you mean?
**ELIZA:** Please elaborate on that.

After just a brief interaction, such behavior results in the immersion-shattering realization that the "understanding" exhibited by this system is really just an illusion. In most task-oriented interactions, immersion does not play a major role. It can also be explicitly undesired in some situations, e. g., during interaction with a dialogue-enabled route-planning application in a moving car.

The appearance of the character is also a major factor for its acceptance, depending on the application. A naturalistic rendition will generate different expectations than a comic-like character. Figure 5 shows three types of virtual characters: Ms Dewey, the front-end of a Microsoft search engine prototype, Mr Kaiser from *VirtualHuman*, and *Smartakus*, the system agent of the *SmartKom* system. While the effect was not verified formally, anecdotal evidence suggests that with the more naturalistic Ms Dewey, users assumed (wrongly) that they could use natural language input, and were disappointed. However, faced with the "cuteness" and simple depiction of *Smartakus*, users had lower expectations and were more forgiving of speech recognition and understanding failures, since their mental model of *Smartakus* takes into account that he is "only a computer character".

Another straightforward requirement for a natural and comfortable interaction is a decent reaction time of the virtual characters. For task-oriented systems, a rule-of-thumb is that a reaction should not take more than about 0.1 seconds to be perceived as instantaneous; delays below 1.0 seconds are noticed as a delay, but still preserve the feeling of a relatively free interaction (Miller, 1968). This does not mean that a character needs to produce an *answer* in that time, but it should be recognizable that the system received an input and is working on it. This can be signaled via a short acknowledgement by the character, or via body language (e.g., gaze and posture) while the input is processed by the dialogue manager.

## 5.3. Habitability

The notion of *habitability* of a dialogue system's interaction was coined by Arne Jönsson (1997). It refers to the problem that the user interacting via natural language input does not know *a priori*

*Figure 5. Different degrees of realism in virtual characters: Ms Dewey (taken from now defunct website www.msdewey.com), Mr Kaiser, and Smartakus.*

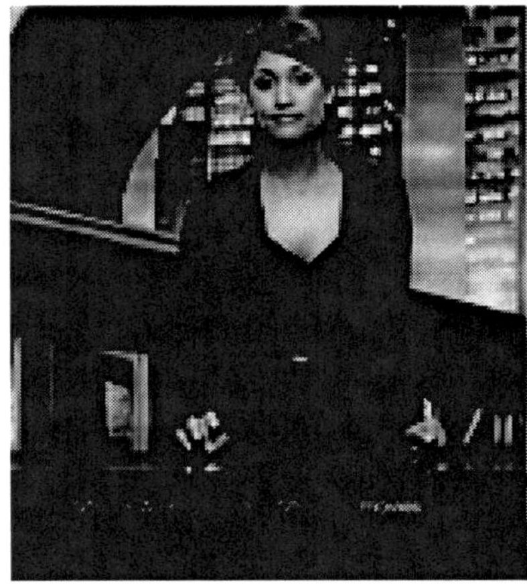
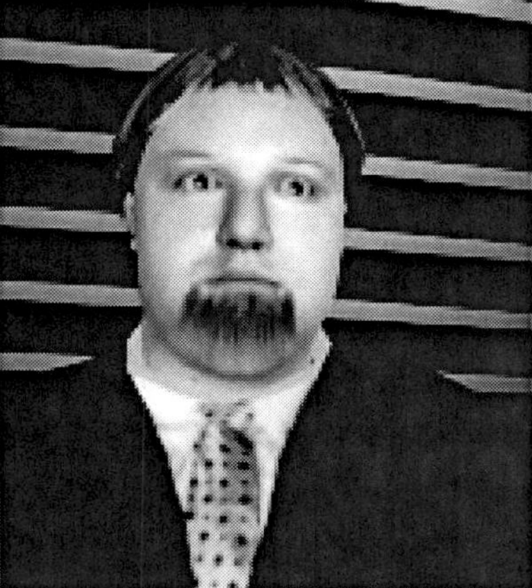
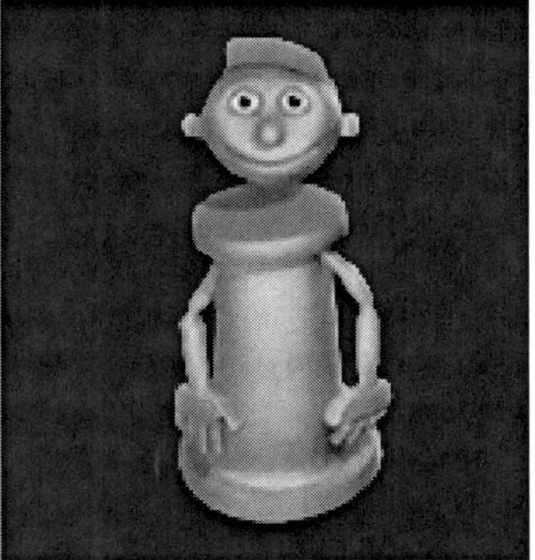

what kind of utterances can be processed by the system. If the system's vocabulary or grammar are too limited and unknown to the user, s/he will frequently be forced to guess what to say to convey his/her intention, and be frustrated by repeated feedback like "I didn't understand you, could you please reformulate". The same can happen if the actual capabilities of the system are unclear, or dependent on context in non-obvious ways. A habitable system will employ some means to ensure that the user can feel comfortable that he will be understood correctly, and to convey what is possible in the interaction overall. The system should *"clearly show the user which actions it is able to perform, which initiatives it can respond to, which it cannot respond to, and why this is the case."* (Jönsson, 1993). How can habitability be achieved without extensively training the users?

One solution for this problem, which was used in early adventure games, is to offer only a limited set of interactions that the user can learn before using the system or look up during the interaction in, e.g., a help menu, but such a method is not comfortable to use and might also conflict with storytelling goals by unintentionally giving away story details *("why is 'open hidden trapdoor' there in the input list?")*. The other extreme, trying to understand every input, is not feasible with current state-of-the-art speech recognition. A suitable "middle road" is to cover some sensible set of inputs, and to give the user the chance to know or find out what they are. The dialogue designer can collect test data with users during development, use collected input on previous similar systems, or use data obtained from "Wizard of Oz" experiments even before the realization of the system has begun.

An interesting and powerful, but in many cases too elaborate technique that can be used is the principle of *no generation without interpretation*: if everything the system produces as "spoken" output also constitutes a valid input, this can help the user to quickly get a feeling for the capabilities of the system by simply interacting with it, and adapting the inputs accordingly. That technique can be applied to the grammatical structure as well as the vocabulary of the output. Its comprehensive application also has downsides: if the system uses more elaborate language and uncommon vocabulary for storytelling effect, "no generation without interpretation" can result in rather baroque grammar rules and an overabundance of lexical entries. Fortunately, taking a middle road of selectively preferring outputs that could also be understood, or incorporating rare vocabulary occurring prominently in the story into the system's lexicon already yields benefits for the dialogue designer.

Habitability is also improved if the system deals gracefully with errors (application failures as well as understanding problems), offers help for inexperienced users, or has means to dynamically adapt to different interaction styles. Additionally, systems can to a certain degree support the user's imagination by adhering to the *principle of least surprise* via consistent dialogue design: even when the system cannot achieve human competence in conversation, it should be possible to predict from past interactions which kind of utterances will probably be understood by the system. For interactive narratives, habitability is possibly even more important than for task-oriented systems, because a lack of it can have a strong adverse effect on immersion of the user or destroy it altogether.

## 5.4. Turn Taking and Floor Management

When more than two participants are present, the distribution of the right to speak – also called *floor management* in dialogue research – becomes more complicated. The basic problem is that speech is an exclusive channel, i.e., if more than one participant speaks at the same time, the quality of the communication channel deteriorates sharply, or can even break down altogether.

Other modalities of communication are not exclusive, e.g., it is not problematic if several participants use gestures at the same time. In a multimodal system, there exist several different communication channels which may possess different degrees of exclusivity, so several communication strands can occur simultaneously on different channels. As in human-human communication, the gesture channel can be used during the turn of another participant to indicate a request for the permission to speak. If one participant has the right to use the speech channel, s/he "holds the floor".

There are several ways for a participant to obtain the floor. The most "polite" way is that either the current speaker explicitly assigns the floor to someone (and subsequently finishes speaking him/herself), or a speaker ends his/her contribution – "releases the floor" – allowing any other participant to pick up the thread of the conversation, or start a new topic. In any case, it is commonplace in natural communication to send signals that one wants to obtain the floor. This can be done by, e.g., seeking eye contact, waving a hand etc. This creates a social obligation for the speaker to consider releasing the turn as soon as it is convenient (although the strength of the obligation can vary greatly according to the social situation).

In *VirtualHuman*, the characters use gestures to signal the desire to speak (see Figure 6) and may repeat them after some time if they do not get the turn upon the first try. Gestures can be produced by characters at any time, while speech output is limited to one character at a time.

*Figure 6. Two virtual characters "fighting" for the right to talk*

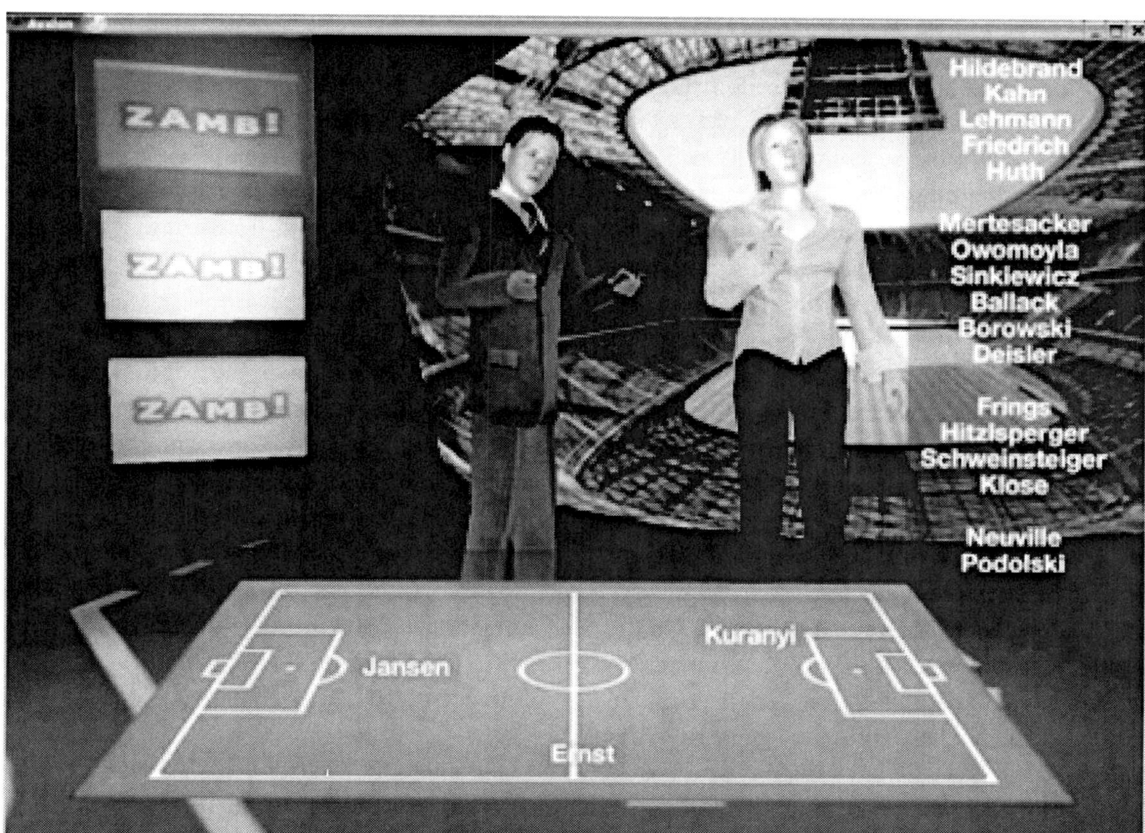

It is of course possible to avoid asynchronous contributions by virtual characters and the floor management problems between them by system design, at the cost of some "naturalness". However, it is not that easy to do the same for the users, if they are free to interact at any time. How to deal with the phenomena of "barge-in" (the user interrupts during a system utterance) and "barge-before" (the user interrupts while a system utterance is being generated) is still an active field of research.

## 5.5. Realization Scheduling

There is a fundamental difference between users and virtual characters with regard to how they are informed about the dialogue contributions and other events in the scenario. Characters send and receive their messages in a semantically-encoded form, while human users generate multimodal input messages (microphone, mouse, etc.) and receive multimodal output messages (via the screen, loudspeakers, etc.). To bridge the gap between human users and virtual characters, the human input must be converted to semantic messages for the characters, but in addition to this, the contributions of characters must also be conveyed in *two* forms: as semantic messages for other characters, and as multimodal (output) messages to be explicitly *realized* for the users in human-observable form.

The question is at what point should a virtual character react to an utterance? Theoretically, the character could react almost instantly, when the realization has just started and the user has not had any chance to know what the reaction is about, since processing a semantic message can be very fast. Clearly, this is not a good approach. On the other hand, waiting until the whole utterance is completely realized also is not very natural. In human interaction, an addressee generally has understood the gist of what a dialogue partner is saying well before the end of the utterance.

In *VirtualHuman*, a "trick" is used to make character reaction times seem more natural. Before realization, the TTS module computes the exact duration of the generated speech output. The different gestures are contained in a gesture lexicon, the *gesticon* that (among other data) also specifies the duration of each gesture. A scheduler module uses this information to create a realization schedule with artificial delays. Based upon experimentation, it was decided to use a heuristic assumption that gestures are recognized immediately, while spoken utterances are understood after two thirds of their duration. Clearly, this is only a rough measure that can sometimes yield bad results, and will be completely off the mark for very long utterances, for example. Fortunately, the utterances occurring in that system are relatively short, and the effect can be improved by applying the heuristic one sentence at a time.

Figure 7 illustrates the principle using the example of a dialogue between the moderator and one of the expert characters that is accompanied with gestures. After the moderator's utterance is "understood", there is a short delay while the expert processes the content. Next, the expert decides to answer, but first has to obtain the floor. This request is denied, since there still is an ongoing utterance; the expert accordingly produces a turn-grabbing gesture: she raises a hand; the moderator will react with a gaze immediately – while speaking – via the parallel "direct mapping" of the dialogue act created by this action. After the utterance is finished, there is a short pause, and then the expert again tries to obtain permission to speak, which is granted, whereupon she can proceed with her utterance. The effect of this scheduling procedure creates a quite natural impression of a smooth transition of speaking turns with "natural" pauses.

## 5.6. Perception Filtering

In the interactive narrative *Clue* that was realized as a student project using the same framework as *VirtualHuman*, an issue with unwanted "om-

*Figure 7. Different realization times for speech and gestures*

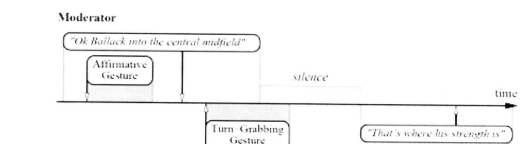

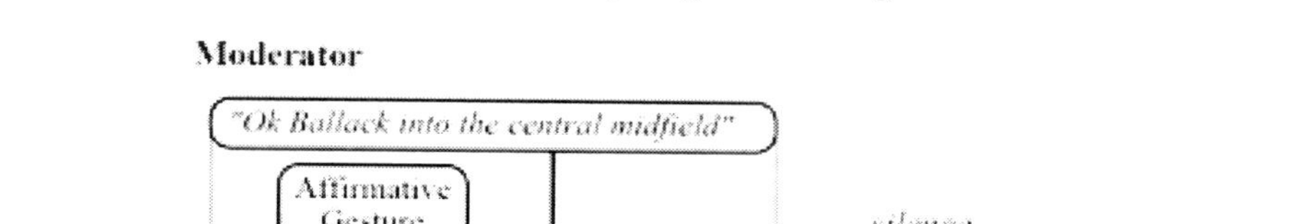


nipresence" appeared. The setup for this system includes four virtual characters that move around in several interconnected rooms to try to solve a murder that occurs at the beginning of the story (actually, one of the characters is the murderer, who obviously tries to cover up evidence instead). There is no previously fixed storyline, and an element of chance influences the selection of the problem-solving strategy each character adopts at different stages of the interaction. The result is an "emergent" narrative that can lead to several different endings.

In the original *VirtualHuman* scenario, the representations of utterances and events are broadcast to all virtual characters (and realized for the users). The individual character then has to determine whether it should produce a reaction. In this modified version, when characters are located in different rooms, it is not plausible that everyone should be able to perceive everything that happens all the time. A straightforward way to address this would be, for example, to send the respective messages only to characters in the same room; however, for *Clue*, it was decided to aim for a more generalized solution called *perception filtering*.

Each character is assigned an individual environmental filter that determines whether messages are perceived or ignored based on their content and context. Provided the messages contain the relevant information, some of the possibilities for such filtering are:

- *Distance-based*: the difficulty to understand a speaker that is far away can be modeled by a probability function that is exponentially deteriorating with distance. This requires information about the spatial positions of speaker and hearer.
- *Orientation-based*: a character can be restricted to only "visually" perceive events that are within its field of view.
- *Noise-based*: if there is background noise, this can lower the probability of understanding a message (alternatively, random errors can be introduced via a probability measure).
- Other environmental factors that can contribute are, e.g., darkness, "impairment" of the character, or any logical condition (e.g., a character is unable perceive an object in a closed container).

This technique allows a more fine-grained control over the perception of the participants. Factors such as the affective state of the characters can also be used to influence a perception filter: for example, if a character is in a state that lowers concentration – such as, being enraged – the filter can adjust the perception threshold dynamically in real-time, and even take into account the "amount" of rage. In *Clue*, a simple distance-based and a condition-based filter were implemented.

## 6. FUTURE RESEARCH DIRECTIONS

The described area of dialogue system research is very much in motion, with lots of issues to be addressed. This section gives a list of some of the most important challenges:

- *Better support for the (possibly non-technical) dialogue designer:* this involves adopting a knowledge base and story representation that is expressive enough and yet computationally feasible. Also, it is difficult and cumbersome to actually write down the knowledge for characters; especially for dialogue designers that ideally should rather be creative writers instead of computer scientists or ontology experts. Therefore, a potentially very useful area of research is the development of editing tools that allow bridging the gap between the (abstract and non-technical) creation of story structure and content and the technical realization of the story. This includes all kinds of secondary questions, such as "how can the story writer ensure that the user does not jeopardize the story development by unforeseen actions?" Some approaches concerning dialogue designer support were mentioned in the background and action planning sections.
- *Increased reusability:* there is still no generally accepted paradigm for dialogue specification that allows for easy re-use. The same is true for the specification of storylines or character traits. As a consequence of this, new dialogue systems and interactive narratives still tend to be constructed "from scratch" each time. Some progress has been made for knowledge base construction: upper-level ontologies such as SUMO (Niles & Pease, 2001) provide a starting point for domain definitions.
- *Better testing possibilities:* the search space of possible inputs in a non-trivial dialogue system is generally very large and may even be infinite. To make matters worse, the system's reaction to an input is not necessarily always the same, but may be dependent on the whole history of previous inputs and sometimes an element of chance (mainly in the case of storytelling). Therefore, to validate the correctness of such a system will be quite time-consuming and difficult or, in the worst case, impossible. Several methods to alleviate this are in use, such as controlled user tests (both on completed systems and in "Wizard-of-Oz" setups that can already be employed in the design stage) and automatic "noise" tests, but there is definitely a lot of room for improvement. A current effort in this area is described in (Scheffler et al., 2009).
- *Better – but realistic – reasoning capabilities:* believable characters should have the capability to understand and react to a wide range of user utterances and actions, even if they are out-of-context or otherwise unexpected. However, improvements in this regard can come at a crippling price in terms of computational tractability. The dialogue designer must decide what the characters should be capable of, and find a balance between the extremes of rigidly scripted behavior and, e.g., using fully-fledged theorem proving (which can be very powerful, but also very resource-hungry) to determine the course of action. If ontological knowledge representations are used, a possibility is to use subsets of full predicate logic such as description logics (DL) that are designed to be more "computation-friendly" (Nardi & Brachman, 2002).

- *Improved character groups:* an interesting and challenging topic is modeling larger and heterogenous groups of characters. In such groups, the behavior is influenced by a multitude of factors, such as roles, social status, or how well interacting members know each other. Dialogues may be nested and intertwined in many ways. Characters can cooperate to achieve joint tasks, which involves whole new types of interaction (e.g., negotiation and planning dialogues). Some challenges of managing character groups are analyzed in (Traum, 2004).
- *Parallel execution:* the simultaneous management of tasks and conversation threads is still a big challenge. Most current systems lack mechanisms for dynamic task suspension and reuptake and, correspondingly, a sophisticated scheduling and prioritization regime. This is especially important if a system has to mediate between multiple back-end applications, and of course in the case of multi-party interaction, where conversation strands concerning different topics may be interleaved or temporarily suspended. This problem was analyzed for robot conversations in (Lemon et al., 2002).

Apart from these rather specific challenges, it would in our opinion be very beneficial to aim for more intensive interdisciplinary collaboration with fields like theater science, literature science, and psychology in the development of interactive narratives. Dialogue systems tend to be designed and written mainly by more technically-minded people without involvement of storytellers or dramatists – a fact which, among other things, has to do with the lack of accessible tools mentioned above. Often, this is showing in the results in a negative way. On the other hand, some concepts from other disciplines have been included in interactive narratives with good results, e.g. the psychological OCEAN model for affective modeling (Gebhard, 2007) or Propp's analysis of the structure of the folk tale (Garzotto & Rizzo, 2005).

## CONCLUSION

This chapter provided a rough overview of several important aspects of virtual character design and examined some implementation issues that are relevant for providing a convincing interaction. To sum up the lessons learned from *VirtualHuman* to a few rules of thumb:

- **Design the knowledge base incrementally and iteratively**. It is a good idea to start building a large dialogue specification, as well as character models, by beginning with a rough and partial model and subsequently refining it. To avoid having to change the program each time, the knowledge base should be as declarative as possible.
- **Invest in character modeling**. This includes their background knowledge, but also their affective state. Believable motivations and emotions add a lot of color to the characters – but they need to have ways to express them, too.
- **Identify, use and reuse building blocks for activities, interactions, and dialogue acts**. Many character subtasks are quite similar, can be hierarchically ordered, and their basic structure will reappear in different places of the interaction. You should avoid having to remodel them time after time.
- **Make the system "habitable"**. A system that leaves the user guessing what to say is a frustrating system. *Wizard-of-Oz* experiments are a good source of information for this, even when the system is not implemented yet.
- **Do not let the story get out of control.** Use techniques like a "virtual director",

preventing actions detrimental to the story goals, or changing their outcome.

- **Look out for dialogue phenomena that make the interaction more natural**, comfortable, or convincing, and seek ways to emulate them. Examples for relevant techniques are perception filtering, realization scheduling, and floor management.

## REFERENCES

Alexandersson, J., & Becker, T. (2001). Overlay as the basic operation for discourse processing in a multimodal dialogue system. In *Proceedings of the IJCAI Workshop on Knowledge and Reasoning in Practical Dialogue Systems* (pp. 8–14), Seattle, WA.

Crawford, C. (1999). Assumptions underlying the Erasmatron interactive storytelling engine. In M. Mateas & P. Sengers (Eds.), *Proceedings of the AAAI Fall Symposium: Narrative Intelligence* (pp. 112–114). Menlo Park, CA.

Doyle, P. (2002). Believability through context using knowledge in the world to create intelligent characters. In *Proceedings of the First International Joint Conference on Autonomous Agents and Multiagent Systems* (pp. 342-349). New York, NY.

Garzotto, F., & Rizzo, F. (2005). The MUST tool: Exploiting Propp's theory. In P. Kommers & G. Richards (Eds.), *Proceedings of World Conference on Educational Multimedia, Hypermedia and Telecommunications 2005* (pp. 3887-3893). Chesapeake, VA, USA.

Gebhard, P. (2007). *Emotionalisierung interaktiver virtueller Charaktere - ein mehrschichtiges Computermodell zur Erzeugung und Simulation von Gefühlen in Echtzeit*. PhD Thesis, University of the Saarland, Saarbrücken, Germany.

Gebhard, P., Kipp, M., Klesen, M., & Rist, T. (2003). Authoring scenes for adaptive, interactive performances. In *AAMAS '03: Proceedings of the 2nd International Joint Conference on Autonomous Agents and Multiagent Systems* (pp. 725–732). New York, NY.

Gholamsaghaee, E. (2006). *Adapting JSHOP to a dialog framework with an ontological domain description*. Bachelor's Thesis, University of the Saarland, Saarbrücken, Germany.

Göbel, S., Becker, F., & Feix, A. (2005). INSCAPE: Storymodels for interactive storytelling and edutainment applications. In Subsol, G. (Ed.), *Virtual storytelling: Using virtual reality technologies for storytelling* (pp. 168–171). Berlin, Germany: Springer. doi:10.1007/11590361_19

Grice, H. P. (1975). Logic and conversation. In P. Cole & J. Morgan (Eds.), *Syntax and semantics, volume 3: Speech acts* (pp. 41-58). New York, NY: Academic Press.

Hall, L., Woods, S., & Aylett, R. (2006). FearNot! Involving children in the design of a virtual learning environment. *International Journal of Artificial Intelligence in Education, 16*(4), 327–351.

Hulstijn, J. (2000). Dialogue games are recipes for joint action. In Poesio, M., & Traum, D. R. (Eds.), *Formal semantics and pragmatics of dialogue (Gotalog '00)* (pp. 99–106). Gothenburg, Sweden: Gothenburg University.

Jönsson, A. (1993). *Dialogue management for natural language interfaces – an empirical approach*. PhD Thesis, Linköping Studies in Science and Technology, No 312, Linköping, Sweden.

Jönsson, A. (1997). A model for habitable and efficient dialogue management for natural language interaction. *Natural Language Engineering, 3*(2), 103–122. doi:10.1017/S1351324997001733

Lemon, O., Gruenstein, A., Battle, A., & Peters, S. (2002). Multi-tasking and collaborative activities in dialogue systems. In *Proceedings of the 3rd SIGdial Workshop on Discourse and Dialogue (vol. 2),* (pp. 113-124), Philadelphia, PA, USA.

Löckelt, M. (2005). Action planning for virtual human performances. In *Proceedings of the 3rd International Conference on Virtual Storytelling,* (pp. 53-62), Strasbourg, France.

Löckelt, M. (2008). *A flexible and reusable framework for dialogue and action management in multi-party discourse.* PhD Thesis, Saarbrücken University, Germany.

Mateas, M., & Stern, A. (2003). Façade: An experiment in building a fully-realized interactive drama. In *Game Developers Conference, Game Design track (Online Proceedings)*, San Jose, CA.

Miller, R. B. (1968). Response time in man-computer conversational transactions. In. *Proceedings of the AFIPS Fall Joint Computer Conference, 33*, 267–277.

Nardi, D., & Brachman, R. J. (2002). An introduction to description logics. In Baader, F. (Eds.), *The description logic handbook* (pp. 5–44). Cambridge, UK.

Niles, I., & Pease, A. (2001). Towards a standard upper ontology. In *Proceedings of the 2nd International Conference on Formal Ontology in Information Systems (FOIS-2001)* (pp. 2-9), Ogunquit, ME: ACM.

Pfleger, N. (2007). *Context-based multimodal interpretation: An integrated approach to multimodal fusion and discourse processing.* PhD Thesis, University of the Saarland, Germany.

Rao, A. S., & Georgeff, M. P. (1991). Modeling rational agents within a BDI-architecture. In J. F. Allen, R. Fikes, & E. Sandewall (Eds.), *Proceedings of the 2nd International Conference on Principles of Knowledge Representation and Reasoning* (pp. 473-484). San Mateo, CA: Morgan Kaufmann Publishers Inc.

Riedl, M. O., & Stern, A. (2006). Failing believably: Toward drama management with autonomous actors in interactive narratives. In *Proceedings of the 3rd International Conference on Technologies for Interactive Digital Storytelling and Entertainment,* (pp. 195-206), Darmstadt, Germany.

Scheffler, T., Roller, R., & Reithinger, N. (2009). SpeechEval – evaluating spoken dialog systems by user simulation. In A. Jönsson, et al. (Eds.), *Proceedings of the 6th IJCAI Workshop on Knowledge and Reasoning in Practical Dialogue Systems,* (pp. 93-98). Pasadena, CA, USA.

Schiel, F., & Türk, U. (2006). Wizard-of-Oz recordings. In Wahlster, W. (Ed.), *SmartKom: Foundations of multimodal dialogue systems* (pp. 541–570). Berlin, Germany: Springer. doi:10.1007/3-540-36678-4_34

Swartout, W. R., Gratch, J., Hill, R. W., Hovy, E., Marsella, S., Rickel, J., & Traum, D. R. (2006). Toward virtual humans. *AI Magazine, 27*(2), 96–108.

Swartz, L. (2003). *Why people hate the paperclip: Labels, appearance, behavior, and social responses to user interface agents.* Honor's Thesis, Stanford University, CA.

Traum, D. R. (2000). 20 questions on dialogue act taxonomies. *Journal of Semantics, 17*(1), 7–30. doi:10.1093/jos/17.1.7

Traum, D. R. (2004). Issues in multi-party dialogues. In Dignum, F. (Ed.), *Advances in agent communication* (pp. 201–211). Berlin, Germany: Springer. doi:10.1007/978-3-540-24608-4_12

Traum, D. R., & Larsson, S. (2003). The information state approach to dialogue management. In Smith & Kuppevelt (Eds.), *Current and new directions in discourse & dialogue* (pp. 325–353). Dordrecht, The Netherlands: Kluwer.

## KEY TERMS AND DEFINITIONS

**Action Planning:** The task of devising an ordered sequence of actions to reach some goal. This requires taking into account the current situation as well as the preconditions and consequences of the available actions to determine when an action is permitted and useful. Additional conditions may apply, e.g. restrictions from requiring the right to speak (cf. the section on floor management).

**Building Block:** A structural unit of interaction that appears in different contexts and can be reused to model dialogues. Building blocks come in different hierarchical levels, e.g., communicative acts such as "Question", communicative patterns such as "Question&Answer", or larger structural units such as a "Discussion".

**Communicative Act:** Generalization of "Dialogue Act", a concept from linguistic theory that describes spoken utterances as actions with consequences like physical acts. Communicative acts also include acts in other modalities, such as gestures or facial expressions.

**Director:** A special character or entity in an interactive narrative responsible for the control of the story. It assigns sub-goals to other characters to drive the story forward and should be able to counter events that threaten the desired outcome of the narrative.

**Goal:** A state of the world that one or more agents strive to realize through their actions, often represented as a set of conditions that must be fulfilled. The conditions can also recursively contain sub-goals.

**Habitability:** Expresses the confidence the user can have that her actions are understood by the system, and which consequences they will have, without referring to a manual, learning a special "system language", or using a help system.

**Information State:** A representation of the current state of the interaction and the "world" of the system. In most cases, the information state is represented in terms of the knowledge base formalism, but it is dynamically updated to reflect new information during the dialogue (knowledge bases are usually static).

**Interactive Narrative:** A system with the primary purpose of conveying a story with the participation of the user, who does not have to be cooperative. The main emphasis usually lies on the story being well-told and engaging instead of reaching the goal quickly; "the journey is the reward".

**Knowledge Base:** A declarative representation of entities, relations and other facts or rules pertaining to the domain of the system. Can be encoded in, e.g., an ontology (or another formal representation mechanism) and allows the system to draw logical inferences.

**Task-Oriented System:** A system that concentrates on completing a task or solving a problem in cooperation with the user. The goal and the intermediate steps are generally well-defined and unambiguous, and the interaction focuses on reaching the goal in an efficient manner.

# Chapter 8
# Extending Conversational Agents for Task-Oriented Human-Computer Dialogue

**Pierre Andrews**
*University of Trento, Italy*

**Silvia Quarteroni**
*University of Trento, Italy*

## ABSTRACT

*We present the role of conversational agents in two task-oriented human-computer dialogue applications: Interactive Question Answering and Persuasive Dialogue. We show that conversational agents can be effectively deployed for interaction that goes beyond user entertainment and can be successfully used as a means to achieve complex tasks. Conversational agents are a winning solution in Persuasive Dialogue because, combined with a planning infrastructure, they can help manage the parts of the dialogue that cannot be planned a priori and are primordial to keep the system persuasive. In Interactive Question Answering, conversational approaches lead users to the explicit formulation of queries, allow for the submission of further queries and accomodate related queries thanks to their ability to handle context.*

## 1. INTRODUCTION

Conversational agents are automatic systems able to interact with users via natural language. As a discipline, conversational agency has been introduced in 1966 by Joseph Weizenbaum's program ELIZA (Weizenbaum, 1966) with the purpose of "fooling" users into believing that they were conversing with a real human.

DOI: 10.4018/978-1-60960-617-6.ch008

Traditionally, conversational agents are used as "chatbots" for small-talk applications, such as the Eliza emulator series or AliceBot[1]. Indeed, chatbots encode a large amount of knowledge to maintain variety and enjoyability of the conversation; however, they rarely contain mechanisms to control the dialogue flow or perform complex reasoning. This is prohibitive for task-oriented dialogue, where more structured conversations are required and advanced reasoning abilities are needed to dynamically generate knowledge presented to the user.

In this chapter, we present the role of conversational agents in two task-oriented human-computer dialogue applications: Interactive Question Answering and Persuasive Dialogue. We argue that conversational agents can be effectively deployed for interaction that goes beyond user entertainment and can be successfully used as a means to achieve complex tasks.

Our first illustration of conversational task-oriented dialogue is Interactive Question Answering (IQA), addressing the needs of users searching for information on the Web and their requests for clarification. We illustrate how an IQA system that denotes reasoning abilities can handle the dialogue context through a conversational interface and support dynamic information retrieval for the user.

The second task-oriented application of conversational agents we propose is Persuasive Dialogue (PD), where users engage in natural language conversation and interact with a system attempting to change their beliefs. This task requires the conversational agent to keep initiative in the dialogue and thus to control its flow more tightly than in conventional chatbots. Both applications show how conversational agents can be extended to include more complex dialogue management techniques on top of existing conversational mechanisms.

This chapter is structured as follows. Initially, we provide a background for automatic task-oriented dialogue approaches and the Persuasive Dialogue and Interactive Question Answering technologies. We then illustrate the use of conversational agents first in Interactive QA and then in Persuasive Dialogue and address their evaluation in both domains. Finally, we discuss future trends and draw our conclusions on these two pioneering-stage technologies.

## 2. BACKGROUND

A number of extensive analyses have been carried out, e.g. (Sinclair & Coulthard, 1975), (Churcher, Atwell, & Souter, 1997) and (Lewin et al., 2000), to identify the main types of human conversation based on their features and objectives. Among these, task-oriented dialogue (one subclass of which is information-seeking dialogue) is the most widely reproduced in the context of human-computer systems. Indeed, both Interactive Question Answering and Persuasive dialogue can be considered as forms of task-oriented dialogue.

Since we argue that conversational agents can be effectively used for task-oriented dialogue, the remainder of this section outlines the main features and challenges of modelling and reproducing this type of interaction and discusses related work specifically in the fields of Persuasive Dialogue and Interactive Question Answering.

### Salient Features of Human Task Oriented Dialogue

Amongst the salient features of human task-oriented dialogue, the *overall structure* is the most noticeable: as observed by (Sinclair & Coulthard, 1975) or (Kitano, 1991), such dialogues usually have an opening, a body and a closing. Hence, they may be represented according to a hierarchical discourse grammar where the dialogue is a set of transactions, composed by exchanges, in turn made of moves, whose elementary components are dialogue acts.

In this framework, that has dominated the computational approaches to dialogue to the present, utterances are considered as dialogue acts as they aim at achieving an effect such as, for instance, obtaining information, planning a trip or driving an unmanned vehicle. This can also be seen in a goal oriented manner where each dialogue act tries to achieve a goal linked to the dialogue's task, thus enabling planning approaches to task oriented dialogue management (Field & Ramsay, 2006).

Another aspect characterizing task-oriented dialogue is *mixed initiative*, which refers to who is taking control of the interaction: when one of the interlocutors is a computer system, the literature typically distinguishes between user-, system- and mixed-initiative (Kitano, 1991). In mixed-initiative dialogue, the system must be able to take control in order to confirm information, clarify the situation, or constrain user responses.

Furthermore, human task-oriented dialogues often involve more information than required, a feature known as *over-informativeness* (Churcher, Atwell, & Souter, 1997). This usually enables dialogue to be more pleasant as the users do not need to ask for all desired pieces of information. For instance, given the question: "Do you have the time?", one would rather reply with the time than with "yes" or "no".

A further key aspect is *contextual interpretation*: indeed, human interaction relies on the conversation participants sharing a common notion of context and topic (Grosz & Sidner, 1986). Such common context is used by participants to issue and correctly interpret rhetorical phenomena such as ellipsis, anaphoric and deictic references (such as "he/his" or "this/that"). Finally, *grounding* (Cahn & Brennan, 1999) is the phenomenon by which speakers engage in a collaborative, coordinated series of exchanges that instantiate new mutual beliefs and make contributions to the common ground of a conversation.

The above features call for an efficient representation in both IQA and PD in order to meet the naturalness and persuasive requirements of both these domains. However, recreating these features in an artificial, human-machine setting is often complex due to a number of issues as identified in (Lewin et al., 2000). Among these issues, the management of *turn-taking* is difficult for an automated system as it is not always clear whether to reply to the user or wait for more input.

In fact, this is linked to the need for fluidity of a dialogue and the need to implement a system that is able to quickly deal with a limited set of data to generate an utterance. Humans rely on subtle cues in the language, tone and expressions which are not always accessible to a computer system (in particular in textual based dialogue) or require heavy resources to process. Similarly, *understanding the user input* is an issue due to the complexity and ambiguity of natural language, in particular in dialogue where many things are not said and shortcuts are often taken following social rules. In fact, most systems prefer to perform a shallow processing of the user's utterance to extract its salient features: modality, the main topic, or the current dialogue act.

At the other end of the dialogue processing pipeline, *utterance generation* implies the construction of replies understandable by humans and contextual to the current dialogue state. Indeed, this relates to the *over-informativeness* and *contextual interpretation* requirements discussed above. The system needs to identify the data to integrate in the utterance and construct a correct grammatical structure to present them. In complex natural language generation systems, this is divided in three phases: text planning – or content selection –, sentence planning, and linguistic – or surface – realisation (Reiter & Dale, 1997); in basic data retrieval systems, a reply may simply be a timetable or other type of structured information.

It is not only important to understand a single user input and generate an understandable answer, but the general consistency of the dialogue has to be controlled. Choosing the dialogue goals and the order of their presentation usually requires *planning*, which generates interesting dialogue management issues. In particular, the system has to take into account – and understand – the *user's intention* in the dialogue. In complete and complex systems, this implies managing the user's goals, beliefs and knowledge linked to the current task.

A number of issues are also linked to managing the *knowledge* required by the dialogue, but also to planning, as the system needs to be able to *maintain the context* of the dialogue. This allows for dealing with special language constructions – like ellipsis – where part of the content is omitted in the user input. The system must also be able to keep trace of the *topics under discussion* to be sure to "talk" about the correct topic in the utterances to come.

Finally, grounding and *clarification* are also part of the issues in reproducing human-human conversation. Indeed, the system should be able to understand when it makes sense to ask the user for explicit confirmation of a given utterance, when implicit confirmation should be sought to avoid lack of fluidity in dialogue (e.g. "Where would you like to search for a Chinese restaurant?") and also when no confirmation at all should be asked.

## Modelling Interactive Question Answering

Question Answering systems aim at returning natural language answers given natural language questions. Hence, QA systems can be seen as information retrieval systems with the added challenge of applying complex natural language processing techniques in order to pinpoint the answer down to the sentence or phrase level rather than the document level.

Question Answering is a nearly 50 year old technology, its first applications being natural language interfaces to small databases. Applications of QA techniques have seen a growing commercial success since the 90s. AskJeeves, now Ask.com[2], was a popular search engine launched in 1996; however, despite its claim to support natural language queries, it is not clear to what extent deep linguistic answer extraction techniques were applied. More recently, Wolfram Alpha[3] has been released as a semantic search engine; its capabilities include the navigation of relations between concepts, multimedia answer extraction and mathematical computation. Although Wolphram Alpha relies on a large body of knowledge to be matched to the user's query, it seems to lack the QA system ability to compute an answer «on-the-fly».

Indeed, state-of-the-art QA systems are able to find relevant answers to virtually any type of question, including definitions and procedures; moreover, current QA is open-domain, i.e. the source of relevant documents are typically either very large corpora – as proposed in the TREC[4] and CLEF[5] evaluation campaigns – or the Web (Kwok, Etzioni, & Weld, 2001).

The standard algorithm applied by a state-of-the-art QA system can be summarized in three main phases. First, in the question processing phase, the natural language question issued by the user is analyzed in order to determine its expected answer type and to create a query suitable for the underlying IR engine. Then, in the document retrieval phase, relevant documents are sought and retrieved using the IR engine; finally, in the answer extraction phase, relevant documents are mined for answers. Typically, the answer returned by a QA system is either a sentence or a small phrase concisely responding to the user's question.

One traditional issue of QA systems is the lack of context: the scope of the interaction covers a single question/answer pair (or "adjacency pair"). However, users often tend to search for specific information in the context of a wider information need: for instance, students researching a particular topic will pose subsequent questions related to the same topic. Unfortunately, standard QA systems are not able to handle related queries, hence they do not allow the use of anaphora and ellipsis, and furthermore they do not support any feedback from the user concerning his/her satisfaction.

In the last decade, a new research direction has been proposed, which involves the integration of Question Answering systems with dialogue interfaces in order to encourage and accommodate the submission of multiple related questions and handle the user's requests for clarification in a less artificial setting (Maybury, 2002). Indeed, there has been an increasing interest towards information-seeking dialogue applications of Question Answering, or Interactive Question Answering, in the aim of respecting the salient features characterizing task-oriented interaction, namely mixed initiative, grounding and contextual interpretation.

IQA systems are still at an early stage and often relate to closed domains (Small et al., 2003; Jönsson & Merkel, 2003; Kato et al., 2006; Kirschner & Bernardi, 2009). Our work focuses specifically on approaches to Question Answering dialogue management based on chatbots, as opposed to Finite-State or plan-based dialogue managers. A similar approach is reported for Question Answering systems in (Galibert, Illouz, & Rousset, 2005), although without full evaluation, in (Quarteroni & Manandhar, 2009), and finally in (Basili, De Cao, Giannone & Marocco, 2007) and (Kirschner & Bernardi, 2009), for a closed domain.

## Modelling Persuasive Dialogue

Computer dialogue is now used at production stage for applications such as tutorial dialogue, that helps teaching students (Freedman, 2000), task-oriented dialogue, that achieves a specific limited task such as booking a trip (Allen et al., 2000), and chatbot dialogue (Levy et al., 1997) that is used within entertainment and help systems.

None of these approaches use persuasion as a mechanism to achieve dialogue goals. However, research towards the use of persuasion in Human Computer Interaction has spawned around the field of natural argumentation (Norman & Reed, 2003). Similarly research on Embodied Conversational Agents (ECA) (Bickmore & Picard, 2005) is also attempting to improve the persuasiveness of agents with persuasion techniques; however, it concentrates on the visual representation of the interlocutor rather than the dialogue management. Previous research on human computer dialogue has rarely focused on persuasive techniques, with the exception of (Guerini, Stock, & Zancanaro, 2003). The dialogue management system presented in the following persuasive dialogue section applies a novel method, taking advantage of persuasive and argumentation techniques to achieve persuasive dialogue.

According to the cognitive dissonance theory (Festinger, 1957), people try to minimise the discrepancy between their behaviour and their beliefs by integrating new beliefs or distorting existing ones. We thus approach persuasion as a process shaping user beliefs to eventually change their behaviour.

The presented dialogue management system has been developed to address well-known limitations of current dialogue systems, in particular the impression of *lack of control* when interacting with a purely task-oriented dialogue system (Farzanfar et al., 2005). This issue is due to the fact that the system follows a plan built *a priori* to achieve the particular task, so that the user's dialogue moves are dictated by the planner and the plan operators and can rarely deviate from such preset plan.

The *lack of empathy* of computers is also a problem in human-computer interaction for applications such as health-care, where persuasive dialogue could be applied (Bickmore & Giorgino, 2004). The system does not respond to the user's personal and emotional state, which sometimes lowers the user's implication in the dialogue. However, existing research (Klein, Moon, & Picard, 1999) shows that a system that gives appropriate response to the user's emotion can lower frustration. In human-human communication, these limitations reduce the effectiveness of persuasion and we show that, by integrating a reactive component to the dialogue manager, inspired by "friendly" chatbot dialogue managers, we can improve the effectiveness of the dialogue's persuasion.

## Automatic Task-Oriented Dialogue Models

Broadly speaking, dialogue management models are attached to two categories: on the one side, pattern-based approaches such as the historical Eliza (Weizenbaum, 1966) or AliceBot systems[6], and on the other side plan-based approaches (Cohen, 1996; Zhe & Boucouvalas, 2002). We discuss existing approaches by considering their strong and weak points in the context of our application domains.

First, Finite-State (FS) approaches provide the simplest method for implementing task-oriented dialogue management. Here, the dialogue manager is represented as a Finite-State machine, where each state models a separate phase of the conversation, and each dialogue move encodes a transition to a subsequent state (Sutton, 1998). Hence, dialogue follows a «scripted» grammar used as a control mechanism; the system proceeds by first identifying the user's dialogue act from the utterance, then by making the appropriate transition, and finally by choosing one of the outgoing arcs to determine the appropriate response. The advantage of state-transition graphs is mainly that users are forced to respond in a predictable way, as the system holds the initiative for most of the time.

However, they allow very limited freedom in the range of user utterances: since each dialogue move must be pre-encoded in the models, there is a scalability issue when addressing open domain dialogue. To compensate the lack of flexibility of FS approaches, a number of systems have taken form-filling (or frame-based) approaches, e.g. (Gorin, Riccardi, & Wright, 1999), where the main advantage with respect to FS approaches is that users can supply more information than requested in the same turn, increasing the user's initiative and reducing the number of system turns needed to perform a task. However, the main issue with these approaches remains their brittleness and "scripted" nature, by which the difficulty in handling unpredicted user behaviour results in the tendency to code system-directed prompts that leave little room to user initiative.

As opposed to FS approaches, plan-based approaches offer a sophisticated strategy for dialogue management; indeed, plan-based theories of communicative action (Cohen, 1996) assume that the speaker's dialogue acts are part of a plan, and the listener's job is to uncover and respond appropriately to the underlying plan rather than just to the utterance. VERBMOBIL (Alexandersson, Reithinger, & Maier, 1997), TRIPS (Allen, Ferguson, & Stent, 2001) and TRAINS (Allen et al., 2000) are examples of plan-based approaches. Within plan-based approaches, a well-established dialogue management model is the Information State approach (Ginzburg, 1996).

Information State (IS) comprises the topics under discussion and common ground in the conversation and is continually queried and updated by rules fired by participants' dialogue moves. The IS theory has been applied to a range of closed-domain dialogue systems, e.g. (Bos et al., 2003). More recently, Hidden Information State approaches have been introduced (Young et al., 2009) in the context of reinforcement learning-based dialogue manager design. However, there does not appear to be a suitable implementation of the IS approach for open domain dialogue.

In contrast to the two approaches to task-oriented dialogue described above, reactive dialogue managers (or chatbots) like Eliza (Weizenbaum, 1966) are mainly based on pattern matching techniques that generate a new answer based on the user input. They are thus purely reactive to what the user says and do not include mechanism for managing the overall dialogue structure or a long dialogue context, thereby they are rarely used in task-oriented dialog. Reactive dialogue management systems rely on a large database of patterns to match all the possible inputs from the user. Even assuming that such a knowledge base could be automatically learned from a dialogue corpus as in (Vrajitoru, 2003), it would need substantial development and tailoring to the particular subject to be discussed in the dialogue. The fact that these systems cannot be used in applications where the user is led to accomplish the goals shared with the system is a limitation to their application domain. Yet, some systems, starting from Eliza the psychotherapist (Weizenbaum, 1966), are able to simulate language and dialogue constructions that the users assimilate to human discourse. A recent trend in reactive dialogue management systems is their use on company web sites to suggest information to the user, although with no claim on efficiency and relevance.

The different requirements discussed earlier for the modelling of IQA and PD make it difficult to single out one of these models as the most eligible for such applications. In fact, features from each of the three models are required. For PD, planning is required for guaranteeing the persuasive goal achievement, but the user has to feel in control of the dialogue and receive a number of social cues for the persuasion to be effective and thus some reactive approach is also required. For IQA, reactive dialogue features are desirable as they ensure the necessary conversational abilities of the dialogue system; however maintaining and efficiently accessing the information state, i.e. the conversation context and query history, is vital.

A solution might be an approach similar to (Stent, 2002), proposing a form of hybrid management based on conversational acts where *Discourse Reasoning* takes care of understanding the user, reasoning about the possible reactions and generating tailored utterances to maintain the discourse context, while *Problem Solving* performs long-term reasoning about the task to achieve in the dialogue and the general behaviour of the agent.

To the best of our knowledge, there are rare examples of systems trying to mix the reactive approach with a structured dialogue approach to both control the achievement of dialogue goals and leave enough freedom in the dialogue for reacting to the user and making the dialogue smoother. In the following sections, we propose two of these hybrid approaches where we extend a reactive approach to manage task and goal oriented dialogue in the fields of Interactive QA and persuasive dialogue.

## 3. CONVERSATIONAL AGENTS FOR INTERACTIVE QUESTION ANSWERING

As Interactive Question Answering is a recent technology, one of the main points under discussion concerns the dialogue management models that best support it. Since an IQA system is a task-oriented dialogue system where the core task is the Question Answering one, a black-box view of such a system consists of a core QA module with a dialogue interface with which the user converses in natural language and the general structure of such a conversation is centered around <question,answer> adjacency pairs.

To conduct this type of conversation, an IQA system must fulfill a number of desiderata. First, the system must be able to identify user utterances containing queries, then handle these by accessing the standard QA system forming its backbone, and finally produce a conversational output, either presenting answers when the user has issued queries or maintaining the conversation when the user's utterance is simply conversational. The abilities of the dialogue interface to a QA system should include recognition of follow-up queries, i.e. queries referring to previous conversation, and the ability to seek and obtain feedback about the quality of answers.

For the purpose of IQA, plan-based approaches that model and update user beliefs seem unnecessary. On the other hand, simpler finite-state approaches are unsuitable to support context-handling phenomena such as ellipsis and clarification. In the following section, we show how conversational agency is suitable to model adjacency pairs in task-oriented information-seeking dialogue thanks to its <pattern,template> structure. We also illustrate how a conversational agent can efficiently handle dialogue phenomena that typically occur in human task-oriented dialogue.

## Advantages of Conversational Agents for Question Answering

Conversational agents are a valuable choice for interactive QA as they allow handling the salient features of task-oriented dialogue introduced above as follows. Concerning *overall structure* and *mixed initiative,* conversational dialogue articulated in <pattern,template> pairs seems ideal to model the <question,answer> adjacency pairs of IQA conversation.

In such a scenario, the dialogue initiative as well as the decision of when to issue a request for information is left entirely at the user's command. However, there is also room for system initiative in clarifying the current conversation as required in some information-seeking dialogue situations. As mentioned earlier, the system must be able to constrain user responses and to take control at times during the conversation in order to confirm given information or clarify the situation.

We propose a solution where the patterns used by a conversational system are oriented to Question Answering conversation so that the user is encouraged to formulate information requests rather than engage in small talk. For instance, a pattern of the type: *HELLO ** may be matched by a template such as: "*Hello,* ***what is your question?***". This way, a user utterance starting with "Hello" will trigger an invitation to formulate a specific question. On the other hand, in this setting the user can take the initiative for most of the dialogue, for instance by ignoring the system's requests for feedback and directly formulating a follow-up question. This happens for instance in turn **User2** of the following interaction example:

**User**: "What is a thermometer?"
**System**: "I found the following answers:... Are you happy with these answers?"
**User**: "How does it measure the temperature?"
**System**: "Do you mean how does a thermometer measure the temperature?"
**User**: "No, how does a digital thermometer measure the temperature?"

*Contextual interpretation* of the user's utterances can be handled by a follow-up question resolution module designed to take care of ellipsis and anaphoric references in questions, as described in the remainder of this section. In terms of *grounding* and *clarification,* the management of misunderstandings is possible in our approach thanks to user and system clarification dialogue moves. A system clarification request may be fired when the current user utterance is not recognized as a question according to the set of question patterns known to the system. For example, the pattern *I NEED ** may fire a response such as "*Is that a question you want me to look up?*". If the user confirms that his/her utterance is a question, the system will proceed to clarify and answer it; otherwise, it will acknowledge the utterance. Symmetrically, the users can be supported when entering a request for clarification of the system's latest utterance at any time they find the latter unclear.

Finally, *over-informativeness* is possible in this solution as patterns enable the user to respond to the system by providing more information than a simple acknowledgment. For instance, in the above sample conversation, the system resolves the pronoun "it" using the noun "thermometer" (turn System2), which is incomplete given the context provided by the QA system results; the user answers the system's request for clarification and corrects the system at the same time in turn User3.

The next section outlines the main design guidelines we have followed in order to achieve the above-mentioned desirable features within an interactive QA system.

## Designing an Interactive Question Answering System

The design of an IQA system presents two main challenges: first, a state-of-the-art QA system must be available to form the backbone of the conversational agent; secondly, the conversational interface must be task-oriented, hence not only a reactive layer, but also a number of task-oriented functions must be encoded, including reference resolution modules, follow-up detection and QA interfacing.

While the design of a state-of-the-art QA system is not the subject of this chapter, we here describe our general method to make a standard QA system interactive. We summarize the design of an IQA system as an iterative process consisting of four general phases. Initially, a detailed conversation scenario must be devised to represent the general algorithm followed by the conversational QA system. Based on the above scenario, the dialogue moves combined into tasks by the dialogue manager must be fixed. Then, the coverage and efficiency of the scenario and of the dialogue moves must be verified within an exploratory experiment, such as a Wizard-of-Oz (WOZ) experiment; here, prospective users are confronted with a human-directed version of the system which they believe to be fully automatic and conversations are monitored in terms of efficiency and user satisfaction. Finally, a dialogue manager can be designed, implemented and evaluated based on the observations from the WOZ experiment. If needed, the design cycle may restart with revised hypotheses.

The next sections discuss the above steps in further detail.

## Dialogue Scenario and Moves

The most general conversational scenario an IQA system should be able to carry out consists of the following steps:

1. An optional reciprocal greeting;
2. An utterance *u* from the user to be analyzed in search of a question *q*;
3. Any question *q* is analyzed to detect whether it is related to previous questions or not;
4. If *q* is unrelated to the preceding questions, it is submitted to the back-end QA system; otherwise, it is resolved according to the conversational context (i.e. previous dialogue history) and submitted to the QA system;
5. As soon as the QA system's results are available, an answer a is provided;
6. The IQA system enquires whether the user is interested in a follow-up session; if this is the case, the user can enter a query again. Else, the system acknowledges;
7. Whenever the user wants to terminate the interaction, a final greeting is exchanged.

The above scenario is based on a sequence of adjacency pairs of the form greeting-greeting, question-answer. Nested dialogue pairs such as the system's request for clarification and the user's reply or acknowledgment can be found within the question-answer pairs. Moreover, at any time the users may issue a request for clarification when they do not understand the system's utterance, in which case the system replies with a clarification.

Based on the scenario, a taxonomy of dialogue acts (or moves) must be adopted to represent the fundamental conversational building blocks. Following well-known dialogue annotation schemes, such as DAMSL (Core & Allen, 1997), TRAINS (Traum, 1996) and VERBMOBIL (Alexandersson et al., 1997) we propose a taxonomy where dialogue acts fall into three main categories: *core*, addressing the fundamental communicative tasks (ask, answer), *feedback* (clarification requests, acknowledgements of the interlocutor's utterance, follow-up proposal and grounding request), and *conventional* or conversation management moves (greet, quit).

It may be noted that as IQA is an information-seeking type of dialogue, it is characterized by the two conversant roles of information seeker (user) and information provider (system). This results in the user and system making a different use of dialogue acts: for instance, the *ask* move is typically a user move, while the *answer* move is typically a system move. Moreover, the feedback moves of follow-up proposal (*follow-up*) and grounding (*ground*) are information provider moves. In contrast, conventional moves such as *greet* and *quit* and the feedback move of *clarification-request* are shared by participants, as the initiative is mixed and the user is free to leave the conversation or ask for clarification at any point.

## Wizard-of-Oz Experiment

Once the fundamental building blocks of the conversation have been devised, a Wizard-of-Oz experiment should be designed in order to test the coverage of an IQA conversation conducted by using the above dialogue acts in the context of a given dialogue management strategy. To this end, a number of task-oriented scenarios must be defined and "canned" or ready-made dialogue moves must be prepared.

Tasks are to be executed by real users, through an interface they believe to be the chatbot. In (Quarteroni & Manandhar, 2009), we proposed six tasks to be followed in pairs to six or more persons in such a way that each individual task would be performed by at least two different users. The tasks reflected the intended typical usage of the system, such as: "Find out who painted Guernica and ask the system for more information about the artist". Users then were asked to interact with what they believed to be an automatic chat agent via a popular commercial chat interface, while the system developer conducted the conversation at the other end by selecting the most appropriate dialogue acts and, consequently, a pre-compiled natural language prompt to return to users via the interface.

The outcome of the WOZ experiment can be mined both in terms of user satisfaction questionnaires and in terms of conversation log analysis; its results serve to update the original architecture of the DM as well as to provide a baseline of the user expectations concerning a so far unknown system.

## Dialogue Manager Design

Based on the scenario and on the revised hypotheses provided by one or more WOZ experiments, a full-fledged dialogue manager may be designed. Generally speaking, the DM is the core of a dialogue component in constant interaction with a standard QA system. In the architecture we propose, the dialogue component's query module submits queries to the standard QA component, performing document retrieval and answer extraction from the Web; results are then returned to the user via the dialogue interface, as illustrated in Figure 1.

We structure the dialogue component according to three modules: a question recognition module able to interpret multiple/follow-up questions, a query management module and a conversational, "chat" module to manage interaction that is not directly oriented to query interpretation and result presentation.

As chatbot dialogue follows a pattern-matching approach, dialogue management is virtually stateless: when a user utterance is issued, the chatbot's strategy is to look for a pattern matching it and fire the corresponding template response. The main focus of attention in terms of dialogue manager design must therefore be directed to the dialogue tasks invoking external resources, such as handling multiple and follow-up questions, and tasks involving the QA component. We briefly outline algorithms for these tasks below.

**Handling multiple questions.** As soon as the dialogue manager identifies a user utterance as a question (using the question recognition patterns), it tests whether it is a multiple question. In (Quarteroni & Manandhar, 2009) for instance, since the core QA component is not able to handle multiple questions, these are detected and broken into simple questions. For this, the system uses a shallow syntactic parser to look for the presence of "and" which does not occur within a noun phrase.

*Figure 1. High-level architecture of an interactive QA system*

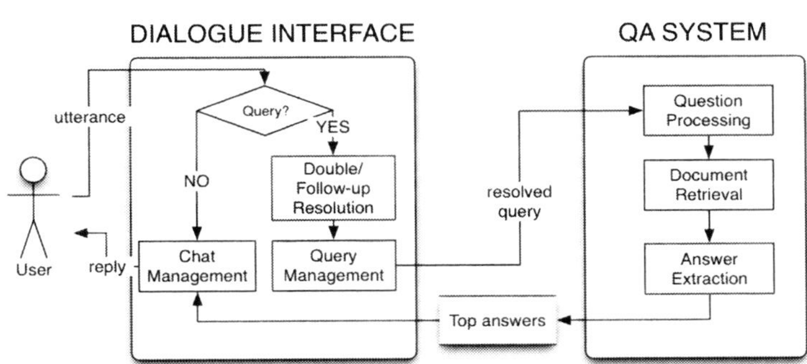


**Handling follow-up questions.** After detecting and handling multiple questions, the next task accomplished by the dialogue manager is the detection and resolution of follow-up questions, a vital task in handling QA dialogue as outlined in (Yang, Feng, & Di Fabbrizio, 2006). For the detection of follow-up questions, the algorithm in (De Boni & Manandhar, 2005) may be adopted. The latter uses as features the presence of pronouns and of word repetitions with respect to previous queries in the current question.

If a question is identified as a follow-up question according to the former algorithm, the following resolution strategy is applied:

1. If it is elliptic (i.e. contains no verbs), its keywords are completed with the keywords extracted by the QA component from the previous question for which there exists an answer. The completed query is submitted to the QA component.
2. If it contains pronoun/adjective anaphora (i.e. contains references to entities in the previous questions in the form of pronouns or adjectives), a shallow syntactic parser is used to find the first compatible antecedent in the previous questions in order of recency. The latter must be a noun phrase compatible in number with the referent.
3. If it contains anaphora in the form of noun phrases, the most recent noun phrase within the list of preceding questions that contains all the words in the referring noun phrase is used in the query to replace such referring noun phrase.

When no antecedent can be found, a clarification request is issued by the system until a resolved query can be submitted to the core QA module. In any case, when the QA process is terminated, the answers (or a message directing the user to an answer page) are returned and a follow-up proposal or an enquiry about user satisfaction may be issued.

## Implementation

We propose to use AIML, the Artificial Intelligence Markup Language, to implement an interactive Question Answering system and extend it to interface its reactive layer with core QA functionalities. In particular, we adopt the Java-based AIML interpreter Chatterbean[7], which allows to define custom AIML tags and to achieve a seamless integration between the QA module and the chat interface. Here, the Chatterbean tag set is augmented with two AIML tags: <query>, to invoke the core Question Answering module, and <clarify>, to support the tasks of follow-up detection and reference resolution.

Moreover, as the Chatterbean context implementation allows to instantiate and update a set of variables, represented as context properties, several of these have been defined, including:

- The user's ID, that is matched against a list of known user IDs to select a profile for answer extraction;
- The current query, which is used to dynamically update the stack of recent user questions. The stack is used by the clarification request detection module to perform reference resolution, following the algorithm exposed above;
- The resolved question, i.e. the current query as resolved during follow-up handling (or the current query if no follow-up is detected);
- The topic of conversation, i.e. the keywords of the last question issued by the user that received an answer. The topic variable is used to clarify elliptic questions, by augmenting the current query keywords with those in the topic when ellipsis is detected.

Figure 2 illustrates an interactive QA system accessible online. The interactive interface consists of a main window with a left panel where the chat takes place and a right panel where results are visualized. As in an instant messaging application, users write in a text field and the current session history as well as the interlocutor replies are visualized in an adjacent text area.

## 4. CONVERSATIONAL AGENTS FOR PERSUASIVE DIALOGUE

In the recent years, research in persuasive technology (Fogg, 2003) and natural argumentation (Norman & Reed, 2003) has become a popular solution for several automatic-counseling tasks. In health-care in particular, personal counselors are important to help people achieve health and life style goals – such as regularly taking medications, eating more healthy food or doing regular physical exercise. Having such counselors for everyone is however very expensive, and thus research in automated techniques to provide personalised, ubiquitous counseling agents to achieve these tasks is flourishing.

A proposed solution for implementing such counseling agents is to use interactive persuasive (or argumentative) dialogue (Cassell & Bickmore, 2002). In such a dialogue, the computer tries to change the users' belief on some issue through a dialogue introducing new information about the issue. For instance, when promoting healthy eating habits, the computer tries to find the users' "barriers" (e.g. "Vegetables are hard to cook", "Fresh fruits do not last long") that stop them from eating healthier food and propose solutions and counter-arguments to these issues.

Each user's belief attached to a "barrier" has to be tackled during the dialogue and thus represents what we call "persuasive goals". Dialogues of this kind are structured in a set of rhetorical exchanges showing argument/counter-argument pairs where one party introduces one of its beliefs and the other party tries to refute such belief with an argument. This argument/counter-argument can continue with a number of sub-arguments about rebuttal beliefs which are hard to predict a priori in the dialogue plan, where only the high level beliefs to be introduced by the system can be computed based on the a priori knowledge of the user's beliefs.

It appears from the study of the state-of-the-art of persuasive communication and argumentation that a different dialogue framework is needed to achieve persuasiveness. For the dialogue to be persuasive, the dialogue management system needs to guarantee the involvement of the user in the conversation as persuasiveness is strongly influenced by the perception of the user. This implies that trust, credibility and a sense of relationship have to be maintained by the system. To achieve these requirements, we have set the hypothesis that a novel method is needed to manage social cues

*Figure 2. An interactive question answering interface*

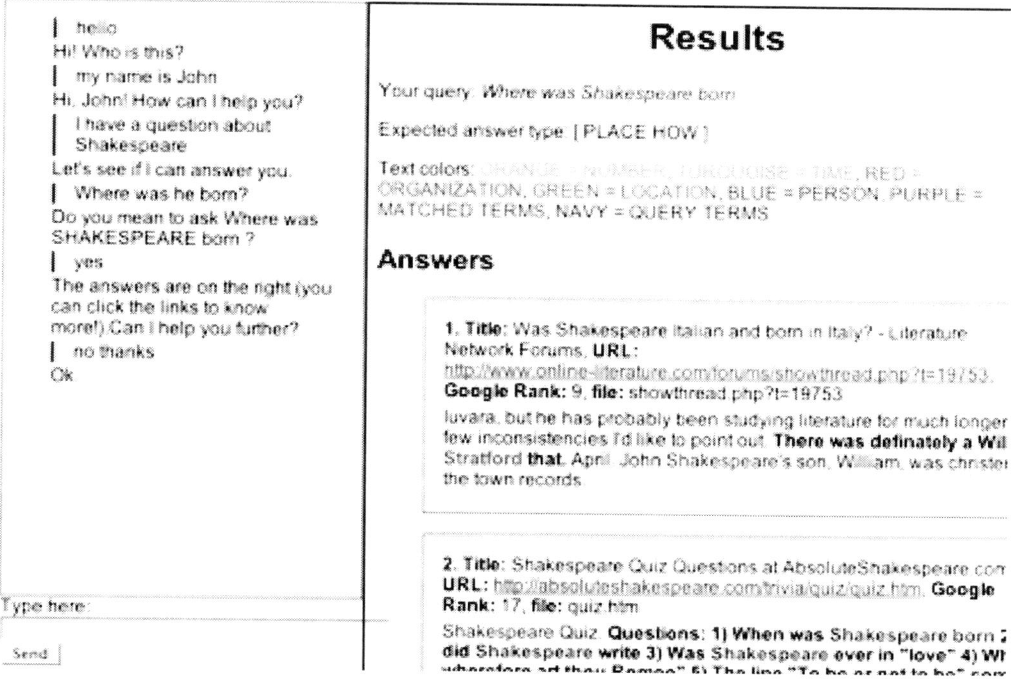


and render the dialogue more natural to improve the persuasiveness.

A persuasive dialogue framework needs to achieve consistency and guarantee the completion of persuasive goals; this requires the ability to reason a priori about the dialogue path and what knowledge the system will introduce during the dialogue to argue with the user. The argumentation strategies have to be chosen to support the goals and fit the user's knowledge. The three-tier planner for tutoring dialogue discussed in (Zinn, Moore, & Core, 2002) provides a dialogue management technique close to the requirements of persuasion planning: a top-tier generates a dialogue plan, the middle-tier generates refinements to the plan and the bottom-tier generates utterances. Mazzotta, de Rosis, & Carofiglio (2007) also proposes a planning framework for user-adapted persuasion where the plan operators are mapped to natural language (or Embodied Conversational Agents) generation. The novel framework design proposed here also adopts such planning approach to manage the dialogue long-term goals and ensure the consistency of the argumentation.

The knowledge required by such planning systems becomes, however, difficult to manage if the framework needs to include a mechanism to react to the user's counter-arguments as well as social cues management. In fact, these reactive parts of the dialogue are inherently difficult to plan a priori. This observation leads to the design of a novel dialogue management framework for persuasion. The intent of this framework can be compared to the work presented by (Stent, 2002) where the author describes a dialogue management system based on the TRIPS architecture (Allen, Ferguson, & Stent, 2001), which proposes to separate discourse reasoning from problem solving.

In preliminary research, different strategies have been studied to achieve persuasive dialogue. In particular, Gilbert et al. (2003) propose a road-map for the development of an argumentative machine, where the system needs a deep understanding of the user's argument content, which involves understanding the type of the argument to choose a tailored counter argumentation. However, such deep understanding of the argument construction and goals is still impossible with the current state of the art in natural language understanding.

A novel framework design is proposed to provide the flexibility needed to react to the user and use social cues while guaranteeing the achievement of persuasive goals. This novel framework, henceforth named the EDEN Framework, has been developed following one main hypothesis:

Managing direct reactions to the user's utterances outside of the dialogue plan improves persuasiveness.

This hypothesis was founded on the reasons described previously as well as observations made during the iterative framework development:

- Persuasion requires the system to show empathy to the user. It needs to provide utterances for chit-chat and for empathizing which cannot be planned a priori.
- When defining the planning component of the system, it appeared highly impractical for domain authoring to include all possible argumentation related reactions at the planning level.
- Predicting the user's beliefs is impossible; in particular the counter-arguments used during the dialogue cannot be predicted without extended knowledge of the user. Relying on the planner for managing this part of the dialogue requires complex online planning or constant re-planning.
- The design of the dialogue management framework is also constrained by the experimental needs of computer science research. Validating the hypothesis requires iterative development and testing of the framework, and ease of testing the framework on different domains.

These requirements led to the design of a modular framework where each independent layer could be replaced easily and where the domain authoring was separated from the dialogue management logic.

## Hybrid Dialogue Design

The EDEN Framework is designed as a modular system composed of five main components (see Figure 3):

- **The Knowledge Model** is common in dialogue systems and is split here between:
  - *The User Model* that stores the system's knowledge about the user's beliefs and monitors the user's belief change to allow for a dynamic handling of argumentative strategies.
  - *The Domain Model* that describes the knowledge of the domain in the *argumentation model* and how utterances should be generated for this domain in the *reaction model*.
- **The Reasoning Component** is divided in two independent layers providing the tools to achieve the reactivity and continuity required by our hypothesis:
  - *The Long Term Planning* layer is responsible for keeping the dialogue on track and achieving the persuasive goals.
  - *The Reactive Strategies* layer performs short-term reasoning and is directly responsible for dealing with the reactions to the user.
  - *The Generation Module* realises the natural language form of the content selected by the reactive layer.

This approach to dialogue management differs from standard layered approaches such as (Zinn, Moore, & Core, 2002) as it introduces a new layer between the dialogue reasoning module

*Figure 3. The EDEN framework architecture*

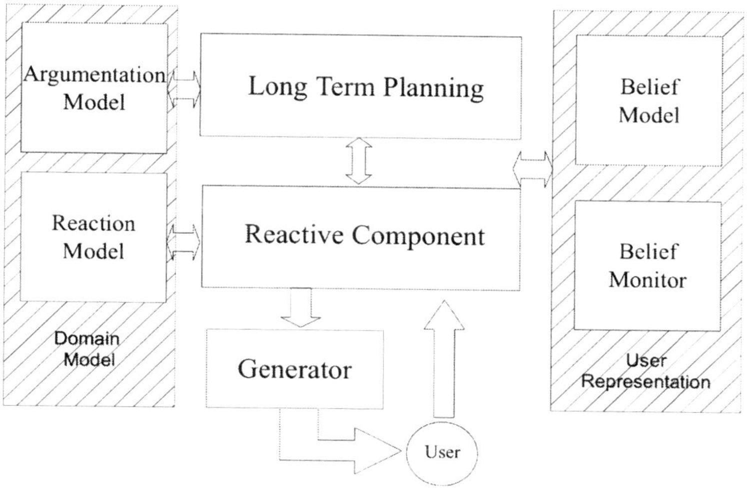

Argumentation Model
Long Term Planning
Belief Model
Reaction Model
Reactive Component
Belief Monitor
Domain Model
Generator
User Representation
User

and the generation layers. The EDEN Framework uses a planning component to select the dialogue content but delegates the exact utterance content selection to the reactive layer. The reactive layer adds flexibility to the plan and helps keeping a simple planning approach by leaving the discourse level reasoning out of the long-term knowledge structure.

## Planning Arguments

The planning component is responsible for content selection and high-level structure planning of the dialogue. The planner uses an argumentation hierarchy and the knowledge of the user's beliefs and preferences to select the arguments to present during the dialogue.

The argumentation hierarchy is based on the standard support hierarchies for studying argumentation where clauses presenting beliefs are linked together to show the supporting premises to the argumentation's conclusion (Walton, 1996). Figure 4 shows an example of our argumentation hierarchy where nodes represent beliefs that can be introduced during the dialogue and the arrows show a *support* relation between beliefs. In practice this encodes the fact that a belief cannot be introduced before its supporting premises (subsuming it in the hierarchy) are introduced and accepted by the user.

A graph-plan (Blum & Furst, 1997) algorithm is used to construct a planning graph from the belief relationships given by the argumentation hierarchy and to find the shortest available path in the hierarchy. The planner performs a search for a minimum set of ordered operations to go from the current belief state (what it knows about the user) to the goal belief state (what it wants the user to believe eventually). Each operation is an instance of a dialogue operator. A dialogue operator specifies a dialogue segment where reactive dialogue will be implemented to argue about the belief introduced by that operator, which is defined in the planner by:

- The set of beliefs it depends on – i.e. what the user should already believe before using this operation.
- The new belief it introduces to the user.
- The existing beliefs it "removes" from the user.

Three operators are available in the framework to use the argumentation hierarchy nodes:

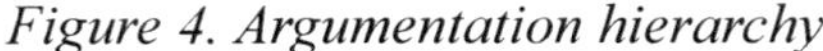
*Figure 4. Argumentation hierarchy*

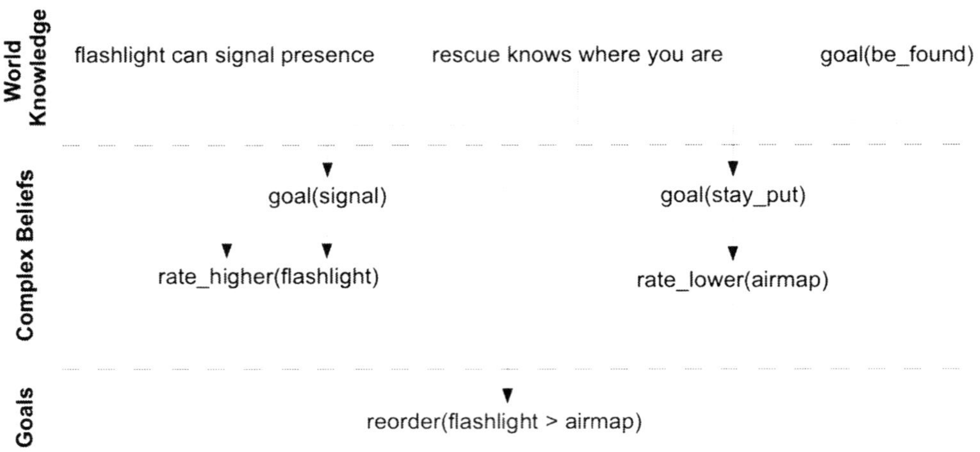


- **ground → F** asserts a simple fact in the user's beliefs
  - *Required Beliefs* none
  - *Introduced Belief* F
- **use_world → F** introduces a fact to the user
  - *Required Beliefs* none
  - *Introduced Belief* F
- **support(A,B,C,...) → D** supports a new belief D with the existing beliefs A, B, C, ....
  - *Required Beliefs* A,B,C,...
  - *Introduced Belief* D

From their planning definition, the **ground → F** and **use_world → F** operators are identical for the planner, they both logically do the same operation of inserting a new belief without support; however the expected reactions from the user during the dialogue is different and their realises in dialogue segments differ.

Figure 5 provides an example of a plan path in the argumentation hierarchy; the planner starts with a set of initial beliefs ($Bel_c$) and tries to find a set of consecutive actions that can be used to introduce the goal beliefs ($Bel_n$ and $Bel_o$). Each arrow is thus an action applying one of the operators discussed earlier to beliefs available in the user's beliefs. We can see that to get from the initial beliefs state, the planner has to go through three different belief states [$Bel_C$] → [$Bel_D$, $Bel_E$, $Bel_F$, $Bel_G$] → [$Bel_H$, $Bel_I$, $Bel_J$] → [$Bel_K$, $Bel_L$, $Bel_M$] → [$Bel_N$, $Bel_D$], each separated by an actions stage defining a set of actions to extend the user's beliefs. We can see that the set of actions to introduce $Bel_N$ and $Bel_O$ are mostly independent, except that to introduce $Bel_K$, the support operator requires $Bel_I$ and $Bel_H$ and thus the path to $Bel_I$ is required to introduce both goal beliefs.

When the plan represented by such path is realised in a dialogue with the user, each arrow will be used to generate a new argument that has to be agreed upon by the user before going to the next actions stage as this one depends on the new beliefs introduced by the actions in the current stage.

## Reactive Model

The Planning Component selects arguments and provides a structure for the segments of the dialogue. This content ordering will not be changed in the rest of the dialogue unless the selected plan fails. The Reactive Component is responsible

*Figure 5. Dialogue plan to introduce beliefs*

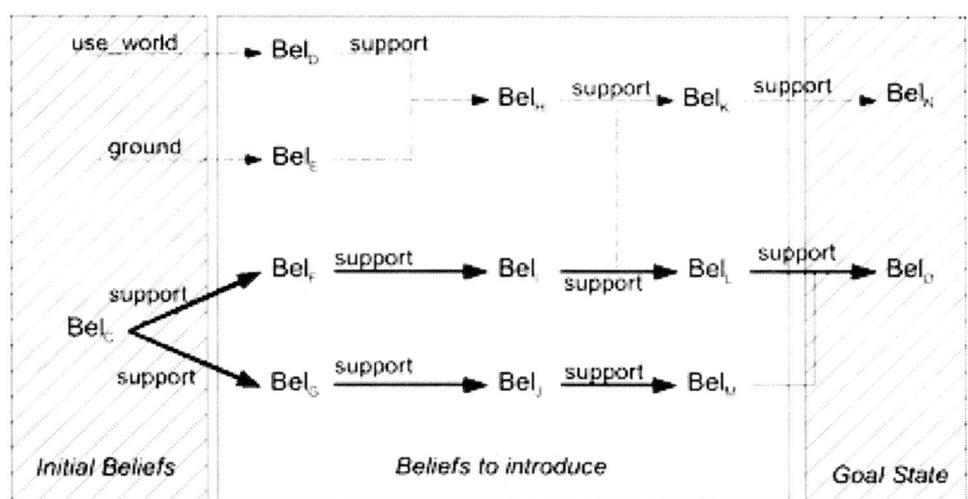


for planning and structuring the content of each dialogue segment according to the user's reactions and the communicative goals provided in the plan structure.

The main difference between the EDEN Framework and state-of-the-art planned or finite-state approaches, such as (Mazzotta, de Rosis, & Carofiglio, 2007), is that each plan step is not directly mapped to one utterance generation. The selected operations are applied as constraints to the possible reactions used for the defense of arguments during the dialogue.

The planner is responsible for high-level dialogue structuring and content selection by creating consecutive communicative goals. The realisation of these goals in natural language utterances is delegated to the lower layers of the EDEN Framework:

1. The reactive layer has the control over the structure of the dialogue segments. The user can react in many ways to the argument presented in each segment, the reactive component uses the constraints provided by the communicative goals to react within the argument by activating context specific reactions. The reactive content is thus able to select content for each specific utterance tailored to the argument and to the user's reaction.
2. The generator is then responsible for the natural language realisation of the content selected by the reactive component.

Reactions are structured into a search tree similar to the one in Figure 6, where a top-down search is performed to find the best utterance to use for the current plan step and context. The pruning of possible reactions for the current dialogue stage is thus similar to a pattern matching system.

Each node of the tree represents one input token or a wildcard matching as many input tokens as possible. The tree is divided in four layers: a branch of the *dialogue segment matching* layer defines a matching pattern used to match dialogue plan steps. When a plan operator is matched, a sub-tree in the *Context Matching* layer is selected. This tree defines a set of patterns matching the last utterance of the system, setting a context for the reactions. Matching a specific plan operator and dialogue context selects a sub-tree from the Utterance Matching layer. The latter defines reactions to particular inputs by the user and is linked to leaves representing generation templates.

*Figure 6. Activation tree*

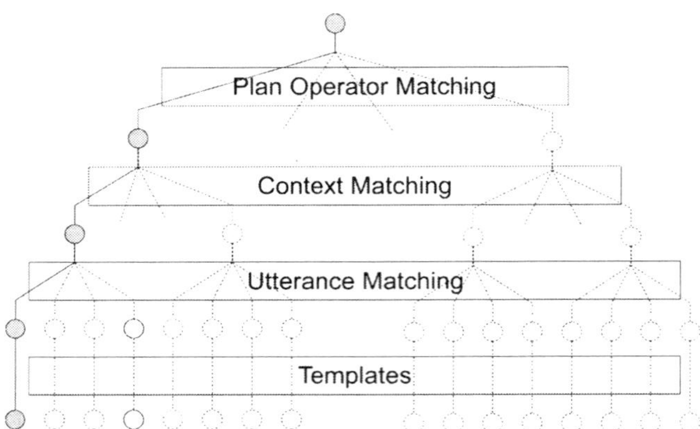


This contextual matching process can happen multiple times as the reactive component will try to implement as best as possible each actions defined by the plan to introduce the required beliefs. The reactive component can thus decide to continue arguing on one particular belief to introduce it to the user, or, if the user is not open to this new belief, ask the planner to provide a new plan where this belief is not required. This might produce a dialogue as in the following example (from the Desert Survival Scenario discussed in Section 5):

**System**: *don't you agree that we should stay close to the plane wreckage? So the rescue can find us.*

*[from plan step: support([goal(be found), rescueknowwhereyouare], goal(stayput))]*

**User**: *I guess you are right.*

*[agreement]*

**System**: *I think the flashlight could be useful as it could help us at night, let's rank it higher.*

*[from plan step: support([can(helpatnight, flashlight)], rate higher(item(flashlight)))]*

**User**: *How is that? We are not going to move during the night.*

*[disagreement]*

**System**: *well, if we want to collect water, it will be best to do things at night and not under the burning sun.*

*[defense in the same plan step]*

**User**: *I see. It could be useful then.*

*[agreement]*

## 5. EVALUATION

Evaluating dialogue systems is a practice that has not reached a stable, agreed-upon level. In particular, this is due to the fact that task-oriented dialogue evaluation is related with the value or cost of fulfilling the system task(s), a measurement that depends both on domain-independent and on domain- or task- dependent factors.

The most common domain-independent factor taken into account in dialogue evaluation is user satisfaction as an estimator of quality collected through a tailored questionnaire, for example in (Walker et al., 1997).

The presence of a task-specific, numerical estimator of the dialogue performance in the context of a specific task is also a fundamental component of dialogue evaluation. In the case of IQA, this should correspond to the accuracy of the core QA system, which can be measured in terms of answer precision and recall as in TREC- and CLEF-style evaluation campaigns. In the case of PD, the persuasiveness of the system has to be evaluated; while this is often dependent on the application domain, we use a standalone application based on the recommendations from (Andrews & Manandhar, 2009) to evaluate the users' change in beliefs during the dialogue.

In IQA in particular, the main term of comparison to evaluate the impact of interactivity consists of a non-interactive version of the system. General and specific aspects of user satisfaction must be polled in order to assess the qualitative difference in experience and accuracy as registered by end users.

In the PD case, we want to evaluate the impact of adding reactivity to the system, which helps particularly in generating social cues, "chit-chat" and keeping the dialogue smooth and not frustrating for the user. As discussed earlier, our hypothesis is that such difference will make the system more persuasive for the same amount of beliefs presented. To evaluate our hypothesis, we thus compare the full dialogue system with planning and reactive part to a purely planning based system.

## Evaluating IQA

While core QA evaluation is not the subject of this chapter, we discuss how to measure the impact of an interactive QA system on user satisfaction. Clearly, the ability of an IQA system to handle related queries must be measured and compared with respect to the performance of a standard QA system. In our experiments, nine series of related questions were chosen from the 2007 TREC QA evaluation campaign[8]. For instance, Series ID 266 was selected with the following questions: 1) "When was Rafik Hariri born?" 2) "To what religion did he belong (including sect)?" 3) "At what time in the day was he assassinated?"

Twelve participants were invited to find answers to the questions using both a standard and an interactive version of the same QA system. At the end of the experiment, users responded to the user satisfaction questionnaire reported in Table 1 by using a five-point Likert scale.

The results obtained from the questionnaire for the standard and interactive versions are reported in columns "Standard" and "Interactive" of Table 1, respectively. We believe that the evidence we collected from the experiment, both quantitative (the questionnaire replies) and qualitative (user comments), suggests interesting interpretations.

First, a good overall satisfaction appears with both versions of the system (Q8), with a slight difference in favor of the interactive version. The standard and interactive versions of the system seem to offer different advantages: while the ease of use of the standard version was rated higher (Q5) – probably because the system's requests for reformulation added a challenge to participants used to a search engine-style interaction – users felt that they obtained more information using the interactive version (Q1).

Concerning interaction comfort, users seemed to feel that the interactive version understood better their requests than the standard one (Q2); they also found it easy to reformulate questions when the former asked them to (Q6). These findings suggest that even a simple chat interface can be very useful in terms of user satisfaction. However, while the pace of interaction was judged slightly more appropriate in the interactive case (Q3), interaction was considered faster when using the standard version (Q4). Unfortunately, in both cases the interaction speed rarely appears adequate, as also registered from user comments. This partly explains the fact that users seemed more ready to use again the standard version of the system (Q7); some users clearly stated so, saying e.g. "I would

*Table 1. Evaluation questionnaire and results: average ± standard deviation*

| Question | Standard | Interactive |
|---|---|---|
| Q1 Did you get all the information you wanted using the system? | 4.1 ± 1.0 | 4.3 ± 0.7 |
| Q2 Do you think the system understood what you asked? | 3.4 ± 1.3 | 3.8 ± 1.1 |
| Q3 How easy was it to obtain the information you wanted? | 3.9 ± 1.1 | 3.7 ± 1.0 |
| Q4 Was it difficult to reformulate your questions when you were invited to? | N/A | 3.9 ±0.6 |
| Q5 Do you think you would use this system again? | 3.3 ± 1.6 | 3.1 ± 1.4 |
| Q6 Overall, are you satisfied with the system? | 3.7 ± 1.2 | 3.8 ± 1.2 |
| Q7 Was the pace of interaction with the system appropriate? | 3.2 ± 1.2 | 3.3 ±1.2 |
| Q8 How often was the system sluggish in replying to you? | 2.7 ± 1.1 | 2.5 ± 1.2 |
| Q9 Did you prefer the standard or the interactive interface? | 41.7% | 58.3% |

be very interested in using the system again once it reaches industrial speed".

An interesting outcome of the evaluation was the "preference" question, Q9: 7 out of 12 users (58.3%) said that they preferred the interactive version. The reasons given by users in their comments were mixed: while some of them were enthusiastic about the chatbot's small talk features and felt that the interface interacted very naturally, others clearly said that they felt more comfortable with a search engine-like interface and that the design of the interactive prototype was inadequate.

However, most of the critical aspects emerging from our overall satisfactory evaluation depend on the specific system we have tested rather than on the nature of interactive QA, to which none of such results appear to be detrimental. We believe that the search-engine-style use and interpretation of QA systems are due to the fact that QA is still a very little known technology. It is a challenge for both developers and the larger public to cooperate in designing and discovering applications that take advantage of the potentials of interactivity.

## Evaluating Persuasion

Current practical research on computer persuasion concentrates on Embodied Conversational Agents. For example, (Bickmore & Picard, 2005) use an ECA to persuade university students to walk more and improve their physical condition. The authors create an evaluation that follows the students over a long period of time and uses a pedometer to assess the evolution of the users' behaviour and hence the persuasiveness of the system. However, in such a setup, it is difficult to guarantee the independence of the behaviour change from external elements not controlled in the experiment; therefore, an atomic evaluation protocol is used, where the dialogue is the only element influencing the change of behaviour as the persuasion is directly evaluated at the beginning and at the end of a dialogue session.

This protocol follows the belief change metric introduced by (Andrews & Manandhar, 2009) within the desert survival scenario, which is a negotiation scenario used in team training. The team is put in a scenario where members are stranded in the desert after a plane crash and the participants have to negotiate a ranking of the most eligible items (knife, compass, map, etc.) that they should keep for their survival. For the evaluation of the dialogue system, a similar scenario is presented to the participants: the user has to choose a preferred initial ranking of items and then goes through a discussion with the dialogue system that tries to persuade the user to change the ranking (see Figure 7). At the end of the dialogue, the user has the opportunity to change the choice

*Figure 7. The dialogue interface with item ranking on the right*

abort dialogue (only click if the system seems to be irresponsive)

Hi there, I am Paul.

looks like we should discuss on this ranking.

I have some basic camping knowledge, it might help.

Well Pierre, I think I' ll never feel safe taking the plane in the future.

Do you want to discuss this ranking then?

**yes, why not**

Our survival is our priority Pierre , we should agree on organising ourself the best possible way, do you want to hear about my desert survival insights?

**what insight?**

well, I think the jack knife is less useful than the air map, that we could use to start a fire

**Type your message here:**

**Your Ratings**

This is your current ranking of the item. If you change your mind, you can drag and drop items to their new ranking.

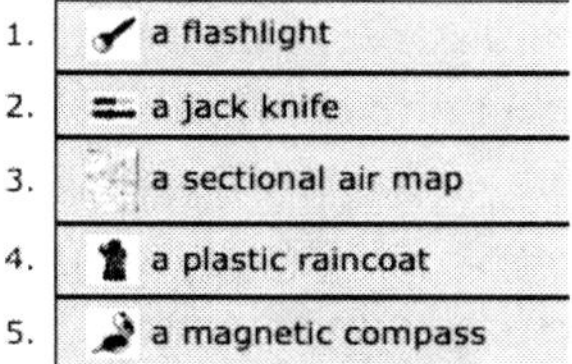

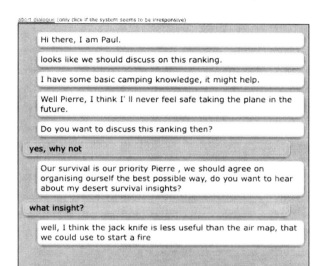

to a final ranking. This change in ranking is used to measure the persuasion with the metric proposed by (Andrews & Manandhar, 2009), which shows how many swaps in the ranking the user did towards the system's ranking.

To compare the novel hybrid dialogue system with the state of the art, an experiment is conducted where each participant faces two dialogue systems consecutively:

- The *full* system, which is the architecture described in the PD section, with hybrid planning and reactive dialogue management.
- The *"limited"* system, which is a dialogue manager trying to solve the same task, only with planning and without a reactive component.

The order in which the full and limited systems are presented is randomly chosen. The procedure for both system is exactly the same for the users, who are not told that two different systems are used and do not know in which order the systems are presented. In our experiment, an informal questioning of the participants showed that they did not realise that they were facing different types of systems. Sixteen participants took part in the online evaluation and faced both systems. The participants group was of mixed gender and age (from 20 to 59) and had a variety of backgrounds. As we discuss in this section, even with such a small number of participants, some interesting features of the persuasive dialogue were observed.

The main hypothesis of this research is that the EDEN Framework design eases the persuasion and achieves better results than a standard planning design. Indeed, a first observation of the results shows that the full dialogue system achieves a significant improvement of persuasiveness. While the participants in the limited system perform on average only 0.44 swaps *away* from the system's goal ranking – with a worst case of 4 swaps away –, when using the full system, the users go towards the system's goal ranking, with an average of 1.44 swaps – with a maximum of 8 swaps. Hence, the EDEN Framework achieves 8.25% stronger persuasion than the purely planned system. The reasons that could explain such increase in persuasiveness are detailed in the following sections.

The study of research in Persuasive Communication (Stiff & Mongeau, 2002) was used to set the hypothesis that human-computer dialogue would be more persuasive if the system is able to make the user feel more comfortable by increasing the empathy of its response and using strategies to lower the user's frustration. The users' answers to the questionnaire statement "In this conversation, the other user interacted with you the way you expected it would." show an interesting evaluation from the participants. The answers to this statement, while showing no significant difference between systems, have an impact on the dialogue persuasiveness, in particular with the *full* system there is a strong correlation between the participants' perception of the system and the resulting persuasiveness. Indeed, the participants that thought the computer system behaved as they had expected change more their mind than the participants that were unhappy with the system interaction.

## 6. FUTURE RESEARCH DIRECTIONS

Interactive QA and automatic persuasive dialogue are two relatively young disciplines in which great progress can yet be made. A common point of improvement is in the technical area, where HCI studies are yet to be optimized. From the linguistic research viewpoint, a better control of context, including improved anaphora and follow-up resolution are required as current algorithms for English only reach 70-80% accuracy depending on the text and domain, while little work exists for languages with fewer available resources.

In IQA in particular, a thorough study of the potentials and limitations of a conversational dialogue manager to address open-domain QA are still missing. In particular, the "search engine bias" of textual IQA, resulting in users addressing a natural language system by using keywords, is still detrimental to the technology. A possible way to overcome this is to look in the direction of spoken QA interfaces. These would prove particularly beneficial for types of question answering that involve breaking the text of the answer or explaining it step by step, as advocated in (Quarteroni & Saint-Dizier, 2009).

In persuasive dialogue, it is thus important to avoid the frustration generated by standard task oriented dialogue (Klein, Moon, & Picard, 1999). We have proposed a first step towards designing a more reactive system to tackle this issue, however this kind of applications of computer dialogue is quite novel and there is still work to be done in modelling and monitoring the users' beliefs and in providing more freedom to the user in the dialogue while still guaranteeing the achievements of dialogue goals.

Another important task for persuasive dialogue is the management of difficult to model human traits, such as personality variations between users that will affect the type of persuasive strategies needed but also the management of emotions of the users (amongst which frustration with the system) to implement persuasive strategies that do not fully rely on logical demonstrations but also on personal and emotional aspects.

## 7. CONCLUSION

We have introduced two hybrid dialogue management approaches that combine a reactive, conversational layer with a task-oriented dialogue layer in the context of Interactive Question Answering and Persuasive Dialogue.

Our results show that although Interactive Question Answering systems are well received in terms of user satisfaction, some users seem to prefer more traditional information retrieval paradigms and value the advantages of interactivity at a lesser extent. We believe that this is due partly to cultural reasons (the search engine-like, non-interactive model of information retrieval biasing users), and partly to the fact that the follow-up resolution mechanism of the interactive version is not always accurate, generating errors and delaying the delivery of results. Moreover, a chat interface raises expectations concerning what the system can understand; when these are not met - e.g. when the system asks for reformulation at a frustrating frequency - user satisfaction decreases.

Moreover, persuasiveness requires that the system does not alienate the users by forcing their choices. In particular, if such a system is to be used on a long-term basis for applications requiring multiple dialogues, the dialogue will need to keep the user involved in the interaction by preserving trust and by avoiding coercion. Our experiments show that the proposed hybrid framework can be more persuasive than a standard planning approach. This is linked to the presence of a new, layered approach that allows a better management of discourse level reactions as well as simpler integration of reactive argumentation strategies. The Desert Survival Scenario experiment results show that the proposed dialogue model and framework achieve better persuasiveness without influencing the perception of the users.

## REFERENCES


Alexandersson, J., Reithinger, N., & Maier, E. (1997). *Insights into the dialogue processing of VERBMOBIL*. Saarbrücken, Germany.

Allen, J., Ferguson, G., & Stent, A. (2001). An architecture for more realistic conversational systems. *IUI '01: Proceedings of the 6th International Conference on Intelligent user interfaces.*

Allen, J. F., Ferguson, G., Miller, B. W., Ringger, E. K., & Sikorski, T. (2000). Dialogue systems: From theory to practice in TRAINS-96. In *Handbook of natural language processing* (pp. 347-376).

Andrews, P., & Manandhar, S. (2009). Measure of belief change as an evaluation of persuasion. *Proceedings of the AISB'09 Persuasive Technology and Digital Behaviour Intervention Symposium.*

Basili, R., De Cao, D., Giannone, C., & Marocco, P. (2007). Data-driven dialogue for interactive question answering. *Proceedings of AI*IA'07.*

Bickmore, T., & Giorgino, T. (2004). *Some novel aspects of health communication from a dialogue systems perspective*. AAAI Fall Symposium on Dialogue Systems for Health Communication.

Bickmore, T. W., & Picard, R. W. (2005). Establishing and maintaining long-term human-computer relationships. *ACM Transactions on Computer-Human Interaction*, *12*, 293–327. doi:10.1145/1067860.1067867

Blum, A. L., & Furst, M. L. (1997). Fast planning through planning graph analysis. *Artificial Intelligence*, *90*, 281–300. doi:10.1016/S0004-3702(96)00047-1

Bos, J., Klein, E., Lemon, O., & Oka, T. (2003). DIPPER: Description and formalisation of an information-state update dialogue system architecture. *Proceedings of SIGDial'03.*

Cahn, J. E., & Brennan, S. E. (1999). A psychological model of grounding and repair in dialog. In S. E. Brennan, A. Giboin, & D. Traum (Ed.), *Working Papers of the AAAI Fall Symposium on Psychological Models of Communication in Collaborative Systems* (pp. 25–33). Menlo Park, CA: AAAI.

Cassell, J., & Bickmore, T. (2002). Negotiated collusion: Modeling social language and its relationship effects in intelligent agents. (in press) *User Modeling and Adaptive Interfaces*.

Churcher, G. E., Atwell, E. S., & Souter, C. (1997). *Dialogue mnagement systems: A survey and overview.*

Cohen, P. (1996). Dialogue modeling. In Cole, R. (Ed.), *Survey of the state of the art in human language technology* (pp. 192–197). Cambridge, UK: Cambridge University Press.

Core, M., & Allen, J. (1997). *Coding dialogs with the DAMSL annotation scheme*. AAAI Fall Symposium on Communicative Action in Humans and Machines, (pp. 28-35).

De Boni, M., & Manandhar, S. (2005). Implementing clarification dialogue in open-domain question answering. *Natural Language Engineering*, 11.

Farzanfar, R., Frishkopf, S., Migneault, J., & Friedman, R. (2005). Telephone-linked care for physical activity: A qualitative evaluation of the use patterns of an information technology program for patients. *Journal of Biomedical Informatics*, *38*, 220–228. doi:10.1016/j.jbi.2004.11.011

Festinger, L. (1957). *A theory of cognitive dissonance*. Standford University Press.

Field, D., & Ramsay, A. (2006). How to change a person's mind: Understanding the difference between the effects and consequences of speech acts. *Proceedings 5th Workshop on Inference in Computational Semantics (ICoS-5)*, (pp. 27-36).

Fogg, B. J. (2003). *Persuasive technology: Using computers to change what we think and do*. Morgan Kaufman Publishers.

Freedman, R. (2000). *Plan-based dialogue management in a physics tutor* (pp. 52–59). ANLP.

Galibert, O., Illouz, G., & Rousset, S. (2005). Ritel: An open-domain, human-computer dialogue system. *Proceedings of INTERSPEECH'05.*

Gilbert, M. A., Grasso, F., Groarke, L., Gurr, C., & Gerlofs, J. M. (2003). The persuasion machine. In Norman, T. J., & Reed, C. (Eds.), *Argumentation machines: New frontiers in argument and computation*.

Ginzburg, J. (1996). *Interrogatives: Questions, facts and dialogue*. Oxford, UK: Blackwell.

Gorin, A. L., Riccardi, G., & Wright, J. H. (1999). *How may I help you? Computational models of speech pattern processing*. Springer.

Grosz, B. J., & Sidner, C. L. (1986). Attention, intentions, and the structure of discourse. *Computational Linguistics*, *12*(3), 175–204.

Guerini, M., Stock, O., & Zancanaro, M. (2003). Persuasion models for intelligent interfaces. *Proceedings of the IJCAI Workshop on Computational Models of Natural Argument.*

Jönsson, A., & Merkel, M. (2003). Some issues in dialogue-based question-answering. *Working Notes from the AAAI Spring Symposium '03.*

Kato, T., Fukumoto, J., Masui, F., & Kando, N. (2006). WoZ simulation of interactive question answering. *Proceedings of IQA'06.* ACL.

Kirschner, M., & Bernardi, R. (2009). Exploring topic continuation follow-up questions using machine learning. *Proc. of NAACL HLT: Student Research Workshop.* Boulder, CO.

Kitano, H. (1991). Toward a plan-based understanding model for mixed-initiative dialogues. *Proceedings of ACL'91* (pp. 25–32). ACL.

Klein, J., Moon, Y., & Picard, R. W. (1999). This computer responds to user frustration. *CHI '99 extended abstracts on Human factors in computing systems - CHI '99.*

Kwok, C. T., Etzioni, O., & Weld, D. S. (2001). Scaling question answering to the Web. In *Proceedings of WWW'01.*

Levy, D., Catizone, R., Battacharia, B., Krotov, A., & Wilks, Y. (1997). CONVERSE: A conversational companion. *Proceedings of 1st International Workshop on Human-Computer Conversation.* Bellagio, Italy.

Lewin, I., Rupp, C. J., Hieronymus, J., Milward, D., Larsson, S., & Berman, A. (2000). *Siridus system architecture and interface report*. Siridus Project.

Maybury, M. T. (2002). *Towards a question answering roadmap*. MITRE Corporation.

Mazzotta, I., de Rosis, F., & Carofiglio, V. (2007). Portia: A user-adapted persuasion system in the healthy-eating domain. *Intelligent Systems, IEEE, 22*, 42–51. doi:10.1109/MIS.2007.115

Norman, T. J., & Reed, C. (2003). *Argumentation machines: New frontiers in argument and computation*. Argumentation Library.

Quarteroni, S., & Manandhar, S. (2009). Designing an interactive open domain question answering system. *Natural Language Engineering*, 73–95. doi:10.1017/S1351324908004919

Quarteroni, S., & Saint-Dizier, P. (2009). *Addressing how-to questions using a spoken dialogue system: A viable approach?* Singapore: KRAQ'09.

Reiter, E., & Dale, R. (1997). Building applied natural language generation systems. *Natural Language Engineering, 3*, 57–87. doi:10.1017/S1351324997001502

Simmons, R. (1965). Answering English questions by computer: A survey. *Communications of the ACM, 8*(1), 53–70. doi:10.1145/363707.363732

Sinclair, J. M., & Coulthard, R. M. (1975). *Towards an analysis of discourse: The English used by teachers and pupils*. Oxford University Press.

Small, S., Liu, T., Shimizu, N., & Strzalkowski, T. (2003). HITIQA: An interactive question answering system- a preliminary report. *Proceedings of the ACL 2003 Workshop on Multilingual summarization and QA* (pp. 46–53). Morristown, NJ: ACL.

Stent, A. (2002). A conversation acts model for generating spoken dialogue contributions. *Computer Speech & Language, 16*, 313–352. doi:10.1016/S0885-2308(02)00009-8

Stiff, J. B., & Mongeau, P. A. (2002). *Persuasive communication* (2nd ed.).

Sutton, S. (1998). Universal speech tools: The CSLU toolkit. *Proceedings of the International Conference on Spoken Language Processing (ICSLP'98).*

Traum, D. (1996). Conversational agency: TRAINS-93 dialogue manager. *Proceedings of the Twente Workshop on Language Technology: Dialogue Management in Natural Language Systems (TWLT 11)*, (pp. 1-11).

Vrajitoru, D. (2003). *Evolutionary sentence building for Chatterbots*. GECCO 2003 Late Breaking Papers, (pp. 315-321).

Walker, M. A., Litman, D. J., Kamm, C. A., & Abella, A. (1997). PARADISE: A framework for evaluating spoken dialogue agents. *Proceedings of the Eighth Conference on European chapter of the Association for Computational Linguistics*, (pp. 271–280).

Walton, D. (1996). *Argument structure: A pragmatic theory*. Toronto Studies in Philosophy.

Webb, N., & Strzalkowski, T. (2006). *Proceedings of the Interactive Question Answering Workshop at HLT-NAACL 2006.* New York, NY: The Association for Computational Linguistics.

Weizenbaum, J. (1966). ELIZA-a computer program for the study of natural language communication between man and machine. *Communications of the ACM, 9*, 36–45. doi:10.1145/365153.365168

Yang, F., Feng, Z., & Di Fabbrizio, G. (2006). A data driven approach to relevancy recognition for contextual question answering. *Proceedings of IQA.*

Young, S., Gasic, M., Keizer, S., Mairesse, F., Schatzmann, J., Thomson, B., & Yu, K. (2009). The iidden information state model: A practical framework for POMDP-based spoken dialogue management. *Computer Speech & Language*, *24*(2), 150–174. doi:10.1016/j.csl.2009.04.001

Zhe, X., & Boucouvalas, A. (2002). *Text-to-emotion engine for real time Internet communication*. International Symposium on CSNDSP.

Zinn, C., Moore, J. D., & Core, M. G. (2002). A 3-tier planning architecture for managing tutorial dialogue. *ITS '02: Proceedings of the 6th International Conference on Intelligent Tutoring Systems*, (pp. 574-584).

## KEY TERMS AND DEFINITIONS

**Activation Structure:** Is a search tree structure that can be used for encoding reaction rules for a reactive dialogue system. It encodes in different layers the contextualisation rules, the single utterance pattern matching and the generation rules. A specific dialogue move can then be matched to a path in this tree to find possible reactions to the latest user input.

**Artificial Intelligence Markup Language (AIML):** Is an XML dialect for creating natural language software agents.

**Dialogue Manager:** The core component of a dialogue system. It maintains the history of the dialog, and is in charge of deploying a dialogue strategy and deciding on the best response to the user.

**Persuasion vs. Argumentation:** Persuasion is a wide term that encompasses many tasks. It is a process that tries to change someone's behaviour, beliefs or attitude towards something. There is number of ways to perform persuasion, in particular, argumentation is a specific dialogue structure that has been studied since the ancient Greeks to improve persuasion through discourse.

**Persuasive Dialogue:** Is a dialogue where an interlocutor tries to change the behaviour of the audience. Computer based persuasive dialogue can take many forms and it is applied to many type of behaviour change tasks. In particular, the current research is focused on health habit changes and counseling to help, for instance, the users stop smoking, eat more healthily or do more physical activities.

**Question Answering (QA):** Is the task of automatically answering a question formulated in natural language. A QA system typically uses a collection of natural language documents (a local text corpus or the Web) as a source for relevant documents from which to extract answers. An Interactive QA system is a system able to perform a Question Answering task in the context of a natural language conversation.

**Wizard-of-Oz:** A research experiment in which users interact with a computer system that they believe to be autonomous, but which is actually being operated or partially operated by an unseen human being.

## ENDNOTES

1 http://www.alicebot.org/
2 http://www.ask.com
3 http://www.wolframalpha.com
4 http://trec.nist.gov/data/qa/
5 http://celct.isti.cnr.it/ResPubliQA
6 http://www.alicebot.org
7 http://chatterbean.bitoflife.cjb.net
8 http://trec.nist.gov

# Chapter 9
# Affective Conversational Agents:
## The Role of Personality and Emotion in Spoken Interactions

**Zoraida Callejas**
*University of Granada, Spain*

**Ramón López-Cózar**
*University of Granada, Spain*

**Nieves Ábalos**
*University of Granada, Spain*

**David Griol**
*Carlos III University of Madrid, Spain*

## ABSTRACT

*In this chapter, we revisit the main theories of human emotion and personality and their implications for the development of affective conversational agents. We focus on the role that emotion plays for adapting the agents' behaviour and how this emotional responsivity can be conveniently modified by rendering a consistent artificial personality. The multiple applications of affective CAs are addressed by describing recent experiences in domains such as pedagogy, computer games, and computer-mediated therapy.*

## 1 INTRODUCTION

Conversational agents (CAs) represent a higher level of intelligence with respect to traditional spoken interfaces as, especially in the case of embodied conversational agents (ECAs), they foster the so-called "persona effect", which refers to the credibility and motivation of agent based interfaces and its positive effect on the users' attitude towards the system (Lester et al., 1997). However, as Picard (2003) highlights, the more complex the system, the more complex the user's demands and when CAs are highly realistic but fail to sufficiently simulate humans, they may have a negative effect on the users, a phenomenon called

DOI: 10.4018/978-1-60960-617-6.ch009

"uncanny valley" (Beale & Creed, 2009). Thus, it is important to endow CAs with emotional and socially rich behaviours to make more natural and compelling interactions possible and meet the users' expectations.

Emotions provide an additional channel of communication alongside the spoken and graphical exchanges from which very valuable information can be obtained in order to adapt the CAs' behaviour (Ball, 2003). In contrast with the Descartian concept of *rational* intelligence, psychologists have introduced the term *emotional* intelligence to describe the necessary emotional processing to tailor our conducts and cognitions to our environment. To endow CAs with emotional awareness makes it possible to recognize the user's emotions and adapt the agent functionalities to better accomplish his/her requirements. Stern (2003) also provides empirical evidence that if a user encounters a virtual character that seems to be truly emotional, there is also a potential to form emotional relationships with each other.

Additionally, the similarity-attraction principle states that users have a better attitude toward agents which exhibit a personality similar to their own. Thus, personality plays a very important role on how users assess CAs and their willingness to interact with them. In the same way as humans understand other humans' behaviour and react accordingly to it in terms of the observation of everyday behaviour (Lepri et al., 2009), the personality of a CA can be considered as a relatively stable pattern that affects its emotion expression and behaviour and differentiates it from other CAs (Xiao et al., 2005).

## 2 BACKGROUND: HUMAN EMOTION AND PERSONALITY

Many authors in research fields such as psychology, biology and neurology have proposed different definitions of the term *emotion* from a diversity of perspectives, each of which has contributed significant insight into the emotion science. A relevant example is Darwin's evolutional explanation for emotional behaviour (Darwin, 1872), with which he gave evidence of the continuity of emotional expressions from lower animals to humans, and described emotions as being functional to increase the chances of survival. According to Plutchik (2003, chapter 2), one of the implications of these findings is that research in emotion was expanded from the study of subjective feelings to the study of behaviour within a biological and evolutionary context.

Based on the evolutionary perspective, Rolls (2007, chapter 2) states that genes can specify the behaviour of animals by establishing goals instead of responses. According to Rolls, these goals elicit emotions through reward and punisher evaluation or appraisal of stimuli. Due to a process of natural selection, animals have built receptors for certain stimuli in the environment and linked them to responses. Rolls suggests several levels of complexity of such mechanism, in the most complicated, the behaviour of humans is guided by syntactic operations on semantically grounded symbols.

Other authors have adopted a physiological perspective by studying how subjective feelings are temporally related to bodily changes such as heart rate, muscle tension or breathing rate. Some authors, leaded by the seminal work by James (1884), argue that humans feel emotions because they experience bodily changes. According to his theory, it is impossible to feel an emotion without experiencing any physiological change. James' work was fundamental for the development of studies on autonomic physiological changes in relation to emotion. In Section 4 we will describe several methods for emotion recognition based on such physiological autonomous changes.

However, James' theory was refuted by Cannon (1929), who probed that this cause-effect relationship was not possible and pointed out a more plausible sequence of events: the perception of a situation gives rise to an emotion, which is then followed by bodily changes. Cannon was interested not only in the behavioural and physiological correlates of emotion, but also on the neural correlates which indicate how emotions are represented within the brain.

Heath, Cox and Lustick (1974) pointed out that all major parts of the brain participate in emotional states. As described in (Fox 2008, chapter 1) recent research indicates that different brain circuits control different aspects of emotion and many brain areas involved in emotion also participate in a range of other functions. Emotion is highly related to cognition; in Section 3 we will study the implications of such relationships for modelling affect in CAs.

For a long time, introspection has been the main way of emotional research so that psychologists have based their work on self reports of emotions. However, as discussed in (Fox 2008, chapter 2), such subjective reports are generally not reliable. As Freud claimed, emotions are complex inner states subject to repression and modification for conscious as well as unconscious reasons. Thus, it is necessary to have information about the causes of emotion, as they can be elicited by the presence of non conscious stimuli which cannot be described with self reports. As will be addressed in Section 3, the representation of emotion in CAs is usually based on models of the emotions' causes and appraisals.

Several attempts have been made to identify the nature of eliciting situations. For example, Roseman, Spindle and Jose (1990) proposed five types of appraisals of events which determine which particular emotional responses are appropriate. Kentridge and Appleton (1990) suggested that the suitability of emotional responses and expression is assessed by humans to reduce the possibility of an undesirable event or increasing the chances of a desirable event, which demands sufficient cognitive capacities to predict future events.

Additionally, emotional expression is influenced by individual characteristics such as age. For example, Scheibe and Carstensen (2010) corroborate that older individuals regulate their emotions more frequently, especially in the case of negative affect. Personality also affects emotion perception and expression. Although there is no universal definition of personality, it can be described as a complex organization of mental and biological systems that uniquely characterize an individual's behaviour, temperament and emotion attributes.

Fox et al. (2008) argue that personality predicts emotional expression both in general and in particular scenarios, concretely they studied public and private interaction. Larsen and Ketelaar (1991) have detected that extraversion is associated with an increased responsivity to controlled inductions of positive (but not negative affect), whereas neuroticism would be associated with an increased responsivity to controlled inductions of negative (but not positive) affect. In Section 5, several applications of CAs using personality models to modify their emotional behaviour are described.

Additionally, personality does not only influence emotion perception and reaction, but also modulates neural mechanisms of learning (Hooker et al., 2008), which for example has a deep impact on intelligence and academic performance (Rindermann & Neubauer, 2001).

## 3 REPRESENTATION OF EMOTION AND PERSONALITY IN CAS

### 3.1 Basic Emotions and Personality Traits

As explained in (Plutchik 2003, chapter 4), one of the difficulties of reporting and understanding emotion is that we assume that the listener understands the terms we use when describing affect because of similar experiences and through empathy. However, it might not be so, precisely because of the inaccuracy of self reports, for example due to stimuli out of conscious awareness. Additionally, there are words that describe similar states, which are to some extent related by an implicit intensity dimension (e.g. sad and desolated), whereas there are other words which are considered to represent opposites (e.g. sad and happy).

This ambiguity in the language of emotion raised the question of whether there exists a reduced number of primary or basic emotions from which secondary emotions can be obtained by blending them in a similar way as colours can be obtained as a mixture of the basic ones. The underlying idea is that once an emotion is triggered, a set of easily and universally recognizable behavioural and physiological responses is produced. This can be empirically demonstrated by the fact that some emotions seem to appear in all cultures as well as across many animal species (Fox 2008, chapter 4).

Several authors have proposed lists of basic emotions – see (Plutchik 2003, chapter 4) for a comprehensive review – however, there has been no agreement about which emotions are primary or secondary and which features make an emotion fall into any of the two categories.

During the last decades, there have been numerous initiatives in which the main words related to emotion have been acquired and grouped using statistical factor analysis. At the same time, several authors such as Osgood, Suci & Tannenbaum (1957) computed correlations between each pair of emotions so that not only grouping could be made, but also it was possible to measure similarity between the categories. When converted into angular distances, these measures could be employed to arrange emotions in a circle as the one proposed by Conte & Plutchik (1981). This same experiment was carried out by Russell (1994) in other languages different from English, and most of the emotion words felt in similar locations on the circle. Also emotions which are intuitively considered as opposite were found in opposite locations in the circular representation.

Regarding personality, it describes what it is most typical and characteristic of an individual, distinguishing him/her from the rest. According to (Fox 2008, chapter 3), self-report instruments have been used to identify the key personality factors or traits that contribute the uniqueness of a person and explain how people differ from each other. Thus, according to Fox, when using the notion of traits it is assumed that people have a reduced number of core aspects of their personality than can influence how a particular situation might be perceived or appraised.

As explained in (Xiao et al., 2005) most trait theorists assume that all people have a fixed number of basic dimensions of personality. However although a consensus about the number of dimensions would be desirable (Eysenck, 1991), several authors have proposed different criteria. Some authors use a reduced number of traits, for example two in (Eysenck & Eysenck, 1963), whereas others take into account more than a dozen, such as Cattell (1943), who suggests 16 dimensions.

Although thousands of different trait words are used in natural language, only a relatively small number is employed in practice. With the aim of reasoning about personality, personality psychologists have tried to identify the most essential and universal terms. To do so, a similar procedure as in the case of emotions was used in which the typically adjectives for describing personality were collected and grouped using factor analysis (Allport & Odbert, 1936).

However, the most widespread grouping is the Five Factor Model (or Big Five), which has become a standard in psychology. Although slightly different words have been used for the five factors, generally the following terms are employed (McCrae & Costa, 1989):

1. Extraversion vs. Introversion (sociable, assertive, playful vs. aloof, reserved, shy);
2. Emotional stability vs. Neuroticism (calm, unemotional vs. insecure, anxious);

3. Agreeableness vs. Disagreeable (friendly, cooperative vs. antagonistic, faultfinding);
4. Conscientiousness vs. Un-conscientiousness (self-disciplined, organized vs. inefficient, careless);
5. Openness to experience (intellectual, insightful vs. shallow, unimaginative).

The five clusters of personality factors are also referred to as the OCEAN model (Openness, Conscientiousness, Extraversion, Agreeableness and Negative emotionality). Cross-cultural stability of the Five Factor Model has been demonstrated by various authors. For example, McCrae et al. (2005) found scalar equivalence of NEO-PI-R factors (a 240-item measure of the model) for 51 cultures.

## 3.2 Models of Emotion and Personality

The notion of primary emotions allows CAs developers to consider them as discrete categories. An alternative solution is placing them in a continuous case, representing them by coordinates in a space with a small number of dimensions. The typical approach is to use the bidimensional activation-evaluation space (Cowie et al., 2001), which emerged from the circumflex arrangement of emotions proposed by psychologists that was discussed in the previous section.

The first dimension of this space corresponds to the valence of the emotional state. Valence represents whether the emotion is perceived to be positive or negative. As discussed by Plutchik (2003), emotions cannot be considered positive or negative by themselves as, from the adaptive role that emotions play (from the evolutive perspective), no emotion can be considered negative (e.g. fear motivates withdrawal behaviour when a danger is perceived). Thus, valence does not deal with the positive/negative nature of emotion, but rather with the perception of the subject, that is, whether the person perceives the emotion to be positive or negative depending on the stimulus.

The second dimension, activation (or arousal), measures the user disposition to take some action rather than none. This is linked with Darwin's theories which relate emotion with action.

According to Fragopanagos & Taylor (2005), the strength of the drive to act as a result of an emotion is an appropriate complement to the valence rating. However, sometimes it is necessary to contemplate additional dimensions to distinguish between similar emotions; for example, by taking into account the perceived control over the emotion or the inclination to engage.

Emotions can also be represented from a cognitive perspective that describes how users deal with the situation that caused the emotion. Ortony, Collins & Clore (1988) proposed a computationally tractable model of the cognitive basis of emotion elicitation which is known as the OCC model. This model argues that emotions derive from self appraisal of the current situation (consisting of events, agents, and objects) with respect to our goals and preferences. Usually this theory is employed for constructing rules for appraising the situations which generate the different emotion considered, which can be used by CAs to infer the user's emotion or to synthesize its own emotional state.

With respect to personality, most of the computational models that have been used in literature are based on trait theories, that is, on easily distinguishable categories or trait dimensions. Some CAs have implemented sophisticated models of personality which take into account a high number of dimensions, for instance the Cybercafé and Bui's ParleE (Bui et al., 2002) successfully applied the 16 dimensions of personality proposed by Rousseau (1996). However, the most employed is the Five Factor Model.

For example, Read et al. (2007) propose the Personality-Enabled Architecture for Cognition (PAC), which is based on the main five traits and designed to represent individual behavioural variability from personality. Their goal was to create agents who make different choices as a function of differences in their underlying motivational systems. Reithinger et al. (2006) also employ a five factor model of personality, in this case to bias the emotions intensities of the ECAs of the Virtual-Human system. The Virtual-Human system provides a knowledge-based framework to create interactive applications in a multi-user multi-agent setting.

## 4 RECOGNITION OF THE USER AFFECTIVE STATE

Emotion recognition for CAs is usually treated as a classification problem in which the input is the user last response (voice, facial expressions, body gestures…) and the output is the most probable emotional state. Many different machine learning classifiers have been employed for emotion recognition and frequently the final emotion is decided considering the results of several of these classification algorithms (López-Cózar et al., 2008). Some of the classifiers most widely used are K-nearest neighbours (Lee & Narayanan, 2005), Hidden Markov Models (Pitterman & Pitterman, 2006; Ververidis & Kotropoulos, 2006), Support Vector Machines (Morrison, Wang & Silva, 2007), Neural Networks (Morrison, Wang & Silva, 2007; Callejas & López-Cózar, 2008) and Boosting Algorithms (Sebe et al., 2004; Zhu & He, 2008). A detailed review can be found in (Ververidis & Kotropoulos, 2006).

In this chapter we will address the features employed for emotion classification, from which we will focus on physiological, neurological, acoustic, linguistic and visual features as summarized in Figure 1. This is not an exhaustive taxonomy, and there are other authors who also incorporate other sources of information such as dialogue-related (Callejas & López-Cózar, 2008) and cultural and social settings. In fact, according to Boehner et al. (2007) emotions are interactionally constructed and subjectively experienced, so that physiological, neurological and other approaches to emotion which measure emotion "objectively" fail to address how emotions are actually experienced.

### 4.1 Physiological Features

The autonomic nervous system controls the physiological changes associated to emotion sending signals to various body organs, muscles and glands (Fox 2008, chapter 2). These changes can be accounted using different measures such as:

- Galvanic skin response (GSR). There is a relationship between the arousal of emotions and changes in GSR.
- Heart rate and blood pressure. The number of heart bits per minute and the systolic and diastolic blood pressure can be good indicatives of changes in arousal.
- Breathing rate. The number of breaths per minute provides a good measure of physiological arousal.
- Electromyography (EMG). EMG can measure different muscle tension, activity and contractions related to emotion expression.

For example, the Emotion Mirror web-based application used physiological measures in a job interview scenario (Prendinger et al., 2003); finding that the users who interacted with a empathetic agent had lower skin conductance, and thus were less stressed than those that interacted with the non-empathetic agent. The empathetic ECA just mirrored the user emotion. In order to recognize it, they obtained a baseline for the bio-signals during an initial relaxation period and subsequently measured the GSR and EMG values during a job interview.

Lim & Reeves (2010) used physiological measures to compliment subjective reports about likeability of computer games and obtained that different patterns of physiological responses may be observed depending on the perceived agency of a co-player. For example, there was greater skin

*Figure 1. Summary of the main features employed for emotion recognition*

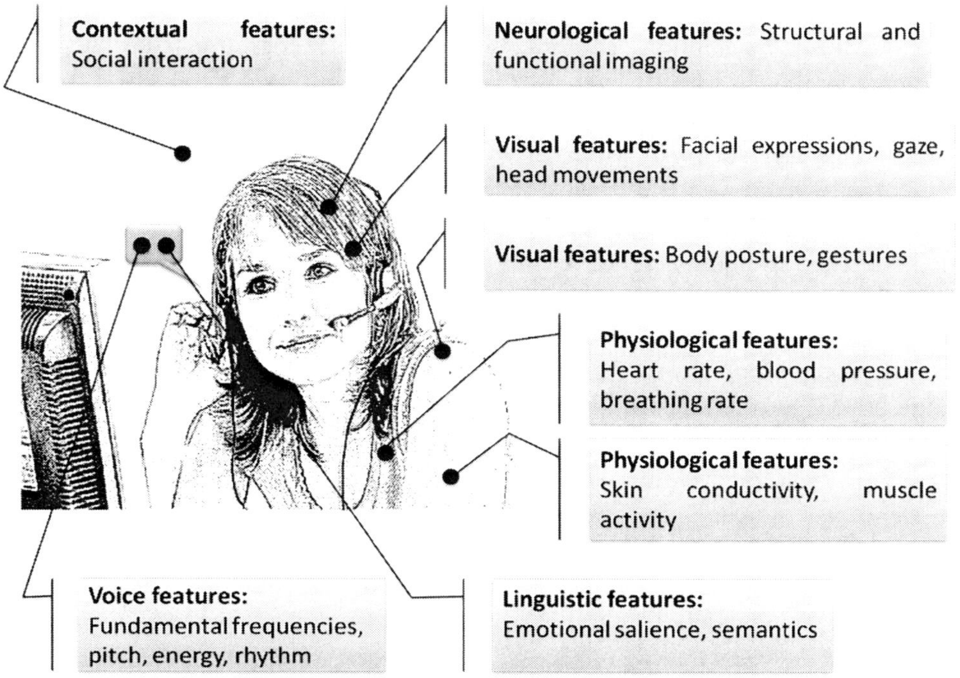

**Contextual features:** Social interaction

**Neurological features:** Structural and functional imaging

**Visual features:** Facial expressions, gaze, head movements

**Visual features:** Body posture, gestures

**Physiological features:** Heart rate, blood pressure, breathing rate

**Physiological features:** Skin conductivity, muscle activity

**Voice features:** Fundamental frequencies, pitch, energy, rhythm

**Linguistic features:** Emotional salience, semantics

conductance activity, and thus more emotional engagement, with CAs controlled by humans (avatars) than with agents, which highlights the importance of providing more humanlike behaviours to CAs, such as for example endowing them with affective awareness and responsivity.

## 4.2 Neurological Features

Neurological features are related to the limbic system. Traditionally, the relationships between emotions and the brain have been discovered to a high extent thanks to the research with animals, usually employing surgery. However, during the last decades there has been a big technological advance which allows to reliably obtaining images of the brain and its activity. A detailed explanation of these methods and its relationship with emotions can be found in (Peper, 2006; Aleman, Swart & Rijn, 2008). We distinguish two main groups:

- Structural imaging methods, such as computerized tomography (CT) or magnetic resonance imaging (MRI).
- Functional imaging methods, such as positron emission tomography (PET), electroencephalography (EEG), functional magnetic resonance imaging (fMRI) or magnetoencephalography (MEG).

Despite their usefulness for measuring brain states, Cowie et al. (2001) claim that research cannot realistically expect brain imaging to identify emotion terms as they are used in natural language, as most of the previous techniques require restricting activity making it impossible to study whether normal activity would interfere with the detection of emotion. The authors argue that recognizing the emotional state of a person implicates subtle features of the ways in which neural systems operate rather than simply detecting whether they are active or not.

## 4.3 Voice Features

Speech is deeply affected by emotions: acoustic, contour, tone, voice quality and articulation change with different emotions. A comprehensive study of those changes is presented in (Cowie et al., 2001). We will distinguish four main groups of features: pitch, formant frequencies, energy and rhythm, a more detailed taxonomy can be found in (Batliner et al., in press).

Pitch depends on the tension of the vocal folds and the sub glottal air pressure (Ververidis & Kotropoulos, 2006), and can be used to obtain information about emotions in speech. As noted by Hansen (1996), mean pitch values may be employed as significant indicators for emotional speech when compared with neutral conditions.

Additionally, the first two formant frequencies (F1 and F2) and their bandwidths (B1 and B2) are a representation of the vocal tract resonances. Speakers change the configuration of the vocal tract to distinguish the phonemes that they wish to utter, thus resulting in shifts of formant frequencies. Different speaking styles produce variations of the typical positions of formants. In the particular case of emotional speech, the vocal tract is modified by the emotional state. As pointed out by Hansen (1996), in stressed or depressed states speakers do not articulate voiced sounds with the same effort as in neutral emotional states.

Energy is also considered a relevant indicative of emotion as it is related to its arousal level (Ververidis & Kotropoulos, 2006). The variation of energy of words or utterances can be used as a significant indicator for various speech styles, as the vocal effort and ratio (duration) of voiced/unvoiced parts of speech change. For example, Hansen (1996) demonstrated that loud and angry emotions significantly increase energy.

With regard to rhythm features, they are based on the duration of voiced and unvoiced segments and previous studies noted that the duration variance decreases for most domains under fast stress conditions (Boersma, 1993).

## 4.4 Linguistic Features

Emotion recognition from linguistic features deals with linguistic changes depending on the emotional state of the user. For this purpose the technique of word emotional salience has gained remarkable attention. This measure represents the frequency of apparition of a word in a given emotional state or category, and is calculated from the analysis of a sentence corpus (Lee & Narayanan, 2005).

Although it is a straightforward method to assign affinity of emotions to words, the probabilities calculated using this approach are highly dependent on the corpus used and have some disadvantages such as not accounting for polysemous words. In order to solve this problem, statistical natural language processing approaches have been used. From the lexical and syntactic perspective, Mairesse & Walker (2007, 2008) have proposed a comprehensive list of features which are indicative of different personality traits, whereas from the semantics perspective, approaches such as Latent Semantic Analysis are usually employed to detect the underlying affective meaning of texts. Semantic analysis of affective expressions is very complicated. This analysis is very complex in the case of unconstrained interactions, for which different strategies must be defined to tackle with ambiguity. For example, Smith et al. (2007) propose an approach to endow CAs with the capability of extracting affect cues from metaphors such as *"you are an angel"* or *"you are a pig"*.

In the ERMIS project (Fragopanagos & Taylor, 2005) a method was introduced which unified the previously described approaches and mapped words in the activation-evaluation space. In this space, the words formed a trajectory which represented the movement of emotion in the speech stream.

When linguistic features are employed, it is important to take into account contextual information such as age and cultural background, as it influences the lexical indicators of emotion and personality. This situation was addressed by Yildirim, Narayanan & Potamianos (in press) who analyzed the effect of age in polite and frustrated behaviour of children during spontaneous spoken dialog interaction with CAs in a computer game.

In other cases, the emotional salience of the linguistic contents can only be disambiguated using acoustic information. De Rosis et al. (2007) claim that rule-based recognition criteria including consideration of the context is necessary to study how the changes in prosody vary the interpretation of affect derived from the linguistic content.

## 4.5 Visual Features

In a conversation, the users convey non-linguistic visual messages which are useful to detect their affective state. Facial expressions, gaze, body posture, and head or hands movements are usually employed for emotion recognition.

The face plays a significant role in human emotion perception and expression. The association between face and affective arousal has been widely studied; a comprehensive review of the main psychological and biological studies on facial expression since Darwin theories is addressed in (Plutchik 2003, chapter 7).

Most studies of automatic emotion recognition focus on six basic facial expressions proposed by Ekman (1994) as universally perceived across cultures. These emotions are: happiness, sadness, anger, fear, surprise and disgust. Usually, in conversational systems facial expression is recognized along with vocal cues in order to differentiate emotional facial expressions and expressions which are caused by articulatory lip movements (Zeng et al., 2007). In (Chibelushi & Bourel, 2003) there is a survey of the main facial expression recognition approaches.

Some authors have focused on specific parts of the face such as gaze or smiles. For example, (Kumano et al., 2009) studied smile as a good indicator of interpersonal emotion in meetings and a cue for attention assessment. Morency, Christoudias & Darrell (2006) built an ECA which, based on the user gaze, could discriminate if he was thinking a response or waiting for the agent to intervene. Bee, André & Tober (2009) used eye-contact between the user and an ECA named Alfred to "break the ice" and determine the user's willingness to engage in an interaction with the agent.

Regarding body gestures, Shan, Gong & McOwan (2007) suggest that using information about body gesture and facial expression allows more accurate emotion recognition. For example, Kapoor & Picard (2005) classified children's affective state of interest when solving puzzles by combining information extracted form face videos, a chair which sensed body posture and the state of the puzzle.

## 4.6 Corpora

In order to train emotion recognizers it is necessary to have a corpus in which all the features used for classification are proportionally present. There are three main approaches for collecting emotional corpora: recording spontaneous conversations, recording induced emotions, and asking actors to simulate emotions. There is a compromise between naturalness of the emotions and control over the collected data: the more control over the generated data, the less spontaneity and naturalness of the expressed emotion, and vice versa.

Spontaneous conversations in the application domain of the emotion recognizer constitute the most realistic approach. However, a lot of effort is necessary for the annotation of the corpus, as it requires an interpretation of which emotion is being expressed in each recording (Callejas & López-Cózar, 2009). Sometimes, the corpus is recorded from human-to-human interaction in the application domain (Forbes-Riley & Litman, 2004). In these cases, the result is also natural but it is not directly applicable to the case in which humans interact with a CA.

Opposite to the previous approach, acted emotions are easier to manipulate and avoids the need for annotation, as emotions conveyed in each recording are known beforehand. The results obtained are highly dependent on the skills of the actors, which implies that the best results are obtained with actors with good drama preparation. When non-expert actors are used, another phase is necessary to discard the recordings that fail to reproduce the required emotion appropriately.

Induced emotions represent a trade-off between the two approaches discussed above. Emotions can be more natural, like the ones elicited when playing computer games (Johnstone, 1996), or easier to manipulate, like the ones induced by making people read texts that relate to specific emotions (Stibbard, 2000).

Due to its complexity, emotion recognition is a study field on its own. There are many researchers trying to find the most representative features for classification, and the most appropriate methods for emotion recognition. Many of them work considering acted emotions, and thus, their results cannot be directly applied to more realistic scenarios where the users behave spontaneously.

Batliner et al. (2004) consider this problem and state that a possible solution, in addition to colleting more data, is taking into account other information sources, such as for example monitoring the user's behaviour. Following this approach, we have obtained good emotion recognition results when considering contextual information about the interaction in an emotionally aware spoken dialogue system (Callejas & López-Cózar, 2008). Concretely, we considered adding information about the user's neutral voice and the dialogue history, which improved both automatic classification and human annotation of a corpus of spontaneous emotions. For illustration purposes, a benchmark with the success rates of different acoustic emotion recognition approaches for nine standard corpora can be found in (Schuller et al., 2009).

## 5 AFFECTIVE RESPONSIVITY AND ADAPTIVITY IN CAS

Picard (2003) poses the question of whether machines have emotions in the same way that humans do, and comes to the conclusion that we can never be sure that we have understood and thus imitated every mechanism involved in human emotion. Hence, we will never be completely confident that machines have emotions. However, she points out the possibility to agree in some value of N known human emotion mechanisms that suffices for a reasonable emotional behaviour.

We are still far from reaching an agreement in which mechanisms are part of this set of N, and every author considers a different mechanism that is relevant for his/her purposes and application domain. Usually, affective applications using CAs follow the so-called "affective loop", which represents the cycle of recognizing the user's emotion, selecting the most suitable action depending on the user state, and synthesizing the appropriate affective response (Höök, 2008, 2009).

Very representative examples of such interactions are interactive storytelling systems, in which expressive ECAs (virtual actors) interact with users involving them in the story. Cavazza, Pizzi and Charles (2009) highlight the importance of affective behaviour of such actors and present the EmoEmma demonstrator, in which an ECA represents Emma Bovary, the main character of Flaubert's novel Madame Bovary. In EmoEmma, the user can address the ECA or respond to her, impersonating her lover. The system recognizes the users' emotions from his utterances, which are analyzed in terms of the current narrative context including the characters' beliefs, feelings and expectations. The recognized emotion influences the ECA behaviour, achieving a high level of realism for the interaction.

Role-playing has also demonstrated being a powerful instrument for exploring social relationships, and to promote intra-psychic self reflection. Imholz (2008) claims that virtual worlds are a very powerful tool for using psychodrama as a therapeutic practice. From her study it seems that role-playing using avatars capable of affective interactions can be very useful for the treatment of affect disorders. However, Nomura (2005) argues that therapeutic agents may be employed just as tools that satisfy the users' desire to talk about themselves while hiding the things concealed in their narratives that would be unmasked by a human therapist. According to this perspective, if the agents are sophisticated enough to explicitly draw things concealed in the users' narratives, they would act contrary to the users' expectations, which may cause abusive behaviours toward the agents.

Many interaction logs show that some users are annoyed by these displays and feel compelled to challenge the agent's assumption of human traits, often expressing their dissatisfaction by verbally abusing the agents (Brahnam, 2005; Brahnam, 2009). Nijholt (2007) offers an interesting solution for the situation in which a CA is attacked because of imperfect behaviour, which is to anticipate it and use humour by endowing the agent with the capability for humorous act generation. The agent can then make fun of its own defects by generating humorous remarks, which is another type of affective behaviour. This way, humour appeals to positive emotion making the interaction between the user and the CA more enjoyable.

In the storytelling application domain, the user influences the agents' emotional state in order to develop the drama. In other applications, the objective is quite the contrary, that is, to endow the agents with persuasion capabilities. This is the case of virtual counsellors such as the one presented in (Schulman & Bickmore, 2009), an ECA which persuades the users to change their attitudes towards exercise. The authors claim that it is important to endow CAs with social dialogue and other relationship-building tactics for successful persuasion. Affective awareness in CAs has a great potential to reach this objective, as shown in (De Rosis et al., 2007), in which an ECA named Valentina adapts its behaviour to the attitude of its users, which makes its dietetic suggestions more effective.

Similarly, in pedagogic application domains, the CAs must be able to recognize the students' emotions. For example, the PrimeClimb agent (Conati & Maclaren, 2009) was able to assess the possible eliciting situations employing the OCC theory to recognize whether the reason for the emotion is something the user has done (e.g. pride or shame depending on his success), or it is because of the agent behaviour (e.g. admiration or reproach). Processing the eliciting situations allows the CA to tailor its responses and reinforce learning in the appropriate way by either making the student feel better towards him/herself and thus more motivated, or by tuning the behaviours which cause a negative effect on the user.

In order to follow the human mechanisms of affective behaviour, the affective response selected by a CA should be tailored to certain personality traits in such a way that personality modifies motivational intensity for decision making. De Sevin (2009) proposed an approach to action selection based on traits with a customizable virtual human and empirically demonstrated that it could be an easy way to test personality traits by tweaking the motivational intensities in order to obtain more distinct and believable virtual humans. For example, Maria & Zitar (2007) compared a regular intelligent agent with a personality-rich one in the domain of an "orphanage care problem", and obtained that the affective agent succeeded in adapting its priorities better based on a model of likes and dislikes.

Additionally, as argued by Ortony (2003), personality is important to build believable emotional agents, as it is needed to ensure situational and individual appropriate internal responses (emotions), external response (behaviours and behavioural inclination), and arrange for sensible coordination between internal and external responses.

Regarding individual responses, the Idolum framework demonstrated an idle-time behaviour of moods and emotions controlled by a consistent personality. In order to be more believable, Idolum took into account aspects of personality, mood and stimuli elements from psychological models such as a time cycle (winter/summer), the weather, or a manic/depressive cycle that can affect its emotional behaviour (Marriot, 2003).

Regarding situational responses, it is necessary to integrate contextual background in affective interactions. For example, Endrass, Rehm & André (2009) were interested in studying differences in communication management between Asian and Western cultures and their implications in developing ECAs. They recorded dialogues with German and Japanese human participants which revealed a different usage of pauses in speech and overlapping speech (Asian conversations contained more pauses and also more overlapping speech). They developed the Virtual Beergarden, a virtual meeting place in which culture-specific ECAs interact rendering the nonverbal behaviour observed with the human subjects. Their study reveals that German subjects seem to prefer communication management in dialogues between virtual agents which rehearse their culture-specific behaviour.

Another important application of affective systems is emotion mirroring (D'Mello et al., 2008). Affective CAs which imitate the user affective state are very useful to treat emotional and personality disorders. For example, in the FantasyA demonstrator of the SAFIRA project (Paiva et al., 2001), the users must interact with 3D conversational agents so that only when the user is able to make the CA portray the appropriate affective expressions, s/he can move to the next level of the game. Other authors (Bickmore & Picard, 2005; McQuiggan & Lester, 2007) have studied the role of empathy in ECAs. However, as stated by Beale & Creed (2009), more research is required still to understand the potential of such agents to help people change their habitual behaviour.

Also affective CAs can be used to simulate human emotion in order to obtain a better understanding of the mechanisms that underlay it. For example, Scheutz (2001) developed a multi-agent environment aimed at studying the role of emotions as motivations for action, and how affective states develop according to the results of the interactions between different types of agents.

An interesting peculiarity of this research domain is that negative emotions and extreme personalities can play a very interesting role. While in other applications it might not be desirable to build negative emotions, in this case, as stated by Becker, Kopp & Wachsmuth (2007), an adequate implementation of a model based on emotion psychology will automatically give rise to negative emotional states which can lead to true understating of human affect.

For example, in the NECA Project (Krenn, 2003), the "socialite" demonstrator was implemented for multi-user web-mediated interaction through CAs that play the role of avatars. These avatars are enhanced with affective reasoning and personality traits and carry out unsupervised interaction with each other in the virtual environment. Similarly the SAFIRA Toolkit for affective computing (Paiva et al., 2001) addressed affective knowledge acquisition, representation, planning, communication and expression with a fuzzy approach. Their goal was to explore the nature of affective interaction which is intentionally made fuzzy, complex and rich to simulate real emotions, which are usually open to interpretation.

Creed & Beale (2008) investigated the psychological impact of simulated emotional expressions in ECAs, accounting for the effect of mismatching the synthesized facial and audio emotional expressions of the agents, for example, by using emotional facial expressions with a synthetic monotone voice. They obtained that mismatched emotions confused the users and altered their perception of the simulated expression which can cause frustration, annoyance and irritation. Their results corroborated the psychological cognitive dissonance theory, which claims that inconsistency between cognitions leads to a negative affective state that can motivate changes in elements of knowledge (Harmon-Jones, 2001).

These results highlight the significance of rendering perfectly tuned multimodal emotional responses. Other authors have also indicated the importance of controlling the visual presence of CAs so that they render the ethnicity and gender which the user perceives as expert in application domains such as education and consumer marketing. For example, Pratt et al. (2007) used ECAs to confirm the theories of neurological activation associated with implicit and explicit prejudicial responses based on stereotyping.

As has been described before, there are many ways in which CAs can show affect, and usually they are tailored to their application domain. Thus, it is very difficult to find a measure to evaluate the "degree of affectiveness" or emotional intelligence of a CA. Some authors take into account the number of modes in which the agent can show an emotional behaviour and the coordination among them. For example, Burleson & Picard (2007) changed the behaviour of a learning companion according to three aspects: the type of intervention (affect support or task support), the level of congruence of the intervention with respect to a learner's frustration, and the presence or absence of social non-verbal mirroring. They considered the agents to show a higher level of emotional intelligence when all these behaviours were coordinated, which also had a positive impact on the students' learning experience.

Other authors evaluate the affective response of their agents focusing on the users' response. On the one hand, this can be done by asking the users to evaluate the agent and provide judgments about their experience interacting with it. For example, Bickmore et al. (2005, 2010) evaluate the behaviour of social agents in the health and adult-care domain by means of self-reported therapeutic alliance and empathy of the patients with the agent. On the other hand, it is possible to measure the affective response of the users by employing any of the different measures described in Section 4, or a combination of several of them to obtain a more reliable assessment (Cavicchio & Poesio, 2008).

## 6 CONCLUSION

Emotions have evolved as a result of biological evolution in the form of complex responses to significant events which involve different physiological, neural, behavioural and cognitive components. This chapter has presented a review of the main emotion theories coming from different study areas, which have tried to progressively understand the nature of emotions and the related concept of personality, which represents the unique characteristics of an individual which have a deep influence on his/her affective experiences.

Many authors have tried to identify the most essential emotional dimensions and personality traits, models which, due to its synthetic nature, are applicable to the computational recognition, treatment and synthesis of emotion and personality. We have discussed the main characteristics of such models for the development of affective conversational agents. As conversation is one of the main components of social behaviours, endowing these agents with the ability to elicitate, imitate and process emotions and personality is essential to obtain more believable and lifelike agents. In the chapter we have described the main methods available to achieve this goal, focusing on the recognition of the user emotional state and the affective adaptability and responsivity of the agents, and presenting some of their most compelling applications.

## ACKNOWLEDGMENT

This research has been funded by the Spanish project HADA TIN2007-64718.

## 7 REFERENCES

Aleman, A., Swart, M., & Rijn, S. (2008). Genetics and imaging in neuroscience brain imaging, genetics and emotion. *Biological Psychology*, *79*(1), 58–69. doi:10.1016/j.biopsycho.2008.01.009

Allport, G. W., & Odbert, H. S. (1936). Trait names: A psycho-lexical study. *Psychological Monographs*, *47*, 171–220.

Ball, E. (2003). A Bayesian heart: Computer recognition and simulation of emotion. In Trappl, R., Petta, P., & Payr, S. (Eds.), *Emotions in humans and artifacts* (pp. 303–332). Cambridge, MA: The MIT Press.

Batliner, A., Hacker, C., Steidl, S., Nöth, E., & Haas, J. (2004). From emotion to interaction: Lessons from real human-machine dialogues. *Lecture Notes on Artificial Intelligence*, *3068*, 1–12.

Batliner, A., Steidl, S., Schuller, B., Seppi, D., Vogt, T., & Wagner, J. (in press). Whodunnit – dearching for the most important feature types signalling emotion-related user states in speech. *Computer Speech & Language*.

Beale, R., & Creed, C. (2009). Affective interaction: How emotional agents affect users. *International Journal of Human-Computer Studies*, *67*(9), 755–776. doi:10.1016/j.ijhcs.2009.05.001

Becker, C., Kopp, S., & Wachsmuth, I. (2007). Why emotions should be integrated into conversational agents. In Nishida, T. (Ed.), *Conversational informatics: An engineering approach* (pp. 49–67). West Sussex, United Kingdom: John Wiley & Sons, Ltd.doi:10.1002/9780470512470.ch3

Bee, N., André, E., & Tober, S. (2009). Breaking the ice in human-agent communication: Eye-gaze based initiation of contact with an embodied conversational agent. *Lecture Notes in Computer Science*, *5773*, 229–242. doi:10.1007/978-3-642-04380-2_26

Bickmore, T., Caruso, L., Clough-Gorr, K., & Heeren, T. (2005). It's just like you talk to a friend – relational agents for older adults. *Interacting with Computers*, *17*(6), 711–735. doi:10.1016/j.intcom.2005.09.002

Bickmore, T., Mitchell, S. E., Jack, B. W., Paasche-Orlow, M. K., Pfeifer, L. M., & O'Donnell, J. (2010). Response to a relational agent by hospital patients with depressive symptoms. *Interacting with Computers*, *22*, 289–298. doi:10.1016/j.intcom.2009.12.001

Bickmore, T., & Picard, R. (2005). Establishing and maintaining long-term human–computer relationships. *ACM Transactions on Computer-Human Interaction*, *12*(2), 293–327. doi:10.1145/1067860.1067867

Boehner, K., DePaula, R., Dourish, P., & Sengers, P. (2007). How emotion is made and measured. *International Journal of Human-Computer Studies*, *65*(4), 275–291. doi:10.1016/j.ijhcs.2006.11.016

Boersma, P. (1993). *Accurate short-term analysis of the fundamental frequency and the harmonics-to-noise ratio of a sampled sound.* Technical Report, Institute of Phonetic Sciences, University of Amsterdam.

Brahnam, S. (2005). Strategies for handling customer abuse of ECAs. *Proceedings of Interact '05 Abuse Workshop*, (pp. 62-67).

Brahnam, S. (2009). Building character for artificial conversational agents: Ethos, ethics, believability and credibility. *Psychology Journal*, *7*(1), 9–47.

Bui, D., Heylen, D., Poel, M., & Nijholt, A. (2002). ParleE: An adaptive plan-based event appraisal model of emotions. *Proceedings of the 25th German Conference on Artificial Intelligence*, (pp. 1-9).

Burleson, W., & Picard, R. (2007). Evidence for gender specific approaches to the development of emotionally intelligent learning companions. *Intelligent Systems*, *22*(4), 62–69. doi:10.1109/MIS.2007.69

Callejas, Z., & López-Cózar, R. (2008). Influence of contextual information in emotion annotation for spoken dialogue systems. *Speech Communication*, *50*(5), 416–433. doi:10.1016/j.specom.2008.01.001

Callejas, Z., & López-Cózar, R. (2009). Improving acceptability assessment for the labelling of affective speech corpora. *Proceedings of 10th Annual Conference of the International Speech Communication Association (Interspeech'09)*, (pp. 2863-2866).

Cannon, W. B. (1929). *Bodily changes in pain, hunger, fear and rage*. New York, NY: Appleton.

Cattell, R. B. (1943). The description of personality - basic traits resolved into clusters. *Journal of Abnormal and Social Psychology*, *38*, 476–507. doi:10.1037/h0054116

Cavazza, M., Pizzi, D., & Charles, F. (2009). Emotional input for character-based interactive storytelling. *Proceedings of the 8th International Conference on Autonomous Agents and Multiagent Systems*, (pp. 313-320).

Cavicchio, F., & Poesio, M. (2008). Annotation of emotion in dialogue: The emotion in cooperation project. *Lecture Notes in Computer Science*, *5078*, 233–239. doi:10.1007/978-3-540-69369-7_26

Chibelushi, C., & Bourel, F. (2003). *Facial expression recognition: A brief tutorial overview. CVonline: Online compendium of computer vision*.

Conati, C., & Maclaren, H. (2009). Modeling user affect from causes and effects. *Proceedings of the 17th International Conference on User Modeling, Adaptation and Personalization (UMAP'09)*.

Conte, H. R., & Plutchik, R. (1981). A circumplex model of interpersonal traits. *Journal of Personality and Social Psychology*, *2*, 823–830.

Cowie, R., Douglas-Cowie, E., Tsapatsoulis, N., Votsis, G., Kollias, S., & Fellenz, W. (2001). Emotion recognition in human–computer interaction. *IEEE Signal Processing Magazine*, *1*, 32–80. doi:10.1109/79.911197

Creed, C., & Beale, R. (2008). Psychological responses to simulated displays of mismatched emotional expressions. *Interacting with Computers*, *20*(2), 225–239. doi:10.1016/j.intcom.2007.11.004

D'Mello, S. K., Craig, S. D., Witherspoon, A. W., McDaniel, B. T., & Graesser, A. C. (2008). Automatic detection of learner's affect from conversational cues. *User Modeling and User-Adapted Interaction*, *18*(1), 45–80. doi:10.1007/s11257-007-9037-6

Darwin, C. (1872). *The expression of the emotions in man and animals*. United Kingdom: John Murray. doi:10.1037/10001-000

De Rosis, F., Batliner, A., Novielli, N., & Steidl, S. (2007). You are sooo cool, Valentina! Recognizing social attitude in speech-based dialogues with an ECA. *Lecture Notes in Computer Science*, *4738*, 179–190. doi:10.1007/978-3-540-74889-2_17

De Sevin, E. (2009). Relation between motivations and personality traits for autonomous virtual humans. *Proceedings of the 8th International Conference on Autonomous Agents and Multiagent Systems*, (pp. 1131-1132).

Ekman, P. (1994). Strong evidence for universals in facial expressions: A reply to Russell's mistaken critique. *Psychological Bulletin*, *115*(2), 268–287. doi:10.1037/0033-2909.115.2.268

Endrass, B., Rehm, M., & André, E. (2009). Culture-specific communication management for virtual agents. *Proceedings of the 8th International Conference on Autonomous Agents and Multiagent Systems*, (pp. 281-287).

Eysenck, H. J. (1991). Dimensions of personality: 16, 5 or 3?—Criteria for a taxonomic paradigm. *Personality and Individual Differences, 12*(8), 773–790. doi:10.1016/0191-8869(91)90144-Z

Eysenck, S. B. G., & Eysenck, H. J. (1963). The validity of questionnaire and rating assessments of extraversion and neuroticism, and their factorial stability. *The British Journal of Psychology, 54*(1), 51–62. doi:10.1111/j.2044-8295.1963.tb00861.x

Forbes-Riley, K., & Litman, D. J. (2004). Predicting emotion in spoken dialogue from multiple knowledge sources. *Proceedings of Human Language Technology Conference - North American chapter of the Association for Computational Linguistics annual meeting*, (pp. 201–208).

Fox, E. (2008). *Emotion science – cognitive and neuroscientific approaches to understanding human emotions*. New York, NY: Palgrave MacMillan.

Fox, H. K., Hui, C. M., Bond, M. H., Matsumoto, D., & Yoo, S. H. (2008). Integrating personality, context, relationship, and emotion type into a model of display rules. *Journal of Research in Personality, 42*(1), 133–150. doi:10.1016/j.jrp.2007.04.005

Fragopanagos, N., & Taylor, J. G. (2005). Emotion recognition in human–computer interaction. *Neural Networks, 18*(4), 389–405. doi:10.1016/j.neunet.2005.03.006

Hansen, J. H. L. (1996). Analysis and compensation of speech under stress and noise for environmental robustness in speech recognition. *Speech Communication, 20*(2), 151–170. doi:10.1016/S0167-6393(96)00050-7

Harmon-Jones, E. (2001). The role of affect in cognitive-dissonance processes. In J. P. Forgas (Ed.), *Affect and social cognition* (212-236). Mahwah, NJ: Lawrence Erlbaum Associates, Inc.

Heath, R. G., Cox, A. W., & Lustick, L. S. (1974). Brain activity during emotional states. *The American Journal of Psychiatry, 131*, 858–862.

Höök, K. (2008). Affective loop experiences – what are they? *Lecture Notes in Computer Science, 5033*, 1–12. doi:10.1007/978-3-540-68504-3_1

Höök, K. (2009). Affective loop experiences: Designing for interactional embodiment. *Philosophical Transactions of the Royal Society Biological Sciences, 354*(1535), 3585–3595. doi:10.1098/rstb.2009.0202

Hooker, C. I., Verosky, S. C., Miyakawa, A., Knight, R. T., & D'Esposito, M. (2008)... *Neuropsychologia, 46*(11), 2709–2724. doi:10.1016/j.neuropsychologia.2008.05.005

Imholz, S. (2008). The therapeutic stage encounters the virtual world. *Thinking Skills and Creativity, 3*(1), 47–42. doi:10.1016/j.tsc.2008.02.001

James, W. (1884). What is emotion? *Mind, 19*, 188–205. doi:10.1093/mind/os-IX.34.188

Johnstone, T. (1996). Emotional speech elicited using computer games. *Proceedings of the 4th International Conference on Spoken Language Processing*, (pp. 1985-1988).

Kapoor, A., & Picard, R. W. (2005). Multimodal affect recognition in learning environments. *Proceedings of MM, 05*, 1985–1988.

Kentridge, R. W., & Appleton, J. P. (1990). Emotion: Sensory representation, reinforcement, and the temporal lobe. *Cognition and Emotion, 4*(3), 191–208. doi:10.1080/02699939008410796

Krenn, B. (2003). The NECA project: Net environments for embodied emotional conversational agents. *Proceedings of Workshop on emotionally rich virtual worlds with emotion synthesis at the 8th International Conference on 3D Web Technology.*

Kumano, S., Otsuka, K., Mikami, D., & Yamato, J. (2009). Recognizing communicative facial expressions for discovering interpersonal emotions in group meetings. *Proceedings of the International Conference on Multimodal Interfaces*, (pp. 99-106).

Larsen, R. J., & Ketelaar, T. (1991). Personality and susceptibility to positive and negative emotional states. *Journal of Personality and Social Psychology*, *61*, 132–140. doi:10.1037/0022-3514.61.1.132

Lee, C. M., & Narayanan, S. S. (2005). Toward detecting emotions in spoken dialogs. *IEEE Transactions on Speech and Audio Processing*, *13*(2), 293–303. doi:10.1109/TSA.2004.838534

Lepri, B., Mana, N., Cappelletti, A., Pianesi, F., & Zancanaro, M. (2009). Modeling the personality of participants during group interactions. *Lecture Notes in Computer Science*, *5535*, 114–125. doi:10.1007/978-3-642-02247-0_13

Lester, J. C., Converse, S. A., Kahler, S. E., Barlow, S. T., Stones, B. A., & Bhogal, R. S. (1997). The persona effect: Affective impact of animated pedagogical agents. *Proceedings of the Special Interest Group on Computer Human Interaction (SIGCHI) Conference on Human Factors in Computer Systems.*

Lim, S., & Reeves, B. (2010). Computer agents versus avatars: Responses to interactive game characters controlled by a computer or other player. *International Journal of Human-Computer Studies*, *68*(1-2), 57–68. doi:10.1016/j.ijhcs.2009.09.008

López-Cózar, R., Callejas, Z., Kroul, M., Nouza, J., & Silovský, J. (2008). Two-level fusion to improve emotion classification in spoken dialogue systems. *Lecture Notes in Computer Science*, *5246*, 617–624. doi:10.1007/978-3-540-87391-4_78

Mairesse, F., & Walker, M. (2007). PERSONAGE: Personality generation for dialogue. *Proceedings of the 45th Annual Meeting of the Association for Computational Linguistics.*

Mairesse, F., & Walker, M. A. (2008). Can conversational agents express big five personality traits through language? Evaluating a psychologically-informed language generator. *Proceedings of the 30th Annual Meeting of the Cognitive Science Society (COGSCI'08).*

Maria, K. A., & Zitar, R. A. (2007). Emotional agents: A modeling and an application. *Information and Software Technology*, *49*, 695–716. doi:10.1016/j.infsof.2006.08.002

Marriot, A. (2003). A facial animation case study for HCI: The VHML-based Mentor system. In I. S. Pandzic & R. Forchheimer (Ed.), *MPEG-4 facial animation* (219-240). West Sussex, UK: John Wiley & Sons Ltd.

McCrae, R. R., & Costa, P. T. (1989). Validation of the five-factor model of personality across instruments and observers. *Journal of Personality and Social Psychology*, *52*, 81–90. doi:10.1037/0022-3514.52.1.81

McCrae, R. R., & Terracciano, A., & 79 Members of the Personality Profiles of Cultures Project. (2005). Personality profiles of cultures: Aggregate personality traits. *Journal of Personality and Social Psychology*, *89*(3), 407–425. doi:10.1037/0022-3514.89.3.407

McQuiggan, S. C., & Lester, J. C. (2007). Modeling and evaluating empathy in embodied companion agents. *International Journal of Human-Computer Studies*, *65*(4), 348–360. doi:10.1016/j.ijhcs.2006.11.015

Morency, L. P., Christoudias, C. M., & Darrell, T. (2006). Recognizing gaze aversion gestures in embodied conversational discourse. *Proceedings of 7th International Conference on Multimodal interfaces (ICMI'06)*, (pp. 18-24).

Morrison, D., Wang, R., & Silva, L. C. D. (2007). Ensemble methods for spoken emotion recognition in call-centers. *Speech Communication*, *49*(2), 98–112. doi:10.1016/j.specom.2006.11.004

Nijholt, A. (2007). Conversational agents and the construction of humorous acts. In T. Nishida (Ed.), *Conversational informatics: An engineering approach* (21-48). West Sussex, UK: John Wiley & Sons Ltd.

Nomura, T. (2005). Narratives and therapeutic conversational agents: Their principle problems. *Proceedings of 10th International Conference on Human-Computer Interaction (INTERACT'05) Workshop on Abuse*, (pp. 58-61).

Ortony, A. (2003). On making believable emotional agents believable. In Trappl, R., Petta, P., & Payr, S. (Eds.), *Emotions in humans and artifacts* (pp. 189–212). Cambridge, MA: The MIT Press.

Ortony, A., Collins, A., & Clore, G. L. (1988). *The cognitive structure of emotions*. New York, NY: Cambridge University Press.

Osgood, C. E., Suci, C. J., & Tannenbaum, P. H. (1957). *The measurement of meaning*. Chicago, IL: University of Illinois Press.

Paiva, A., André, E., Arafa, Y., Botelho, L., Costa, M., & Figueiredo, P. … Vala, M. (2001). SAFIRA - supporting affective interactions in real-time applications. *Proceedings of Conference on Artistic, Cultural and Scientific Aspects of Experimental Media Spaces (CAST)*.

Peper, M. (2006). Imaging emotional brain functions: Conceptual and methodological issues. *Journal of Physiology, Paris*, *99*(4-6), 293–307. doi:10.1016/j.jphysparis.2006.03.009

Picard, R. W. (2003). What does it mean for a computer to have emotions? In Trappl, R., Petta, P., & Payr, S. (Eds.), *Emotions in humans and artifacts* (pp. 213–236). Cambridge, MA: The MIT Press.

Pitterman, J., & Pitterman, A. (2006). Integrating emotion recognition into an adaptive spoken language dialogue system. *Proceedings of the 2nd IEEE International Conference on Intelligent Environments*, (pp. 213-219).

Plutchik, R. (2003). *Emotions and life – perspectives from psychology, biology, and evolution*. Baltimore, MD: American Psychological Association.

Pratt, J. A., Hauser, K., Ugray, Z., & Patterson, O. (2007). Looking at human–computer interface design: Effects of ethnicity in computer agents. *Interacting with Computers*, *19*(4), 512–523. doi:10.1016/j.intcom.2007.02.003

Prendinger, H., Mayer, S., Mori, J., & Ishizuka, M. (2003). Persona effect revisited - using bio-signals to measure and reflect the impact of character-based interfaces. *Proceedings of the 4th International Workshop on Intelligent Virtual Agents*, (pp. 283-291).

Read, S., Miller, L., Kostygine, A., Chopra, G., Christensen, J. L., & Corsbie-Massay, C. … Rosoff, A. (2007). The personality-enabled architecture for cognition (PAC). *Proceedings of the 2nd International Conference on Affective Computing and Intelligent Interaction (ACII'07)*, (pp. 735-736).

Reithinger, N., Gebhard, P., Löckelt, M., Ndiaye, A., Pfleger, N., & Klesen, M. (2006). VirtualHuman - dialogic and affective interaction with virtual characters. *Proceedings of the 8th International Conference on Multimodal Interfaces*, (pp. 51-58).

Rindermann, H., & Neubauer, A. C. (2001). The influence of personality on three aspects of cognitive performance: Processing speed, intelligence and school performance. *Personality and Individual Differences*, *30*(5), 829–842. doi:10.1016/S0191-8869(00)00076-3

Rolls, E. T. (2007). *Emotion explained*. Oxford, UK: Oxford University Press.

Roseman, I. J., Spindle, M. S., & Jose, P. E. (1990). Appraisals of emotion-eliciting events - testing a theory of discrete emotions. *Journal of Personality and Social Psychology*, *59*, 899–915. doi:10.1037/0022-3514.59.5.899

Rousseau, D. (1996). Personality in computer characters. *Proceedings of the Association for the Advancement of Artificial Intelligence (AAAI) Workshop on Entertainment and Artificial Intelligence / A-Life*, (pp. 38-43).

Russell, J. A. (1994). Is there universal recognition of emotion from facial expression? A review of methods and studies. *Psychological Bulletin*, *115*, 102–141. doi:10.1037/0033-2909.115.1.102

Scheibe, S., & Carstensen, L. L. (2010). Emotional aging: Recent findings and future trends. *Journal of Gerontology*, *65*(2), 135–144.

Scheutz, M. (2001). The evolution of simple affective states in multi-agent environments. *Proceedings the Association for the Advancement of Artificial Intelligence (AAAI) Fall Symposium*, (pp. 123-128).

Schuller, B., Vlasenko, B., Eyben, F., Rigoll, G., & Wendemuth, A. (2009). Acoustic emotion recognition: A benchmark comparison of performances. *Proceedings of the IEEE Automatic Speech Recognition and Understanding Workshop*, (pp. 552-557).

Schulman, D., & Bickmore, T. (2009). Persuading users through counseling dialogue with a conversational agent. *Proceedings of 4th International Conference on Persuasive Technology (Persuasive'09)*, (pp. 1-8).

Sebe, N., Sun, Y., Bakker, E., Lew, M. S., Cohen, I., & Huang, T. S. (2004). Towards authentic emotion recognition. *Proceedings of IEEE Conference on Systems, Man and Cybernetics*, (pp. 623-628).

Shan, C., Gong, S., & McOwan, P. W. (2007). Beyond facial expressions: Learning human emotion from body gestures. *Proceedings of British Machine Vision Conference (BMVC'07)*.

Smith, C., Rumbell, T., Barnden, J., Hendley, B., Lee, M., & Wallington, A. (2007). *Don't worry about metaphor: Affect extraction for conversational agents* (pp. 37–40). Proceedings of Association for Computational Linguistics.

Stern, A. 2003. Creating emotional relationships with virtual characters. In R. Trappl, P. Petta & S. Payr (Ed.), *Emotions in humans and artifacts* (333-362). Cambridge, MA: The MIT Press.

Stibbard, R. (2000). Automated extraction of ToBI annotation data from the Reading/Leeds emotional speech corpus. *Proceedings of the International Speech Communication Association (ISCA) Workshop on Speech and Emotion*, (pp. 60–65).

Ververidis, D., & Kotropoulos, C. (2006). Emotional speech recognition: Resources, features and methods. *Speech Communication*, *48*, 1162–1181. doi:10.1016/j.specom.2006.04.003

Xiao, H., Reid, D., Marriott, A., & Gulland, E. K. (2005). An adaptive personality model for ECAs. *Lecture Notes in Computer Science*, *3784*, 637–645. doi:10.1007/11573548_82

Yildirim, S., Narayanan, S., & Potamianos, A. (in press). Detecting emotional state of a child in a conversational computer game. *Computer Speech & Language*.

Zeng, Z., Hu, Y., Roisman, G. I., Wen, Z., Fu, Y., & Huang, T. S. (2007). Audio-visual spontaneous emotion recognition. In Huang, T. S. (Eds.), *AI for human computing* (pp. 72–90). Berlin, Germany: Springer-Verlag.

Zhu, Z., & He, K. (2008). A novel approach of emotion recognition based on selective ensemble. *Proceedings of the 3rd International Conference on Intelligent Systems and Knowledge Engineering,* (pp. 695-698).

## KEY TERMS AND DEFINITIONS

**Affective Computing:** An interdisciplinary field of study concerned with developing computational systems which are able to understand, recognize, interpret, synthesize, predict and/or respond to human emotions.

**Affective Loop:** A cycle that relates emotional expressions with affective responses in human-computer communication. The affective loop consists mainly on four phases: eliciting the emotion, recognizing the user state, selecting the appropriate affective user response and rendering such response.

**Five Factor (or Big Five or ocean) Personality Traits:** A physiological model which considers five basic dimensions or factors (five) of personality which remain stable across the life span: openness, conscientiousness, extraversion, agreeableness and neuroticism (ocean).

**Persona Effect:** A phenomenon which describes the implications of the presence of lifelike agents in interactive systems in the user experience, especially in creating a positive illusion of human-to-human interaction.

**Primary Emotions:** The emotions considered to be the basic ones, being the rest derived as combinations of these basic ones. Different authors consider different sets of basic emotions compiled following disparate criteria such as bodily involvement, biological basis or universal expressions of emotion.

**Similarity-Attraction Principle:** A general psychological statement about interpersonal attraction which says that individuals are more attracted to those who have a personality similar to their own.

**Uncanny Valley Effect:** A metaphor employed to address the region of negative emotional response to lifelikeness in agents/robots which is between a scarcely human behaviour or appearance and the completely human appearance.

# Chapter 10
# Enhancement of Conversational Agents by Means of Multimodal Interaction

**Ramón López-Cózar**
*University of Granada, Spain*

**Zoraida Callejas**
*University of Granada, Spain*

**Gonzalo Espejo**
*University of Granada, Spain*

**David Griol**
*Carlos III University of Madrid, Spain*

## ABSTRACT

*The main objective of multimodal conversational agents is to provide a more engaged and participative communication by allowing users to employ more than one input methodologies and providing output channels that are different to exclusively using voice. This chapter presents a detailed study on the benefits, disadvantages, and implications of incorporating multimodal interaction in conversational agents. Initially, it focuses on implementation techniques. Next, it explains the fusion and fission of multimodal information and focuses on the core module of these agents: the dialogue manager. Later on, the chapter addresses architectures, tools to develop some typical components of the agents, and evaluation methodologies. As a case of study, it describes the multimodal conversational agent in which we are working at the moment to provide assistance to professors and students in some of their daily activities in an academic centre, for example, a University's Faculty.*

DOI: 10.4018/978-1-60960-617-6.ch010

## 1. INTRODUCTION

Conversational agents can be defined as computer programs designed to interact with users *similarly* as a human being would do, using more or less interaction modalities depending on their complexity (McTear, 2004; López-Cózar & Araki, 2005). These agents are employed for a number of applications, including tutoring (Forbes-Riley & Litman, 2011; Graesser et al., 2001; Johnson & Valente, 2008), entertainment (Ibrahim & Johansson, 2002), command and control (Stent et al., 1999), healthcare (Beveridge & Fox, 2006), call routing (Paek & Horvitz, 2004) and retrieval of information about a variety of services, for example, weather forecasts (Maragoudakis, 2007), apartment rental (Cassell et al., 1999) and travels (Huang et al., 1999).

The implementation of the agents is a complex task in which a number of technologies take part, including signal processing, phonetics, linguistics, natural language processing, affective computing, graphics and interface design, animation techniques, telecommunications, sociology and psychology. The complexity is usually addressed by diving the implementation into simpler problems, each associated with an agent's module that carries out specific functions, for example, automatic speech recognition (ASR), spoken language understanding (SLU), dialogue management (DM), natural language generation (NLG) and text-to-speech synthesis (TTS).

ASR is the process of obtaining a sentence (text string) from a voice signal (Rabiner & Juang, 1993). It is a very complex task given the diversity of factors that can affect the input, basically concerned with the speaker, the interaction context and the transmission channel. Different applications demand different complexity of the speech recognizer. Cole et al. (1997) identified eight parameters that allow an optimal tailoring of the speech recognizer: speech mode, speech style, dependency, vocabulary, language model, perplexity, signal-to-noise ratio (SNR) and transduction. Nowadays general-purpose speech recognition systems are usually based on Hidden Markov Models (HMMs).

SLU is the process of extracting the semantics from a text string (Minker, 1998). It generally involves employing morphological, lexical, syntactical, semantic, discourse and pragmatical knowledge. In a first stage lexical and morphological knowledge allow dividing the words in their constituents distinguishing lexemes and morphemes. Syntactic analysis yields a hierarchical structure of the sentences. Semantic analysis extracts the meaning of a complex syntactic structure from the meaning of its constituents. There are currently two major approaches to tackle the problem of spoken language understanding: rule-based (Mairesse et al., 2009) and statistical (Meza-Ruiz et al., 2008), including some hybrid methods (Liu et al., 2006).

The DM is responsible of deciding the next action to be carried out by the agent. One possible action is to initiate a database query to provide information to the user, for example, available flights connecting two cities. Another possible action is requesting additional data from the user necessary to make the database query, for example, date for a travel. A third typical action is confirming data obtained from the user, for example, departure and arrival cities. This last action is very important given the current limitations of state-of-the-art ASR.

Conversational agents can be divided into two types depending on the interaction modalities available: *spoken* and *multimodal*. The former type allows just speech as the interaction modality (McTear, 2004). Typically, these agents are used to provide telephone-based information, and are comprised of the five main technologies mentioned above, i.e., ASR, SLU, DM, NLG and TTS.

Some of these agents support multilingual interaction, thus enabling the same service for users who speak different languages (Glass et al., 1995). Although agents that process only speech are usable in many cases and for many application domains, they are very sensitive to the limitations of the speech recogniser. Even though remarkable advances have been made in the last years, state-of-the-art ASR is not mature enough to enable error-free interaction in real world conditions, i.e. regardless of a diversity of factors that degrade its performance, for example, acoustic conditions, user types, accents, speaking styles and vocabulary size.

Another problem is that the interaction can be adapted only partially to different environments and users, given that there is just one interaction modality available (speech). Because of these reasons, among others, many users do not feel comfortable using these agents and reject using them.

After this brief introduction, the reminder of the chapter is organised as follows. Section 2 discusses benefits and disadvantages of multimodal interaction for conversational agents. Section 3 addresses techniques to implement this type of agent, including Wizard of Oz, system-in-the-loop as well as fusion and fission of multimodal information. The section also describes models for implementing the dialogue management (finite states, frames, models based on Artificial Intelligence, statistical approaches and VoiceXML) and addresses methods to implement Embodied Conversational Agents: FACS, MPEG-4 and XML-based languages.

Section 4 focuses on architectures, addressing Galaxy Communicator, Open Agent Architecture (OAA), Blackboard, R-Flow and others. Section 5 describes tools for implementing automatic speech recognition, spoken language understanding, dialogue management, natural language generation, speech synthesis and embodied conversational agents.

Evaluation methodologies are discussed in Section 6, where we address general evaluation frameworks, types and measures, as well as a number of evaluation techniques (PARADISE, PROMISE, CAS and Wizard of Oz). Section 7 describes our latest work in the development a multimodal conversational agent, termed HADA-DS, the goal of which is to provide assistance to professors and students in some of their daily activities in an academic centre, for example, a University's Faculty. Finally, Section 8 presents the conclusions and outlines possibilities for future research directions.

## 2. MULTIMODAL CONVERSATIONAL AGENTS

Multimodal conversational agents are much more complex than spoken conversation agents. They are based on the fact that human-to-human communication relies on the use of several communication channels to transmit and receive information from the conversation partner, e.g., speech, lip movements, body gestures and gazes (López-Cózar & Araki, 2005).

Humans use all these information channels simultaneously and unconsciously, which enables them to obtain a great performance in understanding messages even in the presence of noise. Imitating this human procedure, multimodal conversational agents can use several input modalities to obtain data from the user, and a number of output modalities to influence several senses of the user simultaneously. This fact poses a number of advantages for the interaction but also some drawbacks, which are discussed in the next section.

### 2.1 Benefits of Multimodal Interaction

Taking into account the modalities available, the interaction can be carried out employing devices such as microphone, keyboard, mouse, camera, touch-sensitive screen, loudspeaker, display, data glove or haptic hardware (Wahlster, 2006). A benefit of having this wide range of devices available is that the user can select the most appropriate devices considering environmental conditions (e.g. in terms of noise) as well as his preferences or needs. For example, handicapped users many not be able to use some modality but yet use another.

The user can also select the interaction modalities considering the type of task to be carried out. For example, while driving a car it is safer to use a modality that allows having the hands and eyes free, for example, speech. On the contrary, in a place requiring silence (e.g. a library) or when providing personal data to the agent, speech may not be the best option. Taking into account the adaptation facilities, there are in the literature agents specifically designed for mobile applications, in which proper adaptation to different acoustic conditions is critical (Johnston et al., 2002; Reithinger & Sonntag, 2005).

Another advantage is that the use of several input modalities in parallel for the input to the agent allows compensating to some extent their respective. For example, speech can be employed to reference objects not displayed on screen, whereas graphics can be used to show on screen the effects of performing actions on specific objects (Kuppevelt & Dybkjaer, 2005).

Many multimodal agents adopt a graphical human-like appearance in order to provide a more natural and friendly interaction to the user. Depending on the portion of body shown on screen, they are usually called Talking Heads or Embodied Conversational Agents (ECAs). These characters provide auditory and visual feedback, which is particularly useful when the interaction takes place in noisy environments. Their complexity varies significantly in terms of sophistication and complexity, from simple cartoon-like to complex animated human faces. These characters are connected to the modules of the conversational agent that generate information by means of the output modalities, for example, speech synthesis, lip movements, facial gestures, and video or images on the display.

We can also find in the literature multimodal conversational agents developed for new computer-based paradigms such as ubiquitous computing, pervasive computing or ambient intelligence (Malaka et al., 2004).

## 2.2 Disadvantages of Multimodal Interaction

In despite of the advantages, enabling multimodal interaction for conversational agents has some drawbacks. For example, some researchers suggest that these agents may impose a greater cognitive load on the user. In fact, there are studies in the literature suggesting that the claimed advantages discussed above are sometimes questionable (Walker et al., 1994; Takeuchi & Nagao, 1995).

In terms of the input to the agents, a problem with using several modalities is that they can provoke ambiguity, contradictions or uncertainty. An example of ambiguity occurs when using a pen on a touch-sensitive screen, the gesture made can be interpreted by several recognisers of the system, e.g. the gesture and the handwriting recognisers, which will create their own recognition hypotheses. Hence, it might not be clear whether the user wanted to make a gesture or write something. An example of contradiction occurs, for example, when interacting with an agent developed for pedestrian navigation, the user says "scroll map to the west" while he draws an arrow on the screen pointing east (Johnston et al., 2002).

Another drawback of multimodal interaction is in terms of the processing of the information captured from the user by means of several modalities. The modalities can cooperate in different ways, and thus can be either processed independently or combined by a process which is typically called *fusion* (Nigay & Coutaz, 1993). Hence, the agent must decide which information chunks correspond to the same input and which ones to different inputs. Making the decision requires implementing complex functions that may consider a number of factors, such as time intervals of the inputs, complementarity of the information chunks and contextual information. Using these different factors, the agents may decide, for example, to combine information chunks provided in parallel if they are complementary and overlapped in time. The problem is that sometimes this decision might be made with some degree of uncertainty.

In terms of the generation of the agent's output, there might be also a problem concerned with the selection of the most appropriate interaction modalities for a given response to be provided to the user. For example, some responses might be provided using a single modality whereas others might be provided using several. Again, the designers of the agent must decide when and how several modalities must be employed in order to enhance friendliness, yet ensuring not over incrementing the cognitive load of the user. In addition, multimodality requires more computational power in order to ensure correct synchronisation of the output modalities, for example, synthesised speech, facial expressions and gestures of the ECAs (Wahlster, 2003).

## 3. IMPLEMENTATION TECHNIQUES

This section firstly describes two implementation techniques typically used for developing conversational agents: Wizard of Oz and System-in-the-loop. Secondly, it addresses two processes called *fusion* and *fission* of multimodal information. Third, it discusses techniques employed to implement the core module of these agents: the dialogue manager. To conclude, it comments briefly three methods employed to implement embodied conversational agents: FACS, MPEG-4 and XML-based languages.

### 3.1 Wizard of Oz

The Wizard of Oz (WOz) is a technique that uses a human called *Wizard* to play the role of the computer in a human-computer interaction (Fraser & Gibert, 1991; Zapata & Carmona, 2007). The users are made to believe that they interact with a computer but actually they interact with the Wizard. This technique has been used in several fields, including test of the software life cycle (Salber & Coutaz, 1993; Fraikin & Leonhardt, 2002), corpus collection (Steininger et al., 2002; Zhang et al., 2005), and spoken or multimodal conversational agents (Mayfield & Burger, 1999; Batliner et al., 2003; Petrelli et al., 1997).

Salber & Coutaz (1993) discussed some requirements of WOz for multimodal conversation agents. They indicated that a multimodal agent is more complex to simulate than an agent based on speech only, which increases the task complexity and the bandwidth necessary for the simulation. For multimodal interaction the authors suggested to employ a multi-wizard configuration, which requires properly organising the work of several wizards. A platform for multimodal WOz experiments must have a high performance and flexibility, and should include a tool to retrieve and manipulate a posteriori data collected during the experiments.

### 3.2 System-in-the-Loop

The system-in-the-loop technique is based on the fact that software systems improve cyclically by means of user interactions. For example, the performance of a speech-based conversational agent can be improved by means of analyses of sentences previously uttered by users. If modifications are needed in the design of the system, the technique is employed again to obtain new experimental results. These steps (collection of data and test of system) are repeated until the system designers are satisfied with the performance. Among others, Van de Burgt et al. (1996) used this technique to implement the SCHISMA system. Concretely, the technique was used to collect user utterances and analyse them in order to improve the performance of the system.

## 3.3 Fusion and Fission of Multimodal Information

The *fusion* of multimodal information is a technique to combine information chunks provided by different input modalities of a conversational agent. The result is a data structure that allows the agent to handle simultaneously different information types. Using this data structure the agent's dialogue manager can decide what to do next. A number of methods have been proposed to represent the combined data. For example, Faure and Julia (1993) employed *Triplets*, which are a syntactic formalism to represent multimodal events in the form: (*verb*, *object*, *location*). The authors found this method very useful to represent speech information combined with deictic information generated by means of gestures.

Nigay & Coutaz (1995) employed *Melting pots* to represent combined information, including timestamps. The authors proposed three criteria for deciding whether to carry out or not the fusion process: complementarily of melting pots, time and context. The pots were combined using either *microtemporal*, *macrotemporal* or *contextual* fusion. The first type combined information chunks produced simultaneously or near in time. The second type combined related information chunks, which were generated either sequentially, in parallel or delayed due to insufficient processing power of the system. The third type combined information chunks considering semantic constraints.

Allen (1995) proposed to use semantic structures called *frames*. The information from each modality was interpreted separately and transformed into frames, the slots of which determined the parameters of the action to be made. Frames contained partial information if some slots were empty. During the fusion the frames were combined, which could fulfil slots. For example, Lemon et al. (2006a) used frames to combine multimodal information in a conversational agent that provided information about hotels, restaurants and bars in a town.

Typed Feature Structures (TFS) have also been used to represent *fusioned* multimodal information. The goal is to employ in the fusion process key aspects regarding three formalisms for information representation: unification-based grammar formalisms, languages for knowledge representation and logic programming (Carpenter, 1992; Emele, 1994). For example, Alexandersson & Becker (2001) used this method in the SmartKom agent to handle speech and gestures to book seats in a cinema.

XML-based languages are other method to represent multimodal information. For example, Wahlster (2001) used an XML-based language called M3L to represent all the information flows between the processing components of the SmartKom agent.

The opposite to the fusion technique is called *fission*. The goal of it is to translate each response of the agent into a set of multimodal actions and coordinate the output across the modalities (Müller et al., 2003). This task is very important for multimodal conversational agents in order to make the information be coherently presented to the user. For example, if an ECA makes a reference to an object shown on the display, the reference and the presentation of the object must be properly synchronised. The reference to the object can be carried out using a variety of modalities, for example, deictic gesture of the ECA or highlighting of the object.

The reference can also be cross-modal, using a spoken message such as *"The image on the left corner of the screen..."*. In this latter case, the reference requires that the modality that makes the reference can access the internal representation of the contents on the display. For example, the SmartKom system (Wahlster, 2006) uses a representation for these contents, which allows the visual objects be part of the discourse representation and thus be referenced using several modalities.

## 3.4 Dialogue Management

The dialogue management is a process that represents the "intelligence" of the conversational agent. It is implemented by means of an agent's component called *dialogue manager*, which analyses the data provided by the different input modalities and decides the next action of the agent, for example, provide information to the user. A number of models can be found in the literature for the implementation of this component. In this section we discuss four of these: finite states, frames, plans and statistical approaches (Allen et al., 2001; McTear, 2004). We also address an XML-based language called VoiceXML for rapid implementation.

### 3.4.1 Finite States

Dialogue management strategy using finite states is determined beforehand and usually represented as a network (McTear, 1998). Nodes represent agent prompts and transitions represent paths in the network considering user responses, so that the interaction is fully structured. The main advantage of this approach is its simplicity, facilitating the development of dialogue managers when the task is straightforward, clearly structured, and there is a small number of types of system responses. The main drawback is that this approach is unsuitable to manage complex dialogues due to the lack of flexibility, since users must follow the paths defined for the different states.

### 3.4.2 Frames

The main objective of using frames for dialogue management is to solve the lack of flexibility of the finite state models. Both methodologies are similar in that they are able to manage tasks based on the filling of a form by requesting data from the user. The main difference is that frame-based model does not require following a predefined order to fulfill the required fields, so that it is possible to use a mixed initiative.

To allow this degree of flexibility, it is necessary to provide the system with three main components: i) a frame that refers to the different concepts and attributes defined for the task; ii) a more complete grammar or language model for the ASR module; iii) an algorithm to control the dialogue and determine the next system action based on the contents of the frame. Additional information can be included in the frame definition, for instance, the use of confidence scores to indicate the data reliability.

Goddeau et al. (1996) present a dialogue manager in the domain of cars using this idea. The defined frame, called E-form (electronic form), includes information about the user preferences. These forms are used for dialogue management in the Bell Labs Communicator system (Potamianos et al., 2003), JUPITER (Zue et al., 2000), ARISE (Den et al., 1999), WITAS (Doherty et al., 1998), COMIC (Catizone et al., 2003), to mention a few examples.

### 3.4.3 Models Based on Artificial Intelligence

We can find in the literature two models based on principles of Artificial Intelligence: *plans* and *agents*. The former takes into account that people plan actions in order to achieve specific goals. Therefore, a dialogue manager implemented using this model must be able to infer user goals and build its own plans to provide the service requested by the user. For example, Cavazza et al. (2008) proposed an agent that generates an 'ideal' plan for the daily activities to be carried out by a human.

Following the same approach, Allen et al. (2007) presented PLOW, an intelligent conversational agent to assist the user in managing his daily tasks, whereas Eliasson (2007) implemented dialogue understanding and action planning in a conversational agent set up in a robot, which was able to plan actions to obey the user.

The model based on agents takes into account that the dialogue manager carries out some reasoning to determine future actions (Turunen, 2004). This model relies on the collaboration of a number of intelligent agents to solve a specific problem or task. It is appropriate for complex tasks, for example, negotiation or troubleshooting, and typically employs mixed initiative for the dialogue management (McTear, 2004).

### 3.4.4 Statistical Approaches

Statistical (or data-based) approaches allow designing automatically the dialogue management strategy by learning a dialog model from a labelled dialogue corpus. The design is much more complicated in the case of the methods discussed above, which requires hand-crafting rules or plans. However, as these models can be trained on corpora of real human-computer dialogue, they explicitly model the variance in user behaviour that hand-written rules cannot cover.

The objective is to build systems which offer more robust performance, improved portability, better scalability and greater scope for adaptation (Schatzmann et al., 2006). Another advantage is in terms of the scalability, as the complexity of the dialogue manager can increase without causing problems for the agent's designer (Schatzmann et al., 2006). The drawback is that they require a considerable amount of data in order to properly compute the probabilities that decide the behaviour of the agent.

A number of techniques have been proposed in the literature following this approach. For example, Levin & Pieraccini (1997) defined a technique for learning dialogue strategies, which can be considered the antecedent of many posterior studies on reinforcement learning (Paek & Horvitz, 2004; Lemon et al., 2006b).

Williams & Young (2007) considered a spoken conversational agent as partially observable Markov decision process (POMDP). This process serves as a basis for optimisation the dialogue management and can integrate the uncertainty of the state of the dialogue in the form of statistical distributions.

Griol et al. (2008) presented a technique to develop a dialogue manager and learn optimal dialogue strategies from a labelled corpus acquired for the specific task. The answers of the conversational agent are generated using a classification process which considers the complete dialogue history. This technique was applied to develop the dialogue manager of an agent that provides railway information using spontaneous speech in Spanish (Griol et al., 2006).

### 3.4.5 VoiceXML

VoiceXML[1] is a standard language to access web applications by means of speech (McGlashan et al., 2004). The language is the result of the joint efforts of several companies and institutions (AT&T, IBM, Lucent, Motorola, etc) which make up the so-called VoiceXML Forum. The language has been designed to ease the creation of conversational agents employing audio, ASR, speech synthesis and recording, and mixed-initiative dialogues. The Florence dialogue manager (Fabbrizio & Lewis, 2004), developed by AT&T Labs, supports mixed initiative as well as different strategies for data confirmation and error correction.

There are two main models for dialogue management in VoiceXML. In the Augmented Transition Networks (ATN), the dialogue flow is represented by a set of states, transitions, conditions and variables. A transition to a specific state is selected when the conditions and prefixed actions have been carried out. The second strategy, called clarification flow controllers, defines the dialogue strategy using a hierarchical tree. The tree includes conditions that describe categories, topics and messages (prompts) to inform the user.

## 3.5 Embodied Conversational Agents (ECAs)

Many studies can be found in the literature regarding the analysis of facial expressions (Tian et al., 2003) and head movements (Morency et al., 2005; Maatman et al., 2005). The knowledge obtained from these analyses has been used as well to represent facial expressions and head movements of the so-called Embodied Conversational Agents (ECAs), which are typically implemented using FACS, MPEG-4 or XML-based languages.

FACS (Facial Action Coding System) is a comprehensive, notational system created by Ekman & Friesen (1978) with the goal to objectively describe facial activity. The system is based on several studies about the activity of facial muscles. It represents facial expressions by means of AUs (*action units)* which model the contraction of muscles (or of a set of them if they are somehow connected). Some AUs can operate in either side of the face, independently of the other side, in which case the user must specify "Left", "Right" or "Both". The combination of AUs can generate more than 7,000 facial expressions (Pelachaud et al., 2004). The direct manipulation of AUs can result difficult for non-experienced users, this is why a number of FACS-based animation toolkits have been developed (Patel & Willis, 1991).

MPEG-4 is a standard for compression of multimedia information that is being used on a variety of electronics products (Malatesta et al., 2009; Tekalp & Ostermann, 2000; Pandzic, 2002). The face models defined in MPEG-4 try to reproduce as faithfully as possible the visual manifestation of speech, the transmission of emotional information by means of the facial expressions, and the face of the speaker.

The standard defines 84 features points (FPs) located in a face model that describes a standard face. These points are used to define FAPs (Facial Animation Parameters) which calibrate facial models when different face players are used. MPEG-4 defines six high levels of expressions with two expression parameters (*viseme* and *expression*): joy, sadness, anger, fear, disgust and surprise. Better results are obtained using other low-level parameters. Each FAP corresponds to a FP and defines low-level deformations applicable to the FP with which it is associated. The FAPs represent a set of standard inputs that the animator can use. However, low-level parameters are not easy to use, and it is preferable to use tools that generate them from scripts written in a high-level language.

Several XML-based languages can be found in the literature to control the behaviour of ECAs. One important characteristic of these kinds of languages is the use of high-level primitives. For example, De Carolis et al. (2002) used AMPL (Affective Plan Markup Language) and DPML (Discourse Plan Markup Language) to control de behaviour of an ECA that has two components: *mind* and *body*. The mind represents the personality and intelligence of the agent, which generates the emotional response to the events occurring in its environment. The body represents the physical appearance. The interaction with the user is carried out using synchronized speech and facial expressions.

Tsutsui et al. (2000) used MPML (Multimodal Presentation Markup Language) to carry out multimodal presentations using ECAs, which can carry out a number of factions such as greet, point and explain. In addition to text and figures, the presentations can contain multimedia elements such as voice. One of the most important advantages of this language is that it is independent of the platform and browser employed by the user. Moreover, the multimedia elements can be played back in a number of tools or players.

Kopp et al. (2006) proposed a language called Behaviour Markup Language (BML), with elements and attributes to describe the behaviour of the conversational agent. For example, the element <head type="nod"/> is used to produce a nod. The elements that can be used are: head, torso, face, gaze, lips, body, gesture, legs and speech.

## 4. ARCHITECTURES

It is important to properly select the architecture to be used for implementing a conversational agent, since it should allow further enhancement of the agent or porting it from one application domain to another. We can find in the literature a number of architectures to implement conversational agents. In this section we discuss some of the most widespread (Galaxy Communicator, Open Agent Architecture, Blackboard and R-Flow) and comment on some other proposals.

### 4.1 Galaxy Communicator

Galaxy Communicator is a distributed, message-based, hub-centred architecture (Seneff et al., 1998). The main components are interconnected by means of a client-server architecture. This architecture that has been used to set up, among others, the MIT's Voyager and Jupiter agents (Glass et al., 1995; Zue et al., 2000).

### 4.2 Open Agent Architecture

The Open Agent Architecture (OAA) architecture was designed to ease the implementation of agent-based applications, enabling intelligent, cooperative, distributed, and multimodal agent-based user interfaces (Moran et al., 1997). The agents can be developed in several high-level languages (e.g. C or Java) and platforms (e.g. Windows and Solaris). The communication with other agents is possible using the Interagent Communication Language (ICL). The cooperation and communication between the agents is carried out by means of an agent called Facilitator. Several authors have used this architecture to implement conversational agents for a variety of application domains, including map-based tourist information (Moran et al., 1997), interaction with robots (Bos et al., 2003), and control of user movements in a 2D game (Corradini & Samuelsson, 2008).

### 4.3 Blackboard

The blackboard architecture was released considering principles of Artificial Intelligence. Its name denotes the metaphor of a group of expert people who work together and collaboratively around a blackboard to solve a complex problem. All the resources available are shared by the agents. Each agent can collaborate, generate new resources and use resources from other agents. A Facilitator agent controls the resources and acts as intermediary among the agents which compete to write in the blackboard, taking into account the relevance of the contribution of each agent.

This architecture has been used to implement a number of conversational agents. For example, Wasinger et al. (2003) used it to represent, analyse and make the fusion of multimodal information in a mobile pedestrian indoor/outdoor navigation system set up in a PDA device. Raux & Eskenazi (2007) implemented a new version of the Olympus framework for the development of conversational agents (Bohus et al., 2007). Within this new framework the information provided by a number of agents is combined and stored in the Interaction State, which is implemented by means of a blackboard.

Huang et al. (2007) also used the blackboard architecture to create the GECA platform, which uses XML messages for the interconnection of the components of a conversational agent. The platform uses a server that handles the management of a number of services, including service naming and message subscription and forwarding.

A variant of the blackboard architecture is the multi-blackboard architecture (Alexandersson & Becker, 2001). It was used, for instance, in the SmartKom conversational agent (Pfleger et al., 2002; Wahlster, 2006) to combine speech with not verbal modalities in order to help processing intelligible multimodal utterances (Kopp & Wachsmuth, 2004). More recently, Huang et al. (2008) have used this architecture to integrate components of an ECA. These components share data in the blackboards by means of a subscribe-publish message passing mechanism. Each blackboard has its own manager, and the architecture includes a server responsible of the message subscription and naming services of the ECA.

### 4.4 R-Flow

R-Flow is an extensible XML-based architecture for multimodal conversational agents (Li et al., 2007). It is based on a recursive application of the Model-View-Controller (MVC) design. The structure is based on three layers: modality independent dialogue control, synchronization of logical modalities and physical presentation. Each one has been codified in different XML-based languages. State-Chart XML (SCXML) is used for dialogue control, SMIL (Synchronized Multimedia Integration Language) and EMMA (Extensible Multimodal Interface Language) based XM-Flow (Li et al., 2006) for modality synchronization and interpretation, and the physical presentation in a generic XML. The prototype presented in (Li et al., 2007) has been developed to manipulate Google map in a multimodal way.

### 4.5 Other Architectures

In addition to the architectures discussed above, which are amongst the most employed, it is possible to find other architectures in the literature. For example, Leßmann & Wachsmuth (2003) used the classical architecture Perceive-Reason-Act for the design of a conversational agent. The *Perceive* module handles the input information, which is collected by sensors (auditory, tactile and visual). The *Act* module generates the output information. Actions can be carried out by means of either *deliberative* or *reactive* behaviour. The component for deliberative behaviour is located in the *Reason* section of the figure. It uses knowledge about the domain updated by perceptions, and generates intentions employing a plan library, which represents what the agent wants to do next. The second way of generating an action is by means of the reactive behaviour, which is reserved for actions that do not need deliberation, for example, making the agent appear more lifelike.

Following a different approach, Wei and Rudnicky (2000) proposed an architecture based on a task decomposition and an expectation agenda. The agenda is a list of topics represented by handlers. A handler encapsulates the knowledge necessary for interacting with the user about a specific information slot. The agenda defines a "plan" for carrying out a specific task, which is represented as a specific order of handlers.

## 5. TOOLS FOR DEVELOPMENT

In this section we focus on tools for developing components of multimodal conversational agents, paying special attention to tools for automatic speech recognition, spoken language understanding, dialogue management, natural language generation, speech synthesis and embodied conversational agents.

### 5.1 Tools for Automatic Speech Recognition

The Hidden Markov Model Toolkit (HTK) was developed by Cambridge University (Young et al., 2000). It is free software for building and using Hidden Markov Models (HMMs). In the community of conversational agents this software is primarily used for ASR, but has been used for a number of applications including character recognition and DNA sequencing. It consists of a set of library modules and tools available in C source form that provide facilities for speech analysis, HMM training, testing and results analysis.

CMU Sphinx (Lee et al., 1990) describes a group of speech recognition systems developed at the Carnegie Mellon University. These include a series of speech recognizers (Sphinx 2 - 4) and an acoustic model trainer (SphinxTrain). Sphinx is a continuous-speech, speaker-independent recognition system making use of HMMs and an n-gram statistical language model. Sphinx 2 focuses on real-time recognition suitable for speech-based applications and uses a semi-continuous representation for acoustic modeling. Sphinx 3 adopted the prevalent continuous HMM representation and has been used primarily for high-accuracy, non-real-time recognition. Sphinx 4 is written entirely in Java with the goal of providing a more flexible framework for research. PocketSphinx has been designed to run in real time on handhelds and be integrated with live applications.

Julius is a two-pass large vocabulary continuous speech recognition software for speech-based applications in Japanese (Lee & Kawahara, 2009). It is based on word 3-gram and context-dependent HMMs, and includes functionalities such as real-time accurate recognition, N-best and word graph outputs, confidence scoring, etc.

Sonic is a large vocabulary continuous speech recognition system developed by the University of Colorado. It is based on continuous density Hidden Markov acoustic models (Pellom & Hacioglu, 2003).

There is a number of proprietary software for ASR, including AT&T WATSON, Windows speech recognition system, IBM ViaVoice, Microsoft Speech API, Nuance Dragon NaturallySpeaking, MacSpeech, Loquendo ASR and Verbio ASR.

## 5.2 Tools for Spoken Language Understanding

The Carnegie Mellon Statistical Language Modeling Toolkit (CMU SLM) is a set of Unix tools designed to facilitate language modeling (Rosenfeld, 1995). The toolkit allows processing corpora of data (text strings) in order to obtain word frequency lists and vocabularies, word bigram and trigram counts, bigram and trigram-related statistics and a number of back-off bigram and trigram language models. Using these tools it is also possible to compute statistics such as perplexity, out-of-vocabulary words (OOV) and distribution of back-off cases.

The Natural Language Toolkit (NLTK) (Bird et al., 2008) is a suite of libraries and programs for symbolic and statistical natural language processing for the Python programming language.

Other tools include Phoenix, designed by the Carnegie Mellon University in combination with the Helios confidence annotation module (Ward & Issar, 1994), and Tina, developed by the MIT based on context free grammars, augmented transition networks, and lexical functional grammars (Seneff, 1989).

## 5.3 Tools for Dialogue Management

A number of toolkits for dialogue management can be found in the literature, which can be classified taking into account the model employed to represent the dialogue management, as was discussed in section 3.4.

### 5.3.1 Dialogue Management Based on Finite States

The Center for Spoken Language Understanding (CSLU) at the Oregon Health and Science University developed a graphical tool called CSLU Toolkit for the design of dialogue managers based on finite states (McTear, 1998).

Another tool for building agents based on finite state systems is the AT&T FSM library. It is a set of Unix tools for building, combining and optimizing weighted finite-state systems (Mohri, 1997). Some conversational agents based on finite states have been created under the SUNDIAL (Müller & Runge, 1993) and SUNSTAR projects (Nielsen & Baekgaard, 1992).

### 5.3.2 Dialogue Management Based on VoiceXML

There are currently many implementations developed in VoiceXML. For example, OpenVXI is a portable open source VoiceXML interpreter available from Carnegie Mellon University and developed by SpeechWorks. It can be used free of charge in commercial applications and also allows the addition of proprietary modifications.

JVoiceXML is an open source VoiceXML interpreter for JAVA. Its main goal is to provide platform-independent implementation of conversational agents that can be used for free.

The OptimSys VoiceXML platform also allows the easy integration with ASR and TTS engines and telephony hardware of your choice.

BeVocal Café is a web-based VoiceXML development environment providing a VoiceXML interpreter that includes speaker verification, voice enrolment, XML data, pre-tuned grammars and professional audio.

Loquendo has developed a VoiceXML Interpreter integrated within the VoxNauta Platform. In addition, Loquendo Café provides developers with resources and tools to learn about creating speech-based applications.

Other tools include the following: Eloquant, HeyAnita, HP OpenCall Media platform, Intervoice's Omvia Media Server, Lucent MiLife VoiceXML Gateway, Motorola VoxGateway, Nuance VoiceXML platform, Vocalocity's platform, and Voxeo VoiceCenter IVR.

## 5.4 Tools for Natural Language Generation

Natural language generation is the process of obtaining texts in natural language from a non-linguistic representation. It is usually carried out in 5 steps: content organization, content distribution in sentences, lexicalization, generation of referential expressions, and linguistic realization. The simplest approach consists in using predefined text messages (e.g. error messages and warnings). Although intuitive, this approach completely lacks from any flexibility.

The next level of sophistication is template-based generation, in which the same message structure is produced with slight alterations. The template approach is used mainly for multi-sentence generation, particularly in applications which texts are fairly regular in structure such as some business reports. Rosetta (Oh & Rudnicky, 2000) is a toolkit developed by the CMU for language generation based on the latter approach.

## 5.5 Tools for Speech Synthesis

Text-to-speech (TTS) synthesizers transform a text string into an acoustic signal. A TTS system is composed of two components: front-end and back-end. The front-end transforms raw text containing symbols such as numbers and abbreviations into their equivalent words. It assigns phonetic transcriptions to each word, divides and marks the text into prosodic units, i.e. phrases, clauses and sentences. The back-end (often referred to as synthesizer) converts the symbolic linguistic representation obtained by the previous component into speech.

Festival (Clark et al., 2004) is a C++ general multi-lingual speech synthesis system developed at Centre for Speech Technology Research (CSTR) at the University of Edinburgh. It is distributed under a free software license and offers a number of APIs as well as an environment for development and research on speech synthesis. Supported languages include English, Spanish, Czech, Finnish, Italian, Polish and Russian.

FreeTTS (Walker et al., 2002) is an open source speech synthesis system written entirely in Java. It allows employing markers to specify when speech generation should not be interrupted, to concatenate speech, and to generate speech using different voices. FreeTTS is based upon CMU Flite (Festival-lite).

Some commercial systems for TTS are Cepstral, Loquendo TTS and Kalliope.

### 5.6 Tools for Embodied Conversational Agents

Xface (Balci, 2005) is an open source toolkit for generating and animating 3D talking heads. The toolkit relies on MPEG-4 Facial Animation Parameters (FAPs) and keyframe-based rendering driven by SMIL-Agent scripting language. All the components in the toolkit are independent of the operating system, and can be compiled with any ANSI C++ standard compliant compiler.

The CSLR's Conversational Agent Toolkit (CAT) (Cole et al., 2003) provides a set of modules and tools for research and development of advanced ECAs. These modules include an audio server, the Sonic speech recognition system, and the Phoenix natural language parser. The CU Animate toolkit (designed for research, development, control and real time rendering of 3D animated characters) is used for the design of the facial animation system.

Microsoft Agent toolkit (Walsh & Meade, 2003) includes animated characters, TTS engines, and speech recognition software. It is preinstalled in several versions of MS Windows and is as an ActiveX control that can be used by web pages. The speech engine is used by means of the Microsoft Speech API (SAPI). New Agent characters can be created using Microsoft's development tools, including the Agent Character Editor. Agents can be embedded in applications with Visual Basic and in web pages with VBScript.

Maxine (Seron et al., 2006) is an open source engine for embodied conversational agents developed by the University of Zaragoza (Spain). It enables interaction with the user by means of different channels, for example, text, voice, mouse and keyboard. The agent can gather information from the user and the environment (noise level in the room, position of the user to establish visual contact, image-based estimate of the user's emotional state, etc.). The agent can interact with the user by means of speech (in Spanish) and has its own emotional state, which depends on the relationship with the user.

Currently there are also several initiatives for the design of conversational agents and chatbots which are able to interact with the user in social networks and virtual worlds (Ieronutti & Chittaro, 2007; Hubal et al., 2008).

## 6. EVALUATION METHODOLOGIES

As conversational agents become more and more complex, it is necessary to develop new evaluation measures and methodologies to test their performance. The definition of new measures and procedures uniquely accepted by the scientific community for the assessment of agents presents many difficulties. In fact, this field can be considered to be still at an early development stage. In this section we firstly address general frameworks for evaluation and discuss evaluation types. Then, we describe briefly well-known approaches for the evaluation of conversational agents: PARADISE, PROMISE, CAS, WOz and simulation of user-agent interactions. Other approaches to the evaluation of multimodal conversational agents can be found in (Cassell et al., 2000; Bernsen, 2002).

### 6.1 General Frameworks for Evaluation

In recent years, various initiatives have been developed to define general frameworks that include the design and evaluation of conversational agents. In the United States one of the main projects was DARPA Communicator (Walker et al., 2001). Some examples in Europe are EAGLES (Expert Advisory Group on Language Engineering Standards) (King et al., 1996) ELSE (Paroubek & Blasband, 1999) and DISC (Bernsen et al., 1998).

Other European institutions that have focused on the study and definition of evaluation techniques are the following:

- COSCODA (Coordinating Committee on Speech Databases and Speech I/O Systems) is concerned with aspects related to the creation of multilingual databases.
- ELRA (European Language Resources Association) is focused on the collection and distribution of linguistic resources.
- SQUALE (Speech Recognition Quality Assessment for Linguistic Engineering) (Young et al., 1997) focused on the adaptation of the ARPA Large Vocabulary Continuous Speech Recognition paradigm (LVCSR) to multilingual contexts.

Two fundamental trends for the evaluation of conversational agents can be considered with regard these initiatives. On the one hand, the definition of quantitative measures to evaluate the quality of the agents (e.g., EAGLES and DARPA Communicator projects). On the other hand, proposals for the definition of qualitative and quantitative measures (e.g. ELSE and DISC projects).

The EAGLES evaluation group proposed a number of quantitative measures, which include: completion task, transaction success, system's response time and conciseness of agent's responses. It also proposed several qualitative measures, such as user satisfaction, agent's adaptation to new users and multimodality features. The group did not only provide insights on what aspects to evaluate, but also on how to carry out the evaluation and report results, setting up a set of parameters and methodology for homogeneous comparison between agents.

Similarly, the DISC project proposed aspects to be evaluated and criteria for evaluation. The methodology was based on templates and considers aspects regarding the life cycle of software.

LINTEST is a tool for the evaluation of conversational agents using dialogue corpora (Degerstedt & Jönsson, 2006). It allows two operation modes: batch and interactive. Using the former the evaluation generates a log file that includes the evaluation results. The latter allows a more detailed evaluation carried out during the interaction.

## 6.2 Evaluation Types and Measures

We can find in the literature many proposals to evaluate conversational agents. For example, Dybkjaer & Bernsen (2000) proposed a set of 15 criteria to ensure the usability of the agents: (1) use of the different modalities, (2) recognition of the user inputs, (3) coverage of user utterances regarding vocabulary and grammars, (4) voice quality of the agent, (5) generation of appropriate responses, (6) agent's feedback, (7) use of different dialogue initiatives for different dialogue tasks, (8) naturalness of the dialogue structure for different tasks, (9) domain coverage, (10) reasoning abilities of the agent, (11) guidance and help for the user during the interaction (12) features on error handling, (13) adaptation to differences between users, (14) existence of communication problems during the interaction, and (15) user satisfaction.

The evaluation measures can be either *objective* or *subjective*. The former are directly obtained from the interaction with the system, not including any kind of assessment made by developers or users. The latter includes an evaluation process typically carried out by the end users of the agent. For example, these measures were employed in the European project Trindi (Larsson et al., 1999).

The evaluation measures can also be classified taking into account how the computing of the evaluation scores is carried out (automatic or manual), or considering the influence on the overall quality of the system (positive or negative measures).

Taking into account the objective of the evaluation, two kinds of evaluation can also be distinguished: *black box* and *crystal box*. The former considers the overall performance of the agent, considering only its inputs and outputs. The latter focuses on the performance of agent's components separately, taking into account inputs and outputs

*Table 1. Measures defined for the evaluation of the different modules of a conversational agent*

| Automatic Speech Recognition |
|---|
| Word Accuracy, Word Error Rate, Word Insertions Rate, Word Insertions Rate, Word Substitutions Rate, Sentence Accuracy |
| **Natural Language Understanding** |
| Percentage of words correctly understood, not covered or partially covered; Percentage of sentences correctly analyzed; Percentage of words outside the dictionary; Percentage of sentences whose final semantic representation is the same as the reference; Percentage of correct frame units, considering the actual frame units; Frame-level accuracy; Frame-level coverage |
| **Dialogue Management** |
| Strategies to recover from errors, to correct/direct user interaction, context management when there are multiple questions and answers associated with a scenario) (% correct responses,% of incorrect answers,% of half-answers, % of times the system works trying to solve a problem,% of times the user acts trying to solve a problem, etc.) |
| **Natural Language Generation** |
| Number of times the user requests a repetition of the reply provided by the system; User response time; Number of times the user does not answer; Rate of out of vocabulary words |
| **Speech Synthesis** |
| Intelligibility of synthetic speech and naturalness of the voice |

of these modules. Table 1 summarizes the most commonly employed measures for the evaluation of the different modules of a conversational agent (San Segundo, 2004).

According to the reference taken for the evaluation of the conversational agent, we can distinguish several types of evaluation. In the *comparative* evaluation, different agents are developed in parallel with the same specifications by different research centers. This evaluation type has been usually used in projects funded by DARPA, e.g., DARPA Communicator. In the *temporary* evaluation the reference is the developed agent, and the goal is to make performance comparisons in several development stages. The *substitutive* evaluation compares the agent with another agent with the same capabilities previously developed, usually employing different technologies. The *initial* evaluation is employed when the reference agent is not available. It makes an estimation of performance *a priori* during the specification phase, and in subsequent evaluations considers the deviation from the expected performance.

## 6.3 PARADISE

PARADISE (PARAdigm for DIalogue System Evaluation) is one of the most employed proposals for globally evaluating the performance of conversational agents (Walker et al., 1998; Dybkjaer et al., 2004). It combines different features in a single function that measures the performance of the agent in direct correlation with user satisfaction. The main assumptions of the approach are two. Firstly, the main goal is to maximise user satisfaction. Secondly, task success and several dialogue costs (objective measures) can be used to predict user satisfaction. These two assumptions are interrelated as shown in the equation in Box 1.

The maximisation of user satisfaction is carried out by minimising dialogue costs and maximising task success. Dialogue costs are quantified by means of efficiency and quality measures. The most commonly used measures on task success are two. The first one is the Kappa factor, which is computed from a confusion matrix of the values of attributes exchanged between the user and the agent. The second measure is completion task, which is computed considering the number of times that the system correctly satisfies the user requests.

## 6.4 PROMISE

PROMISE (PROcedure for Multimodal Interactive System Evaluation) (Beringer et al., 2002) is an extension to multimodality of the PARADISE framework. This paradigm uses methods traditionally employed to evaluate spoken conversational agents, and specific methods to assess the characteristic properties of multimodal conversational agents, as for example, the combination of gestures

*Box 1.*

$$User\ Satisfaction = \propto N\left(Task\ Success\right) - \sum_{i=1}^{N} \omega_i N(Costs\ of\ the\ dialogue)$$

and speech in the input, the combination of speech and graphics in the output, etc.

According to this procedure, the evaluation is carried out by defining a number of qualitative and quantitative measures (called costs) that have an associated weight. Instead of using a linear regression (as in the case of the PARADISE), PROMISE employs a calculated peer Pearson correlation "user - satisfaction cost", some of these objectives costs and other subjective. For the evaluation, test users interact with the system and fill in a questionnaire which includes subjective costs. Some of these costs are equivalent to those used in the procedure PARADISE, while others are used to treat specifically multimodality and behaviour of non-cooperative users.

The most important efficiency and quality measures defined for these models are the average time needed to complete a task, average time per turn, average number of turns per task, minimum time to complete a specific task, types of confirmations used by the system, number of words correctly recognized per turn, rate of correct semantic concepts, percentage of correctly corrected errors, time employed for the user and the system to answer, number of times that the user does not answer, number of times that the user requires a repetition or ask for help, number of times that the user interrupts the system prompt, etc.

## 6.5 CAS

The CAS (Common Answer Specification) approach evaluates the performance of the conversational agent by comparing the responses of the agent with canonical responses extracted from a database (Boisen et al., 1989). This allows automatic evaluation of the agent once the principles for generating the reference responses have been defined, and a labelled corpus for the specific task is available. In addition, it allows the direct comparison of agents.

However, the evaluation with this approach is very limited since it is carried out at the sentence level only, i.e. comparing each agent's response with the canonical response. Moreover, it is not possible to distinguish between partially correct responses and totally wrong ones. Therefore, it does not allow detecting or correcting errors, or evaluating the quality of the responses. Among others, this approach has been used in the ARPA projects to evaluate agents designed for the ATIS domain (Air Travel Information Systems).

## 6.6 Wizard of Oz

The Wizard of Oz technique (WOz) is usually employed to emulate the system performance, as was discussed in section 3.1 (Fraser & Gilbert, 1991). To do this, the approach typically employs a set of scenarios that define the goals the user must try to achieve during the interaction with the conversational agent. The interaction is stored in log files, containing additional information such as user utterances, speech recognition results, semantic representations obtained, agent responses, and time required by the user to answer each agent's prompt (Webb et al., 2010).

A questionnaire is used to consider the user acceptation of the different functionalities of the agent, for example, quality of synthesised speech, ease for error correction, interactivity and friendliness. Taking into account the dialogue logs and questionnaires, it is possible to compute a set of measures that allow to quantitative evaluation of the agent. Some of these measures include: time required to accomplish the scenario goals, number of user questions correctly answered by the agent and user satisfaction.

## 6.7 User Simulation

A technique that has attracted increasing interest in the last decade for the evaluation of conversational agents is based on the automatic generation of dialogues between the agents and an additional module, called user simulator, which represents user interactions (Zukerman & Litman, 2001; López-Cózar et al, 2003; Schatzmann et al., 2006; Griol et al., 2009). The simulator makes it possible to generate a large number of dialogues in a very simple way. Therefore, this technique reduces the time and effort that would be needed for evaluating an agent each time it is modified in order to improve performance.

The construction of user models based on statistical methods has provided interesting and well-founded results in recent years and is currently a growing research area. In terms of user simulation, the goal is to obtain a probabilistic user model from the analysis of a corpus of human-computer interaction, which can be employed for setting up the user simulator (Pietquin & Dutoit, 2005; Cuayáhuitl et al., 2005; Schatzmann & Young, 2009).

# 7. A CASE OF STUDY: HADA-DS

Our work within the HADA project (Adaptive Hypermedia for Attention to Different User Types in Ambient Intelligence Environments) is concerned with setting up a multimodal conversational agent, termed HADA-DS, to assist professors and students in some of their daily activities within a University's Faculty (López-Cózar et al., 2011). The agent works in three different places of the Faculty: Library, Professors' Offices and Classrooms. Our goal is that by using the agent, professors may interact more easily with devices in their environment, e.g. classroom beamers or lights. Moreover, students may receive different types of information depending on their localisation within the environment.

The agent allows multimodal interaction for the user input, namely, using speech, keyboard or mouse. For example, a student can ask for information about available books on a particular subject by either speaking the subject, selecting it on the screen of his/her mobile device, or writing the subject in a form field. Since the agent's output is multimodal as well, a spoken message for this request may indicate that the requested information is available on the screen. The agent does allow combining data provided by different information sources in just one interaction, but allows combining data provided by the user in different dialogue turns.

Figure 1 shows the architecture of the agent, which is comprised of an XHTML+Voice (X+V) document server connected with the users' mobile devices (tablet PCs, laptop computers and PDAs) by means of wireless connections.

## 7.1 XHTML+Voice Documents

The logic of the agent is implemented by means of a set of X+V documents. Some of these documents are stored in the document server, while others are dynamically created using PHP programs that take into account features stored in the user profile (e.g. user gender and preferred interaction language), as well as data extracted from databases. X+V documents are comprised of forms, the fields of which are filled in with the user input provided via speech, text or mouse clicks. To visualise the documents, users must run in their communication device the Opera browser[2], which enables multimodal interaction using voice, text, mouse clicks and graphics.

*Figure 1. Architecture of the HADA-DS conversational agent*

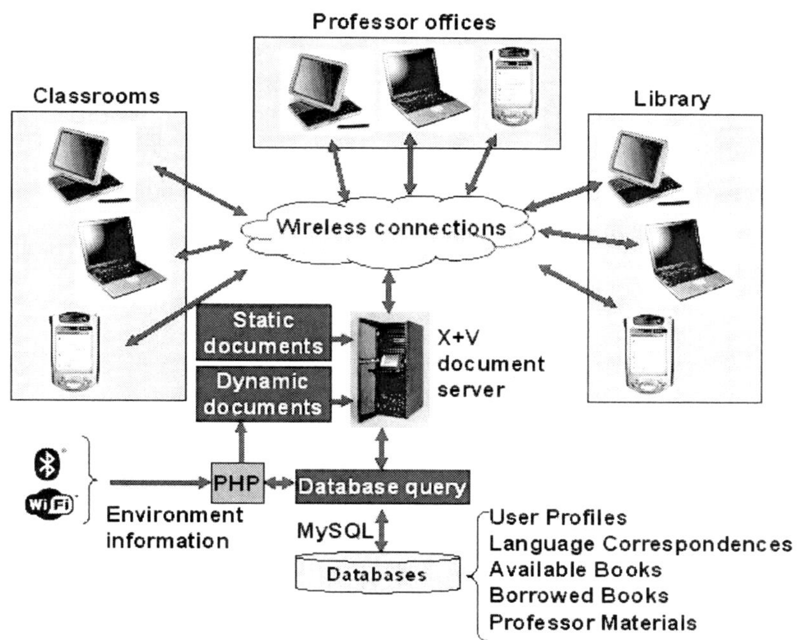


### 7.1.1 Speech-Based Interaction

Automatic speech recognition is carried out by the Opera browser's built-in recogniser. In our setting the recognition is based on a tap-&-talk method, i.e. the user must click and hold a microphone icon or press a key while s/he speaks to the agent. Speech recognition and understanding is carried out using JSGF (Java Speech Grammar Format) grammars that are used either at form or field level. Some of these grammars are static, while others are dynamically created by means of PHP programs that query databases and include the obtained data in the grammars (e.g. book titles). For example, using the grammar to recognise book queries, if a user utters the sentence *I need books about Maths please*, the agent fills in the form field *subject* with the word *Maths*.

The recognition grammars used to handle book queries must be updated as the library catalogue changes, so that they are compiled dynamically using the contents of the *Available Books* database. To update these grammars we have implemented a PHP program that carries out two tasks. Firstly, it queries databases using MySQL functions and obtains data from available books, such as titles, authors or subjects. Secondly, it creates the grammars to recognise complete sentences as well as isolated data items (e.g. title, authors or subjects) using the information gathered in the first step.

In the system output, speech synthesis is carried out by means of sentence patterns included into the <prompt> ... </prompt> labels typically used in VoiceXML[3]. These sentences are transformed into voice by a Text-To-Speech (TTS) process using the Opera browser's built-in speech synthesiser. Some of these sentences are fixed, while others are created at run-time considering the user type (professor or student), the user gender (necessary to create sentences in Spanish appropriately) and data extracted from databases.

### 7.1.2 GUI-Based Interaction

In the system input, the visual interaction is used to obtain data from the user via form fields and selection buttons typically used in XHTML. In the system output, the visual interaction is used to provide data extracted from databases (e.g. list of available books) and information about the current user's name and type.

### 7.1.3 Connection of Both Interfaces

The connection between the speech- and GUI-based interfaces is carried out using event handlers, which are placed at the body section of the X+V documents. We use several types of event handlers available in X+V. For example, when the document used to enter book queries is loaded into the browser, the event onload is thrown and, in response, a VoiceXML form called initial_vform is executed to handle this event.

XHTML+Voice allows that a user utterance can fill in several form fields in one interaction (mixed-initiative interaction strategy). To do so, we use a <vxml:initial name="initial_vform"> ...</initial> section, typically employed in VoiceXML, which allows recognising the user utterance using a form level grammar. Thus, for example, for the book query document the system generates the message *Please enter a book query* and the user can utter a variable number of data items (e.g. authors; authors and publication year; authors, publication year and subjects; etc.). We also use the ev:event="onclick" event, which is thrown when the user clicks on a form field. The handler for this event is VoiceXML code to obtain the value for that particular form field.

### 7.2 Agent's Interaction with the Environment

Our goal is that the agent-user interaction can be carried out in such a way that the location in which the user is interacting at every moment (e.g. in a professor's office) can be taken into account by the conversational agent without the user being concerned. By doing so we expect to enable a more intelligent behaviour of the agent. For example, if a professor says to the agent: *"Switch on the light"* when he is in a room where there are several lights, the agent should ask which light the user is referring to.

Obviously, the agent should not ask this question if the user is a room where there is one light only. To achieve this goal we are using RFID (Radio Frequency IDentification) technology. Each user has one RFID card that identifies him/her, and there are a number of RFID readers in different places of our intelligent environment (Faculty) for user localisation. At the time of writing, we are working in the setting up of a middleware layer, more specifically a *blackboard* (Alamán et al., 2001), to receive information from the RFID readers and the devices in the environment. Using this middleware the agent will operate the devices (e.g. switching them on/off) by changing their status in the blackboard.

## 8. CONCLUSION AND FUTURE RESEARCH DIRECTIONS

In this chapter we have discussed benefits and disadvantages of multimodal interaction for conversational agents. We have addressed implementation techniques, discussing the Wizard of Oz and the System-in-the-loop methods. Moreover, we have discussed the *fusion* and *fission* of multimodal information, and focused on the implementation of the dialogue manager.

Later on, the chapter has addressed Embodied Conversational Agents (ECAs) and agent architectures, focusing on Galaxy Communicator, OAA, Blackboard and R-Flow. It has provided as well a description of tools to develop components of the agents, focusing mainly on automatic speech recognition, spoken language understanding, dialogue management, natural language generation, speech synthesis and ECAs.

We have discussed as well evaluation methodologies, and focused on general frameworks, evaluation types and measures, as well as a number of evaluation techniques (PARADISE, PROMISE, Common Answer Specification, Wizard of Oz and user simulation). Finally, the chapter has discussed our current work in the development of a multimodal conversational agent to assist professors and students in some of their daily activities within a University's Faculty.

The development of multimodal conversational agents is a very active research topic. The design and performance of these agents is very complex, not only because of the complexity of the different technologies involved, but also because of the required interconnection of very different technologies. Hence, additional work is needed in several directions to make these systems more usable by a wider range of potential users. For example, in terms of dialogue management, more studies are needed to set up more adaptive techniques, which learn user preferences and adapt the agent's behaviour accordingly.

The development of *emotional* conversational agents represents another line of research, which relies on the fact that emotions play a very important role in the rational decision-making, perception and human-to-human interaction. From a general point of view, emotionally-dependent dialogue management strategies must take into account that humans usually exchange their intentions using both verbal and non-verbal information. More information on the advances made in this line of research can be read in Chapter 9 of this book.

The development of *social* dialogue strategies is another research direction. It relies on the fact that in human-to-human interaction people do not only speak about topics concerned with the task at hand, but also about other topics and especially at the beginning of the conversation, for example, weather conditions, family or current news. This off-talk typically human dialogue, as can be read in Chapter 6, could also be used to improve the human-computer interaction. Hence, additional efforts must be made by the research community in order to make conversational agents more humanlike by designing dialogue strategies based on this kind of very genuine human behaviour.

## ACKNOWLEDGMENT

This research has been funded by the Spanish project HADA TIN2007-64718.

## REFERENCES

Alamán, X., Haya, P., & Montoro, G. (2001). *El proyecto InterAct: Una arquitectura de pizarra para la implementación de Entornos Activos* (pp. 72–73). Proc. of Interacción Persona-Ordenador.

Alexandersson, J., & Becker, T. (2001). Overlay as the basic operation for discourse processing in a multimodal dialogue system. *Proc. of IJCAI.*

Allen, J. (1995). *Natural language understanding.* The Benjamin/Cummings Publishing Company Inc.

Allen, J., Byron, D., Dzikovska, M., Ferguson, G., Galescu, L., & Stent, A. (2001). Towards conversational human-computer interaction. *AI Magazine*, *22*(4), 27–37.

Allen, J., Chambers, N., Ferguson, G., Galescu, L., Jung, H., Swift, M., & Taysom, W. (2007). PLOW: A collaborative task learning agent. *Proc. of AAAI*, (pp. 22-26).

Balci, K. (2005). XfaceEd: Authoring tool for embodied conversational agents. *Proc. of ICMI*, (pp. 208-213).

Batliner, A., Fischer, K., Huber, R., Spliker, J., & Nöth, E. (2003). How to find trouble in communication. *Speech Communication, 40*, 117–143. doi:10.1016/S0167-6393(02)00079-1

Beringer, N., Kartal, U., Louka, K., Schiel, F., & Türk, U. (2002). PROMISE - a procedure for multimodal interactive system evaluation. *Proc. of LREC Workshop on Multimodal Resources and Multimodal Systems Evaluation*, (pp. 77–80).

Bernsen, N. O. (2002). *Multimodality in language and speech systems - from theory to design support tool* (pp. 93–148). Kluwer Academic Publishers.

Bernsen, N. O., Dybkjaer, L., Carlson, R., Chase, L., Dahlback, N., Failenschmid, K., et al. Paroubek, P. (1998). The DISC approach to spoken language system development and evaluation. *Proc. of the First International Conference on Language Resources and Evaluation (LREC)*, (pp. 185-189).

Beveridge, M., & Fox, J. (2006). Automatic generation of spoken dialogue from medical plans and ontologies. *Biomedical Informatics, 39*(5), 482–499. doi:10.1016/j.jbi.2005.12.008

Bird, S., Klein, E., Loper, E., & Baldridge, J. (2008). Multidisciplinary instruction with the Natural Language Toolkit. *Proc. of the Third ACL Workshop on Issues in Teaching Computational Linguistics*, (pp. 62-70).

Bohus, D., Raux, A., Harris, T., Eskenazi, M., & Rudnicky, A. (2007). Olympus: An open-source framework for conversational spoken language interface research. *Proc. of HLT-NAACL.*

Boisen, S., Ramshaw, L., Ayuso, D., & Bates, M. (1989). A proposal for SLS evaluation. *Proc. of the Workshop on Speech and Natural Language*, ACL Human Language Technology Conference, (pp. 135-146).

Bos, J., Klein, E., & Oka, T. (2003). Meaningful conversation with a mobile robot, *Proc. of EACL*, (pp. 71-74).

Carpenter, R. (1992). *The logic of typed features structures*. Cambridge University Press. doi:10.1017/CBO9780511530098

Cassell, J., Bickmore, T., Billinghurst, M., Campbell, L., Chang, K., Vilhálmsson, H., & Yan, H. (1999). *Embodiment in conversational interfaces: Rea* (pp. 520–527). Proc. of Computer-Human Interaction.

Cassell, J., Sullivan, J., Prevost, S., & Churchill, E. F. (Eds.). (2000). *Embodied conversational agents*. The MIT Press.

Catizone, R., Setzer, A., & Wilks, Y. (2003). Multimodal dialogue management in the COMIC project. *Proc. of EACL Workshop on Dialogue Systems: Interaction, Adaptation, and Styles of Management*, (pp. 25-34).

Cavazza, M., Smith, C., Charlton, D., Zhang, L., Turunen, M., & Hakulinen, J. (2008). A companion ECA with planning and activity modelling. *Proc. of AAMAS.*

Clark, R., Richmond, K., & King, S. (2004). Festival 2 - build your own general purpose unit selection speech synthesizer. *Proc. of 5th ISCA Workshop on Speech Synthesis*, (pp. 173–178).

Cole, R., Mariani, J., Uszkoreit, H., Varile, G. B., Zaenen, A., Zampolli, A., & Zue, V. (Eds.). (1997). *Survey of the state of the art in human language technology*. Cambridge University Press.

Cole, R., Van Vuuren, S., Pellom, B., Hacioglu, K., Ma, J., Movellan, J., et al. Wade-stein, D. (2003). Perceptive animated interfaces: First steps toward a new paradigm for human-computer interaction. *Proc. of the IEEE Special Issue on Multimodal Human Computer Interface*, (pp. 1391-1405).

Corradini, A., & Samuelsson, C. (2008). A generic spoken dialogue manager applied to an interactive 2D game. In E. André, L. Dybkjær, W. Minker, H. Neumann, R. Pieraccini, & M. Weber (Eds.) PIT 2008. *LNCS (LNAI)*, vol. 5078, (pp. 3–13).

Cuayáhuitl, H., Renals, S., Lemon, O., & Shimodaira, H. (2005). Human-computer dialogue simulation using Hidden Markov models. *Proc. of IEEE Workshop on Automatic Speech Recognition and Understanding (ASRU)*, (pp. 290-295).

De Carolis, B., Carofiglio, V., & Bilvi, M. M., & Pelachaud, C. (2002). APML, a mark-up language for believable behavior generation. *Proc. of AAMAS*.

Degerstedt, L., & Jönsson, A. (2006). LinTest, a development tool for testing dialogue systems. *Proc. of the 9th International Conference on Spoken Language Processing (Interspeech/ICSLP)*, (pp. 489-492).

Den, E., Boves, L., Lamel, L., & Baggia, P. (1999). *Overview of the ARISE project* (pp. 1527–1530). Proc. of Eurospeech.

Doherty, P., Granlund, G., Kuchcinski, K., Sandewall, E., Nordberg, K., Skarman, E., & Wiklund, J. (1998). The WITAS unmanned aerial vehicle project. *Proc. of the 14th European Conference on Artificial Intelligence (ECAI)*, (pp. 747-755).

Dybkjaer, L., & Bernsen, N. (2000). Usability issues in spoken language dialogue systems. *Natural Language Engineering*, *6*, 243–271. doi:10.1017/S1351324900002461

Dybkjaer, L., Bernsen, N., & Minker, W. (2004). Evaluation and usability of multimodal spoken language dialogue systems. *Speech Communication*, *43*, 33–54. doi:10.1016/j.specom.2004.02.001

Ekman, P., & Friesen, W. (1978). *Facial action coding system*. Consulting Psychologist Press.

Eliasson, K. (2007). Case-based techniques used for dialogue understanding and planning in a human-robot dialogue system. *Proc. of IJCAI*, (pp. 1600-1605).

Emele, M. C. (1994). The typed feature structure representation formalism. *Proc. of the International Workshop on Sharable Natural Language Resources*.

Fabbrizio, G., & Lewis, C. (2004). Florence: A dialogue manager framework for spoken dialogue systems. *Proc. of International Conference on Spoken Language Processing (ICSLP)*, (pp. 3065-3068).

Faure, C., & Julia, L. (1993). Interaction hommemachine par la parole et le geste pour l'édition de documents. *Proc. International Conference on Real and Virtual Worlds*, (pp. 171-180).

Forbes-Riley, K., & Litman, D. (2011). Designing and evaluating a wizarded uncertainty-adaptive spoken dialogue tutoring system. *Computer Speech & Language*, *25*(1), 105–126. doi:10.1016/j.csl.2009.12.002

Fraikin, F., & Leonhardt, T. (2002). *From requirements to analysis with capture and replay tools. PI-R 1/02*. Software Engineering Group, Department of Computer Science, Darmstadt University of Technology.

Fraser, N., & Gilbert, G. (1991). Simulating speech systems. *Computer Speech & Language*, *5*, 81–99. doi:10.1016/0885-2308(91)90019-M

Glass, J., Flammia, G., Goodine, D., Phillips, M., Polifroni, J., & Sakai, S. (1995). Multilingual spoken-language understanding in the MIT Voyager system. *Speech Communication*, *17*(1-2), 1–18. doi:10.1016/0167-6393(95)00008-C

Goddeau, D., Meng, H., Polifroni, J., Seneff, S., & Busayapongchai, S. (1996). A form-based dialogue manager for spoken language applications. *Proc. of International Conference on Spoken Language Processing (ICSLP)*, (pp. 701-704).

Graesser, A. C., VanLehn, K., Rose, C., Jordan, P., & Harter, D. (2001). Intelligent tutoring systems with conversational dialogue. *AI Magazine*, *22*, 39–51.

Griol, D., Callejas, Z., & López-Cózar, R. (2009). A comparison between dialogue corpora acquired with real and simulated users. *Proc. of the 10th Annual Meeting of the Special interest Group on Discourse and Dialogue (SIGDIAL 2009)*, (pp. 326-332).

Griol, D., Hurtado, L. F., Segarra, E., & Sanchis, E. (2008). A statistical approach to spoken dialogue systems design and evaluation. *Speech Communication*, *50*(8-9), 666–682. doi:10.1016/j.specom.2008.04.001

Griol, D., Torres, F., Hurtado, L., Grau, S., García, F., Sanchis, E., & Segarra, E. (2006). A dialogue system for the DIHANA project. *Proc. of SPECOM*, (pp. 131-136).

Huang, C., Xu, P., & Zhang, X. Zhao, S., Huang, T., & Xu, B. (1999). LODESTAR: A Mandarin spoken dialogue system for travel information retrieval. *Proc. of Eurospeech*, (pp. 1159-1162).

Huang, H., Cerekovic, A., Pandzic, I., Nakano, Y., & Nishida, T. (2007). A script driven multimodal embodied conversational agent based on a generic framework. *Proc. of IVA*, (pp. 381–382).

Huang, H.-H., Cerekovic, A., Nakano, Y., Pandzic, I. S., & Nishida, T. (2008). The design of a generic framework for integrating ECA components. *Proc. of AAMAS*, (pp. 128–135).

Hubal, R. C., Fishbein, D. H., Sheppard, M. S., Paschall, M. J., Eldreth, D. L., & Hyde, C. T. (2008). How do varied populations interact with embodied conversational agents? Findings from inner-city adolescents and prisoners. *Computers in Human Behavior*, *24*(3), 1104–1138. doi:10.1016/j.chb.2007.03.010

Ibrahim, A., & Johansson, P. (2002). Multimodal dialogue systems for interactive TV applications. *Proc. of 4th IEEE Int. Conf. on Multimodal Interfaces*, (pp. 117-122).

Ieronutti, L., & Chittaro, L. (2007). Employing virtual humans for education and training in X3D/VRML worlds. *Computers & Education*, *49*(1), 93–109. doi:10.1016/j.compedu.2005.06.007

Johnson, W. L., & Valente, A. (2008). Tactical language and culture training systems: Using Artificial Intelligence to teach foreign languages and cultures. *Proc. IAAI*, (pp. 1632-1639).

Johnston, M., Bangalore, S., Vasireddy, G., Stent, A., Ehlen, P., Walker, M., et al. Maloor, P. (2002). MATCH: An architecture for multimodal dialogue systems. *Proc. of 40th Annual Meeting of the ACL*, (pp. 376-383).

King, M., Maegaard, B., Schutz, J., & des Tombes, L. (1996). *EAGLES - Evaluation of Natural Language Processing Systems*, (Final report, EAG-EWG-PR.2).

Kopp, S., Krenn, B., Marsella, S., Marshall, A., Pelachaud, C., Pirker, H., et al. (2006). Towards a common framework for multimodal generation in ECAs: The behavior markup language. *Proc. of 6th International Conference on Intelligent Virtual Agents*, (pp. 205-217).

Kopp, S., & Wachsmuth, I. (2004). Synthesizing multimodal utterances for conversational agents. *Computer Animation and Virtual Worlds*, *15*(1), 39–52. doi:10.1002/cav.6

Kuppevelt, J., & Dybkajer, L. (Eds.). (2005). *Advances in natural multimodal dialogue systems*. Springer. doi:10.1007/1-4020-3933-6

Larsson, S., Berman, A., Bos, J., Grönqvist, L., & Junglöf, P. (1999). *A model of dialogue moves and information state revision. Technical Report, D5.1 Trindi*. Task Oriented Instructional Dialogue.

Lee, A., & Kawahara, T. (2009). *Recent development of open-source speech recognition engine Julius. Proc of. Asia-Pacific Signal and Information Processing Association Annual Summit and Conference*. APSIPA ASC.

Lee, K., Hon, H., & Reddy, R. (1990). *An overview of the SPHINX speech recognition system. Readings in Speech Recognition* (pp. 600–610). Morgan Kaufmann Publishers.

Lemon, O., Georgila, K., & Henderson, J. (2006b). Evaluating effectiveness and portability of reinforcement learned dialogue strategies with real users: The TALK TownInfo evaluation. *Proc. of IEEE-ACL*, (pp. 178–181).

Lemon, O., Georgila, K., Henderson, J., & Stuttle, M. (2006a). An ISU dialogue system exhibiting reinforcement learning of dialogue policies: Generic slot-filling in the TALK in-car system. *Proc. of EACL*.

Leßmann, N., & Wachsmuth, I. (2003). A cognitively motivated architecture for an anthropomorphic artificial communicator. *Proc. of ICCM-5*, (pp. 277- 278).

Levin, E., & Pieraccini, R. (1997). *A stochastic model of computer-human interaction for learning dialogue strategies* (pp. 1883–1886). Proc. of Eurospeech.

Li, L., Cao, F., Chou, W., & Liu, F. (2006). XM-flow: An extensible micro-flow for multimodal interaction. *Proc. of MMSP*, (pp. 497-500).

Li, L., Li, L., Chou, W., & Liu, F. (2007). R-Flow: An extensible XML based multimodal dialogue system architecture. *Proc. of MMSP*, (pp. 86-89).

Liu, J., Wang, J., & Wang, C. (2006). Spoken language understanding in dialog systems for Olympic game information. *Proc. of IEEE Int. Conf. on Industrial Informatics*, (pp. 1042-1045).

López-Cózar, R., Ábalos, N., Espejo, G., Griol, D., Callejas, Z. (2011). Using ambient intelligence information in a multimodal dialogue system. *Journal of Ambient Intelligence and Smart Environments*. In printing.

López-Cózar, R., & Araki, M. (2005). *Spoken, multilingual and multimodal dialogue systems: Development and assessment*. Wiley.

López-Cózar, R., de la Torre, A., Segura, J., & Rubio, A. (2003). Assessment of dialogue systems by means of a new simulation technique. *Speech Communication*, *40*, 387–407. doi:10.1016/S0167-6393(02)00126-7

Maatman, R. M., Gratch, J., & Marsella, S. (2005). Natural behavior of a listening agent. *Proc. of IVA*, (pp. 25-36).

Mairesse, F., Gasic, M., Jurcicek, F., Keizer, S., Thomson, B., Yu, K., & Young, S. (2009). Spoken language understanding from unaligned data using discriminative classification models. *Proc. of ICASSP*, (pp. 4749-4752).

Malaka, R., Haeusseler, J., & Aras, H. (2004). SmartKom mobile: Intelligent ubiquitous user interaction. *Proc. of 9th Int. Conf. on Intelligent User Interfaces*, (pp. 310-312).

Malatesta, L., Raouzaiou, A. K., Karpouzis, K., & Kollias, S. D. (2009). Towards modeling embodied conversational agent character profiles using appraisal theory predictions in expression synthesis. *Applied Intelligence*, *30*(1), 58–64. doi:10.1007/s10489-007-0076-9

Maragoudakis, M. (2007). MeteoBayes: Effective plan recognition in a weather dialogue system. *IEEE Intelligent Systems*, *22*(1), 66–77. doi:10.1109/MIS.2007.14

Mayfield, L., & Burger, S. (1999). Eliciting natural speech from non-native users: Collecting speech data for LVCSR. *Proc. of ACL-IALL*.

McGlashan, S., Burnett, D. C., Carter, J., Danielsen, P., Ferrans, J., Hunt, A.,... Tryphonas, S. (2004). *Voice extensible markup language* (VoiceXML). W3C.

McTear, M. F. (1998). Modelling spoken dialogues with state transition diagrams: experiences with the CSLU toolkit. *Proc. of ICSLP*, (pp. 1223–1226).

McTear, M. F. (2004). *Spoken dialogue technology. Toward the conversational user interface*. Springer.

Meza-Ruiz, I. V., Riedel, S., & Lemon, O. (2008). Accurate statistical spoken language understanding from limited development resources. *Proc. of ICASSP*.

Minker, W. (1998). Stochastic versus rule-based speech understanding for information retrieval. *Speech Communication*, *25*(4), 223–247. doi:10.1016/S0167-6393(98)00038-7

Mohri, M. (1997). Finite-state transducers in language and speech processing. *Computational Linguistics*, *23*(2), 269–311.

Moran, D. B., Cheyer, A. J., Julia, L. E., Martin, D. L., & Park, S. (1997). Multimodal user interface in the open agent architecture. *Proc. of ACM*, (pp. 61–68).

Morency, L. P., Sidner, C., Lee, C., & Darrell, T. (2005). Contextual recognition of head gestures. *Proc. of ICMI*, (pp. 18-24).

Müller, C., & Runge, F. (1993). *Dialogue design principles - key for usability of voice processing* (pp. 943–946). Proc. of Eurospeech.

Müller, J., Poller, P., & Tschernomas, V. (2003). A multimodal fission approach with a presentation agent in the dialog system SmartKom. *LNCS*, *2821*, 633–645.

Nielsen, P. B., & Baekgaard, A. (1992). Experience with a dialogue description formalism for realistic applications. *Proc. of International Conference on Spoken Language Processing (ICSLP)*, (pp. 719-722).

Nigay, L., & Coutaz, J. (1993). A design space for multimodal systems: Concurrent processing and data fusion. *Proc. of ACM CHI Conf. on Human Factors in Computing Systems*, (pp. 172-178).

Nigay, L., & Coutaz, J. (1995). A generic platform for addressing the multimodal challenge. *Proc. of ACM CHI*, (pp. 98-105).

Oh, A. H., & Rudnicky, A. (2000). Stochastic language generation for spoken dialogue systems. *Proc. of ANLP/NAACL workshop on conversational systems*, (pp. 27-32).

Paek, T., & Horvitz, E. (2004). Optimizing automated call routing by integrating spoken dialogue models with queuing models. *Proc. of HLT-NAACL*, 41-48.

Pandzic, I. S. (2002). Facial animation framework for the web and mobile platforms. *Proc. of Web3D Symposium*, (pp. 27-34).

Paroubek, P., & Blasband, M. (1999). *A blueprint for a general infrastructure for natural language processing systems evaluation using semi-automatic quantitative black box approach in a multilingual environment.* ELSE project Executive Summary.

Patel, M., & Willis, P. G. (1991). *FACES–The Facial Animation, Construction and Editing System* (pp. 33–45). Proc. of Eurographics.

Pelachaud, C., Maya, V., & Lamolle, M. (2004). Representation of expressivity for embodied conversational agents. *Proc. of Workshop Balanced Perception and Action, 3rd Int. Joint Conf. on Autonomous Agents and Multi-Agent Systems.*

Pellom, B., & Hacioglu, K. (2003). Recent improvements in the CU Sonic ASR System for noisy speech. *Proc. of ICASSP*.

Petrelli, D., De Angeli, A., Gerbino, W., & Cassano, G. (1997). Referring in multimodal systems: The importance of user expertise and system features. *Proc. ACL-EACL*, (pp. 14-19).

Pfleger, N., Alexandersson, J., & Becker, T. (2002). Scoring functions for overlay and their application in discourse processing. *Proc. of KONVENS*.

Pietquin, O., & Dutoit, T. (2005). A probabilistic framework for dialogue simulation and optimal strategy learning. *IEEE Transactions on Speech and Audio Processing, Special Issue on Data Mining of Speech. Audio and Dialog, 14*, 589–599.

Potamianos, A., Ammicht, E., & Fosler-Lussier, E. (2003). Modality tracking in the Multimodal Bell Labs Communicator. *Proc. of IEEE Workshop on Automatic Speech Recognition and Understanding (ASRU)*, (pp. 192-197).

Rabiner, L. R., & Juang, B. H. (1993). *Fundamentals of speech recognition*. Prentice-Hall.

Raux, A., & Eskenazi, M. (2007). A multi-layer architecture for semi-synchronous event-driven dialogue management. *Proc. of ASRU*.

Reithinger, N., & Sonntag, D. (2005). *An integration framework for a mobile multimodal dialogue system accessing the Semantic Web* (pp. 841–844). Proc. of Interspeech.

Rosenfeld, R. (1995). The CMU statistical language modeling toolkit and its use in the 1994 ARPA CSR evaluation. *Proc. of ARPA Spoken Language Systems Technology Workshop*.

Salber, D., & Coutaz, J. (1993). Applying the Wizard of Oz technique to the study of multimodal systems. *Proc. of EWHCI*, (pp. 219-230).

San Segundo, R. (2004). *La evaluación objetiva de sistemas de diálogo. Proc of. Curso de Tecnologías Lingüísticas*. Fundación Duques de Soria.

Schatzmann, J., Weilhammer, K., Stuttle, M., & Young, S. (2006). A survey of statistical user simulation techniques for reinforcement-learning of dialogue management strategies. *The Knowledge Engineering Review, 21*(2), 97–126. doi:10.1017/S0269888906000944

Schatzmann, J., & Young, S. (2009). The hidden agenda user simulation model. *IEEE Trans. Audio. Speech and Language Processing, 17*(4), 733–747. doi:10.1109/TASL.2008.2012071

Seneff, S. (1989). TINA: A probabilistic syntactic parser for speech understanding systems. *Proc. of ACL Workshop on Speech and Natural Language*, (pp. 168-178).

Seneff, S., & Hurley, E. Lau, R., Pao, C., Schmid, P., & Zue, V. (1998). Galaxy-II: A reference architecture for conversational system development. *Proc. of ICSLP*, (pp. 931-934).

Seron, F., Baldassarri, S., & Cerezo, E. (2006). MaxinePPT: Using 3D virtual characters for natural interaction. *Proc. of 2nd International Workshop on Ubiquitous Computing and Ambient Intelligence*, (pp. 241-250).

Steininger, S., Rabold, S., Dioubina, O., & Schiel, F. (2002). Development of the user-state conventions for the multimodal corpus in SmartKom. *Proc. of 3rd International Conference on Language Resources and Evaluation*.

Stent, A., Dowding, J., Gawron, J. M., Bratt, E., & Moore, R. (1999). The CommandTalk spoken dialogue system. *Proc. of 37th Annual Meeting of the ACL*, (pp. 183-190).

Takeuchi, A., & Nagao, K. (1995). Situated facial displays: Towards social interaction. *Proc. of SIGCHI*, (pp. 450-454).

Tekalp, M. A., & Ostermann, J. (2000). *Face and 2-D mesh animation in MPEG-4. Image Communication Journal, Tutorial Issue on MPEG-4 Standard*. Elsevier.

Tian, Y., Kanade, T., & Cohn, J. (2003). Facial expression analysis. In Li, S. Z., & Jain, A. K. (Eds.), *Handbook of face recognition*.

Tsutsui, T., Saeyor, S., & Ishizuka, M. (2000). *MPML: A multimodal presentation markup language with character agent control functions* (pp. 537–543). Proc. of WebNet.

Turunen, M. (2004). *Jaspis - a spoken dialogue architecture and its applications*. Ph.D. Dissertation, University of Tampere, Department of Computer Sciences A-2004-2.

Van de Burgt, S. P., Andernach, T., Kloosterman, H., Bos, R., & Nijholt, A. (1996). Building dialogue systems that sell. *Proc. NLP and Industrial Applications*, (pp. 41-46).

Wahlster, W. (2001). SmartKom: Multimodal dialogues with mobile Web users. *Proc. of International Cyber Assist Symposium*, (pp. 33-40).

Wahlster, W. (2003). *SmartKom: Symmetric multimodality in an adaptive and reusable dialogue shell* (pp. 47–62). Proc. of Human Computer Interaction.

Wahlster, W. (Ed.). (2006). *SmartKom: Foundations of multimodal dialogue systems*. Springer. doi:10.1007/3-540-36678-4

Walker, J. H., Sproull, L., & Subramami, R. (1994). Using a human face in an interface. *Proc. of SIGCHI conference on human factors in computing systems*, (pp. 85-91).

Walker, M. A., Litman, D. J., Kamm, C. A., & Abella, A. (1998). Evaluating spoken dialogue agents with PARADISE: Two case studies. *Computer Speech & Language*, *12*, 317–347. doi:10.1006/csla.1998.0110

Walker, M. A., Passonneau, R., & Boland, J. E. (2001). Quantitative and qualitative evaluation of Darpa Communicator spoken dialogue systems. *Proc. of 39th Annual Meeting of ACL*, (pp. 515-522).

Walker, W., Lamere, P., & Kwok., P. (2002). *FreeTTS: A performance case study*. Sun Microsystems, Inc.

Walsh, P., & Meade, J. (2003). Speech enabled e-learning for adult literacy tutoring. *Proc. of ICALT*, (pp. 17-21).

Ward, W., & Issar, S. (1994). Recent improvements in the CMU spoken language understanding system. *Proc. of ACL Workshop on Human Language Technology* (pp. 213-216).

Wasinger, R., Stahl, C., & Krüger, A. (2003). *Robust speech interaction in a mobile environment through the use of multiple and different media types* (pp. 1049–1052). Proc. of Eurospeech.

Webb, N., Benyon, D., Bradley, R., Hansen, P., & Mival, O. (2010). Wizard of Oz experiments for a companion dialogue system: Eliciting companionable conversation. *Proc. of International Conference on Language Resources and Evaluation (LREC 2010)*.

Wei, X., & Rudnicky, A. (2000). Task-based dialogue management using an agenda. *Proceedings of ANLP/NAACL Workshop on Conversational Systems*, (pp. 42-47).

Williams, J., & Young, S. (2007). Partially observable Markov decision processes for spoken dialogue systems. *Computer Speech & Language*, *21*(2), 393–422. doi:10.1016/j.csl.2006.06.008

Young, S., Adda-Decker, M., Aubert, X., Dugast, C., Gauvain, J., & Kershaw, D. (1997). Multilingual large vocabulary speech recognition: The European SQALE project. *Computer Speech & Language*, *11*, 73–89. doi:10.1006/csla.1996.0023

Young, S., Kershaw, D., Odell, J., Ollason, D., Valtchev, V., & Woodland, P. (2000). *The HTK book*. Microsoft Corporation.

Zapata, C. M., & Carmona, N. (2007). El experimento Mago de Oz y sus aplicaciones: una mirada retrospectiva. *Dyna rev.fac.nac.minas, 74*(151), 125-135.

Zhang, T., Hasegawa-Johnson, M., & Levinson, S. A. (2005). Hybrid model for spontaneous speech understanding. *Proc. of AAAI Workshop on Spoken Language Understanding*, (pp. 60-67).

Zue, V., Seneff, S., Glass, J., Polifroni, J., Pao, C., Hazen, T., & Hetherington, L. (2000). JUPITER: A telephone-based conversational interface for weather information. *IEEE Transactions on Speech and Audio Processing*, *8*(1), 85–96. doi:10.1109/89.817460

Zukerman, I., & Litman, D. (2001). Natural language processing and user modeling: Synergies and limitations. *User Modeling and User-Adapted Interaction*, *11*, 129–158. doi:10.1023/A:1011174108613

## KEY TERMS AND DEFINITIONS

**Automatic Speech Recognition (ASR):** Technique to determine the word sequence in a speech signal. To do this, this technology first detects basic units in the signal, e.g. phonemes, which are then combined to determine words. Some kind of grammatical information is used to determine more precisely the word sequence, by considering that some words are more likely than other taken into account the previous words in the sequence.

**Dialogue Management (DM):** Implementation of the "intelligent" behaviour of the conversational agent. It receives some sort of internal representation obtained from the user input and decides the next action the system must carry out. Typical actions are: i) to query the database module, ii) to generate a prompt to ask the user for additional data, iii) to generate a confirmation prompt to confirm unreliable data obtained from the user, iv) to provide help to the user, etc.

**Embodied Conversational Agent (ECA):** Humanlike computer-generated character that provides auditory and visual feedback for the user, which is particularly useful when the interaction takes place in noisy environments. Its complexity can vary significantly in terms of sophistication and complexity, from simple cartoon-like to complex animated human faces.

**Fission of Multimodal Information:** Opposite to the *fusion* operation, chooses the output to be produced through each output modality and coordinates the output across the modalities in order generate an agent's response appropriately for the user.

**Fusion of Multimodal Information:** Operation that combines the information chunks provided by the diverse input modules of the conversational agent in order to obtain a better understanding of the intention of the user. For example, the combination of acoustic information and visual information obtained from lip movements can enhance notably the performance of ASR systems, especially when processing low quality signals due to noise or other factors.

**Galaxy Communicator:** Distributed, message-based, hub-centred architecture to interconnect the main components of conversational agents. Among others, this architecture that has been used to set up the MIT's Voyager and Jupiter agents.

**HADA-DS:** Multimodal conversational agent in development to assist professors and students in some of their daily activities within a University's Faculty.

**Natural Language Generation (NLG):** Creation of messages in text mode, grammatical and semantically correct, which will be either displayed on screen or converted into speech by means of text-to-speech synthesis.

**PARAdigm for DIalogue System Evaluation (PARADISE):** One of the most employed proposals for globally evaluating the performance of spoken conversational agents. It combines different features in a single function that measures the performance of the agent in direct correlation with user satisfaction.

**PROcedure for Multimodal Interactive System Evaluation (PROMISE):** Extension to multimodality of the PARADISE framework. This procedure uses methods traditionally employed to evaluate spoken conversational agents, and specific methods to assess the characteristic properties of multimodal conversational agents.

**R-Flow:** Extensible XML-based architecture for the implementation of multimodal conversational agents, which is based on a recursive application of the Model-View-Controller design.

**Speech Synthesis:** Artificial generation of human-like speech. Currently, speech synthesis techniques can be classified into voice coding, parametric, formant-based and rule-based approaches. A particular kind of speech synthesis technique is called Text-To-Speech synthesis (TTS), the goal of which is to transform into speech of any input sentence in text format.

**Spoken Language Understanding (SLU):** Technique to obtain the semantic content of the sequence of words provided by the ASR module. It must face a variety of phenomena, for example, ellipsis, anaphora and ungrammatical structures typical of spontaneous speech.

**VoiceXML:** Standard XML-based language to access web applications by means of speech.

**Wizard of Oz (WOz):** Technique that uses a human called *Wizard* to play the role of the computer in a human-computer interaction. The users are made to believe that they interact with a computer but actually they interact with the Wizard.

**XHTML+Voice (X+V):** XML-based language that combines traditional web access using XHTML and speech-based access to web pages using VoiceXML.

## ENDNOTES

1. http://www.w3.org/TR/voicexml20/
2. http://www.opoera.com/
3. http://www.w3.org/TR/voicexml20/

Section 3
# Practices

# Chapter 11
# Embodied Conversational Virtual Patients

**Patrick G. Kenny**
*University of Southern California, USA*

**Thomas D. Parsons**
*University of Southern California, USA*

## ABSTRACT

*Recent research has established the potential for computer generated virtual characters to act as virtual patients (VP) for the assessment and training of novice clinicians in interpersonal skills, interviewing, and diagnosis. These VPs are embodied interactive conversational agents who are designed to simulate a particular clinical presentation of a patient's illness with a high degree of consistency and realism. In this chapter we describe the architecture developed for virtual patients, and the application of the system to subject testing with virtual patients that exhibit a set of clinical conditions called Post Traumatic Stress Disorder (PTSD). The primary goal of these conversational agents was evaluative: can a VP generate responses that elicit user questions relevant for PTSD categorization? The results of the interactions of clinical students with the VP will be discussed. This chapter also highlights a set of design goals for increasing the visual, physical and cognitive realism when building VP systems including the design of the language, scenarios and artwork that is important when developing these characters. Finally, future research directions and challenges will be discussed for conversational virtual patients.*

## 1. INTRODUCTION

The development of the Eliza program by Joseph Weizenbaum (1966) which was capable of engaging humans in a natural conversation and simulated a Carl Rogers empathic psychologist was one of the first conversational agents with a medical theme. Although simple in design and driven by a script called DOCTOR that performed keyword matching and replacement, it was a very powerful mechanism that tricked some people into thinking they were talking to a real psychoanalyst. Today these kinds of conversational programs are more complex with fully embodied characters that exhibit facial expressions, gestures, animation and

DOI: 10.4018/978-1-60960-617-6.ch011

speech. However one of the more challenging aspects that still remain is the conversational dialog.

A general model for conversational agents should account for the intentional and non-intentional aspects of verbal and nonverbal communication as well as the contextually grounded natural biologically based aspects of conversation (Buck, 1994). A further refinement of this understanding may view conversation as something that occurs whenever one agent's (i.e. sender's) behavior influences the behavior of another agent (i.e., receiver).

Our work includes a general theoretical commitment to understanding virtual human conversation as a feedback process, in which interpretation of verbal and nonverbal data (i.e., message reception and production) alone, although potentially useful, are deficient. To make up for the incompleteness of limiting virtual human conversation and to provide more situational context to these two criteria we add psychophysiological information (e.g. heart rate) from the user into the conversational processing as we believe it reflects the conversation found in human agents.

While a full elucidation of this interactionist theory is beyond the scope of this chapter (Buck, 1984, 1989, 1994) we do mention it as the theoretical underpinning of much of what we are trying to do in our work toward an integrated view of virtual and human conversation. Further, our data analytic approach to understanding the utility of virtual human conversation requires that the assessment of the communicative efficacy of the conversational agent's behavior involves the extent to which it reduces uncertainty in the behavior of another (Wilson, 1979). Herein we discuss the development of our virtual patients (VP) and the general assessments that we make when assessing the virtual and human conversation. For our work this involves the integration of verbal communication, nonverbal communication, and contextual factors (e.g., psychophysiological data).

This chapter provides an examination into applying embodied conversational virtual patients for medical simulation and training. These VP's are interactive characters designed to simulate a particular clinical presentation of a patient with a medical illness with a high degree of consistency and realism. This chapter describes the virtual patient architecture used for research and evaluation, the subject testing conducted with VP's that exhibit a clinical condition of Conduct Disorder, Post Traumatic Stress Disorder (PTSD) or assessing racial bias. The development of the characters and dialog for the scenarios will also be addressed. The primary goal of the subject testing was evaluative: can a VP generate responses that elicit user questions relevant for PTSD categorization? The results of the interactions of clinical students with the virtual patient will be discussed along with areas of further research.

## 2. NEED FOR CLINICIAN TRAINING IN CONVERSATION SKILLS

Developing good conversational skills is essential for clinicians to establish good doctor patient relationships. Many undergraduate and postgraduate medical education and training programs have begun to place greater emphasis on the importance of high-quality conversation skills (ACGME; 2007). Traditional approaches to training clinicians in the conversation skills needed for assessment, diagnosis, and interview performance rely upon a combination of classroom learning and role-playing with human standardized patients.

The importance of conversation is reflected in recent requirements for communication evaluation in medical schools. The Accreditation Council for Graduate Medical Education (ACGME; 2007) has emphasized the importance of interpersonal and communication skills in training clinicians. Residents are expected to: 1) create and sustain a therapeutic and ethically sound relationship with the patient; 2) use effective listening skills, eliciting and providing information using effective nonverbal, explanatory, questioning, and writing skills; and 3) work in an efficient manner with others.

However, evaluation studies have revealed methodological deficiencies in many cases (Chant et al., 2002) and limited positive training effects (Hulsman et al., 1999). In an effort to increase interpersonal communication assessment, standardized patients (paid human actors) have been recruited and trained to exhibit the characteristics of an actual patient, thereby affording novice clinicians a realistic opportunity to practice and to be evaluated in a mock clinical environment.

Although a valuable training approach, there are limitations with the use of human standardized patients that can be mitigated through simulation technology. For example, human standardized patients are expensive and cost several thousand dollars per student. Further, given the fact that there are only a handful of sites (for over 130 medical schools in the U.S.) providing standardized patient assessments of the clinician in training's communication ability as part of the U.S. Medical Licensing Examination (USMLE), the current model provides limited availability.

Another concern is the issue of standardization. Despite the expense of standardized patient programs, the standardized patients themselves are typically unskilled actors. As a result of common turnover, administrators face considerable challenges for offering psychometrically reliable and valid interactions with the training clinicians. A related issue is the limited scope that the actors are able to portray. As a result, there tends to be an inadequate array of developmentally, socially, racially and culturally diverse appropriate scenarios.

For example, when a clinician has a pediatric focus and needs access to children, it is difficult for the clinician to pretend that the actor is a child. Finally, many clinical cases (e.g., traumatic brain injury) have associated physical symptoms and behaviors (e.g., dilated pupils, spasms, and uncoordinated movements) that simply cannot be accurately portrayed by human actors.

Additionally, a large part of working with clients is re-visits by the clinician to see how they are progressing. This is rarely performed with the standardized patient actors due to the inconsistency in the population. Virtual patients are not meant to replace actors, but rather augment them with 24/7 availability and more standardized training. An added bonus is the ability to capture multiple forms of data from the participant, for example, the conversation log, speech, body language, facial expressions, gaze and interactions with the patient. This data can be used to evaluate the clinician and build up a more rigorous standardized way of assessing their performance with others that have also used the system from around the country and around the world.

## 2.1 Conversational Characters for Medical Applications

Our response to the difficulties inherent in training clinicians with standardized patients is to use virtual humans as patients. Virtual humans (VH) are developing into powerful interfaces that can enable greatly increased intuitive human like interactions. These virtual human systems consist of characters that have realistic appearances, can think and act like humans, and can express themselves both verbally and non-verbally. Additionally, these virtual humans can listen and understand natural language and track user interactions with speech, vision and biometrics systems. Advances in simulated virtual humans afford the possibility of virtual patients that reduce cost, ensure standardization and faithfully model physical symptoms.

To address the need to teach proper conversational skills requires developing agents that act as patients or clients and can carry out realistic and relevant dialog with a practicing clinician. These conversations are constrained by the mental or physical illness found in the patient. Most questions asked by a clinician will be about the patient's condition, their behavior, symptoms or history; infrequently it will be about general issues like the weather or sports which are more aimed towards relationship building or rapport.

However, proper rapport is crucial towards a better relationship with the client. Dialogs can last 15 minutes in an initial visit that is aimed at medical history gathering to more detailed conversations that can last weeks or months to discuss the problems in a psychological assessment. The dialog can also change over time and issues that were discussed one week should be followed up the next week to assess progress. While the standard interview of a patient takes a form of introduction, discussion of symptoms, assessment and treatment, the dialog that manifests itself in this interview can vary wildly by the type of problems and symptoms the patient is exhibiting.

One thing is certain, humans use many forms of answering the same question, which can vary by many factors such as; personality, emotion or mood. Clinicians perform a method called a differential diagnosis on the patient by asking questions to rule out certain issues and digging down to a set of criteria for the disorder. Fully embodied conversational characters are important for these medical applications as clinicians and physicians need to observe the actions and expressions of the client along with listening to the speech. Studies have shown that this helps to immerse the clinician into the setting and increases the believability of the interaction as a whole by making it more real and natural (Kenny et al., 2007).

Virtual patients are artificially intelligent virtual human agents that control computer generated avatar bodies and can interact with users through speech and gesture in virtual environments (Gratch et al., 2002). Advanced virtual humans are able to engage in rich conversations (Traum et al., 2008), recognize nonverbal cues (Morency & de Kok, 2008), analyze social and emotional factors (Gratch & Marsella, 2004) and synthesize human conversation and nonverbal expressions which are synchronized together to produce realistic actions, facial expressions, lip syncing and gaze (Thiebaux et al., 2008).

Additionally, they can contain underlying physiological models that simulate blood pressure, heart rate, breathing, and blushing (De Melo & Gratch, 2009). Building virtual humans requires fundamental advances in AI, speech recognition, natural language understanding and generation, dialog management, cognitive modeling and reasoning, virtual human architectures and computer graphics and animations. All these technologies need to be integrated together into a single system that can work in unison, be expandable, flexible and plug-and-play with different components.

These VPs will need to be able to exhibit certain behaviors through dialog and physical actions. The focus of this research is to build fully embodied conversational characters capable of exhibiting the full range of human dynamics and behaviors. These characters are referred to as high fidelity characters. The higher the fidelity the closer to human behavior the avatar appears. An example of a lower fidelity agent is one that uses a text interface and does not contain a body. A character with high fidelity input would contain sensors for speech to recognize clinician's voice, for vision to recognize faces or track gestures or postures and biometric readings to record the users heart rate or skin conductance. High fidelity output includes finer grain facial expressions, variability in speech such as intonation or emotion and more expressive body language. The types of conversational agents that we research, design and build as VPs are considered to be high fidelity. High fidelity characters are defined along several dimensions to include these properties:

- **Visual Realism:** The characters should be as realistic as possible in appearance, animation, clothes and other visual aspects.
- **Mental and Physical Behavior Realism:** The characters should contain models that exhibit the proper illness to be displayed, this will in turn drive the conversation. The

mental processes should interact with the physical processes as there is a deep connection between the two.

- **Autonomous Behavior:** The characters need to be able to express themselves and exhibit their own behavior based on underlying models, and attributes. They should not just wait for the user to ask questions and generate responses.
- **Personality, Mood and Emotion:** The characters should contain models of personality, mood and emotion and they should assist in selecting the appropriate conversational style, tone and nonverbal behavior.
- **Social Interaction:** The characters exist in social settings and should have realistic behavior that emulates interpersonal skills. For example, turn taking in conversations, proper gaze and body language.
- **Multi-Modal Input and Output:** The characters should support many forms of input and output, for example, cameras, speech, gestures, biophysiology and sound that should be used by the underlying models when generating the output behavior and conversational dialog.
- **Story Management:** There should be a proper story behind the dialog and character, this will add realism, engage the user more and can help drive or constrain the conversation.

## 2.2 Related Work in Virtual Patients

Virtual patients fulfill the role of standardized patients by simulating a particular clinical presentation with a high degree of consistency and realism and offer a promising alternative to standardized patients (Deladisma et al., 2008; Green et al., 2004; Hayes-Roth et al., 2004, 2009; Hubal et al., 2000; Kenny et al 2007; Lok et al., 2006; Parsons et al., 2008; Stevens et al., 2005).

There is a growing field of research that applies VPs to training and assessment of bioethics, basic patient communication, interactive conversations, history taking, and clinical assessments (Bickmore & Giorgino, 2006; Bickmore et al., 2007; Lok et al., 2006; Parsons et al., 2008; Johnsen et al., 2005). Results suggest that VPs can provide valid and reliable representations of live patients (Kenny et al., 2007; Triola & Feldman, 2006; Andrew et al., 2007; Raij et al., 2007).

Additionally VPs enable a precise presentation and control of dynamic perceptual stimuli that increases ecological validity. Hence, VPs offer the veridical control and rigor of laboratory measures and a verisimilitude that reflects real life situations (Parsons et al., 2009a; Andrew et al., 2007). In addition, some groups have developed complex cognitive models of patients that more deeply simulate a VPs decision making process for a person with gastroesophageal reflux disease (Nirenburg et al., 2009).

## 2.3 Virtual Patients Issues

Virtual patients are a growing area of interest for research and development and application to increase and develop users' interpersonal and diagnostic skills in the medical field. Since it is such a young field there are no common definitions in what constitutes a VP, how they should be used or the best architecture for them. There are no standards in the underlying models, physical or psychological, and how that information should be used, or what attributes or qualities are important for VP characters. There is an enormous amount of research being conducted in the biological fields, neuroscience and brain studies in understanding the cognitive thought processes and how to build models of them (Edelman, 2006). Applying this work to build fully embodied virtual characters and complete architectures that can support them has not been attempted in detail, although it has always been a major goal in the field of Artificial Intelligence.

Most groups focus on creating text based VP systems such as (CASUS, 2010) and CAMPUS (Rudericha et al., 2004) some with very detailed cognitive models (Nirenburg et al., 2009) such as the Maryland Virtual Patients. There are some groups that create systems with 2D like characters, (Bickmore & Giorgino, 2006; Bickmore et al., 2007) and some with 3D characters, (Lok, 2006; Kenny et al., 2007a).

The European electronic virtual patients project (eVIP 2010) is attempting to create a set of standardized clinical cases that can be used by all, however integration of these cases into more complex 3D virtual characters and architectures has not been undertaken. These electronic cases mainly concentrate on the dialog design and not with other attributes like emotion, mood and non-verbal behavior. There is also a great deal of emphasis on creating VPs with physical related illnesses such as stomach problems, eye problems, trauma or military related injuries (Johnston & Whatley, 2005).

The work of our Virtual Patient Simulation Lab focuses is on creating VP's with psychological illnesses such as suicide, depression, post traumatic stress, Alzheimer's and other related disorders. The work here lays out a solution and a modular architecture that supports building complex embodied conversational virtual characters that can be used for medical simulation, interpersonal skills training and diagnosis.

These VPs rely heavily on being dialog driven so that a clinician can have an in-depth conversation with the patient, however they are fully embodied characters that synchronize the dialog with the non-verbal behavior and expressions. The work of the Neuroscience and Simulation Lab enables us to understand and add to the VP architecture with supporting cognitive functions and through assessing how users interact with the system with physiological input and response patterns associated from the users that is feed back to the VP to develop more adaptive VPs to augment the dialog and interaction.

## 3. VIRTUAL PATIENT SYSTEM ARCHITECTURE

Virtual training environments with VP characters are complex systems to construct with many disparate technologies that need to be integrated together to provide the required functionality. The various technologies allow for everything that a person would expect to encounter while interacting with a real human in a real environment, from the dialog and body expressions to real world object interactions like a stethoscope or digital thermometer. The architecture design should be able to support the multiple dimensions of fidelity addressed above.

### 3.1 Virtual Patient Technology

The VP system and architecture we use for research, development, subject testing and evaluation consists of many distributed modules that communicate through message passing. The underlying architecture used to drive the characters can be seen in Figure 1.

While not every module is used in our virtual patient system, the architecture supports building virtual humans of various complexities and has been used to do so (Kenny et al., 2007b). Building large systems like these to drive virtual humans are vast software engineering projects that are hard to manage and develop without proper practices and separating the functionality into distributed modules makes this task easier.

Separate modules allows for easier testing, as this can be performed on individual modules before whole system testing, the modules are easier to upgrade individually and new modules can replace older ones or be added into the architecture easily to add additional functionality. As this current system is a research platform, separating out the functionality into modules allows different researchers to develop components independently without having to use the whole system.

*Figure 1. VP-architecture*

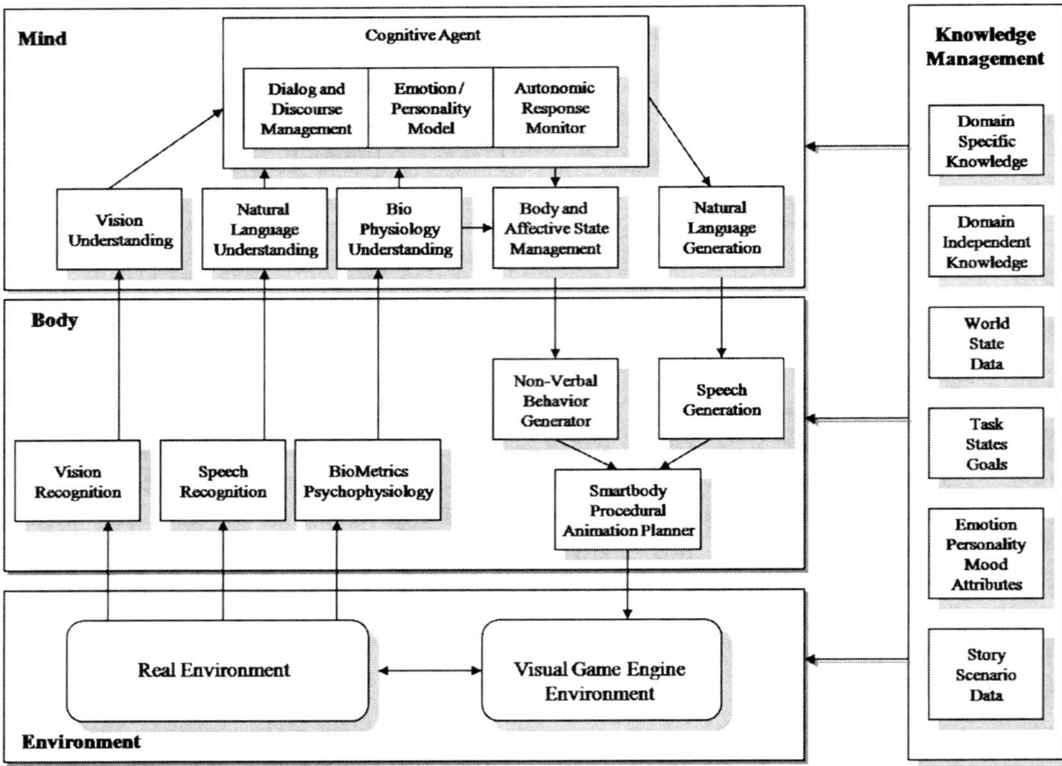


For example, the architecture supports using various Natural Language Understanding Modules. An important requirement for this system is message passing of data and communication between the modules; information should not just be passed in one direction, i.e. from the brain to the body, there should be feedback from lower level modules to higher ones. For example, interruption of speech or gestures if the clinician talks while the patient is responding or if the patients breathing increases then it should cause the heart rate to increase which could cause changes in the selected dialog. The mind should be able to know what the body is doing and vice versa.

The flow of information through the system can be seen in Figure 2 and involves three phases; Input, Reasoning and Output. Data is gathered at each phase and is used to assess the system and evaluate a user's interaction with the character. Each of the modules in the phases requires domain data that is built beforehand. The Interaction works as follows:

### 3.1.1 Input Phase Modules

In the Input phase a user talks into a microphone in plain English (or language). The speech recognition engine records the audio signal which is converted to text string that is passed to a reasoning engine.

Speech Input – For Speech input the SONIC speech recognition engine from the University of Colorado, Boulder (Pellom, 2001) is used. The engine's acoustic and language models are customized for the domain of interest (Sethy et al., 2005). The domain for the virtual patient consists of a corpus 10,000 words of general and specific

*Figure 2. VP-architecture-flow*

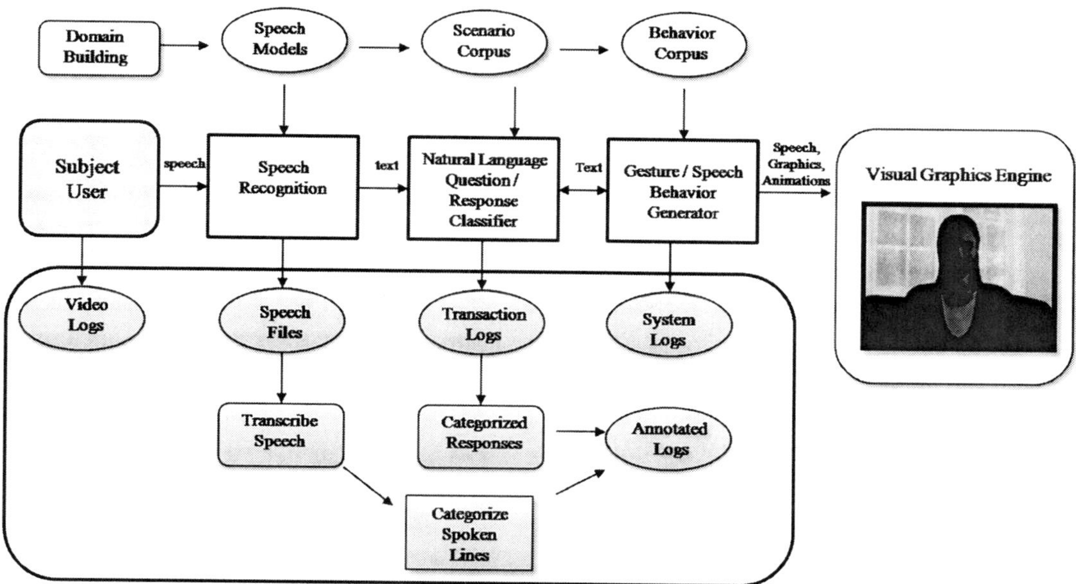


medical terminology. The engine requires no training of a user voice and is a push to talk system.

### 3.1.2 Reasoning Phase Modules

The reasoning phase involves making decisions based on the input data and internal state to generate action states and dialog for the character. The text from the speech engine is used by the natural language understanding system to select an appropriate response text string. This response text is further parsed to select appropriate non-verbal behavior and animations which is then sent to the output phase.

Natural Language Understanding System (NLU) – The NLU contains a corpus of questions and answers. The NLU parses the text string produced by the speech recognition module and uses a statistical text classifier to select the best question that matches the input string (Leuski et al., 2006). The question has an associated answer which is sent to the Non-verbal behavior module. Since the dialog plays a critical role in the characters interaction, the next section will describe this in more detail.

Non-Verbal Behavior Generator (NVBG) – Gestures and postures play a key role in realizing expressive, interpretable behavior in general and communicative intent specifically. For example, they qualify information in the speech such as a shrug when saying, "I don't know." They also emphasize important words by using, for example, a beat gesture (e.g., short chopping movement) synchronized with the word. The timing of gestures to the speech is critical, and small changes can alter an observer's interpretation of the utterance of the speaker. Without gestures, or with poorly timed gestures, a character will look unnatural. The NVBG (Lee & Marsella, 2006) applies rules based on theoretical foundations of movement space to select the appropriate gesture animations, postures, facial expressions, and lip synch timing for the virtual character. Once the NVBG selects the appropriate behavior for the text, it then packages this up into a Behavioral Markup Language (BML) (Kopp et al., 2006) structure and sends it to the procedural animation system, SmartBody in the output phase.

### 3.1.3 Output Phase Modules

The output phase involves the character generating the appropriate gestures, animations and behaviors. A procedural animation system that synchronizes the gestures, speech and lip synching and plays a pre-recorded or generated voice of the text for the character for final output to the screen is accomplished in this phase. The user then listens to the response and interacts more with the character.

Procedural Animation System – This system is called SmartBody and takes as input a message that contains the set of behaviors that need to be executed for the head, facial expressions, gaze, body movements, arm gestures, speech and lip syncing and synchronizes all of this together (Thiebaux et al, 2008). It is capable of using either generated speech or pre-recorded speech. Smartbody is also capable of using controllers that perform specific actions based on rules or timing information, such as head nods. The controllers are seamlessly blended in with the animations specified in the input message. A Motex, which is a looping animation file, can be played for the character to give it a bit of sway, finger tapping, or some repetitive movement.

Speech Generation- The text to speech voice generation is performed by a commercial product called cerevoice, additionally pre-recorded voice has been used for some of the characters. The language models for cerevoice are generated from an actor that speaks a large set of utterances, machine learning techniques are then used to create a dynamic model that is capable of creating any utterance. The output text string is converted into an audio file by the speech synthesis software and is played and synchronized by the Smartbody system when the character speaks. An alternative approach is to use a set of pre-recorded voice files that can be used by the character when it speaks, however this limits the set of utterances and is not dynamic, the advantage is that the voice actor can add more emotion and realism to the recorded voice.

Graphical Game Engine – The game engine is used to visualize the embodied conversational characters, animations of those characters, the environments and objects in the environment, such as chairs, tables, sounds, lighting, and medical devices. This is a commercial game engine, (GameBryo, 2010), with many of the advanced features in computer graphics such as shaders, bump mapping and environmental lighting that enhance the visual realism of the setting and characters.

## 3.2 Dialog and Discourse management for virtual patients

This section describes the Dialog system in more details as it is an important part of interacting with VP characters since a clinical interview relies heavily on the types of questions asked and the responses from the patient. The current VP system uses a classifier system called the NPCEditor for Non-Player-Character Editor, a term used in computer games to represent characters in the game that are not controlled by another human player (Leuski et al., 2006; Leuski & Traum, 2010).

The NPCEditor is a user friendly software package for editing and adding to the corpus of questions and responses, it allows a developer to test the text classifier. The classifier is trained on the set of questions, responses and links between them, and will generate a threshold value that is used for the matching and classification process. This response selection process is based on a statistical text classification approach (Leuski & Traum, 2010). There is no limit to the number of responses or sample questions, but it is advisable to have at least two or three sample questions for each response. The system allows for several response categories described below. Sometimes the system combines the text from different categories to produce the final response.

The category types are as follows:

- **On-Topic:** answers that are relevant to the domain of the conversation. These are the answers the system has to produce when asked a relevant question. Each on-topic answer should have a few sample questions and single sample question can be linked to several answers. The text classifier generally returns a ranked list of answers and the system makes the final selection based on the rank of the answer and whether the answer has been used recently. That way if the user repeats his/her questions, s/he may get a different response from the system.
- **Off-Topic:** answers for questions that do not have domain-relevant answers. They can be direct, e.g., "I do not know the answer", or evasive, e.g., "I will not tell you" or "Better ask somebody else". When the system cannot find a good on-topic answer for a question, it selects one of the off-topic lines.
- **Repeat:** if the classifier selects an answer tagged with this category, the system does not return that answer but replays the most recent response. Sample questions may include lines like "What was that?" or "Can you say that again?" Normally, there is at most one answer of this category in the domain answer set.
- **Alternative:** if the classifier selects an answer tagged with this category, the system attempts to find an alternative answer to the most recent question. It takes the ranked list of answers for the last question and selects the next available answer. Sample questions may include lines like "Do you have anything to add?" Normally, there is at most one answer tagged with this category in the answer set.
- **Pre-Repeat:** sometimes the system has to repeat an answer. For example, it happens when a user repeats a question and there is only one good response available. The system returns the same answer again but indicates that it is repeating itself by playing a pre-repeat-tagged line before the answer, e.g., "I told you already." There is no need to assign sample questions to these answer lines.
- **Delayed:** lines from the system that prompt the user to ask about a domain related thing, e.g., "Why don't you ask me about…" Such a response is triggered if the user asks too many off-topic questions. The system would return an off-topic answer followed by a delayed-tagged answer. That way the system attempts to bring the conversation back into the known domain. This category has no sample questions assigned.

The VP question and response system provides a powerful mechanism to quickly develop domains and build the dialog for the scenarios by experts who are not familiar with the underlying technology. The advantages are that it works quite well even with long utterances and misrecognized speech input. The disadvantages are that the characters do not respond well to follow on questions, to general questions such as "can you tell me more" referring to the context of the last question or response, and the system does not have initiative to ask questions by itself.

Other approaches to natural language processing involve building goal directed agents with dialog managers (Gratch et al., 2002) or cognitive models (Nirenburg et al., 2009). These are effective, but can be quite complex to build. The focus of this current virtual patient research was to build up a corpus of the kinds of questions and interactions that a clinician would have with the system and character and gather data with real clinicians or student clinicians in a bottom up approach before moving on to more complex systems.

## 3.3 Psychophysiology to Enhance Conversational Aspects of Virtual Humans

Cognitive and affective models can enhance conversational aspects of virtual humans in that they enhance human computer interactions through incorporation of the emotional state of the user (Picard, 1997; Lisetti and Schiano, 2000). Current cognitive and affective models found in virtual human research tend to use appraisal models that specify how events, agents and objects are used to elicit an emotional response depending on a set of parameters (e.g., goals, standards and attitudes) representing the subject (Gratch and Marsella, 2001, 2003, 2004).

The appraisal theories that are used draw upon the work of Smith and Lazarus's (1990) cognitive-motivational-emotive theory. As such, they view affect as something that arises from appraisal and coping. By "appraisal", virtual human researchers mean the methods by which persons assess their overall (i.e., events leading to the then current state, the current state itself, and future prospects) relationship with the environment. By "coping", virtual human researchers are referring to that which determines how persons respond to the appraised significance of events. Said researchers argue that best practices in the design of symbolic systems includes appraisal theories of affect that emphasize the cognitive and symbolic influences of affect and the underlying processes that lead to this influence (see Lazarus, 1991). For these researchers, this is a practice that is to be understood as in contrast to models that emphasize lower-level processes such as drives and physiological effects (Velásquez, 1998).

In principle, it is possible to model appraisal processes for conversational aspects of virtual humans using classical symbolic AI techniques (Picard, 1997; Chwelos & Oatley, 1994). However, cognitive and affective models of virtual humans do not generally account for neurophysiological data (Fellous, Armony, & LeDoux, 2003). Further, as Magnenat-Thalmann & Thalmann (2005) have pointed out in their review of virtual human research, virtual human models of emotional responses tend to be generated from a cognitive point of view and do not adequately take into account the psychophysiological response. Although appraisal does play a role in many current theories of emotion, most contemporary psychologists studying emotion emphasize the importance of psychophysiological arousal and that emotions are to be understood as cognitive appraisals and are accompanied by autonomic nervous system activity.

Even though many appraisal models contend that cognitive processes (e.g., sensory perception) present verification for the preeminence of appraisal in emotion, other theorists indicate that appraisal processes occur following perception and represent a separate cognitive process (Izard, 1993). Of course, while most would agree that perception is a necessary part of any sensory experience, it is not known whether perceptual processes are the foundation of cognitive models of emotion or if these emotions are concerned with higher order cognitive appraisals that assign meaning and valence (i.e., intrinsic attractiveness (positive valence) or aversiveness (negative valence) of an event, object, or situation; see Eckhardt, Norlander, & Deffenbacher, 2004).

A major limitation to applying many appraisal models to conversational aspects found in virtual human research is that they follow outdated appraisal models that assert specific patterns of physiological changes that may be observed in affect occurrence after the subjective experience of affect within a conversation. Research in psychophysiology has not supported these cognition first models (Cox & Harrison, 2008). In fact, a common frustration to attempts at developing an adequate scientific approach to emotion has been to focus upon constructing theories of subjective appraisals. Again studies of the neural basis of emotion and emotional learning have instead focused on how the brain detects and evaluates emotional stimuli and how, on the basis of such evaluations, emotional responses are produced (Magnenat-Thalmann & Thalmann, 2005).

Our preferred approach to enhancing conversational aspects of virtual humans is to develop cognitive and emotional virtual human models that include psychophysiological inputs that are sent in real-time interactions from the user (e.g., heart rate, respiration, skin conductance) to the virtual human. The additional input of the user's psychophysiological states offers contextual information to cognitive and emotional models. It is believed that these additional inputs can be developed into affect-sensitive VP interfaces that go beyond conventional virtual human models designed by pure (i.e., devoid of psychophysiological metrics) cognitive appraisal principles.

The resulting affect-sensitive VP interfaces would be similar to brain-based-devices (BBDs) that are being designed based on biological principles and are programmed to alter their behavior to the environment through self-learning (Edelman, 2006). An example of such research is found in work to develop intelligent robots. A series of devices with sensors and computer-simulated brains have been built in Gerald Edelman's (2006) Neurosciences Institute in La Jolla. The brains are modeled on human anatomy, complete with versions of visual cortex, inferotemporal cortex, and hippocampus. They are not pre-programmed, but evolve neuronal connections in response to experience. These devices can learn to recognize patterns and navigate novel environments.

Although the development of such computational models of emotion for conversational aspects of virtual humans can be difficult, researchers (Magnenat-Thalmann & Thalmann, 2005) have pointed out that computational approaches to emotional processing are both possible and practical. It is important to note, however, that there is a tendency of virtual human researchers to rely upon modalities such as facial expression, vocal intonation, gestures, and postures.

Unfortunately, this tendency results in limitations due to "communicative impairments" (both nonverbal and verbal) inherent in the technology. This is very much the case regarding expression of affective states. Although these vulnerabilities place limits on traditional conversational and observational methodologies found in much virtual human research, psychophysiological signals are 1) continuously available; and 2) are arguably not directly impacted by these difficulties. As a result, psychophysiological metrics may proffer an approach for gathering robust data despite potential virtual human technology limitations.

Furthermore, there is evidence that psychophysiological activity of persons immersed in virtual environments is associated with 1) trait differences (immersability; Macedonio, Parsons, & Rizzo, 2007) and 2) state differences (intensity of the environment; Parsons et al., 2009a, 2009b). These findings from virtual reality research reflect the finding that transition from one affective state to another is accompanied by dynamic shifts in indicators of autonomic nervous system activity (Bradley, 2000).

Individual (Parsons et al., 2009a) and cohort (Parsons et al., 2009c) differences have been shown to impact results gleaned from psychophysiological assessments using virtual environments, which reflects the need for psychophysiological assessment of persons interacting with VPs. In addition to extending the validation of VPs, this author's lab uses psychophysiological metrics to develop a psychophysiological interface (Neuroscience and Simulation Interface; NSI) for VPs that can adapt VP scenarios to the user's psychophysiological processing of information.

More specifically, psychophysiological measures such as heart rate, skin conductance responses, facial electromyographic response recordings, respiration, electroencephalographic recordings, and eyetracking can be continuously recorded while subjects interact with the VP. These recordings can be processed in real time to gain information about the user's current state of emotional and cognitive processing. This information can then be relayed to the virtual human in order to change for example, the behavior of the VP. If the user is distressed by the current state of the interaction, a psychophysiological pattern of increased heart rate, increased skin conductance levels, a more rapid rate of respiration, increased corrugator muscle activity, decreased alpha wave activity and diversion of gaze may develop. Allowing for access to this information about the user's current emotional state offers the VP an increased capability to understand the dynamics of the current interaction and develop a context appropriate response or behavior change.

## 4. DESIGN AND EVALUATION OF PATHOLOGIES

One of the challenges of building complex interactive VPs that can act as simulated patients has been in developing the specific mental condition in the domain of interest as it requires breadth and depth of expertise in the psychological domain to generate the relevant material for the character and dialog. This section discusses the domain and scenarios created for the subject testing and evaluation of the characters with real clinicians talking to the automated system. The results are described in the next section.

### 4.1 Domain Building

The domain consists of the story, the dialog, characters and settings and the illness and diagnosis criteria for the medical application. This data is generated through a combination of methods; discussions with subject matter experts, role playing exercises, user testing and textbooks or manuals. For the psychological medical illness that we want to exhibit we refer to the Diagnostic and Statistical Manual on Mental Disorders (DSM IV-TR, 2000). This manual is used by all professional clinicians and lists the criteria for a proper diagnosis for a particular mental disorder.

Building the domain involves developing the proper set of dialog and words that will be uttered by the character for the scenario. It is important to capture the kinds of questions that a clinician will typically ask during an interview or diagnosis session. The questions can vary from introductions and rapport to ones that elicit specific kinds of information. This is initially done through using experts to role play out the scenario, where one expert plays the patient and the other plays the clinician.

The role play scenarios are then transcribed and the set of questions and responses are put into a corpus database. This is an iterative process that will capture about 80 to 90 percent of the dialog. It is still a challenge to predict all the questions that a clinician will ask of a patient. Another method to capture additional questions and to assess the proper responses for questions is to use a Wizard of Oz method (Kelley, 1983), this is where a subject user talks to the virtual character, but the character is controlled by a human selecting appropriate responses from an interface. Similar methods have been used effectively to gather and evaluate spoken user data in tutoring systems (Litman & Silliman, 2004; Litman & Forbes-Riley, 2010).

This corpus is used to customize the engine's acoustic and language models for the domain of interest. In general a language model is tuned to the domain word lexicon. We collect user's voice data during each session, it allows us to go over the data to collect words not recognized to enhance the lexicon and domain corpus and to get word error rates to compare the input speech with the recognized speech from the speech engine.

### 4.2 Artwork and Character Design

The artwork plays a crucial role in defining the characters behavior, attitude and condition. People

*Figure 3. Justin-VP*

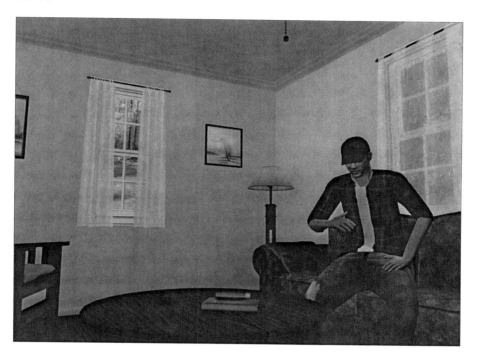

are able to make a judgment about someone within the first few seconds. The VP project involved the development of several characters. For one scenario we developed "Justin", (see Figure 3) a sixteen year old boy that has some kind of mental problem, but we wanted to keep the character design general so that the artwork would not be tied to a specific medical condition, for example giving him a broken arm.

For the boy we wanted a typical teenager with a T-shirt, blue jeans and baseball hat. One must be careful with the design of the character as everything can lead to questions by the users. For example the character has a rip in the pants. This was seen, but not realized until one of the subject testers asked the patient where he got the rip in the pants. Since this was not anticipated, there were no appropriate responses.

Another scenario was the development of "Justina" an adolescent female patient, (see Figure 4). This character was developed with more thought and time and the goals are to increase the realism with successive iterations. The artwork makes use of game technological advances such as shaders that apply graphical properties to the characters to make them look more realistic, like the skin, wrinkles or blushing to increasing the number of polygons and textures to make them look less blocky.

The project also involved the development of a clinical virtual environment that was modeled after a typical clinician's office and was meant to represent a place that would make the patient feel at home. Another important aspect is the animations that the character will use. Since these characters are in seated positions, then most of the gestures will involve hand movement or upper body alterations, head movement and facial expressions. A library is built that is used by the non-verbal generator to apply the appropriate animations for the spoken text and state of the character.

*Figure 4. Justina-VP*

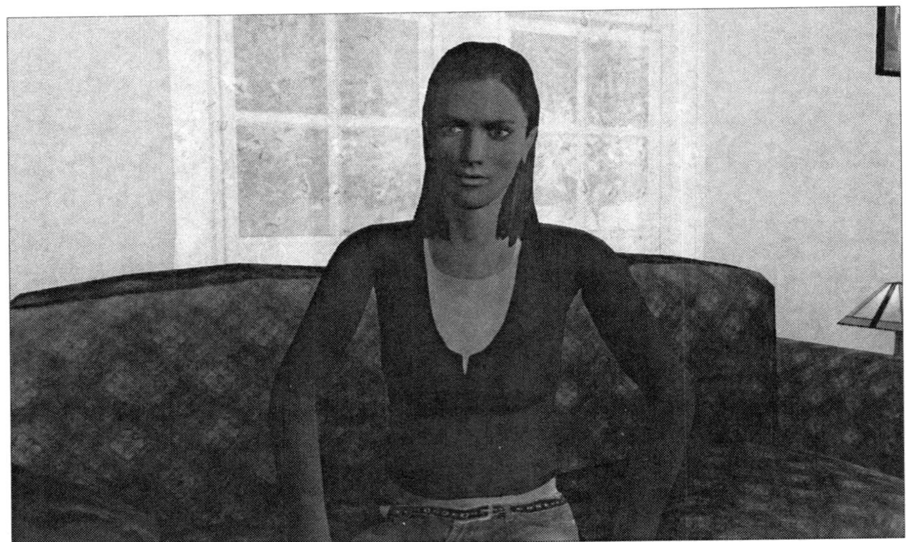

## 4.3 Virtual Patient: Conduct Disorder

The first scenario involved the construction of a natural language-capable VP named "Justin". The clinical attributes of Justin were developed to emulate a conduct disorder profile as found in the Diagnostic and Statistical Manual of Mental Disorders. Justin (see Figure 3) portrays a 16-year old male with conduct disorder who is being forced to participate in therapy by his family.

Justin's history is significant for a chronic pattern of antisocial behavior in which the basic rights of others and age-appropriate societal norms are violated. He has stolen, been truant, broken into someone's car, been cruel to animals, and initiated physical fights. Our goal was to obtain objective data from an initial intake interview by the clinician. An intake interview is where the clinician asks more general questions and tries to get an overview of what the problems are and make an initial diagnosis, not trying to apply therapy or 'cure' the patient.

The trainee's interview questions were guided by the need to determine if the patient is internalizing or externalizing behaviors and for eliciting information regarding the four general symptom categories prevalent in conduct disorder:

- **Aggressive behavior:** fighting, bullying, being cruel to others or animals.
- **Destructive behavior:** arson, vandalism.
- **Deceitful behavior:** repeated lying, shoplifting, breaking into homes or cars.
- **Violation of rules:** running away, engaging in non appropriate behavior for age.

The VP system is designed to provide answers to questions that target each of these categories and will respond to a variety of questions pertinent to these areas. Some responses by the VP may be on target, off target, involve "brush off" responses, and in some cases, they may be irrelevant replies.

The probability of a specific response being emitted is rated to the question asked. For example if the trainee asks: "How are things going at home" or "Are you having any problems at home" or "How are things going?". The system will respond with "My parents think I messed up." Further questions will lead to finding out that the patient has been running away. This will lead to marking one of the above categories true for the diagnosis in the trainees' interview.

In order for the trainee to pass the test will require responses in all of the categories. The total set of questions and responses are extracted from role playing exercises, initial subject testing, interviews with doctors and common sense for specific responses. In total a response set would consist of over 800-1200 lines of text and 200-300 questions. The matching of user questions to an appropriate patient response in the NPCEditor Dialog tool is a manual process performed by a domain designer and can be done over a period of a few days, but requires a few weeks to perfect with lots of testing as there can be many ways to ask the same question that will generate a single response.

## 4.4 Virtual Patient: Trauma Exposure

For the next VP scenario, our lab constructed an adolescent female character called "Justina" that had been the victim of an assault and showing signs of PTSD (see Figure 4). The technology used for this character and the "Justin" character is the same underlying VP architecture. The changes in this scenario were in the speech recognizer and natural language understanding module for the new scenarios to include a more in-depth and larger set of dialogs.

The experience of victimization is a relatively common occurrence for both adolescents and adults. However, victimization is more widespread among adolescents, and its relationship to various problem outcomes tends to be stronger among adolescent victims than adult victims. Whilst much of the early research on the psychological sequelae of victimization focused on general distress or fear rather than specific symptoms of PTSD, anxiety, or depression, studies have consistently found significant positive correlations between PTSD and sexual assault, and victimization in general and violent victimization in particular (Norris et al., 1997).

Although there are a number of perspectives on what constitutes trauma exposure in children and adolescents, there is a general consensus amongst clinicians and researchers that this is a substantial social problem (Resick & Nishith, 1997). The effects of trauma exposure manifest themselves in a wide range of symptoms: anxiety, post-trauma stress, fear, and various behavior problems. New clinicians need to come up to speed on how to interact, diagnose and treat this trauma.

According to the most recent revision to the American Psychiatric Association's DSM Disorders (2000), PTSD is divided into six major categories; refer to the DSM-IV category 309.81 for a full description and subcategories.

1. Past experience of a traumatic event and the response to the event.
2. Re-experiencing of the event with dreams, flashbacks and exposure to cues.
3. Persistent avoidance of trauma-related stimuli: thoughts, feelings, activities or places, and general numbing such as low affect and no sense of a future.
4. Persistent symptoms of anxiety or increased arousal such as hyper vigilance or jumpy, irritability, sleep difficulties or cannot concentrate.
5. Duration of the disturbance, how long have they been experiencing this.
6. Effects on their life such as clinically significant distress or impairment in social or educational functioning or changes in mental states.

Diagnostic criteria for PTSD includes a history of exposure to a traumatic event in category A and meeting two criteria and symptoms from each B (re-experiencing), C (avoidance), and D (hyper vigilance). The duration of E is usually greater than one month and the effects on F (social functioning) can vary based on severity of the trauma. Effective interviewing skills are a core competency for the clinicians, residents

*Table 1. Question / response categorization*

| Category | User Question | Justina Response |
|---|---|---|
| 1(A) Trauma | So, what happened to you that night? | Something really bad happened. |
| 2(B) Re-experience | Do you still think about what happened? | Sometimes I feel like the attack is happening all over again |
| 3(C) Avoidance | Do you go out with your friends? | I just stay away from everyone now. |
| 4(D) Arousal | Do you feel jumpy? | I feel like I have to watch my back all the time. |
| 5(E) Duration | How long has this been going on? | A few months |
| 6(F) Life Effect | Are you upset? | Sometimes I do not do anything but stay in my room and cry. |
| 7(G) Communication | Hi Justina, I'm Doctor.. | Hello |
| 8(H) Other | Button Press | I do not get what you mean. |

and developing psychotherapists who will be working with children and adolescents exposed to trauma. A clinician needs to ask questions in each of these categories to properly assess the patient's condition.

Table 1 is an example of the types of questions asked for each of the DSM criteria for PTSD. Below that is an example dialog between a real student clinician and the automated VP character, "Justina".

Example Interchange between a Clinician and the Virtual Patient "Justina"

**Clinician:** *What, a, what, brings you in the office today?*

**Justina:** *Something bad happened that night*

**Clinician:** *Sorry to hear that, can you tell me what happened?*

**Justina:** *I was in the car with Eddie and he stopped the car and wanted me to kiss him. But when I tried to stop him, he threatened me with a knife.*

**Clinician:** *When did this happen to you Justina?*

**Justina:** *I was so scared*

**Clinician:** *That must have been very tough for you.*

**Justina:** *Yea it still is*

**Clinician:** *Do you find yourself, ah, still being bothered by what happened?*

**Justina:** *Whenever thoughts of the event pop into my head I put my ipod on real loud.*

**Clinician:** *Ah, you mentioned thoughts pop into your head, what kind of thoughts pop into your head?*

**Justina:** *I want to get away.*

**Clinician:** *When you think about it, you feel like you need to get away?*

**Justina:** *That horrible time replays in my mind over and over.*

**Clinician:** *Can you tell me, ah, what happens in your mind when you think of it over and over?*

**Justina:** *Something really bad happened*

## 4.5 Evaluation and Results

The primary goal of the subject testing was evaluative: can a VP generate responses that elicit the proper user questions relevant for categorization and representation of a clinical condition.

Additionally, can the supporting architecture be used as a mechanism to train clinicians and provide a level of fidelity for the VP's that will make it believable by the participants? This was accomplished through evaluation of the users' utterances, and VP responses to those utterances, through assessment of the technology underlying the VP system and through psychophysiological responses to the VP in a bias task.

### 4.5.1 Subject Testing Method

Participants were asked to take part in a study of novice clinicians interacting with a VP system. They were not told what kind of condition the VP had if any. Two recruitment methods were used: poster advertisements on the university medical campus; and email advertisement and classroom recruitment to students and staff.

The VP system consisted of the virtual character "Justin" and "Justina", as seen in Figure 1 and 2, along with a headset for the speech input and mouse button to press and hold when the subject talks and releases when they stop talking. A control station was adjacent to the subject to run the system and log the data. Additionally cameras were setup to record the subjects face and the interaction with the VP from the side for later post processing, analysis and review.

There were two subject testing sessions that were performed, one with "Justin" and one with "Justina". A total of 21 people were involved between both set of subject testing. The sample of participants for Justin included 6 persons, medical clinicians and staff, from the University of Southern California's Keck School of Medicine. A total of 15 people (6 females, 9 males; mean age = 29.80, SD 3.67) took part in the study for Justina.

Ethnicity distribution was as follows: Caucasian = 67%; Indian = 13%; and Asian = 20%. The subject pool was made up of three groups: 1) Medical students (N=8); 2) Psychiatry Residents (N=6); 3) Psychiatry Fellows (N=4), Nurses (N=3). For participation in the study, students were able to forgo certain medical round time for the time spent in the interview and completing questionnaires.

The subject testing followed a standard method of a set of pre-questionnaires, next a 15 minute interactive interview of the character followed by a set of post-questionnaires. The subjects were allowed to ask anything they wanted to the patient using the speech recognition software so as to not put any constraints on how they talked or what they talked about. Since this was an initial pilot study, the goal was also to find out what they would ask the character. The subject testing adhered to the following paradigm:

Pre-Questionnaires

1. Tellegen Absorption Scale (TAS) (Tellegen & Atkinson, 1974).
2. Immersive tendencies questionnaire (ITQ) (Witmer & Singer, 1998).
3. Virtual Patient Pre-Questionnaire (VPQ1).
4. Justina or Justin Pre-questionnaire (JPQ1).

15 Minute Virtual Patient Interview by the clinician with the automated system.

Post-Questionnaires

1. Presence questionnaire (PQ) (Witmer & Singer, 1998).
2. Justina Post-questionnaire (JPQ2).
3. Virtual Patient Post-questionnaire (VPQ2).

The TAS questionnaire aims to measure the subject's openness to absorbing and self-altering experiences. The TAS is a 34-item measure of absorption. The ITQ measures individual differences in the tendencies of persons to experience "presence" in an immersive VE. The VPQ1, VPQ2 scale was developed to establish basic diagnosis competence for interaction with a patient that is intended to be presented as one with PTSD, although no mention of PTSD is on the test. We developed the JPQ1, JPQ2 scale to gather basic demographics and ask questions related to the user's experience and perception of the technology and how well they think the performance will be and was. The PQ is a common measure of presence in immersive virtual reality.

### 4.5.2 Justin Evaluation

Research has been completed to assess the system by 1) experimenter observation of the participants as they communicated with the VP; and 2) questionnaires. To adequately evaluate the system, a number of areas were used as a basis for the evaluation that included:

- **Consistency:** The behavior of the VP should match the behavior one would expect from a patient in such a condition (e.g. verbalization, gesture, posture, and appearance)
- **Adequacy:** The discourse between the VP and the participants should provide adequate verbal and nonverbal communication
- **Proficiency:** The clarity, pace, utility of VPs discourse with the participant
- **Quality:** The quality of the speech recognition of utterances spoken.

Basic usability findings revealed that the VP had high-quality overall system performance. Participants reported that the system 1) simulated real-life experience; and 2) the verbal and non-verbal behavior was satisfactory. However, results also revealed that some participants found aspects of the experience "frustrating". For example, some participants complained that they were receiving un-anticipated responses and the system tended to repeat some responses too frequently. This was due to the speech recognition's inability to evaluate certain of the stimulus words. Further, there were too many "brush off" responses from the VP when participant questions were outside the VP's dialog set.

### 4.5.3 Justina Evaluation

The primary goal in this study was evaluative: can a virtual patient generate responses that elicit user questions relevant for PTSD categorization? Findings suggest that the interactions between novice clinicians and the VP resulted in a compatible dialectic in terms of rapport, discussion of the traumatic event, and the experience of intrusive recollections. Further, there appears to be a satisfactory amount of discussion related to the issue of avoidance. These results comport well with what one may expect from the VP (Justina) system

Assessment of the system was completed with the data gathered from the log files in addition to the questionnaires to evaluate the number and types of questions being asked. Figure 5 is a graph showing that for the 15 minute interview the 15 subjects asked on average, 68.6 questions, lighter color, and responses by the system, darker color for each of the 8 DSM categories.

A summary of relations (measures as effect sizes "r") was developed between each 1) DSM PTSD Category cluster of user questions; and 2) each (corresponding) cluster of responses from the VP representing the same DSM PTSD Category. These are "clusters" of Question/Response pairs that reflect categories used for differential diagnosis. The present focus is on effect sizes that describe the strength of association between question and response pairs for a given diagnostic category. For this experiment an effect size of 0.20 was regarded as small, 0.50 as moderate, and 0.80 as a large effect.

Moderate effects existed between User Questions and VP Response pairs for Category A ($r = 0.45$), Category B ($r = 0.55$), Category C ($r = 0.35$), but only small effects were found for Category D ($r = 0.13$) and Category F ($r = 0.13$). After controlling for the effects of the users openness and feeling of "being with" the virtual environment and character through the TAS, increased effects were found for Category A ($r = 0.48$), Category C ($r = 0.37$), Category D ($r = 0.15$), and Category

*Figure 5. VP-DSM question / responses*

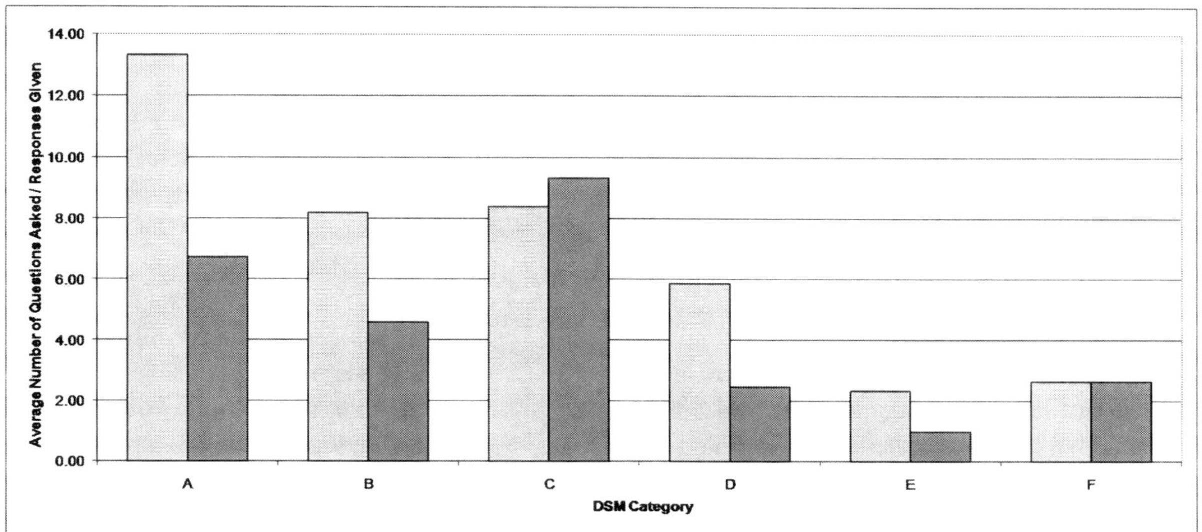


F (r = 0.24). The "believability" of the VP as a relationship showed strong effects existed between the TAS and ITQ (r = 0.78).

### 4.5.4 Virtual Patient: Assessing Bias

As mentioned above, cognitive and affective models can enhance conversational aspects of virtual humans in that they enhance human computer interactions through an incorporation of the emotional state of the user which can increase the believability of the system as a whole. This can be accomplished through evaluation of a user's emotional state in a bias task while interacting with a VP.

In addition to the experiments mentioned above, this author's lab has also run subjects through protocols in which we measured the activation and control of affective bias using 1) psychophysiological startle eye blink responses; and 2) self-reports as human participants interacted with VPs, "Justin and Justina" variations, representing both the human's race and another race (Parsons et al., 2009d. We also assessed the differences in psychophysiological responses of humans interacting with VPs representing same and different sex groups. By measuring eyeblink responses to startle probes occurring at short and long latencies following the onset of the same compared with other ethnicity VPs, we were able to examine affective processes associated with both the activation and potential control of bias.

The initial participant pool included 5 adults at the University of Southern California. Four were Caucasian, one was African-American. Our findings revealed a difference score between the median blink amplitude to African American VPs and Caucasian VPs was determined. A one-way ANOVA was performed to determine if high vs. low external motivation related to physiological responses to different racial groups of virtual patients. The difference score tended to be lower in those with high external motivation to behave in a non-racist manner. Those who were lower in external motivation had a larger difference score between startle amplitudes while looking at African American vs. Caucasian VPs. The larger difference score reflects larger startle amplitudes to African American VPs, suggesting an implicit negative bias towards that group. We are currently running additional subjects to enhance the modeling through the inclusion of other modalities such as facial expression, vocal intonation, gestures, and postures, which may be amalgamated with psychophysiology to increase the complexity of the user representation.

## 5. FUTURE RESEARCH DIRECTIONS

The field of creating conversational virtual patients is an emerging area that requires advanced speech and language understanding and dialog systems that are tied to the underlying physical and mental models for embodied conversational characters. Additionally, developing tools to assist in dialog and scenario building is of a great need as is standardizing clinical cases that can be used by various architectures.

To expand on the VP system architecture additional multi-modal input will allow for powerful sensing for the characters and increase the realism of the interaction. These modules that will be included in the future iterations of the VP architecture include:

- **Bio Physiological Input:** biophysiological input to the system used the Biopac system to capture heart rate, skin conductance and eye blinks. The collected data is used to evaluate the user in performing the tasks with the VP; additionally the input would be feed back into the virtual patient so that it can sense the participant and react accordingly. A version was used to assess racial bias with the VPs (Parsons, 2009b).
- **Vision Input:** The vision input consists of a users head and eye gaze information, i.e. what they are looking at, the orientation of the head and eye blink information that is used to evaluate the user's non-verbal behavior and rapport (Morency & de Kok, 2008).
- **Natural Language Understanding (NLU):** More complex forms of natural language parsing that form a semantic representation by matching it to semantic frames that are part of a large framebank generated from an ontology for the domain can be used to have a better understanding of the dialog by the agent. In addition to the core semantics, these frames could also includes information like speech act and modality intonation and prosidy generated by a more advanced speech recognizer.
- **Natural Language Generation (NLG):** maps an internal semantic representation generated by a Dialog Manager into a surface string. This can be similar to the process used by the NLU, but in reverse order, or based upon a domain dependent grammar. The resultant string sent would contain more complex information to add inflection to the speech or for selection of better animations of specific illnesses, emotions or moods. The reasoning phase could also take into account underlying models of cognition, emotion and personality to generate more autonomous and realistic behavior for the various clinical cases.
- **Intelligent Agent:** reasons about plans and generates actions based on its internal state and the input from the verbal text or other multi-modal devices. Complex agents can be created using a cognitive architecture that reason about plans and actions and integrate models of personality, emotion, mood and specific clinical illness criteria.

According to Fairclough (2009), the next generation of intelligent technology will be characterized by increased autonomy and adaptive capability. Such intelligent systems need to have ample capacity for real-time responsivity (Aarts, 2004). For example, to decrease the intensity of a conversation if a user is becoming too aroused while conversing with a virtual human, or to make the conversation more engaging if the user is bored. The psychophysiological computing approach proffers the VP a means of monitoring, quantifying, and representing user context and adapt in real-time.

We have collected (and continue to collect) quantitative and qualitative results. The VPs fit well into usability testing. Clinicians in training had positive responses to the VP and behaved as they normally would during a clinical encounter. It seems apparent that VPs will play an important role in the future of psychotherapy education for psychiatry residents and psychology trainees. The use of VPs could be implemented in several ways. For example, VPs could be developed to recognize the essential features and common pitfalls of an initial psychotherapy interview so that they could give more specific, relevant, and reliable verbal feedback to the residents involved. In addition, the use of VPs illustrating common problems such as acting out, transference, intrusive questions, or seductive behavior would allow residents to have an experience with these anxiety provoking situations in a simulated setting before they occur in their practice. Finally, performance in VP scenarios could be used as an additional source of data for the assessment of resident competency in the psychotherapy and educational domains.

## 6. CONCLUSION

In this chapter, there was a discussion of the ways in which advanced technologies (i.e., virtual patients) can move beyond traditional approaches to training clinicians in assessment, diagnosis, interviewing and interpersonal communication. The traditional approaches rely upon a combination of classroom learning and role-playing with human patients. Much of this work is done with actors that have been recruited and trained to exhibit the characteristics of an actual patient, thereby affording novice clinicians a realistic opportunity to practice and to be evaluated in a mock clinical environment.

Although a valuable training approach, there are limitations with the use of human patients that can be mitigated through simulation technology. For example, human patients are expensive and cost several thousand dollars per student. Further, given the fact that there are only a few sites providing standardized patient assessments as part of the U.S. Medical Licensing Examination, the current model provides limited availability.

In addition to issues of availability of trained actors, there is the issue of standardization. Despite the expense of standardized patient programs they are typically unskilled actors. As a result of common turnover, administrators face considerable challenges for offering psychometrically reliable and valid interactions with the training clinicians. The limited scope that the actors are able to portray tends to be an inadequate array of developmentally, socially, and culturally appropriate scenarios. For example, when a clinician has a pediatric focus and needs access to children, it is difficult for the clinician to pretend that the actor is a child. Finally, many clinical cases (e.g., traumatic brain injury) have associated physical symptoms and behaviors (e.g., dilated pupils, spasms, and uncoordinated movements) that simply cannot be accurately portrayed by human actors.

In this chapter a series of experiments were described to elucidate the usefulness and effectiveness of an affect-sensitive VP Interface System. This study was our initial prototype of building an interactive VP that was capable of discourse with novice clinicians so that they may establish the VPs clinical history and differential diagnosis. We described the domain, the architecture and the subject testing and evaluation conducted. The primary goal in this study was evaluative: can a virtual standardized patient generate responses that elicit user questions relevant for clinical illness categorization? Findings suggest that the interactions between novice clinicians and the VP resulted in a compatible dialectic in terms of rapport, discussion of the traumatic event, and the experience of intrusive recollections of the event.

While self- report data are widely used in virtual human research, they are susceptible to modification by a participant's awareness of the social desirability of particular responses, reducing the sensitivity of the measures, implicit behavioral and psychophysiological responses are automatic and thus considered less susceptible to self-conscious influences (Schwarz, 1999). A further issue discussed in this chapter was that the current cognitive and affective models found in virtual human research tend to use appraisal models generated from a cognitive point of view and do not adequately take into account the psychophysiological response.

It was contended that a preferred approach to developing cognitive and emotional virtual human models would include psychophysiological inputs from the humans to the virtual humans during interactions. It is believed that these additional inputs can be developed into affect-sensitive VP interfaces that go beyond conventional virtual human models designed by pure (i.e., devoid of psychophysiological metrics) cognitive appraisal principles. The resulting affect-sensitive VP interfaces would be similar to brain-based-devices (BBDs) that are being designed based on biological principles and are programmed to alter their behavior to the environment through self-learning.

In summary, effective interview skills are a core competency for training clinicians. Although schools commonly make use of standardized patients to teach interview skills, the diversity of the scenarios standardized patients can characterize is limited. Virtual Standardized Patient technology has evolved to a point where researchers may begin developing mental health applications that make use of virtual human patients for training.

## REFERENCES

Aarts, E. (2004). Ambient intelligence. A multimedia perspective. *IEEE MultiMedia, 11*(1), 12–19. doi:10.1109/MMUL.2004.1261101

Accreditation Council for Graduate Medical Education. (2007). *ACGME Outcome Project*. Retrieved December 5, 2007, from www.acgme.org/Outcomes

American Psychiatric Association. (2000). *Diagnostic and statistical manual of mental disorders (4th edn, text revision)*. Washington, DC: American Psychiatric Press, Inc.

Bickmore, T., & Giorgino, T. (2006). Health dialog systems for patients and consumers. *Journal of Biomedical Informatics, 39*, 556–571. doi:10.1016/j.jbi.2005.12.004

Bickmore, T., Pfeifer, L., & Paasche-Orlow, M. (2007). Health document explanation by virtual agents. *Lecture Notes in Computer Science, 4722*, 183–196. doi:10.1007/978-3-540-74997-4_18

Bradley, M. (2000). Emotion and motivation. In Cacioppo, J. T., Tassinary, L. G., & Berntson, G. (Eds.), *Handbook of psychophysiology*. New York, NY: Cambridge University Press.

Buck, R. (1984). *The communication of emotion*. New York, NY: Guilford Press.

Buck, R. (1989). Emotional communication in personal relationships: A developmental-interactionist view. In Hendrick, C. D. (Ed.), *Close relationships* (pp. 44–76). Beverly Hills, CA: Sage.

Buck, R. (1994). The neuropsychology of communication: Spontaneous and symbolic aspects. *Journal of Pragmatics, 22*, 265–278. doi:10.1016/0378-2166(94)90112-0

*CASUS Project*. (2010). Retrieved July 23, 2010, from http://www.casus.eu/

Chant, S., Jenkinson, T., Randle, J., Russell, G., & Webb, C. (2002). Communication skills training in healthcare: A review of the literature. *Nurse Education Today*, *22*, 189–202. doi:10.1054/nedt.2001.0690

Chwelos, G., & Oatley, K. (1994). Appraisal, computational models, and Scherer's expert system. *Cognition and Emotion*, *8*, 245–257. doi:10.1080/02699939408408940

Cox, D. E., & Harrison, D. W. (2008). Models of anger: Contributions from psychophysiology, neuropsychology and the cognitive behavioral perspective. *Brain Structure & Function*, *212*, 371–385. doi:10.1007/s00429-007-0168-7

De Melo, C., & Gratch, J. (2009). *Expression of emotions using wrinkles, blushing, sweating and tears*. Intelligent Virtual Agents Conference, Amsterdam, Sep 14-16. *eVIP Project.* (2010). Retrieved July 23, 2010, from http://www.virtualpatients.eu/

Deladisma, A. M., Johnsen, K., Raij, A., Rossen, B., Kotranza, A., & Kalapurakal, M. (2008). Medical student satisfaction using a virtual patient system to learn history-taking communication skills. *Studies in Health Technology and Informatics*, *132*, 101–105.

Eckhardt, C. I., Norlander, B., & Deffenbacher, J. (2004). The assessment of anger and hostility: A critical review. *Aggression and Violent Behavior*, *9*, 17–43. doi:10.1016/S1359-1789(02)00116-7

Edelman, G. M. (2006). *Second nature: Brain science and human knowledge*. Yale University Press.

Fairclough, S. H. (2009). Fundamentals of physiological computing. *Interacting with Computers*, *21*, 133–145. doi:10.1016/j.intcom.2008.10.011

Fellous, J. M., Armony, J. L., & LeDoux, J. E. (2003). Emotional circuits and computational neuroscience. In *The handbook of brain theory and neural networks* (pp. 398–401). Cambridge, MA: The MIT Press.

GameBryo. (2010). *Emergent game technologies.* Retrieved July 23, 2010, from http://www.emergent.net/

Gratch, J., & Marsella, S. (2001). Tears and Fears: Modeling Emotions and Emotional Behaviors in Synthetic Agents, *Fifth International Conference on Autonomous Agents*, Montreal, Canada.

Gratch, J., & Marsella, S. (2004). A domain independent framework for modeling emotion. *Journal of Cognitive Systems Research*, *5*, 269–306. doi:10.1016/j.cogsys.2004.02.002

Gratch, J., Rickel, J., André, E., Badler, N., Cassell, J., & Petajan, E. (2002). Creating interactive virtual humans: Some assembly required. *IEEE Intelligent Systems*, (July/August): 54–63. doi:10.1109/MIS.2002.1024753

Green, N., Lawton, W., & Davis, B. (2004). An assistive conversation skills training system for caregivers of persons with Alzheimer's Disease. In *Proceedings of the AAAI 2004 Fall Symposium on Dialogue Systems for Health Communication*.

Hayes-Roth, B., Amano, K., Saker, R., & Sephton, T. (2004). Training brief intervention with a virtual coach and patients. In B. K. Wiederhold, & G. Riva (Eds.), *Annual Review of Cyber-Therapy and Telemedicine, 2,* 85-96.

Hayes-Roth, B., Saker, R., & Amano, K. (2009). Automating brief intervention training with individualized coaching and role-play practice. *Methods Med Informatics*, in rev.

Hubal, R., Frank, G., & Guinn, C. (2003). Lessons learned in modeling Schizophrenic and depressed responsive virtual humans for training. In *Proceedings of 8th International Conference on Intelligent User Interfaces*.

Hubal, R. C., Kizakevich, P. N., & Furberg, R. (2007). Synthetic characters in health-related applications. *Advanced Computational Intelligence Paradigms in Healthcare*, *2*, 5–26. doi:10.1007/978-3-540-72375-2_2

Hubal, R. C., Kizakevich, P. N., Guinn, C. I., Merino, K. D., & West, S. L. (2000). The virtual standardized patient-simulated patient-practitioner dialogue for patient interview training. In Westwood, J. D., Hoffman, H. M., Mogel, G. T., Robb, R. A., & Stredney, D. (Eds.), *Envisioning healing: Interactive technology and the patient-practitioner dialogue*. Amsterdam, The Netherlands: IOS Press.

Hulsman, R. L., Gos, W. J. G., Winnubst, J. A. M., & Bensing, J. M. (1999). Teaching clinically experienced physicians communication skills: A review of evaluation studies. *Medical Education, 33*, 655–668. doi:10.1046/j.1365-2923.1999.00519.x

Izard, C. E. (1993). Organizational and motivational functions of discrete emotions. In Lewis, M., & Haviland, J. M. (Eds.), *Handbook of emotions*. New York, NY: Guilford Press.

Johnsen, K., Dickerson, R., Raij, A., Lok, B., Jackson, J., Shin, M., … Lind, D. (2005). Experiences in using virtual characters to educate medical communication skills. *IEEE Virtual Reality*.

Johnston, C., & Whatley, D. (2005). Pulse!! - A virtual learning space project. *Studies in Health Technology and Informatics, Medicine Meets. Virtual Reality (Waltham Cross)*, *14*, 240–242.

Kelley, J. F. (1983). An empirical methodology for writing user-friendly natural language computer applications. *Proceedings of the ACM SIG-CHI '93 Human Factors in Computing Systems* (pp. 193-196). New York, NY: ACM.

Kenny, P., Hartholt, A., Gratch, J., Swartout, W., Traum, D., Marsella, S., & Piepol D., (2007b). Building Interactive Virtual Humans for Training Environments in proceedings of *I/ITSEC*, Nov.

Kenny, P., Parsons, T. D., Gratch, J., Leuski, A., & Rizzo, A. A. (2007). Virtual patients for clinical therapist skills training. *Intelligent Virtual Agent Conference, LNAI 4722*, (pp. 197-210).

Kenny, P., Parsons, T. D., Gratch, J., & Rizzo, A. A. (2008b). Evaluation of Justina: A virtual patient with PTSD. *Lecture Notes in Artificial Intelligence*, *5208*, 394–408.

Kenny, P., Parsons, T. D., Pataki, C. S., Pato, M., St-George, C., Sugar, J., & Rizzo, A. A. (2008a). Virtual Justina: A PTSD virtual patient for clinical classroom training. *Annual Review of Cybertherapy and Telemedicine*, *6*, 113–118.

Kenny, P., Parsons, T. D., & Rizzo, A. A. (2009). Human computer interaction in virtual standardized patient systems. *Lecture Notes in Computer Science*, *5613*, 514–523. doi:10.1007/978-3-642-02583-9_56

Kenny, P., Rizzo, A. A., Parsons, T. D., Gratch, J., & Swartout, W. (2007a). A virtual human agent for training novice therapist clinical interviewing skills. *Annual Review of Cybertherapy and Telemedicine*, *5*, 81–89.

Kopp, S., Krenn, B., Marsella, S., Marshall, A., Pelachaud, C., & Pirker, H. … Vilhjalmsson, H. (2006). *Towards a common framework for multimodal generation: The behavior markup language*. 6th International Conference on Intelligent Virtual Agents, Marina del Rey, CA, August 21-23.

Lazarus, R. (1991). *Emotion and adaptation*. New York, NY: Oxford University Press.

Lee, J., & Marsella, S. (2006). *Nonverbal behavior generator for embodied conversational agents*. 6th International Conference on Intelligent Virtual Agents, Marina del Rey, CA.

Leuski, A., Pair, J., Traum, D., McNerney, P. J., Georgiou, P., & Patel, R. (2006a). How to talk to a hologram. In E. Edmonds, D. Riecken, C. L. Paris, & C. L. Sidner, (Eds.), *Proceedings of the 11th International Conference on Intelligent user interfaces(IUI'06)*, Sydney, Australia, (pp. 360–362). New York, NY: ACM Press.

Leuski, A., Patel, R., Traum, D., & Kennedy, B. (2006). Building effective question answering characters. In *Proceedings of the 7th SIGdial Workshop on Discourse and Dialogue*, Sydney, Australia.

Leuski, A., & Traum, D. (2010). NPCEditor: A tool for building question-answering characters. In *Proceedings of The Seventh International Conference on Language Resources and Evaluation*.

Lisetti, C. L., & Schiano, D. (2000). Facial expression recognition: Where human-computer interaction, artificial intelligence, and cognitive science intersect. *Pragmatics & Cognition*, *8*, 185–235. doi:10.1075/pc.8.1.09lis

Litman, D., & Forbes-Riley, K. (In Press, 2010). Designing and evaluating a wizarded uncertainty-adaptive spoken dialogue tutoring system. *Computer Speech and Language*.

Litman, D., & Silliman, S. (2004). ITSPOKE: An intelligent tutoring spoken dialogue system. *Proceedings of the Human Language Technology Conference: 4th Meeting of the North American Chapter of the Association for Computational Linguistics* (*HLT/NAACL*), Boston, MA.

Lok, B., Ferdig, R. E., Raij, A., Johnsen, K., Dickerson, R., & Coutts, J. (2006). Applying Virtual reality in medical communication education: Current findings and potential teaching and learning benefits of immersive virtual patients. *Virtual Reality (Waltham Cross)*, *10*, 185–195. doi:10.1007/s10055-006-0037-3

Macedonio, M., Parsons, T. D., & Rizzo, A. A. (2007). Immersiveness and physiological arousal within panoramic video-based virtual reality. *Cyberpsychology & Behavior*, *10*, 508–516. doi:10.1089/cpb.2007.9997

Magnenat-Thalmann, N., & Thalmann, D. (2005). Virtual humans: Thirty years of research, what next? *The Visual Computer*, *21*, 1–19. doi:10.1007/s00371-004-0243-5

Morency, L. P., & de Kok, I. (2008). *Context-based recognition during human interactions: Automatic feature selection and encoding dictionary*. 10th International Conference on Multimodal Interfaces, Chania, Greece, IEEE.

Nirenburg, S., McShane, M., Beale, S., Jarrell, B., & Fantry, G. (2009). Integrating cognitive simulation into the Maryland virtual patient. *Proceedings from MMVR-09*.

Norris, F. H., Kaniasty, K., & Thompson, M. P. (1997). The psychological consequences of crime: Findings from a longitudinal population-based study. In Davis, R. C., Lurigio, A. J., & Skogan, W. G. (Eds.), *Victims of crime* (2nd ed., pp. 146–166). Thousand Oaks, CA: Sage Publications, Inc.

Parsons, T. D., Cosand, L., Courtney, C., Iyer, A., & Rizzo, A. A. (2009b). Neurocognitive workload assessment using the virtual reality cognitive performance assessment test. *Lecture Notes in Artificial Intelligence*, *5639*, 243–252.

Parsons, T. D., Courtney, C., Cosand, L., Iyer, A., Rizzo, A. A., & Oie, K. (2009c). Assessment of psychophysiological differences of West Point cadets and civilian controls immersed within a virtual environment. *Lecture Notes in Artificial Intelligence*, *5638*, 514–523.

Parsons, T. D., Iyer, A., Cosand, L., Courtney, C., & Rizzo, A. A. (2009a). Neurocognitive and psychophysiological analysis of human performance within virtual reality environments. *Studies in Health Technology and Informatics*, *142*, 247–252.

Parsons, T. D., Kenny, P., Cosand, L., Iyer, A., Courtney, C., & Rizzo, A. A. (2009d). A virtual human agent for assessing bias in novice therapists. *Studies in Health Technology and Informatics*, *142*, 253–258.

Parsons, T. D., Kenny, P., Ntuen, C., Pataki, C. S., Pato, M., & Rizzo, A. A. (2008). Objective structured clinical interview training using a virtual human patient. *Studies in Health Technology and Informatics*, *132*, 357–362.

Pellom, B. (2001). *Sonic: The University of Colorado continuous speech recognizer*. (Technical Report TR-CSLR-2001-01), University of Colorado, Boulder, CO.

Picard, R. W. (1997). *Affective computing*. Boston, MA: The MIT Press.

Raij, A. B., Johnsen, K., Dickerson, R. F., Lok, B. C., Cohen, M. S., & Duerson, M. (2007). Comparing interpersonal interactions with a virtual human to those with a real human. *IEEE Transactions on Visualization and Computer Graphics*, *13*, 443–457.

Resick, P. A., & Nishith, P. (1997). Sexual assault. In Davis, R. C., Lurigio, A. J., & Skogan, W. G. (Eds.), *Victims of crime* (2nd ed., pp. 27–52). Thousand Oaks, CA: Sage Publications, Inc.

Riva, G., Mantovani, F., & Gaggioli, A. (2004). Presence and rehabilitation: Toward second-generation virtual reality applications in neuropsychology. *Journal of Neuroengineering and Rehabilitation*, *1*(9).

Rudericha, F., Baucha, M., Haaga, M., Heida, J., Levena, F. J., Singera, R., … Tönshoffd, B., (2004). CAMPUS – a flexible, interactive system for Web-based, problem-based learning in healthcare. *International Journal of Medial Information*, IOS Press.

Schwarz, N. (1999). Self-reports: How the questions shape the answers. *The American Psychologist*, *54*, 93–105. doi:10.1037/0003-066X.54.2.93

Sethy, A., Georgiou, P., & Narayanan, S. (2005). Building topic specific language models from Web data using competitive models. *Proceedings of EUROSPEECH*, Lisbon, Portugal.

Smith, C. A., & Lazarus, R. (1990). Emotion and adaptation. In Pervin, L. A. (Ed.), *Handbook of personality: Theory & research* (pp. 609–637). New York, NY: Guilford Press.

Stevens, A., Hernandex, J., Johnsen, K., Dickerson, R., Raij, A., & Harrison, C. (2005). The use of virtual patients to teach medical students communication skills. *American Journal of Surgery*, *191*(6), 806–811. doi:10.1016/j.amjsurg.2006.03.002

Tellegen, A., & Atkinson, G. (1974). Openness to absorbing and self-altering experiences ("absorption"), a trait related to hypnotic susceptibility. *Journal of Abnormal Psychology*, *83*, 268–277. doi:10.1037/h0036681

Thiebaux, M., Marshall, A., Marsella, S., & Kallmann, M. (2008). *SmartBody: Behavior realization for embodied conversational agents*. International Conference on Autonomous Agents and Multi-Agent Systems. Portugal.

Traum, D., & Marsella, S. Gratch, J., Lee, J., Hartholt, A. (2008). Multi-party, multi-issue, multi-strategy negotiation for multi-modal virtual agents. 8th International Conference on Intelligent Virtual Agents. Tokyo, Japan: Springer.

Triola, M., & Feldman, M. (2006). A randomized trial of teaching clinical skills using virtual and live standardized patients. *Journal of General Internal Medicine*, *21*, 424–429. doi:10.1111/j.1525-1497.2006.00421.x

Velásquez, J. (1998). *When robots weep: Emotional memories and decision-making*. Presented at Fifteenth National Conference on Artificial Intelligence, Madison, WI, 1998.

Weizenbaum, J. (1966). Eliza -a computer program for the study of natural language communication between man and machine. *Communications of the ACM*, *9*, 26–45. doi:10.1145/365153.365168

Wilson, W. R. (1979). Feeling more than we can know: Exposure effects without learning. *Journal of Personality and Social Psychology*, *37*, 811–821. doi:10.1037/0022-3514.37.6.811

Witmer, B., & Singer, M. (1998). Measuring presence in virtual environments: A presence questionnaire. *Presence (Cambridge, Mass.)*, *7*(3), 225–240. doi:10.1162/105474698565686

## ADDITIONAL READING

Barney, C., & Shea, S. C. (2007). The Art of Effectively Teaching Clinical Interviewing Skills Using Role-Playing: A Primer. *The Psychiatric Clinics of North America*, *30*, 31–50. doi:10.1016/j.psc.2007.03.001

Marsella, S., & Gratch, J. (2003). Modeling coping behaviors in virtual humans: Don't worry, be happy, *Second International Joint Conference on Autonomous Agents and Multi-Agent Systems*, Melbourne, Australia.

## KEY TERMS AND DEFINITIONS

**Discourse:** A formalized written or spoken communication.

**DSM:** Diagnostic and Statistical manual on Mental Disorders book that describes the properties and criteria of mental illnesses.

**Fidelity:** The level of human behavior which the avatar can generate.

**Multimodal interaction:** Provides the user with multiple modes of interfacing with a system.

**Psychophysiological:** Investigates at the way psychological activities produce physiological responses by measuring attributes such as blood pressure, heart rate, respiration, skin conductance, eyeblinks and others.

**Standardized Patient:** An actor trained to exhibit the characteristics of an actual patient.

**Subject Testing:** A method of testing and analyzing participants with an automated virtual patient system through speech, video, and questionnaire analysis.

**Text Classifier:** A statistical algorithm to match user questions to character responses from a corpus of utterances.

**Virtual Patient:** A computer generated character programmed to act like an actual patient.

**Wizard of Oz Testing:** A method to gather domain data with participants in a simulation system by having a person act out the virtual character and typing or saying appropriate responses to the participant who asks questions, like a virtual role play.

# Chapter 12
# A Conversational Personal Assistant for Senior Users

**Deborah A. Dahl**
*Conversational Technologies, USA*

**Emmett Coin**
*ejTalk, Inc., USA*

**Michael Greene**
*newInteractions, Inc., USA*

**Paulette Mandelbaum**
*newInteractions, Inc., USA*

## ABSTRACT

*Senior users could benefit from computer assistance in managing the details of everyday life and maintaining contact with friends and family; however, current computer interfaces can be difficult to use as a consequence of the physical, sensory, and cognitive changes that accompany aging. This chapter describe a multimodal application, which we have called Cassandra, that provides an extremely natural, conversational way for senior users to perform tasks like managing reminders or appointments, medication schedules, shopping lists, and phone calls. We discuss the implications of the characteristics of the target user population on the application design. In addition to describing the application, we will also discuss end user feedback.*

## INTRODUCTION

A long and healthy life is what we wish for ourselves and our loved ones. But we fear the consequences of aging. Beyond any specific infirmity, perhaps our greatest concern is that we will become increasingly vulnerable and dependent. In fact among seniors living independently, there is a greater fear of moving into a nursing home and losing one's independence than of death (Prince Market Research, 2007). In the US 90% of those over 65 want to stay in their homes or move to another independent setting (Prince Market Research, 2007).

Many senior adults experience varying degrees of hearing loss, forgetfulness, problems with word

DOI: 10.4018/978-1-60960-617-6.ch012

retrieval, and slowing in some areas of intellectual functioning. Routine activities become increasingly difficult. The greater need for medical care adds another level of complexity that involves having to navigate the health system and manage medications. In fact, medication non-compliance, often a result of memory decline, is responsible for the deaths of more than 125,000 Americans each year (M-PILL, 2009). Perhaps less obvious is the challenge to one's mental health with the combination of diminished physical mobility and cognitive challenges. This can contribute to a decrease in social interaction, withdrawal, and clinical depression (Ford & Ford, 2009).

Technology has the potential to make a significant impact in some of these areas. This chapter discusses a senior-friendly interface with a set of useful applications aimed at assisting users in managing the details of everyday life and maintaining social connections to friends and family.

We see the following benefits of this type of application:

1. Decreasing social isolation for the many seniors whose mobility has become limited.
2. Useful support in helping the elderly age at home.
3. Delaying the need of some seniors to move into more managed settings.
4. Greater access to seniors and a sense of the senior's status for family members.

The ability to remain independent and age at home has benefits both for the senior who maintains a higher quality of life, to their family, and to society, by reducing some of the substantial costs associated with long-term care (assisted living care for a senior costs about $38,000 per year in the United States, not including medical expenses. Nursing home care is more than twice that amount) (MetLife Mature Market Institute, 2009).

## CONVERSATIONAL ASSISTANCE

Everyday life is becoming increasingly complex for everyone and can become more difficult to manage as one ages. Automated assistance in such simple tasks such as remembering to buy or do things can reduce this complexity. In addition, technology can also help seniors maintain stronger social connections to help combat isolation. Technology in the form of software for computers and smartphones is available to assist in achieving these goals, but it has two major drawbacks for older users:

- First: Current computer interfaces are complex and may be confusing, hard to learn, and intimidating for an inexperienced user.
- Second: Current computers are not always nearby when they need to be consulted, and for many older users, mobility is a concern.

Consequently, we believe that managing the details of everyday life and maintaining social connections can usefully be done with a very simple and portable interface that draws on a range of modalities, including speech, audio and touch. We describe considerations for such an application in this section.

### Multimodal UI Considerations for the Elderly

Multimodality, a key feature of this application, is especially important for older users because of limitations such as decreased ability to see and hear and limitations on mobility caused by conditions like arthritis, Parkinson's, and general muscle decline. On the output side, visual and auditory displays of information can supplement and/or complement each other for users with sensory limitations. Cognitive changes such as increased distractibility and difficulty in focusing attention suggest that it is important to design the user interface so that it accommodates user-initiated digressions from an ongoing task and assists the user in resuming an interrupted task.

For this reason the application places a strong emphasis on seamlessly handling task-switching and task-resuming utterances. For example, the user might be in the middle of working on a shopping list and then say something like "Oh, by the way, could you remind me to call Julie in fifteen minutes?" to change tasks, and then say something like "Where were we?" to go back to the shopping list after the reminder is registered.

In this section we look at how the characteristics of the users as well as the context of use inform the design of our application. We can divide user characteristics into perceptual, motor, cognitive and social characteristics. Perceptual abilities affect system output, motor considerations affect user input, and cognitive and social considerations affect both input and output. We look at each of these in turn.

1. Perception: Clearly, users must be able to perceive the user interface (most typically through vision and/or hearing) in order to use it. One third of people over the age of 65 and half of people over 85 experience some loss of hearing (National Institute on Deafness and other Communication Disorders) Statistics cited in (Arch, 2008) point out that 45.8% of people over the age of 85 experience vision problems that significantly affect their daily lives. So, although hearing and visual losses are not universal with aging, they are very common. Consequently, the design of our application includes the ability to modify the graphical and audio displays through speech to match the user's capabilities.
2. Motor: Motor limitations are common among older people. Arthritis is very common, affecting over 50% of Americans over the age of 65 (Arthritis Foundation, 2008), but there are also specific diseases that affect motor control such as Parkinson's. Possible degradation of the ability to perform fine motor functions due to arthritis or other diseases has led us to emphasize the use of a touch screen rather than a mouse for pointing actions.

Some older users also have mobility problems which require them to use a wheelchair or walker. For this reason, it is important for an application designed for older users to be accessible without requiring the user to get up and go to another room, which may reduce the user's motivation to use it, especially for quick tasks. Ideally, the application should be as ambient as possible.

It is also worth mentioning that motor problems can affect speech, if they affect the user's ability to control the speech articulators. For an application that depends on speech, this is a concern. Minor speech problems can be addressed through speaker-dependent recognition, but this application is probably not appropriate in its current form for users who have severe speech limitations.

3. Cognitive Factors: These include such factors as memory (long term, short term and working), attention, executive function, and learning. These cognitive factors have ramifications for both the system's output and the user's input. On the system side, the user interface must be comprehensible so that the user can know what to do. On the user's side, the system must be able to accommodate, for example, a user who might need more time to formulate a response to the system's questions. As mentioned above, motor limitations can affect user's ability to speak, but other language issues can arise from cognitive limitations. For example, word retrieval problems are commonly reported by the elderly. In general, cognitive factors that need to be taken into account in user interfaces are more subtle than motor and perceptual concerns.

Finally, it is worth pointing out that guidelines designed primarily for making applications accessible by disabled users, such as Web Content Accessibility Guidelines (WCAG) (Caldwell et al., 2007) may also provide helpful insights for user interface design for older users as well as for users with disabilities.

## THE APPLICATION: A CONVERSATIONAL ASSISTANT FOR SENIOR USERS

The application discussed in this chapter consists of two major components. The first component is a generic, application-independent, conversation manager that provides the underlying ability to conduct a conversation. The second component of the application consists of several additional files that contain the information required to perform specific functions. Primarily, these include grammars and the files that define dialogs (step files).

The application discussed in this chapter is a conversational assistant for senior users that helps them manage the details of daily life. We believe that a multimodal, conversational, interface is an ideal approach to providing a usable and effective interface for older users. In contrast to many previous systems, this application is much less task-oriented. Rather than containing a deep knowledge of a complex task and assisting the user in completing that specific task, the system described in this chapter assists the user in navigating among various simple tasks, which we believe is more useful for the kinds of tasks that people need to do in everyday life.

Our system has a general goal of providing a unified face for a number of tasks to assist aging seniors. Consequently our system must address a number of problems in managing several ongoing, possibly unrelated, tasks that are not addressed by earlier systems, such as the TRAINS and TRIPS (Ferguson & Allen, 1998; Allen et al., 2000) systems, Similarly, while the Companions project (Catizone et al., 2010) shares some of our goals, it is looking at more in-depth tasks that are outside of everyday activities.

For example, it is exploring conversational speech interfaces for a suite of functionality such as annotating photographs with a focus on capturing a senior's deeper knowledge of the people, places and relationships they represent. This group also has roots in COMIC (Catizone, Setzer, & Wilkes, 2003). Another previous task-oriented system was Jennifer – virtual co-worker for "hands and eyes busy" logistics tasks, which was a commercial product designed as a wearable synthetic partner for warehouse order fulfillment workers (by one of the authors, (Coin, 2007)). It acted as if it were a member of an order picking team and "read" the details of the order, directing the human to locations and confirming amounts through spoken interaction. It added some other modalities to the mix such as pointing with a small bar-code scanner worn as a ring and RFID via an antenna on the wrist.

Another task-oriented application was the Exhibit/Tour Guide – a question/response system for points of interest, which was a portable application that assisted visitors to an historical site in obtaining information about the site (Santangelo et al., 2006). There was little need for maintaining much context so the pattern detection and response mode of an AIML based system was sufficient.

A more generic system with less of a focus on a specific task was TRIK -- communication training for children, which was a talking and drawing robot for children with communication difficulties (Larsson et al., 2008). TRIK was designed to engage children who had problems interacting with natural speech interactions. The goal was general practice of communication skills in a non-threatening context. This system differs from ours in that the users were not trying to accomplish any specific task, and also because the users are children.

Another relatively generic system was Hearsay – generic voice enhanced web browsing. This system developed at Stony Brook University in collaboration with the Helen Keller Services for the Blind attempts to use voice in addition to mouse/keyboard/touch modalities (Borodin et al., 2007). In the case of Hearsay, the task was to discover navigational and content elements on a web page and provide a voice mode in addition to the expected browser mode. The goal was to browse existing web content by automatically providing a voice modality to the mix. The Hearsay system was not multimodal as it was based on a voice-only interface for blind users.

An underlying principle of our design is the support for multiple domains and the natural movement between them. Our system is assumed to be "always on" and to manage context from a domain and temporal perspective.

The key features of the application described in this chapter are:

1. A multimodal interface that allows the user to speak to the system as well as to control the application by touch and keyboard.
2. The generic conversation manager described above that converses with the user to perform specific tasks.
3. The ability of the conversation manager both to respond directly to the user's requests as well as to proactively bring up its own topics, for example, to remind the user of upcoming events or appointments.
4. Simultaneous visual and audio outputs that reinforce each other in case the user has difficulty hearing or seeing.
5. The ability to respond to integrated multimodal inputs such as "take that off my shopping list," spoken while touching a word on the screen.
6. The ability to assist the user in multitasking by handling interruptions and digressions, and helping the user in resuming an interrupted task.
7. Personalized configuration of the user interface to suit the user's tastes and needs.
8. Pervasive availability since the application is always nearby.

An important point is that the application is a generic conversational platform, not a particular application such as managing schedules. Obviously, to be useful, the platform has to perform specific tasks. As initial tasks that seem to be especially beneficial to older users, and to illustrate the general capabilities of the platform, we have selected managing schedules, shopping lists, and communication with other people.

Figure 1 shows a tree diagram of a set of tasks that might be done by a conversational platform to conduct a personal assistant application. The tasks include general control of the interface, obtaining general information, and specific tasks having to do with the management of everyday activities, such as putting events in one's schedule. The user might decide to digress from any ongoing activity to perform one of the activities in the gray boxes. In that case it would be necessary to preserve the state of the interrupted activity so that the user can return to it if desired. Similarly, the system can also initiate digressions, for example, to accept an incoming phone call or remind the user of an important appointment. These are shown in white ovals in the diagram.

As in the case of a user-initiated digression, the system must maintain the state of any tasks that were ongoing when the digression occurred. It is also important to maintain information about when the digression occurred because different techniques would be used to resume a task that was interrupted only for a minute as opposed to one that was interrupted an hour ago.

## Conversation System Overview

The application is built on the conversation manager (Coin & Qua, 2000), which coordinates all of the input and output modalities including speech I/O, GUI I/O, avatar rendering and lip sync. The architecture is similar to other general architec-

*Figure 1. Tasks for a personal assistant*

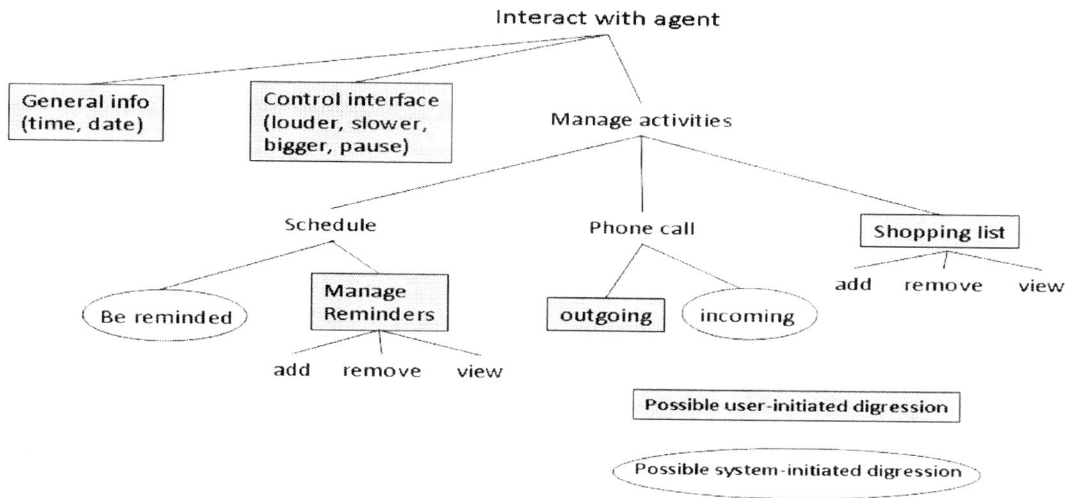


tures for spoken and multimodal dialog systems, for example the DARPA Communicator (Bayer, 2005) and the W3C Multimodal Architecture (Barnett et al., 2008), both of which provide a coordination component that manages interaction among multiple components that provide modality processing services. The conversation manager also marshals external backend functions as well as a persistent memory which is used for short and long term memory as well as application knowledge.

The agent is composed of the following parts:

1. Conversation Manager: The component that orchestrates and coordinates the dialog between the human and the machine.
2. Speech I/O: This system encapsulates speech recognition and pre-and post-processing of data involved in that recognition as well as the synthesis of the agent's voice.
3. Browser GUI: This displays information from the conversation manager in a graphic browser context. It also supports the human's interaction with the displayed data via inputs from the keyboard, mouse and touchscreen.
4. Avatar: This is a server/engine that renders a 3-D image of the avatar/agent and lip-synched speech and represents the conversational agent with which the user interacts. It also manages the performance of gestures (blinking, smiling, etc.) as well as dynamic emotional levels (happy, pensive, etc.). The avatar is based on the Haptek engine (Haptek Inc., 2009). The technical literature clearly supports that seeing a speaking face improves perception of speech over speech provided through the audio channel only (Massaro et al., 2000; Sumby & Pollack, 1956), even in persons with normal hearing. Although there is relatively little previous work on the use of an avatar with older users, Morandell et al., (2008) have shown that using avatars with users in an assisted living situation has valuable benefits such as improvements in user attention, although it did not show effects on memory functions. In addition, research by (Kwon, Gilbert, & Chattaraman, 2010) in an e-commerce application has shown that the use of an avatar on an e-commerce website makes it more likely that older website users will buy something.
5. Conversation definition: The engine itself has no inherent capability to converse. It is rather an engine that interprets a set of

definition files. One of the most important definition file types is the step file. This file represents a high-level limited domain representation of the "happy path" that the dialog should take.

6. External functions: These are functions callable directly from the conversation flow as defined in the step files. They are real routines/programs that can access data in normal programmatic ways such as files, the Internet, etc. and can provide results to the engine's persistent memory that are immediately accessible to the conversation.
7. Persistent memory: The conversation manager maintains a persistent memory. This is a place for application related data, external function parameters and results. It also provides a range of "autonomic" functions that track and manage a historical record of the previous experiences between the agent and the human.

All of these components combine to create the embodiment of a particular synthetic agent. Next, we consider these components in more detail.

## The ejTalker Conversation Engine

The central hub of the system is the conversation manager. It communicates with the other major components via XML (either through direct programmatic links or through socket-based communication protocols). At the highest level, the ejTalker engine interprets step files which define simple state machine transitions that embody the "happy path" for an anticipated conversation. Of course the "happy path" is only an ideal. That is where the other strategies of the ejTalker engine come to bear.

The next level of representation allows the well-defined "happy path" dialogs to be derived from other potential dialog behaviors. The value of this object-oriented approach to dialog management has also been shown in previous work, such as (Hanna et al., 2007). Using an object-oriented approach it is possible to handle "off focus" patterns of behavior by following the step derivation paths. This permits the engine to incorporate base behaviors without the need to weave all potential cases into every point in the dialog. These derivations are multiple and arbitrarily deep as well. This facility supports simple isolated behaviors such as "thank you" interactions, but also more powerfully, it permits related domains to be logically close to each other so that movement between them can be more natural.

Typically, any of the following systems (Audio I/O, Browser GUI, and Avatar) can be used to interact with the human. In our system, we use all three to create a richer experience and to increase communicative effectiveness through redundancy.

## Audio I/O

The ejTalker conversation manager considers the speech recognition and speech synthesis components to be a bundled service that communicates with the conversation engine via programmatic xml exchanges. In our system, the conversation manager instructs the speech I/O module to load a main grammar that contains all the rules that would be necessary for a conversation. It is essential that we can recognize utterances that are off-topic and that have relevance in some other domain. Note that the conversation manager does not directly interface to any specific ASR or TTS component. Nor does it imply any particular method by which the speech I/O module interprets the speech via the SRGS grammars (Hunt & McGlashan, 2004). The conversation engine delegates the active listening to the speech I/O subsystem and waits for the speech I/O to return when something was spoken. The engine expects the utterance transcription as well as a number of digested components such as rules fired and semantic values along with durations, energies, confidence scores etc. and all of this is returned in an xml structure by the conversation engine. In addition, and in the case where the Avatar is not handling the speech output component, the speech I/O module synthesizes what the conversation manager has decided to say.

## Browser GUI

The conversation manager includes an HTML server. It is an integral part of the engine and it is managed via step file definitions. This allows the conversation manager to dynamically display HTML. This is accomplished via AJAX methodology and inserts "inner HTML" into an HTML page that is hosted by the internal HTML server. Additionally, keyboard, mouse, and screen touch actions can be associated with individual parts of the dynamically displayed HTML page that enable acts of "clicking" or "typing" in a text box to generate unique identifiable inputs for the conversation manager. Note these inputs into the engine are treated much the same way as spoken input. All the modalities of input are dealt with at the same point in the conversation engine and are considered as equal semantic inputs. The conversation engages all the modalities equally and this makes acts of blended modalities very easy to support.

## Avatar

The Avatar Engine is a stand-alone server that renders a 3-D model of the avatar head, based on the Haptek engine (Haptek Inc., 2009). When the avatar engine is active, the spoken output from the conversation manager is directed to the avatar directly and not to the speech I/O module. This is because tight coupling is required between the speech synthesis and the visemes that must be rendered in sync with the synthesized voice. The avatar receives an xml structure from the conversation manager which contains what to speak, any gestures that are to be performed (look to the right, smile, etc.), and the underlying emotional base. That emotional base can be thought of as a very high level direction given to an actor ("you are feeling skeptical now," "be calm and disinterested"). It is achieved with a stochastic process across a large number of micro-actions that makes it appear natural and not "looped."

## Conversation Definition

These are a set of files that define the details of what the agent does and what it can react to. There are several types of files that define the conversational behavior. The recognition grammar is one of these files and is integral to the dialog since the step files can refer directly to rules that were fired and/or semantics that were set.

The step file represents a simple two turn exchange between the agent and the human (turn 1: agent speaks, turn 2: human speaks). In its simplest form, the step file begins with something to say upon entry and then it waits for some sort of input from the user which could be spoken or "clicked" on the browser display or other modalities that the conversation engine is prepared to receive. And finally a collection of rules that define patterns of user input and/or other information stored in the persistent memory. When speech or other input has been received by the engine, then the rules in the step with conversational focus are examined to see if any of them match the pattern (fire). If not, the system follows the derivation tree (steps can be derived from other steps) and scans for a more generic rule that might match. If it finds a match then it executes its associated actions. If nothing matches through all the derivation then no action is taken. It is as if the agent heard nothing.

The step also controls other aspects of the conversation. For example, it can control the amount of variability in spoken responses by invoking generative grammars (production SRGS grammar files). Additionally, the engine is sensitive to the amount of exposure the user has had at any conversational state and can react to it appropriately. For example, if the user has never been to a specific section of the conversation, the engine can automatically prompt with the needed explanation to guide the user through, but if the user has done this particular thing often and recently then the engine can automatically generate a more direct and efficient prompt and present the conversational ellipsis that a human would normally provide. This happens over a range of exposure levels.

When displaying HTML, versions of complex elements such as lists or tables display format files that are associated with the raw XML data for those elements with display instructions. These display format files also inform the conversation manager about which fields can be used to identify records or whether the table is numbered and therefore can be referenced by index, etc.

## External Functions

These functions do the actual programmatic work of retrieving, modifying, updating, converting, etc. the information for the conversational system. The conversation definition (i.e., step files) is focused purely on the conversational components of the human-computer encounter. Once the engine has determined the intent of the dialog, the conversation manager can delegate specific actions to an appropriate programmatic function. Data from the persistent memory, or blackboard, (Erman et al., 1980) along with the function name, are marshaled in an XML-Socket exchange to the designated Application Function Server (AFS). The AFS completes the requested function and returns an XML-Socket exchange with a status value that is used to guide the dialog (e.g. "found_item" or "item_missing") as well as any other detailed information to be written to the blackboard. In this way, the task of application development is neatly divided into linguistic and programming components. The design contract between the two is a simple statement of the part of the blackboard to "show" to the function, what the function does, what status is expected, and where any additional returned information should be written on the blackboard.

## Persistent Memory

The conversation manager is built on the premise of a persistent memory, or blackboard. In our system, this memory appears as a very large XML tree. The elements and/or subtrees can be identified with simple path strings. Throughout the conversation, the engine writes and reads to-and-from the blackboard for internal purposes such as parses, event lists, state recency, state specific experience, etc.

Additionally the conversation can write and read data to-and-from the blackboard. Some of these application elements are atomic, such as remembering that the user's favorite color was "red." Some other parts that manage the conversational automaticity surrounding lists will read and write things that allow it to remember what row and field had the focus last. Other parts manage the experience level between the human and the agent at each state visited in the conversation. It records the experience at any particular point in the conversation and it also permits those experiences to fade in a natural way. Importantly, this memory persists for more than just the session. It can persist indefinitely which is important for any agent that will develop a relationship over time with the human.

Figure 2 represents the components of our system. User interaction modalities are at the top of the diagram. The user can speak to the system and listen to its replies as well as touch or click the browser display screen, or use the keyboard. All of those interactions are sensed by the corresponding hardware. The adjunct tech layer represents various self-contained functionality in software systems that translate between the hardware layer and the ejTalker conversation manager. In our system, these include a number of third-party technologies. The conversation manager is encapsulated in that it communicates

Figure 2. Conversational system architecture

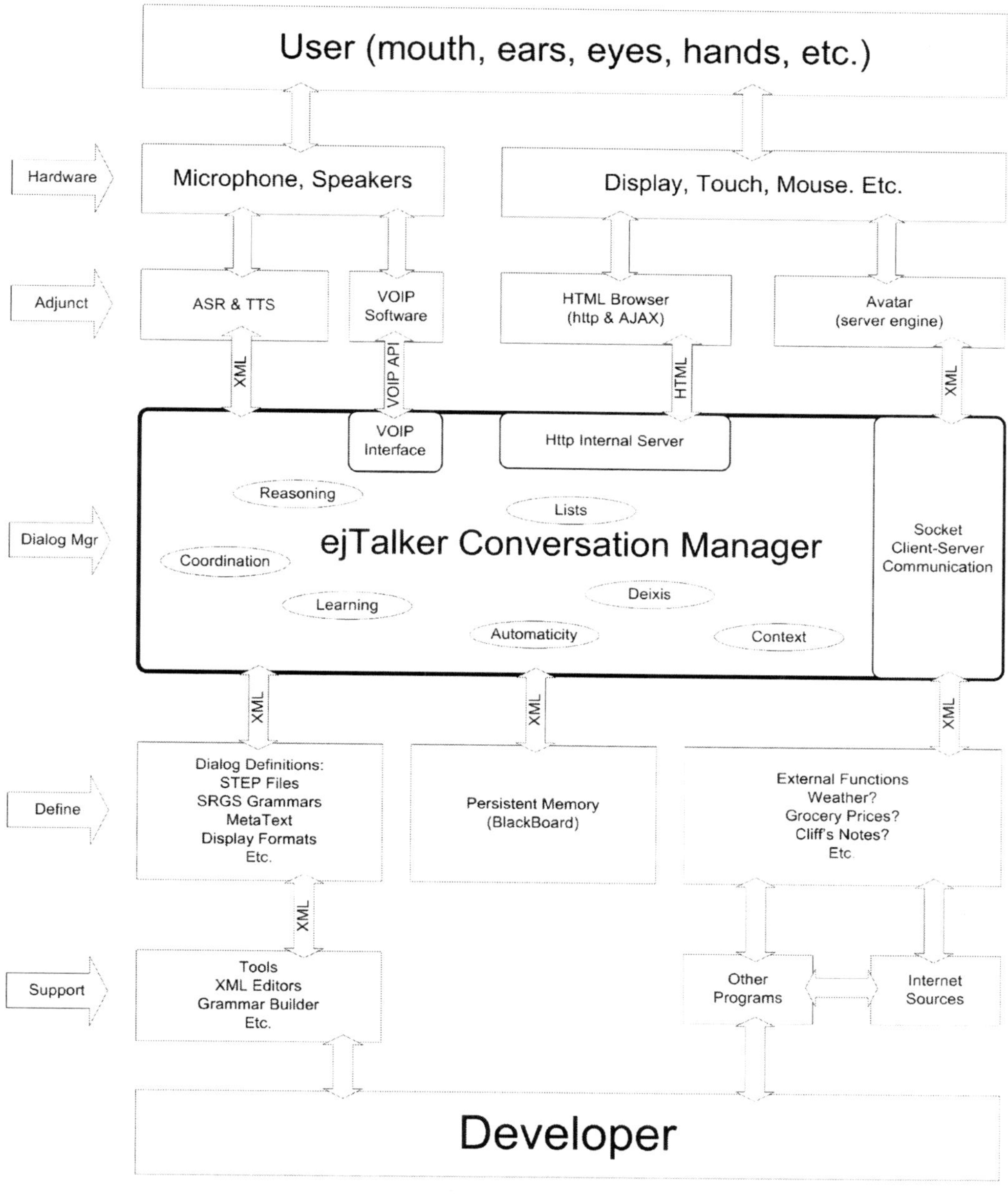


solely with the outside world via XML exchanges and anything it knows or records is structured as XML in its persistent memory (the blackboard).

The system behavior is defined by step files (as well as grammars, display formats and other files). These are also XML files. External functions communicate with the conversation manager via a simple XML-based API. These XML functions are invoked when corresponding "rules" in the step files "fire." The developer activity is at the bottom of the diagram and represents standard XML editing tools and conventional programming IDE's (for the external functions) as well

*Figure 3. Screenshot of the shopping list application*

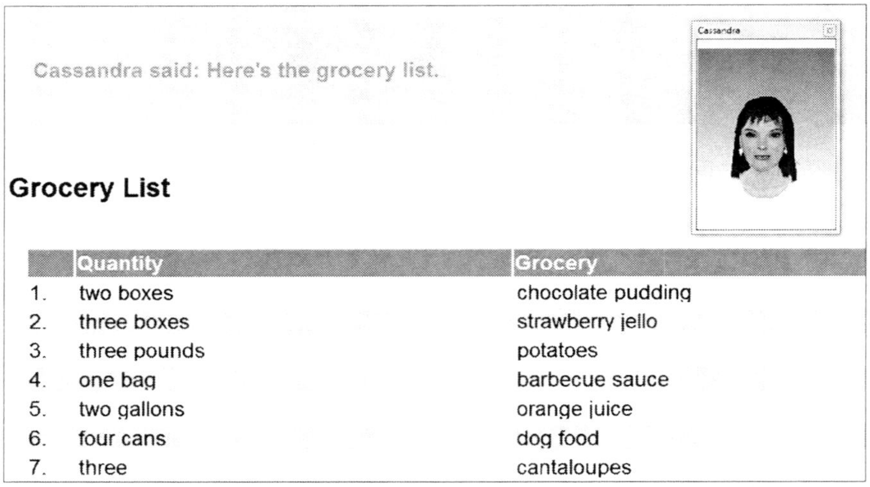

Cassandra said: Here's the grocery list.

Cassandra

**Grocery List**

| | Quantity | Grocery |
|---|---|---|
| 1. | two boxes | chocolate pudding |
| 2. | three boxes | strawberry jello |
| 3. | three pounds | potatoes |
| 4. | one bag | barbecue sauce |
| 5. | two gallons | orange juice |
| 6. | four cans | dog food |
| 7. | three | cantaloupes |

as specialized debugging and evaluation tools specific to the ejTalker conversation engine.

## Platform Considerations

The basic client platform requirements are

1. The ability to run a web browser.
2. A touchscreen.
3. The ability to capture audio at a sufficiently high quality for speech recognition. The audio capture client does not necessarily have to be the same device as the device that runs the web browser and the touchscreen.

Speech recognition needs to be available, either on the client device or on a server. One possible configuration is a Windows 7 tablet touchscreen laptop, running a Firefox web browser, and using Windows Speech Recognition. In this configuration, the conversation manager also runs locally on the laptop. A screen shot of this configuration is shown in Figure 3. While this configuration is simple, and provides portability for the speech interface, it does not provide very good pervasiveness for the graphical part of the interface because the laptop is too big and heavy to be conveniently moved around as the user moves to different locations.

Another, more portable, configuration runs the conversation manager and speech recognizer on a server on a local area network, with the graphical display on a smartphone, and with the microphone wirelessly connected to the server. This configuration is shown in Figure 4. The smartphone is very portable, but the screen is small. We believe that speech input and output will compensate to some degree for the small size of the visual display, but the usability of the smartphone display with a speech interface for older users remains an open question. The eventual graphical client will undoubtedly be a compromise between portability and the available size of the visual display. As the space of small, wireless, and web-enabled devices continues to expand, we believe that many options will continue to become available for the graphical client component of the hardware architecture.

## A Sample Dialog

Although managing a shopping list seems to be a simple application, we can see from the following dialog that a natural multimodal interface to this

*Figure 4. Shopping list application running on a smartphone*

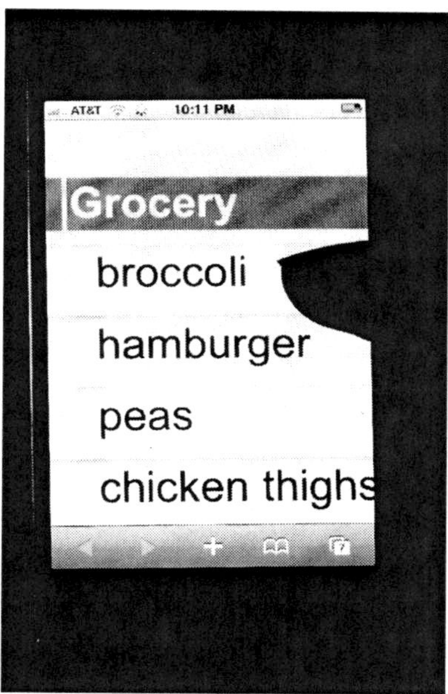


application introduces the possibility of some interesting behavior.

**User:** Show my shopping list.
**Computer:** "Here's the shopping list" (shows the list).

The user interface shows the information redundantly — by voice, by text and by showing the list. This reinforces the information.

**User:** Add milk to my shopping list
**Computer:** I added milk to the list (shows the list with milk).
**User:** Is dog food on my list?
**Computer:** No, dog food isn't on the list.
**User:** Add it.
**Computer:** I added dog food to the list (shows the list with dog food).

The computer correctly interprets the pronoun, "it", but reinforces its understanding by saying "dog food." If the computer just said "I removed it from the list," it would be harder for the user to notice an error.

**Computer:** You asked me to remind you — start cooking dinner.

The computer proactively tells the user about a reminder that was set earlier.

**User:** Ok.
**User:** (switching the task to the shopping list after the reminder digression and touching the word "bananas" on the display, which is an item on the list) Remove that.

The computer interprets a deictic reference to the item that the user is pointing to, and removes "bananas" from the shopping list.

Interestingly, a wide range of applications can be usefully conceptualized in terms of list, or more generally table, management. So, for example, an application that involves managing a list of reminders would make use of many of the same capabilities as an application for managing shopping lists. In both applications the user would want to add and remove items by voice and by touching, as well as check to see if items are on the list (Coin, 2010).

## Components Underlying this Dialog

The conversation manager described above is the central component that makes this kind of a dialog possible. For actual applications, it must be supplied with domain-specific information. This includes:

1. The step file(s) that define the pattern-action rules the dialog manager follows in conducting the dialog.
2. Speech recognition grammar(s) written in a modified version of the SRGS format (Hunt & McGlashan, 2004).

3. The blackboard that contains the system's memory from session to session, including such things as the user's shopping list.
4. Some applications may need non-conversation-related functions, referred to earlier as AFS functions. An example of this might be a voice-operated calculator. This kind of functionality can be supplied by an external server that communicates with the dialog engine over sockets.
5. A basic HTML file that defines the graphical layout of the GUI display and is updated by the conversation engine using AJAX calls as needed.

The following section describes a rule from a step file for shopping list management and part of the blackboard that supports the shopping application.

## Description of the Major Components of the step File

The overall arc of the conversation is defined by the step file. It consists of an administrative section <head> and a functional section <body> much like an HTML page. An important part of the <head> section is the <derivedFrom> element which points to a lineage of other STEP files from which this particular step file inherits behaviors (this inheritance is key to the depth and richness of the interactions that can be defined).

The <body> section represents two "turns" beginning with the <say> element which defines what the agent says, gestures and emotes. This is followed by a <listen> section which can be used to restrict what the agent listens for, but in very open dialog such as ours, the "listen" is across a larger grammar to allow freer movement between domains.

The last major component of the <body> is the <response> section and it is where most of the mechanics of the conversation take place. This section contains an arbitrary number of rules each of which may have an arbitrary number of cases. The default behavior is for a rule to match a pattern in the text recognized from the human's utterance. In actual practice, the source string to be tested as well as the pattern to be matched, can be complex constructs assembled from things that the conversation engine knows— things that are in its persistent memory. If a rule "fires," then the corresponding actions are executed.

Usually this involves calling some sort of internal or external function, generating something to "say" to the human, and presenting some visual elements for multimodal display. Note that the input pattern for a "rule" is not limited to speech events and rules can be based on any input modality that the engine is aware of. In this application the engine is aware of screen touches, gestures, mouse and keyboard interaction in addition to speech. (Box 1)

The following example illustrates the concept of inheritance of basic conversation capabilities that are inherited by other more specific dialogs. This inherited step supports a user request for the system to "take a break," and is available from almost every other dialog. Notice that even this step is derived from other basic steps. (Box 2)

## Blackboard

A wide variety of information is represented on the blackboard, including dynamic, user-specific information such as a user's grocery list. In this example the <currentList> node has a number of attributes that are automatically maintained by the conversation manager to keep track of context. (Box 3)

## Initial User Reactions

Although the application has not been formally tested with users, a mockup presenting the system's functionality has been shown to 80 seniors, with a median age of approximately 75 years in 10 senior centers in New York City (Greene, 2010),

*Box 1.*

```
<step>
  <name>groceryListDomain</name>
  <head>
     <purpose>Manage a Grocery List</purpose>
     <derivedFrom>niBase.XML</derivedFrom>
     <author>Emmett Coin</author>
     <date>20100221</date>
  </head>
  <body>
     <say>
        <text>Cool! Let's work on your grocery list.</text>
     </say>
     <listen>
     </listen>
     <response>
        <rule name="show">
           <pattern input="{R:ejShowCMD:ejExist},{S:ejListCategory:}">
              TRUE,ejGroceryList
           </pattern>
           <examplePattern>
              <ex>show my shopping list</ex>
           </examplePattern>
           <action>
              <function>
                 <AFS function="list.display">
                    <paramNode>
                       <listFormatName>shoppingListFormat1.XML</listFormatName>
                        <dataLocation>grocery/currentList</dataLocation>
                    </paramNode>
                    <resultNode>grocery</resultNode>
                 </AFS>
              </function>
              <presay>
                 <text>Here's the shopping list.|</text>
              </presay>
              <displayHTML>
                 <information type="treeReference">
                    grocery/display/form/div
                 </information>
                 <ejSemanticFeedback>Show my shopping list.</ejSemanticFeedback>
              </displayHTML>
           </action>
           <goto>groceryListDomain.XML</goto>
        </rule>
<!-- in the full STEP there are many more rules to service: -->
<!--       deixis, deletion, verifying, etc. -->
     </response>
  </body>
</step>
```

*Box 2.*

```
<step>
  <name>ejBase</name>
  <head>
    <objectName>CassandraBase</objectName>
    <purpose>Foundation for all application STEP objects</purpose>
    <version>3.05</version>
    <derivedFrom>ejTimeBase.XML|reminderListDomain.XML</derivedFrom>
    <author>Emmett Coin</author>
    <date>20090610</date>
  </head>
  <body>
    <listen>
      <grammar>ejBase</grammar>
    </listen>
    <response>
      <rule name="baseCommand">
        <pattern>[W:command] CASSANDRA</pattern>
        <examplePattern>
          <ex>Take a break Cassandra</ex>
        </examplePattern>
        <action>
          <function>
            <AFS server="INTERNAL" function="agent.command">
              <paramNode>system/asr/vars</paramNode>
              <resultNode>system/program/request</resultNode>
            </AFS>
          </function>
        </action>
        <branch>
          <!-- other case sections service Help, log off, louder, softer,
           etc. behaviors -->
          <case id="*BREAK*|*HOLD*|*WAIT*">
            <action>
              <presay>
                <text emotion="ejSkeptic">Okay, I'll take a break.  To wake
                 me up, say "Cassandra, let's continue."  </text>
              </presay>
            </action>
            <call>ejOnBreak.XML</call>
          </case>
          <!-- other case sections service Help, log off, louder, softer,
           etc. behaviors -->
        </branch>
      </rule>
    </response>
  </body>
</step>
```

*Box 3.*


```
<currentList open="TRUE" format="shoppingListFormat1.XML" lastIn-
dex="8" listName="grocery1" dataPath="grocery/currentList" rowFo-
cus="3" fieldFocus="GROCERY" focusRecord="4" focusPath="description"
focusValue="milk" pathClicked="units">
                    <item>
                         <description>green beans</description>
                         <ejTUID>1</ejTUID>
                    </item>
                    <item>
                         <description>cream</description>
                         <ejTUID>2</ejTUID>
                    </item>
                    <item>
                         <description>milk</description>
                         <ejTUID>3</ejTUID>
                    </item>
               </currentList>
```


in order to find out their reactions. In general the seniors were very positive about the application and appreciated the potential benefits that the application might provide. However, there were a number of concerns voiced that would have to be addressed in order to make the application acceptable to users.

Concerns having to do with the application itself included the importance of being able to easily increase the volume of the audio and the size of fonts presented, as well as a wide tolerance in the touch interface for users who have problems with fine motor control. In addition, the users were concerned that setup of the application might be complex. Although these concerns can be addressed with careful attention to the design of the application, the seniors also voiced additional concerns that go beyond the application itself to its context of use. These included a concern that an assistant such as the one described in this chapter might lead to a negative impact on the senior's own ability to perform these functions for themselves. Another concern was that a conversational assistant might lesson the users' connection with people. These broader concerns could be addressed through adding features to the application to practice doing various functions for themselves and to encourage them to maintain contact with other people

## CONCLUSION

We have described a multimodal application that is designed to improve the lives of older users by helping them manage tasks of daily living and assisting them in maintaining social connections. The multimodal interface accommodates users' limitations caused by the normal aging process and makes the application easier to use than current complex computer interfaces. The system is based on a general-purpose conversation manager that improves the usability and convenience of the system by providing a natural multimodal interface as well as general capabilities such as pausing and resuming interrupted tasks.

## FUTURE DIRECTIONS

There are a number of crucial questions that need to be addressed through testing with actual users.

This is a key next step. Clearly, an important question is whether the level of accuracy of speech recognition is adequate for these users, or they will find it difficult to accomplish their goals. Speech recognition errors are inevitable. We need to know to what extent speech recognition errors are tolerated by users, and how easy they are to fix.

Having to repeat an occasional utterance once or twice is common in conversations between people, so it would be expected that occasionally needing to repeat an utterance would not be too burdensome for users. On the other hand, an actual misrecognition of key information is much more irritating, because the error will have to be corrected. Research by (Fink, Schwarz, & Dahl, 2009) found that speech recognition errors did not have an impact on user satisfaction in a speech therapy application, but that research did not address user satisfaction in an application designed for daily use.

Another major area of testing is usability of the actual application. The questions that need to be answered include how intuitive is the user interface to use, and will users find it easy to learn.

We also need to consider usability in a broader context. Usability is not just a matter of how easy it is to make the application work. Usability, especially for an application that is designed to become an intrinsic part of daily life, must take into account contextual usability, or usability in the context of all the other things that the user might be doing (Nicoll, 1995).

An application that requires the user to set aside a dedicated period of time, go into a quiet room away from other people, boot up their computer, and use the application without interruptions will have very different contextual usability requirements from an application that needs to be accessed quickly in a few seconds without materially interrupting whatever else they are doing. For this reason, our application will have to be tested in users' homes while they are carrying out their normal activities. The question of whether users will want to talk to the application while they are around other people is another important question that will be addressed by testing in the home.

Many of the features commonly anticipated within the emerging ubiquitous computing environment will have significant implications in the evolution of our senior-friendly conversationally based assistant. The first trend relates to the shift away from the standard keyboard as the primary input mechanism to the computer/network. With the iPad, the first of what will probably be a wide array of different sized touch-based computers, we see the nascent forms of multimodal, though largely touch based, computing. With physical keyboards no longer required and the cost of screens continuing to plummet, it is easy to imagine intelligent picture frames (now thought of as tablet computers) being placed throughout the house.

Concurrently, it is likely that other input/output devices such as microphones, cameras and speakers will also proliferate thereby allowing for true multimodal interactions throughout one's living quarters. The system will be "aware of the senior's location," and capable of accurately hearing his/her speech throughout the house or communicating when it having trouble doing so. In a sense, dispersed input/output devices will enable conversational applications to have "mobility" and be more of a real time and fully present assistant. The person will not need to be sitting in a limited spot in order for the network to "intelligently" respond to a command or request. For those seniors who have difficulty moving around, this robust sensing environment with availability in all places of the home will be extremely helpful.

In the presentations and focus groups we have conducted, Cassandra's potential medical alerting capabilities were consistently mentioned as a feature that people found quite useful. However, for most seniors, the biggest impact that our senior friendly virtual assistant will have relates to obtaining socially related services from the rapidly growing intelligent network. Our conversational assistant will make it easier for seniors to stay in touch, reminding them about their last interactions with family and friends and making it much easier to initiate contact through voice enabled calling, transcribed email or texts and reading of incoming communications.

Social networking sites are already rapidly gaining interest among seniors and will probably become a major component in their lives. Memoir creation will also be enhanced through interactive dialog. There will be many options but more importantly beyond the usefulness of specific features, the overall access to people and ease of social interactions will enhance the senior's sense of connectedness and directly combat isolation. We believe this will promote better health and dramatically impact the lives of many of our elders.

## REFERENCES


Allen, J., Byron, D., Dzikovska, M., Ferguson, G., Galescu, L., & Stent, A. (2000). An architecture for a generic dialogue shell. *Natural Language Engineering*, *6*(3-4), 213–228. doi:10.1017/S135132490000245X

Arch, A. (2008). *Web accessibility for older users: A literature review*. Retrieved from http://www.w3.org/TR/wai-age-literature/

Arthritis Foundation. (2008). *Arthritis prevalence: A nation in pain*. Retrieved from http://www.arthritis.org/media/newsroom/media-kits/Arthritis_Prevalence.pdf

Barnett, J., Dahl, D. A., Kliche, I., Tumuluri, R., Yudkowsky, M., & Bodell, M. (2008). *Multimodal architecture and interfaces*. Retrieved from http://www.w3.org/TR/mmi-arch/

Bayer, S. (2005). Building a standards and research community with the Galaxy communicator software infrastructure. In Dahl, D. A. (Ed.), *Practical spoken dialog systems* (*Vol. 26*, pp. 166–196). Dordrecht, The Netherlands: Kluwer Academic Publishers.

Borodin, Y., Mahmud, J., Ramakrishnan, I. V., & Stent, A. (2007). *The HearSay non-visual Web browser.* Paper presented at the W4A 2007.

Caldwell, B., Cooper, M., Reid, L. G., & Vanderheiden, G. (2007). *Web content accessibility guidelines* 2.0. Retrieved May 30, 2010, from http://www.w3.org/TR/2007/WD-WCAG20-20071211/

Catizone, R., Setzer, A., & Wilkes, Y. (2003). *Multimodal dialogue management in the COMIC project.* Paper presented at the Proceedings of EACL 2003 Workshop on Dialogue Systems: Interaction, adaptation, and styles of management.

Catizone, R., Worgan, S., Wilks, Y., Dingli, A., & Cheng, W. (2010). A world-hybrid approach to a conversational companion for reminiscing about images. In Wilks, Y. (Ed.), *Artificial companions in society: Scientific, economic, psychological and philosophical perspectives*. Amsterdam, The Netherlands: John Benjamins.

Coin, E. (2007, February 21, 2007). *Today and the future of wearable agents.* Paper presented at the SpeechTEK West, San Francisco.

Coin, E. (2010, April 22-23). *Table talking.* Paper presented at the Mobile Voice Conference, San Francisco.

Coin, E., & Qua, J. (2000, July 3-5, 2000). *A fundamental architecture to integrate conversation management engines with conversation development and evaluation tools.* Paper presented at the Third Workshop on Human-Computer Conversation, Bellagio, Italy.

Erman, L. D., Hayes-Roth, F., Lesser, V. R., & Reddy, D. R. (1980). The HEARSAY-II speech understanding system: Integrating knowledge to resolve uncertainty. *Computing Surveys*, *12*, 213–253. doi:10.1145/356810.356816

Ferguson, G., & Allen, J. (1998, July). *TRIPS: An intelligent integrated problem-solving assistant.* Paper presented at the Fifteenth National Conference on Artificial Intelligence (AAAI-98), Madison, WI.

Fink, R. B., Schwarz, M., & Dahl, D. A. (2009). *Using speech recognition for speech therapy: MossTalkWords 2.0.* Paper presented at the American Speech-Language-Hearing Association, New Orleans, LA, USA.

Ford, G. S., & Ford, S. G. (2009). Internet use and depression among the elderly. *Phoenix Center Policy Papers, 38*. Retrieved from www.phoenix-center.org

Greene, M. (2010). *User reactions to senior-friendly interfaces*. Paper presented at the SpeechTEK.

Hanna, P., O'Neill, I., Wootton, C., & Mctear, M. (2007). Promoting extension and reuse in a spoken dialog manager: An evaluation of the queen's communicator. *ACM Transactions in Speech and Language Processing*, *4*(3), 7. doi:10.1145/1255171.1255173

Haptek Inc. (2009). *Haptek*. Retrieved from www.haptek.com

Hunt, A., & McGlashan, S. (2004). *W3C speech recognition grammar specification* (SRGS). Retrieved from http://www.w3.org/TR/speech-grammar/

Kwon, W. S., Gilbert, J., & Chattaraman, V. (2010). *Effects of conversational agents in retail websites on aging consumers' interactivity and perceived benefits.* Paper presented at the Proceedings of the 28th ACM Conference on Human Factors in Computing Systems CHI 2010 Workshop Senior-Friendly Technologies: Interaction Design for the Elderly, Atlanta, GA, USA.

Larsson, S., Ljunglof, P., Muhlenbock, K., & Thunberg, G. (2008). *TRIK: A talking and drawing robot for children with communication disabilities.* Paper presented at the Proc. NordiCHI'08 Workshop: Designing Robotic Artefacts With User- and Experience Centred Perspectives.

M-PILL. (2009). *M-Pill.* Retrieved from http://www.m-pill.com/index.php?browse=compliance

Massaro, D. W., Cohen, M. M., Beskow, J., & Cole, R. (2000). Developing and evaluating conversational agents. In Cassell, J., Sullivan, J., Prevost, S., & Churchill, E. (Eds.), *Embodied conversational agents* (pp. 287–318). Cambridge, MA: MIT Press.

MetLife Mature Market Institute. (2009). *Market survey of long-term care costs.* Retrieved from http://www.metlife.com/assets/cao/mmi/publications/studies/mmi-market-survey-nursing-home-assisted-living.pdf

Morandell, M. M., Hochgatterer, A., Fagel, S., & Wassertheurer, S. (2008). *Avatars in assistive homes for the elderly: A user-friendly way of interaction? HCI and usability for education and work.* Berlin / Heidelberg, Germany: Springer.

National Institute on Deafness and other Communication Disorders. (n.d.). *Hearing loss and older adults*. Retrieved May 30, 2010, from http://www.nidcd.nih.gov/health/hearing/older.asp

Nicoll, D. W. (1995). *Contextual usability: A methodological outline of contextual usability and quality function deployment in the development of advance media products.* TechMaPP Working Paper, Department of Psychology, University of Edinburgh.

Prince Market Research. (2007). *Aging in place in America*. Retrieved from http://clarityproducts.com/press-news/

Santangelo, A., Augello, A., Gentile, A., Pilato, G., & Gaglio, S. A. (2006). *Chat-Bot based multimodal virtual guide for cultural heritage tours*. Retrieved from http://ww1.ucmss.com/books/LFS/CSREA2006/PSC4614.pdf

Sumby, W. H., & Pollack, L. (1956). Visual contribution to speech intelligibility in noise. *The Journal of the Acoustical Society of America*, *26*(2), 212–215. doi:10.1121/1.1907309

## KEY TERMS AND DEFINITIONS

**AJAX:** Asynchronous JavaScript and XML; a technology for allowing data to be updated from a server without having to reload an entire HTML page.

**Avatar:** an animated rendering of a conversational agent.

**Cognitive Factors:** User characteristics having to do with intellectual functions such as memory, attention and learning.

**Conversational Agent:** A synthetic character that interacts with the user to perform activities in a conversational manner, using natural language and dialog.

**Conversation Manager:** A system component that coordinate the interaction between the system and the user. Its central task is deciding what the next steps in the conversation should be based on the user's input and other contextual information.

**Multimodal Dialog Systems:** Dialog systems where the user can choose to interact with the system in multiple modalities, for example speech, typing, or touch.

**Multimodality:** Use of multiple input modes in an application, such as speech, typing, touch, and handwriting.

**Pervasive Availability:** Describes an application that is continually available no matter what the user's location is.

**STEP File:** A declarative XML representation of a dialog used in the ejTalker system.

**Task-Switching:** interrupting an ongoing task to engage in another task. A task-switching utterance tells the system to move to a different task, saving task state and data so that the interrupted task can be resumed.

**Task-Resuming:** returning to a task that was previously interrupted. A task-resuming utterance instructs the system to resume an interrupted task, restoring task state and data as needed. Meta-utterances about the state of the resumed task may be useful in reorienting the user to the task state.

# Chapter 13
# A Companionable Agent

**Roberta Catizone**
*University of Sheffield, UK*

**Yorick Wilks**
*University of Sheffield, UK*

## ABSTRACT

*Companions are agents devised to accompany users day by day building long-term relationships with them. They do not only assist users for particular tasks in sporadic times, but they provide more support and have more information to adapt themselves to each users' needs. Currently, these agents and their possibilities are being researched as a part of an EU project, which is described in this chapter.*

## INTRODUCTION

We describe a system developed as part of an EU project that aims to change the way we think about the relationships of people to computers and the Internet by developing a virtual conversational 'Companion'. This will be an agent or 'presence' that stays with the user for long periods of time, developing a relationship and 'knowing' its owners preferences and wishes. The Companion communicates with the user primarily through speech, but also using other technologies such as touch screens and sensors.

This chapter describes the functionality and system modules of the Senior Companion (SC), one of two initial prototypes built in the first two years of the project. The SC provides a multimodal interface for eliciting, retrieving and inferring over personal information from elderly users by means of conversation about their photographs.

The Companion, through conversation, elicits their life memories and reminiscences, often prompted by discussion of their photographs; the aim is that the Companion should come to know a great deal about its user, their tastes, likes, dislikes, emotional reactions etc, through long periods of conversation. It is assumed that most life information will soon be stored on the Internet (as in the [Memories for Life] project) and we are linking the SC directly to photo inventories

DOI: 10.4018/978-1-60960-617-6.ch013

in Facebook, a matter we discuss in more detail below. The overall aim of the SC is to produce a coherent life narrative for its user from these materials, although its short-term goals, reported here are to assist, amuse, entertain and gain the trust of the user. The Senior Companion uses a hybrid approach to dialogue management as well as intelligent adaptation of the user's emotional state which plays an important part in gaining the user's trust.

The technical content of the project is to use a number of types of machine learning (ML) to achieve these ends in original ways, initially using a methodology developed in earlier research: first, by means of an Information Extraction (IE) approach to deriving content from user input utterances (Catizone et al., 2002); secondly, using a training method for attaching Dialogue Acts (DA) to these utterances (Webb et al., 2008) and lastly, using a specific type of dialogue manager (DM) that uses Dialogue Action Forms (DAF) to determine the context of any utterance, and a stack of these DAFs as the virtual machine that models the ongoing dialogue by means of a shared user and Companion initiative and generates appropriate responses (Catizone et al., 2003).

The SC is not a robot and could be embodied in a screen, a handbag or a mobile phone while retaining the same "personality": it is more a very high level conversational internet agent, dedicated to a single user over the long term.

This chapter is organized as follows: firstly, it describes the current SC prototype's functionality. Next, it sets out the SC architecture and modules, focusing on the Natural Language Understanding module and the Dialogue Manager and the short term plans to enhance Dialogue Management performance with direct Internet access and initial ML experiments. Finally, it describes the experimental work done by linking the DM to emotional considerations.

## 2. THE SENIOR COMPANION SYSTEM

The Senior Companion (SC) prototype (Wilks, 2007, 2008; Wilks et al., 2008) was designed to make a rapid advance in the first two years of a project so as to be the basis for a second round of prototypes embodying more advanced ML. This strategy was deliberately chosen to avoid a well-known problem with experimental AI systems: that a whole project is spent in design so that a prototype never emerges until the very end, which is then never fully evaluated and, most importantly, nothing is ever built upon the experience obtained in its construction.

The central function of the SC is engaging the user in discussion about their photographs: where and when they were taken, details about the people in them and their relationship to the user and each other. The SC extracts and stores facts obtained from the user's input and is able to pick up discussion with the user where the system left off in later user sessions. In addition to allowing reminiscing, the SC also permits the user to do basic photo management including selecting particular images or groups of images by pointing and organizing the photos by means of a dialogue.

Once a photo is loaded, it is processed with face recognition software to identify any faces in it. The recognition software, OpenCV[1], provides positional information by identifying the face coordinates and this information is exploited in the Dialogue Manager by making explicit reference to the position of people in the photograph (the person on the left, right, center, etc.) as well as recognizing when there are groups of people. The system discusses properties of the photo as well as properties and relationships of the people in the photos.

The SC also contains a news reading feature which adds an interesting accompaniment to the photo domain and demonstrates the ability of the system to handle more than one kind of application at a time, and news has, of course, an unconstrained vocabulary. It is taken via RSS feeds from the BBC news website and includes news from three popular categories: politics, sports and business, and the user can choose between them, stop and start the feed by speaking etc. The system can also tell jokes on request, from a potentially endless internet source.

The following is the middle part of a sample dialogue generated by the system when discussing a group photo from a vacation in Zanzibar, and after the system had already stored from an earlier conversation that the user had a daughter Zoe. One of the people in the photo has been tagged as 'doctor' using Facebook:

**SC:** What is your relationship to the doctor?
**User:** There is no relationship.
**SC:** Please tell me how you know the doctor
**U:** Uh, he is a friend.
**SC:** How old was the doctor when this photo was taken?
**U:** I am not sure but I think about 30.
**SC:** How do you know Octavia?
**U:** She is my daughter.
**SC:** Aha! We see. Octavia's sister is Zoe.
**SC:** How old was your daughter Octavia when this photo was taken?
**U:** Octavia was 19 years old.
**SC:** What was the occasion of this photo?
**U:** This was another family holiday.
**SC:** Where was this photo taken?
**U:** This photo was taken in Tanzania.
**SC:** Have you ever been to Zanzibar?
**U:** Yes, I have.
**SC:** Great place, we hope you saw the beaches. When was this photo taken?
**R:** Last year.

It is a key feature of the SC that it can make simple inferences from family relationships it already knows (e.g. that daughters of the same parent are siblings) and that it can access real-time information about places to show that it has some knowledge of what is being talked about, in this case the beaches on Zanzibar, and how this is done is discussed below. This real time access to unconstrained place information on the Internet is an attempt to break out of classic Artificial Intelligence (AI) systems that only know the budget of facts they have been primed with.

This basic system provides the components for future development of the SC, as well as its main use as a device to generate more conversation data for machine learning research in the future. Key features of the SC are listed below followed by a description of the system architecture and modules:

- A visually appealing multimodal interface (Figure 1) with a character avatar to mediate the system's functionality to the user.
- Interacts with the user with multiple modalities – speech and touch.
- Includes face detection software for identifying the position of faces in the photos.
- Accepts pre-annotated (XML) photo inventories as a means for creating richer dialogues more quickly.
- Engages in conversation with the user about topics within the photo domain: when and where the photo was taken, discussion of the people in the photo including their relationships to the user.
- Reads news from three categories: politics, business and sports.
- Tells jokes taken from an internet-based joke website.
- Retains all user input for reference in repeat user sessions, in addition to the knowledge base that has been updated by the Dialogue Manager on the basis of what was said.
- Contains a fully integrated Knowledge Base for maintaining user information which contains:
    - Ontological information which is exploited by the Dialogue Manager and

*Figure 1. The senior companion interface*

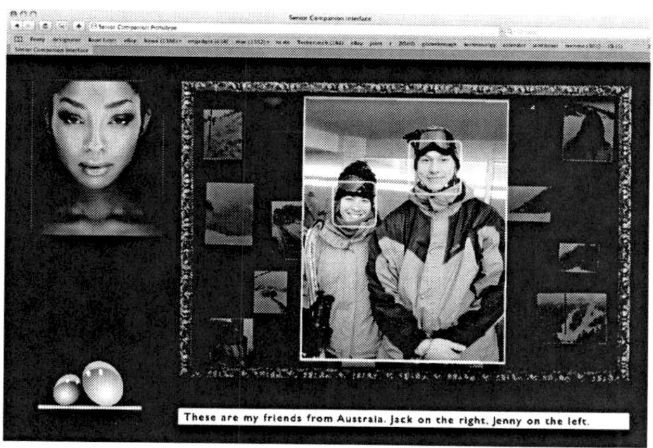

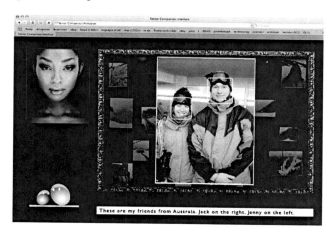


provides domain-specific relations between fundamental concepts.

- ◦ A mechanism for storing information in a triple store (Subject-Predicate-Object)-the Resource Description Format (RDF) Semantic Web format---- for handling unexpected user input that falls outside of the photo domain, e.g. arbitrary locations in which photos might have been taken.
- ◦ A reasoning module for reasoning over the Knowledge Base and world knowledge obtained in RDF format from the internet; the SC is thus a primitive Semantic Web device (see Wilks, 2008)

- Contains basic photo management capability allowing the user in conversation to select photos as well as display a set of photos with a particular feature.

## 3. SYSTEM ARCHITECTURE

In this section we will review the components of the SC architecture. As can be seen from Figure 2 below, the architecture contains three abstract level components – Connectors, Input Handlers and Application Services – together with the Dialogue Manager and the Natural Language Understander (NLU).

**Connectors** form a communication bridge between the core system and external applications. The external application refers to any modules or systems which provide a specific set of functionalities that might be changed in the future. There is one connector for each external application. It hides the underlying complex communication protocol details and provides a general interface for the main system to use. This abstraction decouples the connection of external and internal modules, makes changing and adding new external modules easier. At this moment, there are two connectors in the system – Napier Interface Connector and CrazyTalk Avatar Connector. Both of them are using network sockets to send/receive messages.

**Input Handlers** are a set of modules for processing messages according to message types. Each handler deals with a category of messages where categories are coarse-grained and could include one or more message types. The handlers separate the code handling inputs into different places and make the code easier to locate and change. Three handlers have been implemented in Senior Companions system – Setup Handler, Dragon (ASR) Events Handler and General Handler. The Setup Handler is responsible for

Figure 2. Senior companion system architecture

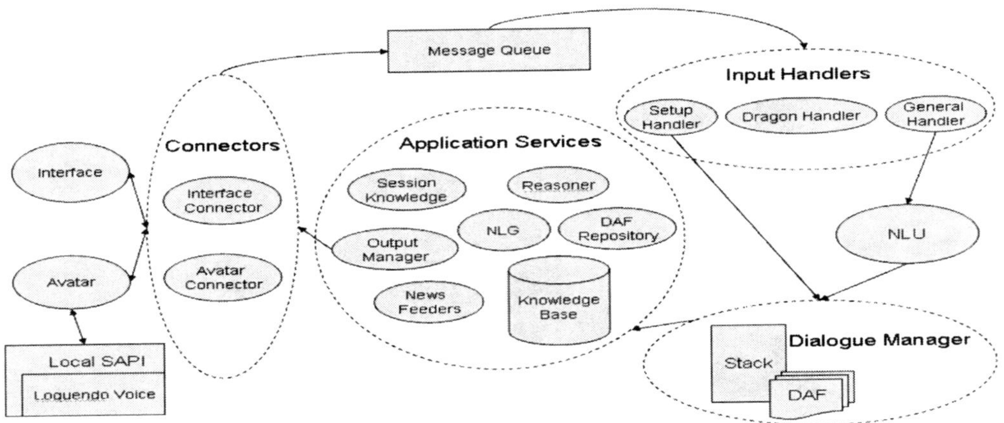

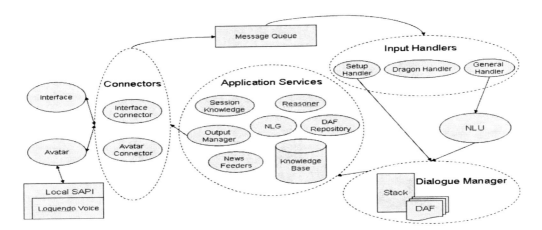


loading the photo annotations if any, performing face detection if the annotation file is missing and checking the Knowledge Base to see if the photo that is being processed has been discussed in earlier sessions. Dragon Event Handler deals with dragon speech recognition commands sent from the interface while the General Handler processes user utterances and photo change events of the interface.

**Application Services** are a group of internal modules which provide interfaces for the Dialogue Action Forms (DAF) to use. It has an easy-to-use high-level interface for general DAF designers to code associated tests and actions as well as a low level interface for advanced DAFs. It provides the communication link between DAFs and the internal system and enables DAFs to access system functionalities. Following is a brief summary of modules grouped into Application Services.

**News Feeders** are a set of RSS Feeders for fetching news from the internet. Three different news feeders have been implemented for fetching news from BBC website Sports, Politics and Business channels. There is also a Jokes Feeder to fetch Jokes from internet in a similar way. During the conversation, the user can request news about particular topics and the SC simply reads the news (using TTS) downloaded through the feeds.

**DAF Repository** is a list of DAFs loaded from files generated by the DAF Editor. A fresh copy of a DAF can be obtained by passing the DAF name to this module.

**Natural Language Generation (NLG)** is responsible for randomly selecting a system utterance from a template. An optional variable can be passed when calling methods in this module. The variable will be used to replace special symbols in the text template if applicable. For example, a template utterance "How do you know $?" will be returned as "How do you know John?" if passing variable "John" when calling the generation method of this module.

**Session Knowledge** is the place where global information for a particular running session is stored. For example, the name of the user who is running the session, the list of photos being discussed in this session, the list of user utterances, etc.

**Knowledge Base** is the data store of persistent knowledge. It is implemented as an RDF triplestore using a Jena implementation. The triplestore API is a layer built upon a traditional relational database. The application can save/retrieve information as RDF triples rather than table records. The structure of knowledge represented in RDF triples is discussed later.

**Reasoner** is used to perform inference on existing knowledge in the Knowledge Base (example in next section).

**Output Manager** deals with sending messages to external applications. It has been implemented in a publisher/subscriber fashion. There are three different channels in the system – the text channel, the interface command channel and the avatar command channel. Those channels can be subscribed by any connectors and handled respectively.

The original work behind the SC was based on a closed world where the user converses with the system. The SC initiates further conversation and in so doing elicits the discovery of tacit knowledge from the user.

Whilst conducting the initial tests, the limitations of this approach immediately became evident. As soon as the user interacted with the SC, the conversation quickly went through unexpected paths which required more knowledge than was stored within the knowledge-base. For example, when an elderly person is speaking with the SC about an old photograph taken during WWII, the person would easily recall events of the period. Our Hybrid-World approach tackles this issue. Initially, it makes use of a closed-world where all the information is stored in the Knowledge Base, but the system's second version was able to access open internet knowledge, initially in unstructured (text) format, which we convert to, or locate in, RDF format. Before discussing this we shall discuss the SC's basic process for extracting content from dialogue input.

## 4. DIALOGUE INPUT UNDERSTANDING AND INFERENCE

Every utterance is passed through the Natural Language Understanding (NLU) module for processing. This module uses a set of well-established natural language processing tools such as the GATE (Cunningham, et al., 1997) system. The basic processes carried out by GATE are: tokenizing, sentence splitting, POS tagging, parsing, semantic tagging and Named Entity Recognition.

These components have been further enhanced for the SC system by adding new and improved gazetteers. These include new locations and family relationships. The Named Entity (NE) recognizer is a key part of the NLU module and recognizes the significant entities required to process dialogue in the photo domain: PERSON NAMES, LOCATION NAMES, FAMILY RELATIONS and DATES.

Apart from the gazetteers mentioned earlier and the hundreds of extraction rules already present in GATE, new extraction rules using the JAPE rule language were also developed for the SC module. These included rules which identify complex dates, family relationships, negations and other information related to the SC domain. The following is an example of a simple rule used to identify relationship in utterances such as "Mary is my sister":

Using the rule in Box 1 with the example mentioned earlier, the rule interprets person1 as referring to the speaker so, if the name of the user speaking is John (which was known from previous conversations), it is utilized. Person2 is then the name of the person mentioned, i.e. Mary. This name is recognized by using the gazetteers we have in the system (which contain about 40,000 first names). The relationship is once again identified using the almost 800 unique relationships added to the gazetteer. With this information, the NLU module identifies Information Extraction patterns in the dialogue that represent significant content with respect to a user's life and photos.

The information obtained (such as Mary=sister-of John) is passed to the Dialogue Manager (DM) and then stored in the knowledge base (KB). The DM filters what to include and exclude from the KB. In this example, Mary is the sister of John, so the NLU knows that *sister* is a relationship between two people and is a key relationship. The NLU also discovers syntactical information such as the fact the both Mary and John are nouns.

*Box 1. Macro: RELATIONSHIP_IDENTIFIER*

```
(
({Token.category=="PRP$"}|{Token.category=="PRP"}|{Lookup.majorType=="person_
first"}):person2
({Token.string=="is"})
({Token.string=="my"}):person1
({Lookup.minorType=="Relationship"}):relationship
)
```

Even though this information is important, it is too low level to be of any use by the SC with respect to the user, i.e. the user is not interested in the part-of-speech of a word. Thus, this information is discarded by the DM and not stored in the KB. The NLU module also identifies a Dialogue Act Tag for each user utterance based on the DAMSL set of DA tags and prior work done jointly with the University of Albany (Webb et al., 2008).

The KB is a long-term store of information which makes it possible for the SC to retrieve information stored between different sessions. The information can be accessed anytime it is needed by simply invoking the relevant calls. The structure of the data in the database is an RDF triple, and the KB is more commonly referred to as a triple store.

In mathematical terms, a triple store is nothing more than a large database of interconnected graphs. Each triple is made up of a subject, a predicate and an object. So if we had to take the previous example, Mary sister-of John; Mary would be the subject, *sister-of* would be the predicate and John would be the object. If we had to imagine this graphically, Mary and John would be two distinct points in a 3D space and the sister-of relationship would be the line (or relationship) that joins these two points in space.

There are various advantages to using this structure; first, the relationship between different objects is explicitly defined using the predicates in the triples. The second advantage is that it is very easy to perform inferences on such data. So if in our KB, we add a new triple which states that Tom is the son of Mary, we can easily infer (by using the previous facts) that John is the uncle of Tom. The inference engine is an important part of the system because it allows us to discover new facts beyond what is elicited from the conversation with the user.

```
Uncle Inference Rule:

(?a sisterOf ?b),
(?x sonOf ?a),
(?b gender male) -> (?b uncleOf ?x)

Triples:

(Mary      sisterOf     John)
(Tom       sonOf        Mary)

Triples produced automatically by AN-
NIE (the semantic tagger):

(John      gender       male)

Inference:

(Mary      sisterOf     John)
(Tom       sonOf        Mary)
(John      gender       male)
->
 (John uncleOf Tom)
```

This kind of inference is already used by the SC and we have about 50 inference rules aimed at producing new data on the relationships domain. This combination of triple store, inference engine and inference rules makes a system which is weak but powerful enough to mimic human reasoning in this domain and thus give the SC minimal appearance of intelligence.

For our prototype we are using the JENA Semantic Web Framework for the inference engine together with a MySQL database as the knowledge base. However, this knowledge of family relationships is not enough to cover all the possible topics which can crop up during a conversation. In such circumstances, the DM switches to an open-world model and instructs the NLU to seek further information online.

## 5. THE HYBRID-WORLD APPROACH

When the DM requests further information on a particular topic, the NLU first checks with the KB whether the topic is about something known. At this stage, we have to keep in mind that any topic requested by the DM should already be in the KB since it was preprocessed by the NLU when it was mentioned in the utterance. So, if the user informs the system that the photograph was taken in Paris, (in response to a system question asking where the photo was taken), the utterance is first processed by the NLU which discovers that "Paris" is a location using its semantic tagger ANNIE (A Nearly New Information Extraction engine)[Annie]. The semantic tagger makes use of gazetteers and IE rules in order to accomplish this task. It also goes through the KB and retrieves any triples related to "Paris". Inference is then performed on this data and the new information generated by this process is stored back into the KB.

Once the type of the information is identified, the NLU can use various predefined strategies: In the case of locations, one of these strategies would be to seek for information in Wiki-Travel or Virtual Tourists. The system already knows how to query these sites and interpret their output by using predefined wrappers. A wrapper is essentially a file, which describes where a particular piece of information is located. This is then used to extract that information from the webpage. So a query is sent online to these sites and the information retrieved is stored in the triple-store and this information is then used by the DM to generate a reply.

In the previous example, the system managed to extract the best sightseeing spots in Paris. The NLU would then store in the KB triples such as [Paris, sight-seeing, Eiffel Tower] and the DM with the help of the NLG would ask the user "I've heard that the X is a very famous spot. Did you see it when you were there? "In this case, X will be replaced by the "Eiffel Tower".

On the other hand, if the topic requested by the DM is unknown or the semantic tagger is not capable of understanding the semantic category, the system uses a normal search engine. A query is sent to the search engines and the top pages are retrieved. These pages are then processed using ANNIE and the different attributes are analyzed. The standard attributes returned by ANNIE include information about Dialogue Acts, Polarity (i.e. whether a sentence has positive, negative or neutral connotations), Named Entities, Semantic Categories (such as dates and currency), etc. The system then filters the information collected by using generic patterns and generates a reply from the resultant information. So if the user is talking about cats, the system searches for cats online. It processes the pages and its current strategy is to identify all the statements by using Dialogue Acts. So in our example, the system would retrieve the following statements:

1. "Cats may be the most popular pet in the world"
2. "Cats recover quickly from falls"
3. "Some people do not like Persian Cats"

These statements are then checked for polarity and only the most polarity-distinct statements are kept (i.e. if the statements are prevailingly negative then the system will give a negative answer, and so on). The polarity checking is performed by using a list of words with negative or positive connotations and counting which words prevail in the sentence.

A sentence with a prevailing number of positive words is considered a positive sentence. The opposite occurs for negative words. In this example, the first two statements are prevailingly positive because of words such as "popular" and "recover" so the answer returned will be a positive one. The NLU would then select one of these two statements at random, send it to the DM and using the NLG, it would reply "You know that I have heard that X" where X is replaced with "cats may be the most popular pet in the world". ANNIE's polarity methods have been shown to be an adequate implementation of the general word-based polarity methods pioneered by Wiebe and her colleagues (see e.g. Akkaya et al., 2009).

## 6. CONCLUSION

In synthesis, this hybrid world approach allows us to focus on the closed world of images that exists between the user and the system but, when necessary, the system is allowed to venture cautiously in the open world, thus enriching the user experience. This is, as we noted, an important step towards breaking down the traditional closed-world assumptions of practical AI systems.

Initial experimental results show that on average the system adopts the open world approach 20% of the time. The open world approach adds facts to the database only when the topic under discussion is known to the system. So, in the previous example where the system asks whether the user visited the Eiffel Tower, a positive or negative reply will be stored in the database and used during later conversations.

However, when the topic is unknown such as in the case of the cats, the response of the SC is quite generic thus the conversation is not stored. During interactions with the system, it was noticed that the use of an open world approach (even when the subject was unknown by the system) produced a rather more realistic conversation than a system without the open world model. Users reported that they were amazed by the system possessed so much knowledge about the topic being discussed. We believe that the hybrid world model is potentially useful as a way of improving the interaction between the user and such systems. More detail on the expectations for the future of Companions is provided in Chapter 17.

## ACKNOWLEDGMENT

This work was funded by the Companions project www.companions-project.org) sponsored by the European Commission as part of the Information Society Technologies (IST) programme under EC grant number IST-FP6-034434.

## REFERENCES

Akkaya, C., Wiebe, J., & Mihalcea, R. (2009). Subjectivity word sense disambiguation. In *Proc. EMNLP.*

Catizone, R., Setzer, A., & Webb, N. (2002). Scaling-up information extraction. In *Proceedings of the Workshop on Event Modelling for Multilingual Document Linking, Language Resources and Evaluation Conference (LREC 2002),* Las Palmas, Canary Islands.

Catizone, R., Setzer, A., & Wilks, Y. (2003). Multimodal dialogue management in the COMIC project. In *Proc. Workshop on Dialogue Systems: interaction, adaptation and styles of management, European Chapter of the Association for Computational Linguistics* (EACL), Budapest, Hungary.

Cunningham, H., Humphreys, K., Gaizauskas, R., & Wilks, Y. (1997). GATE-a TIPSTER based general architecture for text engineering. In *Proceedings of the TIPSTER Text Program (Phase III) 6 Month Workshop*. DARPA, Morgan Kaufmann, CA.

Webb, N., Liu, T., Hepple, M., & Wilks, Y. (2008). Cross domain dialogue act tagging. In *Proceedings of the Sixth International Conference on Language Resources and Evaluation (LREC-08)*. Marrakech, Morocco.

Wilks, Y. (2007). Has there been progress on talking sensibly to computers? *Science*, 318.

Wilks, Y. (2008). The Semantic Web and the apotheosis of annotation. In *Proc. IEEE Intelligent Systems*. (May/June)

Wilks, Y., Catizone, R., & Mival, O. (2008). The companions paradigm as a method for eliciting and organising life data. In *Proc. Workshop on Memories for Life, British Computer Society*, London, March.

## INTERNET SITES

Annie:http://gate.ac.uk/sale/tao/splitch6.html#chap:annie

Memories for Life. http://www.memoriesforlife.org/

## KEY TERMS AND DEFINITIONS

**Conversational Internet Agents:** Computer programs accessible over the Internet that attempt to understand what is said and engage in a conversation—usually thought more intelligent than chatbots.

**Dialogue Action Forms:** Network structures used by the COMPANIONS project that attempt to capture the structure of a conversation and to model the alternative paths it can take.

**Dialogue Acts:** A way of categorizing utterances to and by a conversational agent so as to capture their "force" over and above their meaning—e.g. whether they are trying to get someone to do something or just to state a fact.

**Dialogue Manager:** An algorithm at the core of a computer conversation system that decides what the computational agent should say next.

**Extensible Markup Language (XML):** Is a set of rules for encoding documents in machine-readable form.

**Natural Language Generation:** A technology for assembling from parts the utterance that a computer will utter to reply to something a human has said.

**Natural Language Understander:** A technology by which a computational system attempts to decide the meaning of a text it has been fed.

**Ontological Information:** Information stored in a structure in a computer that expresses the relationship of concepts e.g. that aluminium is a metal.

**Semantic Web:** A new technology that aims to construct an Internet where the system of the web itself understands to some degree what it contains, differently from the world wide web that only contains texts and images but has no way of knowing what they express.

## ENDNOTE

1 http://opencv.willowgarage.com/wiki/

# Chapter 14
# Humanizing Conversational Agents:
## Indisys Practical Case Study in eHealth

**J. Gabriel Amores**
*Intelligent Dialogue Systems (Indisys), Spain*

**Pilar Manchón**
*Intelligent Dialogue Systems (Indisys), Spain*

**Guillermo Pérez**
*Intelligent Dialogue Systems (Indisys), Spain*

## ABSTRACT

*This chapter describes an eHealth human-like conversational agent called Maria embedded in the Web page of the Health Department of the Junta de Andalucía in Spain. Although this implementation is based on a strong theoretical background, a more practical approach has been preferred for the real-world case hereby described. Maria has been designed to perform several major tasks: she can arrange a doctor's appointment, reply to queries pertaining to many varied subdomains, and navigate through the Web page. One of Maria's most remarkable features is the successful application of advanced design and humanizing techniques which endow her with unusual skills and an enticing personality. Maria has been developed by Intelligent Dialogue Systems (Indisys) within a larger scale Web development project conducted by Sadiel SA.*

## 1 INTRODUCTION

Conversational Agents (CAs) can be defined as "communication technologies that integrate computational linguistics techniques with the communication channel of the Web to interpret and respond to statements made by users in ordinary natural language" (Lester et al., 2004). Embodied Conversational Agents (ECAs) are empowered with a human representation that shows some degree of empathy with the user as the dialogue goes on.

DOI: 10.4018/978-1-60960-617-6.ch014

The fact of adding explicit anthropomorphism in Conversational Agents has some effects over the solution designed:

- A number of the user interactions are actually social dialogue or "small-talk", where the users interact with the ECA informally (Robinson et al., 2008).
- Users may perceive the combination of embodied characters with advanced natural language processing techniques and social dialogue strategies positively. But on the other hand, if the language understanding performance or the social dialogue strategies behave poorly, users perceive the solution worse than the equivalent text-only chatbot without any character (De Angeli, Johnson, & Coventry, 2001; Schulman & Bickmore, 2009).

Deploying high-quality, intelligent ECAs which actually serve the purpose for which they were designed continues to be a challenge in a society which perceives computers as incredibly powerful machines for which natural language should be such a trivial task. In particular, failing to be successful in the first interactions seems to have a negative, long term impact on users, who are usually not very permissive. This situation becomes more critical as the linguistic coverage of the ECA is highly ambitious, which is the case of the application at hand.

Natural language processing for commercial ECAs applications shows some peculiarities. Usually, customers and service providers come to an agreement on the set of questions and services that the final users may request from the ECA. Customers demand optimal performance and fast reaction time over the previously agreed domain.

Throughout this chapter we will try to demonstrate how an adequate combination of design issues, solid theoretical background, and efficient computational techiques can actually produce the desired result. Since this is a commercial application, the project description provided is eminently practical and in terms of the different stages and components in the implementation.

Each section therefore provides relevant background on the specific issues discussed in that section, only to continue explaining how that research has been implemented in Maria. The chapter is organized as follows. Section 1 introduces the chapter. Section 2 describes the context of online ECAs. Section 3 focuses on the design principles which have guided the development of Maria. Section 4 describes the application from the perspective of eHealth and natural language complexity. Section 5 outlines how the design principles and the natural language complexity described in Sections 3 and 4 are reflected in the functional components of the system's architecture. Finally, Section 6 concludes with an analysis of the application's performance, user's perception and statistics of use after its first 2 months of deployment.

In the context of the type of applications described in this chapter, the "humanizing" process of ECAs is understood in terms of the overall outcome rather than just the specific humanizing techniques described in forthcoming sections. Maria's level of humanization is reached only through the combination of state-of-the-art Natural Language Processing and Dialogue Management technology described in Section 4, with the additional design and cognitive strategies illustrated in Section 3. It is therefore important to portray the solution in terms of all its components and implementation levels in order to understand its complexity and potential for further development.

## 2 RELATED WORK

Since the first appearance of ELIZA (Weizenbaum, 1966), a naïf rule-based system that simulated a psychotherapist, a huge number of different chatbots has been published on the web. The holy grail of these applications has always been the Turing

*Table 1.*

| | | |
|---|---|---|
| **Generation 1** | **Agent** | Primitive cartoon character |
| | **RoR**[1] | Poor search results |
| | **Interaction** | Mostly text based Q&A |
| **Generation 2** | **Agent** | Moving animated gif |
| | **RoR** | Better search results; basic decision tree |
| | **Interaction** | Mostly text input with some voice delivery |
| **Generation 3** | **Agent** | Human form assistant but still animated |
| | **RoR** | Good search results; reporting |
| | **Interaction** | Text-Text, Text-Speech, Speech-Text |
| **Generation 4** | **Agent** | Excellent photographic human image |
| | **RoR** | Great search results; high level accuracy; built-in dashboard; Often including mobile solutions. |
| | **Interaction** | Text-Text, Text-Speech, Speech-Text, Speech-Speech |
| **Generation 5** | **Agent** | 3D human image |
| | **RoR** | Great search results; high level accuracy; built-in dashboard; Mobile solutions; user feedback requests. |
| | **Interaction** | Text-Text, Text-Speech, Speech-Text, Speech-Speech; Mobile solutions |

test (Turing, 1950), considered as the proof of real intelligence in artificial systems. In 1991, the Loebner prize (http://loebner.net/Prizef/loebner-prize.html) was founded with the noble objective of promoting the research and development of these systems. This well recognized competition awards bronze, silver and gold medals, the lattest being reserved for the first system capable of passing the Turing test. No system has ever been awarded the gold medal yet. The Loebner prize has helped disseminate systems like the "PC Therapist" (winner in 1991, 1992, 1993 and 1995) or ALICE (winner in 2000, 2001 and 2004).

From an industrial point of view, ECAs are usually referred to as "Virtual Assistants", VAs, (aka "Digital Assistants"), although it could be argued that not all VAs can be considered ***conversational***. VAs may or not be embodied, may or not handle natural language, and may or not manage dialogue at any level. Sometimes VAs are just advanced search engines that may or not be sugar-coated with an animated agent.

What seems to be crystal clear is that the market for online conversational agents is growing all around the world. Acording to the Gartner Group (Jacobs, 2010), the eServices market will grow 20% just in 2010. As of today, online VAs can be found in almost every first-world country and every sector. A growing demand implies more investment on further research and, hopefully, more long-lusted scientific breakthroughs in the area and performance boosts.

The Gartner Group classifies VAs into 5 generations according to the criteria in Table 1 (Jacobs, 2010).

According to this classification, Maria would be a combination of Generation 2 (text input only), Generation 3 (animated human agent), Generation 4 (great search results; high-level accuracy and built-in dashboard) and Generation 5 (user feedback requests).

This classification, although useful from a commercial point of view, can be however rather misleading from the scientific research point of view. Many of the research key features are not directly taken into account in the classification but rather considered as additional "*key factors*":

- Multimodal interactions.
- Speech recognition performance.
- Intelligence, dialogue management and natural language understanding.
- Animation quality, video output, streaming, rendering, etc.
- Humanization and user perception.

Unfortunately, there is no classification at hand that defines the level of "*humanization*" a VA or an ECA has reached. As we will see in forthcoming sections, different levels of intelligence as well as other human-like features implemented in Maria have a positive impact on user acceptance and willingness to use the system. As to measuring the level of humanization of a VA, the challenge is still to be overcome.

## 3 DESIGN ISSUES

User Centered Design (UCD) is one of the most representative design methodologies in industry and has significantly extended during the last few years. Nonetheless, it is not quite as widespread as it could be expected. Advanced design methodologies as well as other disciplines such as VUI design, or Human Factors and Usability testing are largely underestimated.

Indisys, however, has developed its own UCD-based approach: the "*Holistic Approach Design*" or HAD where UCD (*User Centered Design*), HCD (*Human Centered Design*), ACD (*Activity Centered Design*) and even TCD (*Technology Centered Design*) are integrated in a symbiotic relationship (Manchón, 2009). 'User motivation' in data collection and closeness to real world situations are of great relevance. HAD stands for the synthesis and refinement of previous approaches, combining their advantages into a more balanced solution, contributing to the expansion of human-aware methodologies.

Additionally, another important aspect of the framework hereby presented is the "Humanization" of conversational agents and the cognitive strategies applied to achieve optimal results. In this section we will also analyze the impact these considerations have on the design of an ECA.

Maria is an excellent example of the successful application of the design methodology hereby described.

### 3.1 Holistic Approach Design

HAD stands for the synthesis and refinement of previous approaches, combining their advantages into a more balanced solution, together with the addition of some relevant considerations.

Recent surveys in the field (Mao & Vredenburg, 2001; Mao et al., 2005) indicate that the most critical indicator of good UCD is "Customer satisfaction", followed by other important indicators such as "Ease of use" and "Impact on sales". The top five most important commonly used UCD methods used in industry are: iterative design, usability evaluation, field studies, task analysis and informal expert review. These methods are followed closely by focus groups, formal heuristic evaluation, and user interviews. Nonetheless, it seems that UCD is not as extended nor as well-regarded as it should be.

The main objectives of the compilatory approach hereby described are:

1. Optimizing design for focus-groups of users.
2. Analyzing a range of user models to optimize adaptation.
3. Optimizing design to achieve top efficiency.
4. Exploiting technology without imposing the way to use it.
5. Re-using existing methodologies to distil the most appropriate solution.
6. Ensuring objective results evaluation.

7. Applying the spiral-design cycle and Extreme Programming strategies to ensure robust test cases.
8. Minimizing post-launch tuning.
9. Reusable results.
10. Above all, focusing on real-world situations.

This set of requirements can be understood as the application of all principles of UCD in its broader sense (analogous to HCD) (Iivari & Iivari, 2006), together with a profound understanding of the activities and tasks to be performed (ACD). Although the focus of TCD can be considered out-of-fashion, the spirit of this approach is also recycled here. TCD focuses on technology as a goal in itself rather than as the means to perform a task or activity.

Processing speed, efficiency and robustness are all important qualities, but when they surpass what makes a difference in terms of the human user behind it, progress in these areas becomes stale in terms of usability (Manchón, 2009). However, it is also true that once we humans become familiar with a technology and '***accept it***', we are more willing to adapt to the technology if the gain is appealing enough. Therefore, improving the technology beyond what a standard user would be capable of using it for could indeed be useful for very advanced users. This may become more evident in the case where the technology is used for professional purposes, when efficiency may be a plus and training may not be a problem.

Another remarkable feature of the design methodology used here is the emphasis placed on '*user motivation during data collection*'. Although UCD and HCD both focus on user issues such as profile, tasks, goals, skills, etcetera, as far as the literature goes, motivation is analyzed in terms of the focus group applications are designed for. However, user motivation during the data collection process has never been in the priority list, to the best of our knowledge.

Beyond the application of specific techniques to data collection and so on, HAD has much more to offer. An additional key aspect of the Indisys's ECA designed under HAD is the concept of adding not only 'intelligence' but also 'cleverness', 'social acceptance' and 'user trust'. It is in the application of these considerations that Cognitive Science, Psychology and Sociology studies come into play in the development of intelligent conversational agents.

In Maria's case, *HAD* has been applied to its full extent: iterative spiral design cycle, exhaustive user requirements and task/activity analysis, real and artificial corpora generation and analysis, a formalized expert review process, and a formal heuristic evaluation. The application was reviewed and corrected until the internal quality threshold was reached. Then naïve-subject usability and human factors testing was performed. Nonetheless, once the application is deployed, additional data was collected and analyzed for fine-tuning. Linguistic, Cognitive Science and Sociology strategies are conjoined to optimize efficiency, flexibility, robustness and naturalness, according to the specific needs and priorities of the application domain.

Although this is obviously an effort-intensive and costly process, we have nonetheless corroborated that it endows the systems with a high level of robustness only to be enhanced by continuous fine-tuning.

Fortunately, industry is slowly waking up to these concepts and understanding their importance and the need of highly qualified and specialized professionals to do the job. Indisys is pioneering this movement in the field of intelligent ECA.

## 3.2 Humanizing Design

Another important aspect of the framework hereby presented is the "Humanization" of conversational agents and the cognitive strategies applied to achieve optimal results. The psychological and HCI research in this area confirms that:

1. Virtual characters provide a more natural and humanlike interaction between human users and automated systems (Isbister & Nass, 2000; Manchón et al., 2007)
2. Endowing that character with human traits such as personality, name, expressiveness, etc., enhances the user experience (Isbister & Nass, 2000; Reeves & Nass, 1996; Thomas & Johnston, 1981).
3. Intelligence and/or cleverness are key to increase the user satisfaction (Manchón, 2009).

Developing well-rounded, clear and consistent personalities (Cassell, McNeill, & McCullough, 1998) to achieve best results and engage the user in the communication process has proven to be of enormous importance. Indisys's virtual humans have been endowed with additional degrees of intelligence, achieving a remarkable humanlike conversational ability, and optimizing the user experience.

The effective use and implementation of the research results in neighboring areas such as Social Intelligence, Emotional Intelligence and Cognitive Ergonomics have a noticeable impact on the quality and capabilities of the conversational agents hereby depicted and therefore represent a step forward in the race towards humanlike dialogue systems.

'Social Intelligence', 'Social Cognition' or 'Interpersonal Intelligence' (Gardner, 1983; Gardner, 1993; Gardner, 1999) can be defined as the intelligence behind the individual and/or the group behavior in a complex society. Recent proposals discuss a number of factors relevant in social intelligence such as Situational Awareness, Presence, Authenticity, Clarity, and Empathy (Albrecht, 2005); other approaches from neuroscience research point at the importance of two factors: Social Awareness and Social Facility. The former includes empathy, attunement, empathic accuracy, and social cognition; the latter includes synchrony, self-presentation, influence, and concern. When designing the personality and behavior of Maria, the following factors have been taken into account: Situational Awareness, Self presentation, Attunement, Clarity and Empathy (Manchón, 2009).

'Emotional Intelligence' could be defined as the ability to manage emotions. This implies detecting, appraising and in the case of one's self, displaying emotions suitably (Bos & Gabsdil, 2000; Goleman, 1995). There is no consensus about the definition of Emotional Intelligence, the way to measure it or its true nature. Nonetheless, what has been prioritized in the implementation of this character is the fact that the ability to understand, manage and display emotions correctly in any given situation generates an appearance of intelligence or appropriateness, which enhances the impression of humanlike communication.

The main goal of cognitive ergonomics is adapting artificial entities or settings to the cognitive abilities or limitations of human beings, mostly in order to optimize the human performance at all possible levels (Cañas, & Waern, 2001; Cañas, 2003; Long, 1987). In Maria's case, the application of cognitive ergonomics has been focused on bringing human-computer interaction as close as possible to human-human interaction, and exploiting the advantages of artificial entities to lighten the user's cognitive effort to communicate (Manchón, 2009). This is achieved for instance by using human-human collaborative strategies during communication, such as the effort speakers make to adapt to their interlocutor when they are speaking; this is particularly the case where the virtual character is providing a service and the human interlocutor is requesting the service.

Additionally, the inclusion of cultural and/or general knowledge in intelligent systems also increases the perception of intelligence from the users' perspective (Manchón, 2009).

In Maria's case, the main humanizing strategies have been applied. Her looks evoke the style of a typical Andalusian woman and her expressions range from happiness to anger, including surprise, doubt, fear, embarrassment and disgust.

*Figure 1. Functional components*

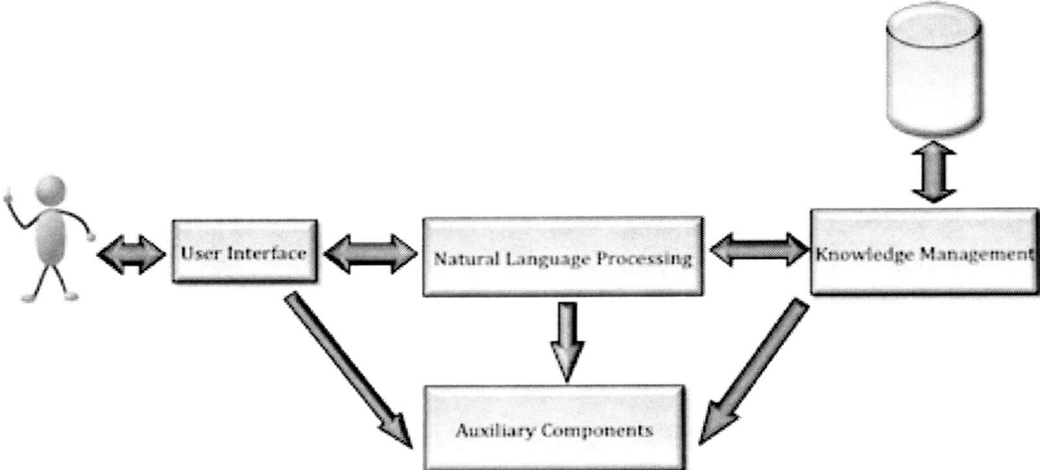


Her ability to display an emotional response to the user's actions grants her an emotional dimension, which is reinforced by the empathy she is also able to convey if necessary. Her synthetic voice is synchronized with her lip movement, and her body language is very natural: she breaths, blinks, moves, nods, looks around, etc.

Maria has also been endowed with a rather sober personality, which does not prevent her however from surprising the user occasionally. Her ability to understand chitchat-like inputs and other out-of-domain questions, terms and observations grants her more humanlike depth, which in turn makes users more at ease with her overall. Her likes and dislikes also provide a means for users to profile her, to form and opinion on her at a similar level at which humans relate to other humans. She also projects a sense of belonging somewhere, being born and relating to family and friends, which are features that make us humans 'normal', as opposed to social outcasts or detached artificial entities.

Every humanizing detail contributes to building Maria's image as a valid interlocutor (Fiske & Taylor, 1991; Cassell, McNeill, & McCullough, 1998; Cantor & Mischel, 1979), a social actor (Reeves & Nass, 1996), a reliable service provider and therefore, a valuable asset in any company or organization.

## 4 FUNCTIONAL COMPONENTS

Indisys conversational agents rely on a modular architecture designed to allow for flexible configuration in different application domains, different languages and even different interaction modalities. Every component has a separate language and domain independent execution layer, and a specification layer based on plain text configuration files. (Figure 1)

The modules can be classified into four different groups: Natural Language, Knowledge Management, User Interface and Auxiliary Components. This section provides a short description of each of those modules.

### 4.1 NL Components

These submodules manage all interactions and therefore constitute the core of the system. The NLU (Natural Language Understanding) module generates the semantic representations of the user's utterances; the Dialogue Manager keeps track of the dialogue history and runs dialogue strategies; and finally, the Natural Language Output module generates the NL outputs of the system.

## 4.2 Natural Language Understanding

Incoming user sentences are processed in two phases:

- Lexical Analysis: during this phase the lexical analysis submodule proposes lexical units for the input according to a predefined dictionary. In Maria's case, this dictionary contains over one million Spanish terms.
- Grammatical Analysis: in this phase, a unification based context free parser, analyzes the whole sentence and provides the dialogue manager with its semantic representation. This module is mainly based on LFG (Bresnan, 1982). Two different structures are generated: the C-structure and the F-structure. The former consists of a language-dependent parsing tree, and the latter is a set of language independent attribute-value pairs.

Other approaches include a third, semantic analysis phase. However, in the solution hereby described the semantic information is embedded into the lexical and grammatical configuration, and therefore, no explicit semantic layer is necessary. The F-Structure constitutes the semantic representation of the input sentence.

In terms of computational complexity, this submodule is the most time and resource consuming. However, processing time remains below 100 milliseconds in the worst-case scenario (very long sentences, recursive rules, etc.). It is therefore negligible compared to the network latency.

## 4.3 Dialogue Manager

According to (Amores, Pérez, & Manchón, 2010) there are up to eight non mutually exclusive types of dialogue manager approaches:

- Dialogue Grammars: where the dialogue structure is analyzed in a similar way as a sentence structure is parsed with a syntactic parser.
- Finite State Machines: the dialogue structure is modeled as a states transition network where the nodes are the turns and the arcs are the user options
- Frame Models: similar to the finite state approach but with a higher degree of flexibility. This approach makes use of slot filling templates.
- Plan-Based: these modules try to identify the global goal of the user, hidden behind the dialogue acts.
- Conversational Games: a combination of Plan-Based and Dialogue Grammars.
- Collaborative Models: both participants share the information trying to reach a common understanding.
- Stochastic Approaches: this family of dialogue managers includes those that try to get dialogue patterns out of a Corpus of tagged dialogues applying Machine Learning techniques. The ones that have claimed best results are based on Reinforcement Learning (Henderson, Lemon, & Georgila, 2005) and POMDP (Williams & Young, 2007).
- Information State Update (ISU) Approach: the idea of information state update for dialogue modeling is centered on the information state (IS). Within the IS, the current state of the dialogue is explicitly represented. "*The term Information State of a dialogue represents the information necessary to distinguish it from other dialogues, representing the cumulative additions from*

*previous actions in the dialogue, and motivating future action*" (Larsson & Traum, 2000).

Maria's dialogue manager component used can be considered mainly an ISU based one, but has several features typically included in some of the other approaches. A set of update dialogue rules are defined for every subdomain within the application. These rules can be triggered by an incoming input sentence or by another dialogue rule. The dialogue rules transform the Information State with the new incoming information, increasing the system knowledge as the dialogue goes on.

## 4.4 Natural Language Output

Although a full, template-based natural language generation submodule (Amores, Pérez, & Manchón, 2006) has been integrated with our system for other scenarios, the prompts provided by Maria were canned text included in an external database. The reason why this natural language section was placed outside of the system was that the medical doctors team needed to have instant access to the answers and be able to easily modify them at any time (e.g. the legislation regarding abortion and anti-conceptive pills changed during the course of the project, and needed appropriate revision).

An additional functionality included in this module regards the random selection of possible outputs in order to avoid a monolithic and tedious repetition of frequently ocurring messages, such as *Hello, Sorry, I don't quite understand*, and enhance flexibility and naturalness.

## 4.5 Knowledge Management Components

These submodules connect the system with external knowledge sources, such as the customer databases or web services. Also within this group, an indexation submodule parses the customer web page and indexes all concepts (not just the terms) within the web site.

Maria is connected to an Andalusian government database with over four million users. This enables the Virtual Assistant to help users schedule, cancel or modify their doctor appointments.

Regarding the indexation of the web site, the process is divided into two stages: offline and online.

- During the offline phase, the system crawls the site, segmenting every sentence in every web the crawler pulls. These sentences are then parsed by the NLU module, which in turn logs the parsing results and links them to the hosting web page.
- During the online phase, the Virtual Assistant accesses the indexation database through the Knowledge Manager and pulls the web pages where the concepts the user is interested in appear.

This process endows the indexation with a semantic layer, enabling the system to associate concepts (and not only isolated terms) to URLs.

## 4.6 User Interface Components

The User Interface level encompasses the graphical agent as well as a number of additional elements. Figure 2 shows the different components:

The usability of the Agent is maximized by including a whole range of facial expressions that improves the empathy with the user. The Virtual Assistant is also empowered with different animations as well as voice and lip synchronization.

One of the key concerns in Maria's graphical interface design is usability. In order to optimize both accessibility and usability, a number of aspects have been carefully analyzed and improved through various rounds of testing. Font size control, information visualization, help tips and a full range of facial expressions and animations have been implemented, achieving a higher level

*Figure 2. User interface*

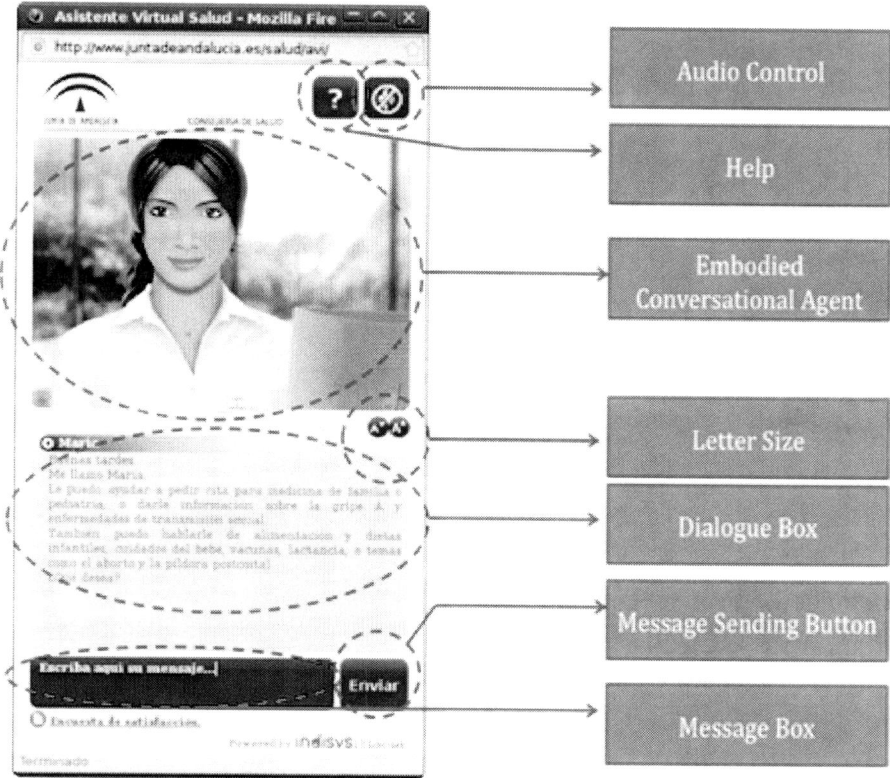


of usability. Voice and lip synchronization has also been carefully designed. These abilities and features have a significant impact on the user's perception and sense of shared empathy, as has already been mentioned.

Figure 3 illustrates some of the expressions Maria may choose to disclose throughout the interaction with the user.

Both user sessions and security measures are also managed at User Interface level. One of the security measures implemented is for example a specific anti-denial-of-service mechanism that prevents massive attacks from stopping the service. Other measures prevent man-in-the-middle situations or even internal hacker attacks.

## 4.7 Auxiliary Components

These submodules provide additional functionalities:

- Logging: All the conversations as well as the main relevant checkpoints in each dialogue are stored in a database. Additionally, important technical data such as response time, origin IP address, etc. are logged.
- Alarms: Whenever and unusual situation takes place, the system registers an alarm. Depending on its severity, it can just be loaded in the database or sent by email to the support team.
- Monitoring: A web based tool provides real-time reports to customers, including both general information such as the num-

*Figure 3. Maria's range of facial expressions*

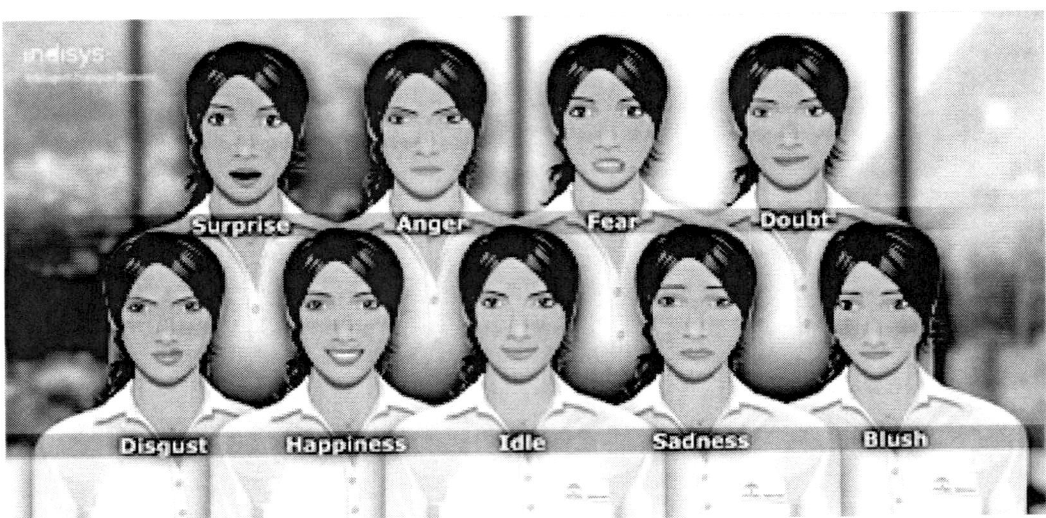


ber and temporal distribution of dialogues, and domain-specific information such as the distribution of users' requests.

## 5 NATURAL LANGUAGE COVERAGE

From a natural language understanding point of view, Maria has been designed to take part in a wide range of conversations: she can arrange a doctor's appointment, respond to 'personal' questions, engage in 'chit-chat' exchanges, identify who is who in the institution she works for, and reply to domain-specific questions regarding a set of pre-defined topics, such as sexually transmitted diseases, child care, the post-coital pill, abortion, eating habits, vaccination, swine flu, child nutrition, and breastfeeding. Just in-domain questions result in more than 400 hundred possible scenarios.

Most of these dialogue types go beyond the FAQ type of interaction, and require an adequate management of expectations. For example, child vaccination protocols vary depending on the age and previous vaccination history. In this particular example, seven different expectations must be managed in order to provide the exact vaccination advice. A similar type of complex scenario involving the management of many different scenarios takes place when the end user wishes to request, modify or delete a doctor's appointment: personal identification, doctor's speciality, date, and time of appointment must all be managed appropriately.

In addition, the user may wish to use the virtual assistant as an alternative, more user-friendly, search interface for the Institution's web page. Finally, if the user's input is not understood as part of any of the abovementioned scenarios, a search for near possible concepts in all the parent and subsidiary web pages will be launched.

At the end of the dialogue session, the user may also engage in a self-evaluation dialogue for a specific set of diseases, or fill in a customer satisfaction survey before leaving the application.

Thus, the natural language understanding module consists of five sub-grammars and lexicons:

1. General purpose lexicon and grammar for indexation purposes (web page search).
2. Maria's Personality.
3. Chit-chat.
4. Domain-specific, customer defined questions.
5. Appointments scheduling, modification and cancelation.

*Table 2. Sample dialogue*

| | |
|---|---|
| **User** | I have a few questions regarding child care |
| **Maria** | I may provide some pedriatic advice, such as caring of the umbilical cord, the heel prick test, bathing care, or Phenylketonuria.<br>Please, be more precise. |
| **User** | What is Phenylketonuria? |
| **Maria** | Phenylketonuria (PKU) is an inherited error of metabolism caused by a deficiency in the enzyme phenylalanine hydroxylase. Loss of this enzyme results in mental retardation, organ damage, unusual posture and can, in cases of maternal PKU, severely compromise pregnancy. |
| **User** | I am impressed! |
| **Maria** | Thank you. Is there anything else I can do for you? |
| **User** | What's your name? |
| **Maria** | My name is Maria. What else can I do for you? |
| **User** | Hello Maria, my name is Ann. |
| **Maria** | Hello Ann, Is there anything else I can do? |
| **User** | Is it correct to use soap whenever I bath my baby? |
| **Maria** | At an early state, it is only recommended to use soap if the baby is dirty, twice or three times a week. |
| **User** | How do I know which vaccines are due now? |
| **Maria** | Okay, Let me ask you some questions. Has the baby been vaccinated previously? |
| **User** | Yes |
| **Maria** | Does the baby have the vaccines which correspond to its age? |
| **User** | Dunno |
| **Maria** | I am afraid that in this case, the appropriate thing to do would be to go to your Health Center.<br>Would you like to see the child vaccination calendar? |
| **User** | Yes, please. |
| **Maria** | (Shows the vaccination calendar's web page) |
| **User** | Can I drink coffee and coke if I am breastfeeding? |
| **Maria** | Having one or two drinks with caffeine a day should not affect your baby. However, it should be taken into account that newborns and infants cannot eliminate caffeine as quickly as older children, and it might cause sleeplessness or uneasiness. Have you observed whether your baby is more uneasy after you have taken a drink with caffeine? |
| **User** | No. |
| **Maria** | Not to worry then, you may have two drinks with caffeine a day. |
| **User** | All right. Let's talk about something else. |
| **Maria** | Yes, What can I do for you? |
| **User** | My fifteen-year-old daughter wants to start a diet. What should I do? |
| **Maria** | Miracle diets in adolescents should be avoided. The goal should be to change her dietary habits, which should naturally result in lossing weight.<br>Let's see. Let me ask you a few questions.<br>Is her weight adequate for her sex and height? |
| **User** | Yes. |
| **Maria** | Do you want some advice on how to change her dietary habits? |
| **User** | Yes, please. |
| **Maria** | It is advisable not to reduce the number of calories drastically; replace unhealty foods with others like fruit and vegetables; avoid sugary and carbonated drinks; do some work out; eat slowly; have three meals a day and two smaller meals; do not skip any meal.<br>Do you suspect any eating disorder? |
| **User** | Yes |
| **Maria** | I recommend that you visit a specialist. |
| **User** | You are smart! |
| **Maria** | Thanks for the compliment, … |

Table 2 displays a dialogue session with Maria. Each of the dialogue samples above use a different syntax, lexical register and pragmatic context.

From a grammatical point of view, the application can parse a wide variety of linguistic constructions, such as question types (Wh-, Yes/No), statements, conditional constructions, cause-effect constructions, final clauses, right-node raising, coordination, topicalization, comparative constructions, negation, etc.

The application is also capable of dealing with complex linguistic phenomena such as anaphora and contextual resolution, and distinguishes between simple and complex commands. On top of this linguistic complexity, the application is equipped with a spell-checker and is capable of understanding usual, language-dependent short-message syntax and vocabulary, without punctuation or capitalization constraints. This capability increases linguistic ambiguity as well.

With such a wide variety of semantic domains and linguistic constructions at hand, avoiding ambiguity and overlapping is not a trivial task. The amount of context-free grammatical productions (around 7,300) and the size of the lexical database (20,000 lexical entries) in the domain give an idea of the complexity of the natural language understanding module.

Context-free productions in the domain contain semantic labels. An ontology of domain specific actions defines the range of functionality predefined in the application. Additionally, a general purpose set of context-free productions with syntactic labels are used to parse utterances outside of the domain. It is the parser's task to decide whether the input belongs to the domain or not. If the text input has been understood as belonging to the domain, an in-house semantic representation is returned by the parser and passed on to the dialogue manager. It is this intermediate natural language understanding module which makes our application particularly powerful.

The in-domain dialogue manager module comprises more than 200 different language-independent dialogue rules, many of which may be reused in other domains.

Maria is in a constant process of updating, both in terms of new functionality, and linguistic coverage in the existing domain. In order to prevent loss of coverage, it is tested over more than 4,600 different dialogues covering the questions in the client domain. Other tests are also carried out for other domains such as personality and chit-chat.

The development of such a complex and wide coverage application calls doubt on how non-rule-based approaches (especially statistics) would perform. In the domains at hand, just a subtle difference in the input sentence may lead to different responses from the dialogue manager. For example, the following two input sentences will receive a different answer from Maria:

- *Can I vaccinate if the previous dose of a different vaccine caused reaction?*
- *Can I vaccinate if the previous dose of this vaccine caused reaction?*

## 5.1 Cooperativeness and Coverage Convergence

Perhaps one of the most difficult problems in ambitious, broad-coverage dialogue systems is not failing the user's expectations, while preserving the system's ability to engage in mixed initiative dialogues. On the one hand, only a set of predefined questions which the client considers more likely to be issued will receive a specific answer by Maria. On the other, health is a vast domain, and the case load is immeasurable. How can these two extremes converge?

A number of strategies have been designed which try to minimize this gap, but a 100% fail safe strategy is, to our knowledge, beyond the current technology.

a. Opening: Maria introduces herself and sets the scene of the types of questions she can deal with.

*I may help you schedule an appointment with pediatrics or GP, or give you information about swine flu (NH1N1), or sexually transmitted diseases.*

*I can also provide information related to child nutrition and food habits, newborns care, vaccination, breastfeeding, or topics such as abortion and the postcoital pill.*

*How can I help you?*

This narrows the domain somehow, but the user may still want to use the system as a general purpose search engine, such as *Give me the telephone of Marbella's hospital*.

b. Close extrapolation:

In the child care subdomain, Maria has a specific answer for a question like *What should I do if the umbilical cord bleeds copiously?* First, she will enquire about the texture of the blood, and depending on the answer, she will provide a different advice.

Now consider a question like *What should I do if my nose bleeds?* for which no specific answer has been provided. In this case, Maria will combine information from related questions, and perform a closer search in the web portal:

*I don't have specific information about bleeding in that body part. Let me search the web.*

c) Guiding the user:

Also within the subdomain of child care, Maria may reply to some questions related to newborn baths. However, the user's question may be underspecified, as in *Bathing cares*. In this case, Maria replies cooperatively, showing hyperlinks of questions for which she has a reply:

*I am afraid I don't have specific information about that.*

*At present I may reply to related questions such as:*

- *How should I care my baby if he has been circumcisized?,*
- *What should I do if my baby has diaper irritation?,*
- *How should I bath my baby's head?,*
- *Steps to follow when cleaning the teat of the bottle*

User's underspecification may go a step forward, as in *I need some pediatric advice*. In this case, Maria will try the user to narrow his/her question to some of the subtopics she can handle:

*I can provide some pediatrics-related information such as how to care a baby's umbilical cord, what is the heel test, and when should it be done, what is Phenylketonuria, or cares when bathing a newborn.*

*Please, be more precise.*

## 6 USER AND CLIENT PERCEPTION

This section provides an analysis of the preliminary data collected during the first two months of service. It is important to highlight that, in order to allow for a period of fine-tuning, no specific dissemination activities for public awareness of Maria had been put in place at this point. This process will ensure optimal performance once the gross of the population becomes aware of the new service.

The data collected so far may give us an idea of the initial system's performance, and users' level of satisfaction and perception. Additionally, preliminary statistics on users' interests and service requests are available. This information will be used to improve Maria's performance and coverage in future versions. The system's performance as well as the users' level of satisfaction is expected to increase as the application is fine-tuned.

Figure 4 shows the distribution of daily accesses in the first two months, starting on March 10th 2010. After the expected peak during the first few days due to limited dissemination and post-launch testing, the average number of dialogues has preliminary settled on around 200 dialogues per day.

Analyzing the distribution of dialogues as a function of the hour, it can be shown how, as expected, the number of users decreases during the night hours. It is also noticeable how the number of dialogues is clearly higher during the morning and decreases in the afternoon.

From a performance point of view, it must be highlighted that up to 92% of the inputs have been parsed by Maria, that is, an appropriate answer has been provided to the user. Only 8% of the inputs were not understood by Maria.

In terms of user interests, Figure 6 shows how 45% of the user inputs are in-domain utterances (34% of doctor appointments, 11% of

*Figure 4. Daily accesses during the first two months*

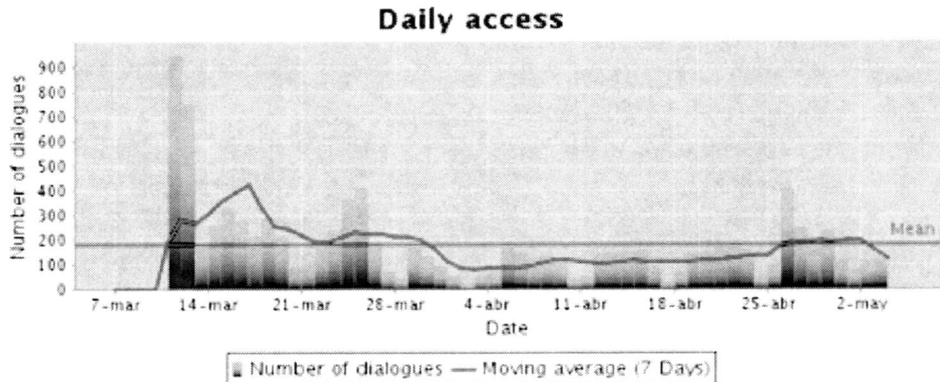


*Figure 5. Distribution of dialogues per hour and "check points"*

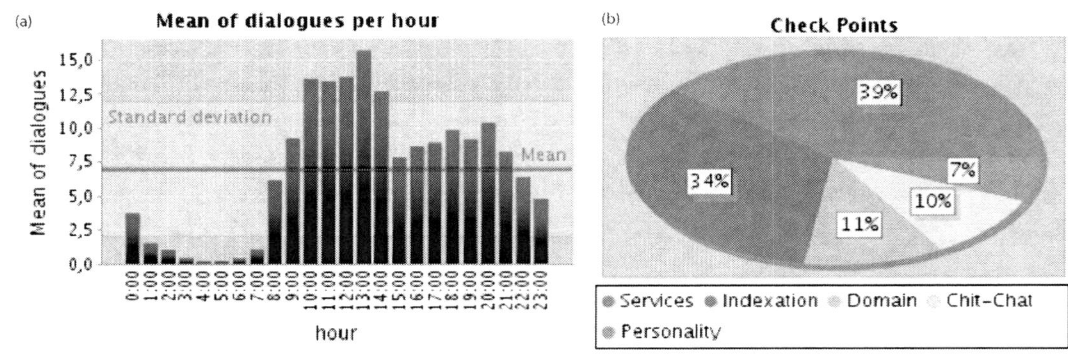


general questions), while 17% engages in social dialogues with the Assistant (10% Chit-Chat and 7% Personal questions).

The remaining 39% of the inputs are classified as "indexation results" which corresponds to out-of-domain user inputs, for which Maria has provided relevant matches available in the customer's site.

Users were also encouraged to perform a user satisfaction survey before leaving the application. The current data proves that only 3.4% of the users actually filled in the survey. Users usually need motivation to fill in surveys; we can consider that, in general, and without any additional incentive available, users have more of a tendency to fill in surveys when they are either very pleased or very unpleased with the service provided. Although 3.4% is a small percentage, the results can be considered quite positive.

## 7 CONCLUSION

This chapter has introduced Maria, an embodied conversational agent in Spanish, which has been deployed in the web page of the Regional Government of Andalucia's Health portal.

Maria's success is the result of advanced user-centered design and humanization strategies, efficient computational techniques and a sound theoretical background. The combination of these three aspects ensures the scalability of

*Figure 6. User requests distribution*

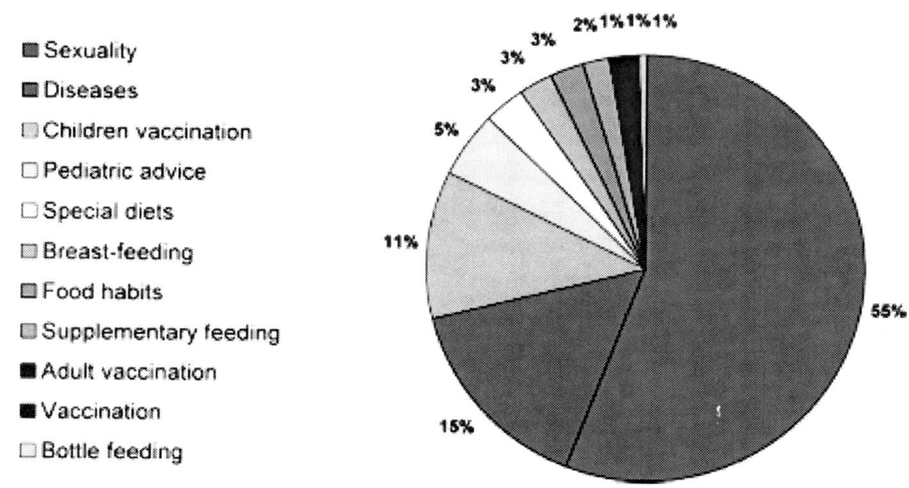


*Figure 7. User satisfaction survey*

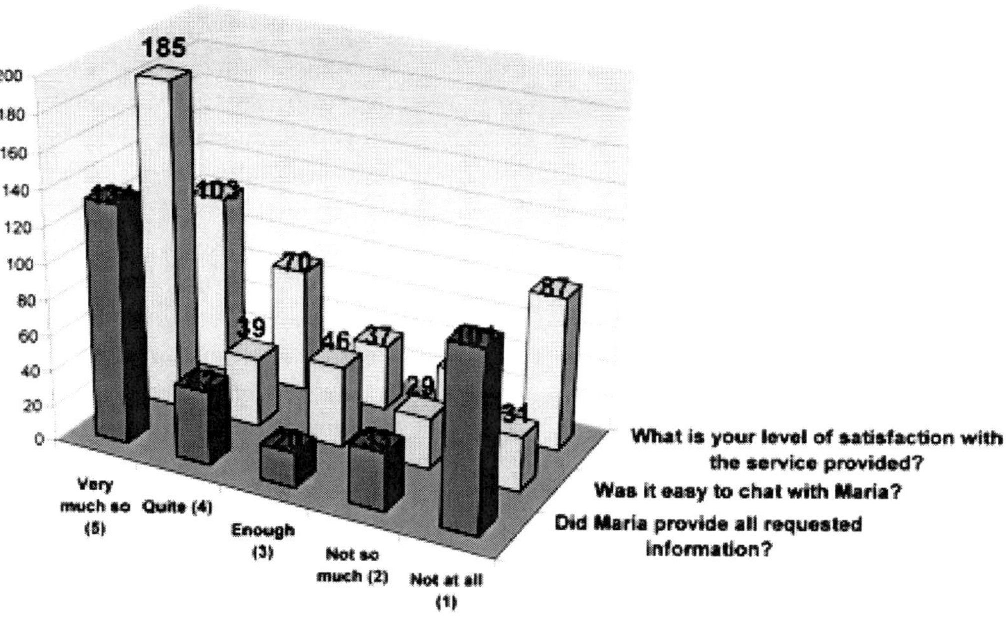

the system with new services and questions from the health domain. Even though Maria has only been in service for three months, she has been already awarded numerous compliments and recognitions from users and institutions. Intelligent conversational agents like Maria will surely contribute to closer, friendlier, and more efficient web services for the general public, especially in e-government scenarios.

We have seen throughout this chapter different aspects that define Maria as an amicable, accessible, efficient and human-like online service that brings the e-administration closer to citizens of all ages, cultural levels and computer skills. Maria represents therefore a step forward in Human-Computer Interfaces in general and e-government applications in particular.

This successful experience opens up the path for a legion of well-trained and humanlike intelligent ECAs that may in time achieve great results in the wide spreading of highly specialized information and services. These advanced ECAs' pseudo-human traits and conversational intelligence have proven effective in the arduous ordeal of overcoming some major human-computer interactions barriers.

To the best of our knowledge, there is no ECA Maria can be fully measured up to. There are a few health-related virtual assistants already in place, but since the content coverage and services provided are significantly inferior in quantity and complexity to those offered by Maria, and no in-depth technical description of such solutions is available, proper contrastive evaluation is hardly possible.

## 8 FUTURE RESEARCH DIRECTIONS

Giving the continuous advancements made available through the ongoing research activities in this area, several improvements are currently available in ECA and will hopefully be gradually incorporated into Maria:

- **3D characters:** research in HCI underlines the importance of intelligence and human-like, natural interaction, as well as depth and coherence in the character's personality and behavioral design (Manchón, 2009). Another relevant feature is the graphical interface quality and the concordance between the quality of the graphical character and the intelligence users perceive (De Angeli et al., 2001). The newest applications in this area are starting to offer higher quality 3D characters. These new characters, however, do not always represent and advancement in the overall human-computer communication process. While the graphical character's quality increases, the system latency imposed by much heavier interfaces often make some ECA difficult to interact with in real time and rather unnatural. Indisys's research in this area has been able to generate 3D photo-realistic agents. This new 3D characters are nonetheless very light-weight which allows for highly efficient and real time interaction, bringing users deeper into the illusion of a human-human video-conference, and increasing user satisfaction, trust and willingness to interact with the system.
- **Multilinguality:** as of today, Maria is only available in Spanish. Additional languages (Catalan, Basque, Galician, English, French, etc.) are already possible with Indisys's multilingual technology. It is only a matter of time that Maria becomes available to a wider range of users. This feature could be available both under explicit request (*"please, speak in English"*) and also upon automatic language identification.
- **Mobile Virtual Assistants:** another relevant and recent breakthrough is the integration of the 3D and intellligent ECA in the mobile environment. Given the processing limitations of mobile devices, there

*Figure 8. Indisys 3D agents*

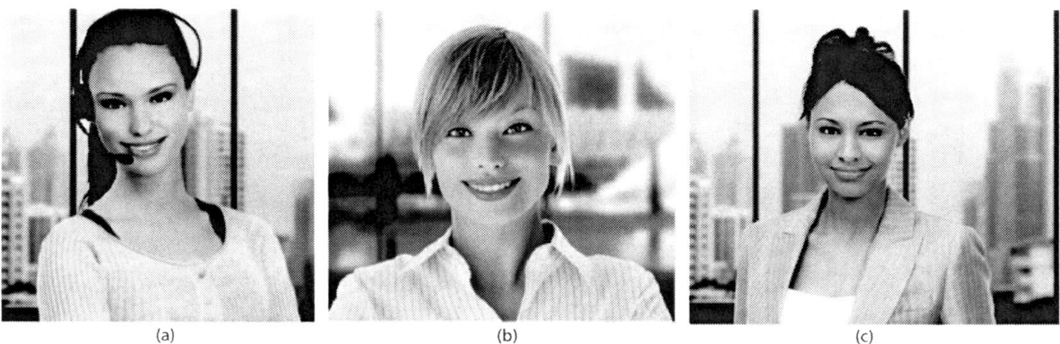


is usually a decrease in the quality of the graphical agents in order to minimize the impact on the overall system performance. Indisys has been able to integrate high-quality 3D and photo-realistic characters in Android-based mobile devices, with no performance decrease.

Yet, many challenges lie ahead and therefore much research in this area is still necessary:

- **Usability in mobile devices:** although the integration of these solutions in the mobile world is already a fact, there are still pending issues in terms of the usability of these interfaces in mobile devices. The limitations in screen size raises information visualization issues; the keyboard size and typing strategies are also relevant; the language users employ in mobile devices also raise some issues regarding natural language processing, spelling correction and message ambiguity.
- **Speech input:** adding speech input as one of the functionalities of the Virtual Assistants is already a fact. Indisys, for instance, already has a speech-enabled application on Android. However, there are still a number of important limitations. The limiting factors are manifold: ASR still lacks the desirable robustness and the trade-off between performance and coverage would impose a significant coverage reduction; the jittering effect on online communications significantly penalizes performance; users need good quality microphones that guarantee sufficient voice quality; ASR technology significantly increases the solution cost.
- **Improvements in Natural Language Processing:** this is a never ending research area, with plenty of well founded proposals. Two of them are currently under evaluation for future application:
    - Reinforcement Learning at dialogue level: recent works show how the dialogue management can be improved by using Reinforcement Learning techniques (Henderson et al., 2005), and more specifically POMDP approaches (Williams & Young, 2007) when the systems chooses and applies the dialogue policy. The corpus of real interactions that is currently being built as users access Maria will provide valuable insight and structured data that could be used for this purpose in the near future.
    - Reranking parsing results: choosing the correct semantic interpretation of the user's utterances is crucial to improve customer satisfaction. Some

*Figure 9. Mobile virtual assistants*

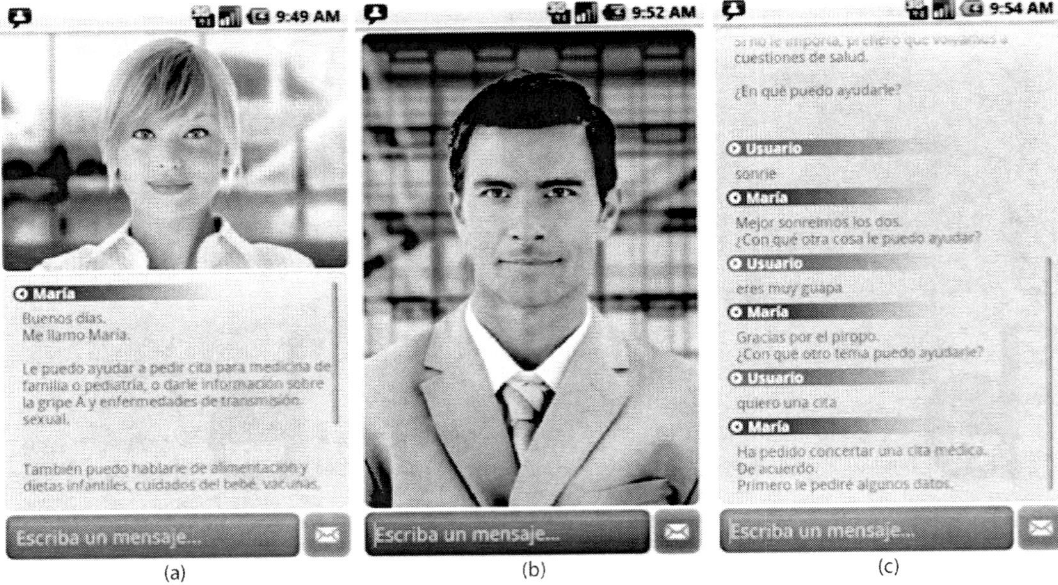


authors (Charniak & Johnson, 2005; Riezler et al., 2002) propose reranking the parsing results using a Maximum Entropy approach. In Collins and Koo (2003), a similar strategy using boosting algorithms is proposed. All these approaches could potentially be applied in the near future.

## 9 REFERENCES


Albrecht, K. (2005). *Social intelligence: The new science of success*. Retrieved from http://eu.wiley.com/WileyCDA/WileyTitle/productCd-0787979384.html

Amores, J. G., Pérez, G., & Manchón, P. (2006). Reusing MT components in natural language generation for dialogue systems. *Procesamiento de Lenguaje Natural*, *37*, 215–221.

Amores, J. G., Pérez, G., & Manchón, P. (Coords.). (2010). *Gestión de diálogo multilingüe y multimodal*. Sevilla: Secretariado de Publicaciones de la Universidad de Sevilla.

Bos, J., & Gabsdil, M. (2000). First-order inference and the interpretation of questions and answers. In M. Poesio & D. Traum (Eds.), *Proceedings of Goetalog. Fourth Workshop on the Semantics and Pragmatics of Dialogue*.

Bresnan, J. (Ed.). (1982). *The mental representation of grammatical relations*. Cambridge, MA: The MIT Press.

Cañas, J. J. (2003). *Ergonomía cognitiva: Alta dirección*, vol. 227.

Cañas, J. J., & Waern, Y. (2001). *Ergonomía cognitiva*. Madrid, España: Editorial Médica Panamericana.

Cantor, N., & Mischel, W. (1979). Prototypes in person perception. *Advances in Experimental Social Psychology*, *12*, 3–52. doi:10.1016/S0065-2601(08)60258-0

Cassell, J., McNeill, D., & McCullough, K. E. (1998). Speech-gestures mismatches: Evidence for one underlying representation of linguistic and nonlinguistic information. *Pragmatics & Cognition*, 6.

Charniak, E., & Johnson, M. (2005). Coarse-to-fine n-best parsing and MaxEnt discriminative reranking. In K. Knight (Ed.) *Proceedings of the 43rd Annual Meeting of the Association for Computational Linguistics* (pp. 173–180). Ann Arbor, MI: Association for Computational Linguistics.

Collins, M., & Koo, T. (2003). Discriminative reranking for natural language parsing. *Computational Linguistics*, *31*(1), 175–182.

DeAngeli, A., Johnson, G., & Coventry, L. (2001). The unfriendly user: Exploring social reactions to Chatterbots. In K. Helander & Tham (Eds.), *Proceedings of International Conference on Affective Human Factor Design* (pp. 257-286). London, UK: Asean Academic Press.

Fiske, S. T., & Taylor, S. E. (1991). *Social cognition*. New York, NY: McGraw-Hill, Inc.

Gardner, H. (1983). *Frames of mind. The theory of multiple intelligences*. New York, NY: Basic Books.

Gardner, H. (1993). *Multiple intelligences: The theory into practice*. New York, NY: Basic Books.

Gardner, H. (1999). *Intelligence reframed: Multiple intelligences for the 21st century*. New York, NY: Basic Books.

Goleman, D. (1995). *Emotional intelligence - why it can matter more than IQ*. Bantam Books.

Henderson, J., Lemon, O., & Georgila, K. (2005). Hybrid reinforcement/supervised learning for dialogue policies from communicator data. In *Proceedings of International Joint Conferences on Artificial Intelligence Workshop on Knowledge and Reasoning in Practical Dialogue Systems.*

Iivari, J., & Iivari, N. (2006). Varieties of user-centeredness. *Proceedings of the 39th Hawaii International Conference on System Sciences.*

Isbister, K., & Nass, C. (2000). Consistency of personality in interactive characters: Verbal cues, non-verbal cues, and user characteristics. *International Journal of Human-Computer Studies*, *53*, 251–267. doi:10.1006/ijhc.2000.0368

Jacobs, J. (2010). *Key considerations for virtual assistant selection*. (Gartner ID: G00201581).

Larsson, S., & Traum, D. (2000). Information state and dialogue management in the TRINDI dialogue move engine toolkit. *Natural Language Engineering*, *6*, 323–340. doi:10.1017/S1351324900002539

Lester, J., Branting, K., & Mott, B. (2004). Conversational agents. In Singh, M. P. (Ed.), *The practical handbook of Internet computing*. London, UK: Chapman & Hall.

Long, J. (1987). Cognitive ergonomics and human-computer interaction. In Warr, P. (Ed.), *Psychology at work. Harmondsworth*. Middlesex, UK: Penguin.

Manchón, P. (2009). *Towards clever human-computer interaction*. Doctoral dissertation, University of Seville, Spain.

Manchón, P., Del Solar, C., Amores, G., & Pérez, G. (2007). Multimodal interaction analysis in a smart house. *In Proceedings of the 9th international Conference on Multimodal interfaces (Nagoya, Aichi, Japan, November 12 - 15, 2007)*. ICMI '07.

Mao, J., & Vredenburg, K. (2001). User-centered design methods in practice: A survey of the state of the art. In D. A. Stewart & J. H. Johnson (Eds.), *Proceedings of the 2001 Conference of the Centre for Advanced Studies on Collaborative Research, 12*.

Mao, J., Vredenburg, K., Smith, P., & Carey, T. (2005). The state of user-centered design practice. *Communications of the ACM, 48*(3), 105–109. doi:10.1145/1047671.1047677

Reeves, B., & Nass, C. (1996). *The media equation: How people treat computers, television and new media like real people and places*. Stanford, CA: CSLI Publications.

Riezler, S., King, T. H., Kaplan, R. M., Crouch, R., Maxwell, J. T., & Johnson, I. M. (2002). Parsing the Wall Street Journal using a lexical-functional grammar and discriminative estimation techniques. In P. Isabelle (Ed.), *Proceedings of the 40th Annual Meeting of the Association for Computational Linguistics* (pp. 271-278). Philadelphia, PA: Association for Computational Linguistics.

Robinson, S., Traum, D., Ittycheriah, M., & Henderer, J. (2008). What would you ask a conversational agent? Observations of human-agent dialogues in a museum setting. In N. Calzolari, K. Choukri, B. Maegaard, J. Mariani, J. Odjik, S. Piperidis, & D. Tapias (Eds.), *Proceedings of the Sixth International Language Resources and Evaluation* (pp. 1125-1131). Marrakech, Morocco: European Language Resources Association (ELRA).

Schulman, D., & Bickmore, T. (2009). Persuading users through counseling dialogue with a conversational agent. In S. Chatterjee & P. Dev (Eds.), *Proceedings of the 4th International Conference on Persuasive Technology Persuasive '09, vol. 350, 25*. New York, NY: ACM Press.

Thomas, F., & Johnston, O. (1981). *The illusion of life: Disney animation*. New York, NY: Norton.

Turing, A. (1950). Computing machinery and intelligence. *Mind, 236*, 433–460. doi:10.1093/mind/LIX.236.433

Weizenbaum, J. (1966). ELIZA - a computer program for the study of natural language communication between man and machine. *Communications of the ACM, 9*, 36–45. doi:10.1145/365153.365168

Williams, J., & Young, S. (2007). Scaling POMDPs for spoken dialog management. *IEEE Audio. Speech and Language Processing, 15*, 2116–2129. doi:10.1109/TASL.2007.902050

## ADDITIONAL READING

Bickmore, T. W. (2003). *Relational agents: Effecting change through human--computer relationships*, Unpublished doctoral dissertation. Massachusetts Institute of Technology

Cassell, J. (2000). Embodied conversational interface agents. *Communications of the ACM, 43*(4), 70–78. doi:10.1145/332051.332075

Cassell, J. (2000). Embodied Conversational Agents: Representation and Intelligence in User Interfaces. *AI Magazine, 12*(4), 67–84.

Cassell, J., Sullivan, J., Prevost, S., & Churchill, E. (Eds.). (2000). *Embodied Conversational Agents*. Cambridge, Mass: The MIT Press.

Dybkjær, L., Bernsen, N. O., & Minker, W. (2004). Evaluation and usability of multimodal spoken language dialogue systems. *Speech Communication, 43*, 33–54. doi:10.1016/j.specom.2004.02.001

Ekman, P., & Friesen, W. V. (1977). *Manual for the facial action coding system. Technical report*. Palo Alto, CA: Consulting Psychologist Press, Inc.

Gasson, S. (2003). Human-centered vs. user-centered approaches to information systems design [JITTA]. *The Journal of Information Technology Theory and Applications, 5*(2), 29–46.

Gattass, M., Lucena, P. S., & Velho, L. (2002). Expressive talking heads: A study on speech and facial expression in virtual characters. *Scientia, 13*(2), 1–12.

Georg, G., Cavazza, M., & Pelachaud, C. (2008). Visualizing the importance of medical recommendations with conversational agents. In: H. Prendinger, J. Lester, & M. Ishizuka. *Intelligent Virtual Agents: 8th International Conference, IVA 2008*, (pp. 380-393). Springer Publishing Company.

Gibbon, D., Mertins, I., & Moore, R. (Eds.). (2000). *Handbook of Multimodal and Spoken Dialogue Systems*. Norwell, MA: Kluwer Academic Publishers.

Grosz, B. J., & Sidner, C. L. (1986). Attention, intentions, and the structure of discourse. *Computational Linguistics, 12*(3), 175–204.

Jokinen, K., & McTear, M. (2010). *Spoken dialogue systems*. Toronto, Canada: Springer.

Jurafsky, D., & Martin, J. H. (2009). *Speech and Language Processing* (2nd ed.). London: Pearson Education.

Larsson, S. (2002). *Issue-based Dialogue Management*. Unpublished doctoral dissertation. Gothenburg University.

Larsson, S., & Traum, D. (2000). Information state and dialogue management in the trindi dialogue move engine toolkit. *Natural Language Engineering, 6*(3-4), 323–340. doi:10.1017/S1351324900002539

López-Cózar Delgado, R., & Araki, M. (2005). *Spoken, Multilingual and Multimodal Dialogue Systems Development and Assessment*. West Sussex, UK: John Wiley & Sons Ltd. doi:10.1002/0470021578

Mairesse, F., & Walker, M. (2007). PERSONAGE: Personality generation for dialogue. In J. Carroll (Ed.) *Proceedings of the 45th Annual Meeting of the Association for Computational Linguistics (ACL)* (pp. 496–503). Prague: The Association for Computational Linguistics.

Manchón, P. (2006). *Gabriel Amores, Guillermo Pérez*. Malaga, Spain: User-Centered Design in Smart Natural Language Multimodal Interfaces. Mobile Europe.

Manning, C., & Schütze, H. (1999). *Foundations of Statistical Natural Language Processing*. Cambridge, Mass: The MIT Press.

McTear, M. (2004). *Spoken dialogue technology: toward the conversational user interface. University of Ulster, Northern Ireland*. Springer.

Norman, D. (1988). *The Design of Everyday Things*. New york: Currency Doubleday.

Norman, D. (2004) HCD Harmful: A Clarification. Retrieved May 15th, 2010, from http://www.jnd.org/dn.mss/hcd_harmful_a_clari.html

Norman, D. A. (1998). *The invisible computer*. Cambridge, MA: MIT Press.

Oviatt, S. (2003). User-centered modeling and evaluation of multimodal interfaces. *Proceedings of the IEEE. 91*(9).

Oviatt, S., Coulston, R., & Lunsford, R. (2004). When Do We Interact Multimodally? Cognitive Load and Multimodal Communication Patterns. In R. Sharma, T. Darrell, M. P. Harper, G. Lazzari & M. Turk. *Proceedings of the Sixth International Conference on Multimodal Interfaces* (ICMI 2004), (pp. 129-136). New York: ACM Press.

Pelachaud, C., Martin, J. C., André, E., Chollet, G., Karpouzis, K., & Pelé, D. (Eds.). (2007): *Intelligent Virtual Agents, 7th International Conference Lecture Notes in Computer Science*. New York: Springer.

Pelachaud, C., & Poggi, I. (2002). Multimodal Embodied Agents. *The Knowledge Engineering Review*, *17*(2), 181–196. doi:10.1017/S0269888902000218

Pérez, G. (2009) *Contribuciones a los Sistemas de Diálogo Multimodales*. Unpublished doctoral dissertation: Universidad Politécnica de Madrid

Pervin, L. A., & John, O. P. (Eds.). (1997). *Personality Theory and Research*. New York: Wiley.

Prendinger, H., Lester, J., & Ishizuka, M. (Eds.). (2008). *Intelligent Virtual Agents, 8th International Conference*. Lecture Notes in Computer Science. New York: Springer.

Ruttkay, Z., Kipp, M., Nijholt, A., & Vilhjálmsson, H. (Eds.). (2009). *Intelligent Virtual Agents, 9th International Conference Lecture Notes in Computer Science*. New York: Springer.

Schmidt, C. T. A. (2005). Of Robots and Believing. *Minds and Machines*, *15*, 195–205. doi:10.1007/s11023-005-4734-6

Searle, J. R. (1969). *Speech Acts: An essay in the philosophy of language*. Cambridge University Press.

Zipf, G. K. (1949). *Human behaviour and the principle of least effort: An introduction to human ecology*. Cambridge, MA: Addison-Wesley.


## KEY TERMS AND DEFINITIONS

**Activity Centered Design (ACD):** Pays special attention to the multiple dimensions of human engagement with the world. Critical to understanding these processes of engagement for use in the field of HCI is the mediating role that is played by cultural artifacts or tools and their transformative power.

**Dialogue Systems:** A dialog system is a computer system intended to converse with a human, with a coherent structure.

**Embodied Conversational Agent (ECA):** Graphically embodied agents which aim to unite gesture, facial expression and speech to enable face-to-face communication with users.

**Human Centered Design (HCD):** Tries to overcome the poor design of software products by emphasizing the needs and abilities of those who are to use the software.

**Human Computer Interaction (HCI):** Is the study of interaction between people (users) and computers.

**Information State Update (ISU) Approach:** A dialogue modelling framework characterised by the following components: a specification of the contents of the information state of the dialogue; the datatypes used to structure the information state; a set of update rules covering the dynamic changes of the information state; and a control strategy for information state updates.

**Natural Language Understanding (NLU):** Is a subtopic of natural language processing in artificial intelligence that deals with machine reading comprehension.

**User Centered Design (UCD):** A design philosophy and a process in which the needs, wants, and limitations of end users of an interface given extensive attention at each stage of the design process.

## ENDNOTE

1 RoR: Relevance of Response

# Chapter 15
# Design and Development of an Automated Voice Agent: Theory and Practice Brought Together

**Pepi Stavropoulou**
*University of Athens, Greece*

**Dimitris Spiliotopoulos**
*University of Athens, Greece*

**Georgios Kouroupetroglou**
*University of Athens, Greece*

## ABSTRACT

*Sophisticated, commercially deployed spoken dialogue systems capable of engaging in more natural human-machine conversation have increased in number over the past years. Besides employing advanced interpretation and dialogue management technologies, the success of such systems greatly depends on effective design and development methodology. There is, actually, a widely acknowledged, fundamentally reciprocal relationship between technologies used and design choices. In this line of thought, this chapter constitutes a more practical approach to spoken dialogue system development, comparing design methods and implementation tools highly suited for industry oriented spoken dialogue systems, and commenting on their interdependencies, in order to facilitate the developer's choice of the optimal tools and methodologies. The latter are presented and assessed in the light of AVA, a real-life Automated Voice Agent that performs call routing and customer service tasks, employing advanced stochastic techniques for interpretation and allowing for free form user input and less rigid dialogue structure.*

## INTRODUCTION

Automated Voice Agents are systems capable of communicating with users by both understanding and producing speech within a specific domain. They engage in humanlike spoken dialogues, in order to route telephone calls, give traffic information, book flights, solve technical problems and provide access to educational material among others.

DOI: 10.4018/978-1-60960-617-6.ch015

Depending on their design, the speech understanding and dialogue management technology involved, they may be of two basic types:

- Directed Dialog Systems: ranging from finite state-based to frame-based systems (McTear, 2004). The former systems are very simple and inflexible menu-driven interfaces, where the dialogue flow is static, specified in advance, no deviations from that flow are allowed, and only a limited number of words and phrases provided by the user can be understood. The latter systems are more advanced interfaces, where the interaction is not completely predetermined and a more elaborate vocabulary can be handled. While both types of systems are primarily system-directed, frame-based systems allow for a modest level of mixed-initiative by handling over-specification in user's input; that is the user can provide more items of information than those requested by the system at each dialogue turn.
- Open-ended natural language conversational systems: mixed-initiative systems, where both system and user can take control of the dialogue introducing topics, changing goals, requesting clarifications, establishing common ground. Equipped with sophisticated speech and language processing modules, they can handle long, complex and variable user input in an attempt to approximate natural human-human interaction as close as possible.

The two types of systems to a significant extent reflect the differences in trends and directions followed by the spoken dialogue industry compared to spoken dialogue research during the last decades. As commercial dialogue systems aim primarily at usability and task completion (Pieraccini & Huerta, 2008), focus was placed on ways to restrict users' input, in order to amend for speech technology limitations and reach industrial standards for useful applications. As a result, industry opted for more directed dialogue systems, which are the most commonly used on the market today.

Furthermore, the need for cost reduction, ease of development and maintenance has led to the development of reusable dialogue components and integration platforms promoting modularity and interoperability. Accordingly, VoiceXML (McGlashan et al., 2004; Larson, 2002) has become an industry standard for building voice applications, which exploits the existing and universally accepted web infrastructures eliminating the need for specific application protocol interfaces (APIs) designated to speech technology integration. Based on the Form Interpretation Algorithm it incorporates a frame-based architecture, providing an industry-feasible trade-off between naturalness and robustness.

Research, on the other hand, aims primarily at naturalness and freedom of communication (Pieraccini & Huerta, 2008). In an attempt to handle almost unrestricted user input and allow for a fully mixed initiative, conversational interface, focus has been on dialogue manager architectures exploiting inference and planning as part of a truly conversational agent. Speech act interpretation (Allen, 1995, Chapter 17; Cohen & Perrault, 1979; Core & Allen, 1997; Allen et al., 2007) and conversational games (Kowtko et al., 1993; Pulman, 2002), discourse structure (Grosz & Sidner, 1986; Stent et al., 1999; Fischer et al., 1994) and prosody manipulation (Hirschberg et al., 1995; Noth et al., 2002) are only some of the topics in an ongoing research for building natural language interfaces.

Furthermore, accessibility issues have gained attention, being important not only for the visual impaired (Freitas & Kouroupetroglou, 2008) but also to people with various disabilities (Fellbaum & Kouroupetroglou, 2008). In particular, spoken dialogue systems are considered as key technological factors for the universal accessibility strategies of – for example – public terminals, information kiosks and Automated Teller Machines (ATMs) (Kouroupetroglou, 2009).

Nevertheless, the emerging need to support complex, demanding domain applications such as education, help desk or customer care, along with the evolution and level of maturity accomplished by the current speech and natural language understanding technology have led to a significant number of commercially developed and deployed mixed initiative systems and the introduction of more free style automated voice agents, indicating some level of convergence between the two fields, research and industry.

Building on practices and experiences from developing such a system, this chapter comprises a more pragmatic approach to Automated Voice Agents, focusing on practical spoken dialogue systems, presenting techniques, tools and resources for effective design and implementation, assessing them in the light of a real life customer care and call routing application, commenting on best practices and suggesting ways to best utilize these practices.

We follow the typical lifecycle of an automated voice agent and focus on the requirements analysis and design phase, as well as the development of the Automatic Speech Recognition (ASR) and Natural Language Understanding (NLU) modules.

In the following sections we first give a brief overview of previous related work. Next we present the main features and architecture of an automated voice agent, before going on to describe AVA, the real-life application at hand. Illustration of the main steps in an agent's lifecycle follows, and design and implementation phases are subsequently discussed in detail. Final section summarizes key concepts throughout the process.

## RELATED WORK

The field of spoken dialogue systems is one of the fastest growing areas over the last decades. With regards to field textbooks, Cohen et al. (2004) is a thorough, well organized presentation of the complete spoken dialogue interface development process and methodology based on extensive real word experience. A sample application is presented as means to observe how development and design principles can be applied in practice. Harris (2005) is another comprehensive guide to spoken dialogue system development grounded on an in depth grasp of relevant literature, and focusing particularly on development process and design. Hempel (2008) is a collection of articles on system quality and usability issues with reference to multimodal systems as well.

Weinschenk & Barker (2000) and Balentine & Morgan (1999) provide a set of practical design principles and guidelines for building a Voice User Interface (VUI). Pitt & Edwards (2003) is another practical approach focusing on menu and prompt construction applying the proposed principles on real life applications involving road traffic information and a voice mail system.

McTear (2004) is an introduction to technical (among other) aspects of spoken dialogue systems, illustrating development of applications with particular software and toolkits. Huang et al. (2001) is a standard guide to spoken language system technology (including signal processing, speech recognition and synthesis techniques as well as Natural Language Understanding (NLU) algorithms and dialogue management strategies). Finally, Jurafsky & Martin (2000, Chapter 19) introduce algorithms and architectures for dialogue managers in conversational agents.

There is a significant number of practical (Dahl, 2004) and more advanced (Pellom et al., 2001; Allen et al., 1995, 1996, 2001; Wahlster, 2000; Sidner, 2004, among others) system descriptions. Here reference will be made to call routing and customer care related spoken dialogue applications. Riccardi et al. (1997) and Gorin et al. (1997) describe the Automatic Speech Recognition (ASR) and Understanding components of the HMIHY call routing system, which utilize phrase based language modeling and a classifier that uses salient text fragments as features in order to associate user utterances to predetermined call types.

Walker et al. (2002) report on automatically predicting problems in human-machine dialogues for improved error recovery also within the HMIHY system. Chu-Carroll & Carpenter (1999), Garfield & Wermter (2002, 2006) and Zitouni et al. (2003) also place attention on advanced NLU techniques – such as vector based classifiers and recurrent neural networks – for such systems. Lee & Chang (2002) describe an operator assisted call router that integrates a generic ASR module with an information retrieval module based on keyword extraction from existing company documentation with descriptions of routing destinations (i.e. departments), thus eliminating the need for collecting and transcribing actual call recordings.

Williams & Witt (2004) compare menu driven directed dialogue strategies to open ended, free form "how may I help you" strategies for use in automated call routing. Finally, Gupta et al. (2006) touch upon subjects such as system scalability and minimization of development effort describing the NLU component of VoiceTone, a system that provides automated customer care services in addition to call routing.

In the vein of theorized practice, this chapter presents a real life call routing and customer care information provision application focusing on design, ASR and NLU implementation and the reciprocal relationship among the three, building on a more general, theoretical perspective.

## THE AUTOMATED VOICE AGENT

As mentioned in the introductory section, Automated Voice Agents are programs capable of communicating with users by both understanding and producing speech within a specific domain. Figure 1 illustrates the Automated Voice Agent architecture. The Automatic Speech Recognition (ASR) component converts acoustic user input into text, and passes the text string to the Natural Language Understanding (NLU) component for semantic interpretation.

In addition, a Dual-Tone Multi-Frequency (DTMF) recognizer may be used to allow for DTMF input as well. Next, the Dialogue Manager (DM) evaluates and/or disambiguates the semantic information from the NLU module based on processes such as dialogue history and context interpretation. Depending on input evaluation the DM plans and proceeds to execute certain dialogue actions such as database queries or system prompt formulation. For prompt formulation, the DM output is converted to a well formed written ut-

*Figure 1. Automatic voice agent main component layout*

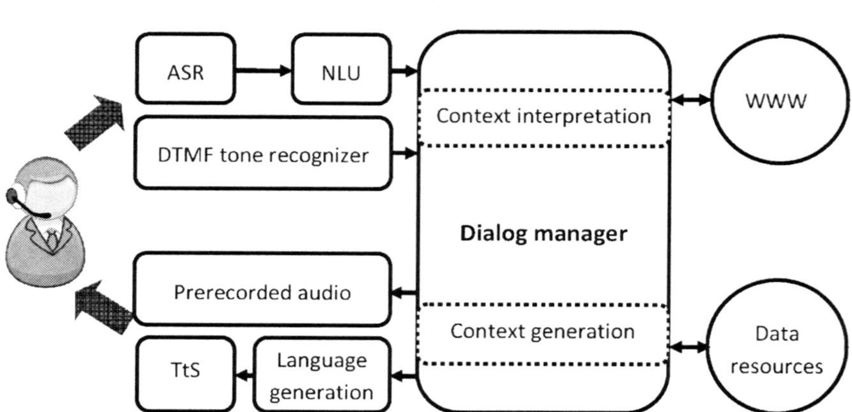

terance by the Natural Language Generation (NLG) module, and then the Text to Speech (TtS) Synthesizer converts the written utterance to speech. In most commercial spoken dialogue systems pre-recorded prompts are used instead.

The main feature of an agent is personification (Harris, 2005). Personification refers to a primitive, inherent human disposition to assign human attributes to non human entities, or in this case, a personality to the automated voice agent. There are certain parameters, design and implementation choices, that affect the personality ascribed to the agent. In particular:

- The kind of language used, namely the vocabulary, syntax, prosody and style, the agent's gender or dialect may cause the agent to appear calm, pleasant, helpful, interesting or encouraging. For example, simple syntax (e.g. use of simple coordination structures rather than subordination) and avoidance of jargon may cause the agent to appear more informal and helpful. Variation in the wording of prompts and tone may make the agent sound more interesting. Use of prosody to convey emotion increases the level of perceived conversation engagement.
- The range of functions, the capabilities and limitations of the agent, the dialogue initiative handling, the interaction style, the choice on grounding and error recovery strategies may cause the agent to appear competent, trustworthy, dependable, credible, co-operative, intelligent, sensible, helpful or knowledgeable. For example, mixed-initiative strategies are usually signs of intelligent behavior. In contrast, an agent that sequentially asks for pieces of information already given just sounds brainless. Changing dialogue strategies (e.g. backing off to a more conservative directed dialogue strategy when the dialogue is problematic) may be considered a sign of co-operative and helpful behavior.

Given the reciprocal relationship between design and available technology, a successful voice agent, one that sounds smart, pleasant and helpful, depends both on effective design methodologies and adequate speech and language technology tools. At the same time business requirements should be met and cost/time constraints should be taken into consideration. Figure 2 illustrates these interactions.

*Figure 2. Design considerations and interactions in building an automate voice agent*

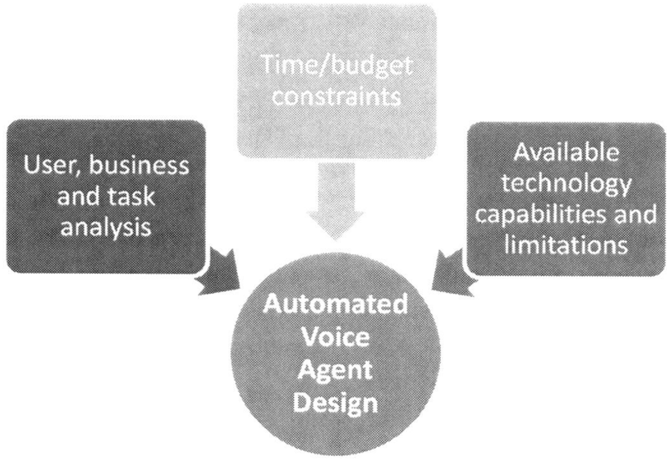

In the next sections we present AVA, an Automated Voice Agent for a customer care system, with the aim to address the following question: how do our tools and techniques affect design, implementation and evaluation choices, and how can we make the best choice possible?

## AVA: AN AUTOMATED VOICE AGENT FOR CUSTOMER CARE

AVA is an automated voice agent built for a Customer Care call centre of a Mobile Telephony company. She performs two major tasks: a) appropriate routing of the client's call to one of 17 dedicated queues, and b) database information retrieval for speech-based automated self-service modules. For both tasks she needs to identify and correctly categorize the caller's request as one of the approximately 100 services and respective thematic categories provided by the Customer Care department.

In addition, AVA displays the following key features (among others): a) recognition and understanding of free style user input. If there is under-specification and ambiguity in the user's input, AVA should formulate an appropriate question, in order to determine how the call should be handled, b) support of mixed dialogue initiative in the following sense: on one hand AVA should be able to handle over-specification; on the other hand, the callers should be able to shift goal at almost any time during the interaction. For example, if the users have already chosen a particular self service, and within the self service sub-dialogue they decide that they want a different service after all, AVA should be able to understand this new request and handle the call accordingly.

As is often the case with automated voice agents, AVA replaces an existing DTMF system. A DTMF system is static and menu driven and so providing coverage for a complex domain such as customer care eventually results in a large and complicated menu hierarchy. Consequently, the caller is forced to spend precious time navigating through various levels of this hierarchy before finally being transferred to a human agent; efficiency decreases, while user dissatisfaction increases.

Furthermore, even with an overcomplicated menu hierarchy, no exact mapping is guaranteed between the user's request and the menu options offered. The result is an increase in the number of hang ups and misroutings. As AVA replaces the old DTMF system, there is no longer need for dysfunctional, complex menus, a lot more services can be handled and the interaction becomes more natural, efficient and effective.

Spiliotopoulos et al. (2009) compare DTMF systems to spoken language interfaces performing usability testing on a real life paradigm involving both types of systems, showing a great increase in user satisfaction and system efficiency when using a spoken dialogue interface. In particular, the average call duration was 25 and 44 seconds for the spoken dialogue and the DTMF system respectively, while user satisfaction score was 9 percentage points higher for the former compared to the latter.

As is, AVA poses three major challenges with regards to design, implementation and maintenance considerations respectively. The first one involves building on the existing user's mental model and breaking down the customer care domain into a service hierarchy that reflects the user's point of view. A second interdependent challenge involves the automatic recognition of the user input to open-ended questions covering a large range of responses, and mapping it to one or more services. The latter requires, among other things, a large set of typical caller utterances for training the statistical models for speech recognition and interpretation. The third challenge involves minimizing the cost and need for support in a constantly changing domain. These challenges are analysed and addressed in the following sections.

*Figure 3. Testing methodology to develop automated voice agents*

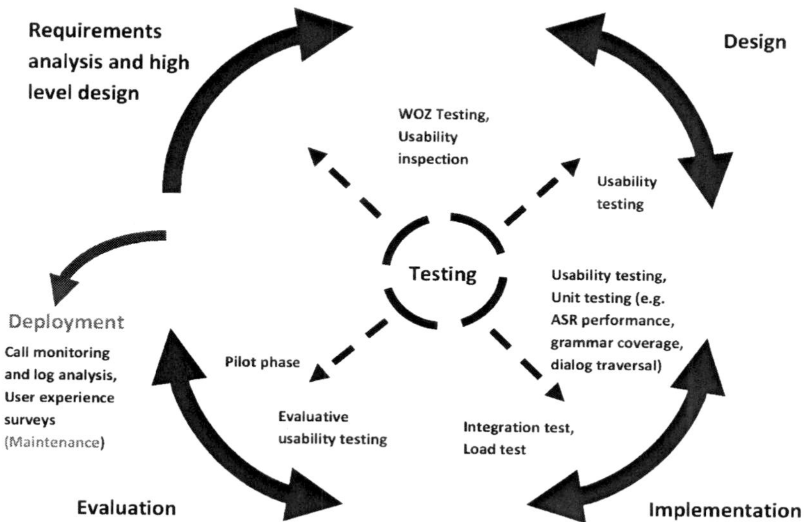


## THE AUTOMATED VOICE AGENT'S LIFECYCLE

Figure 3 shows the basic steps in the process of building an automated voice agent. The adapted phases from Cohen et al. (2004) are the following:

- Design phase, which is further divided into a) the requirements analysis and high level design, where the basic system functionality is analysed and defined and key design decisions are made, and b) detailed design, which results in a complete, detailed specification of the dialogue.
- Implementation phase during which the system components – the Automated Speech Recognition (ASR) Module, the Natural Language Understanding (NLU) Module, the Dialog Manager (DM), the Language Generation Module and the Text to Speech Synthesizer (TtS) – are developed. As an alternative to having a generation module and a TtS synthesizer, static prompts may be pre-recorded and used. Integration with third party software systems is completed. At the end of the implementation phase there should be a fully integrated, working prototype.
- Evaluation and Tuning phase. Final usability tests are performed with the (nearly) finished product aiming primarily at application fine tuning, since important design choices should have already been made and evaluated during the previous steps. Pilot phase is a significant part of the whole tuning process. It is because of the abundance of in service realistic data available for training, testing and tuning purposes, when the market-ready system is released to real users.
- Deployment: the final production system is released to the entire user population.
- Maintenance and quality assurance monitoring.

As Kouroupetroglou & Spiliotopoulos (2009) note, testing is an important, inherent part of all phases rather than the evaluation phase alone (for example it can be in the form of usability testing or usability inspection during the design phase, unit testing and usability testing during the implementation phase (cf. following sections)), essentially turning the process of building an automated voice agent into an iterative design, (re)test, redesign and (re)implement procedure.

Therefore, even though the steps are depicted in the sequence they principally apply (cf. Figure 3), in practice there is no clear cut line distinguishing among phases, which typically blur into each other. Figure 3 further illustrates the main tests available at each phase, analysed in the following sections. For a more detailed description of how each test applies within the automated voice agent development lifecycle readers may refer to Cohen et al. (2004).

## DESIGN PHASE

First in an automated voice agent's lifecycle come the requirements analysis and the design phase. During these phases the developer needs to analyze the *users' characteristics* (demographics, linguistic characteristics, domain and task knowledge, frequency of use, experience with similar systems), the *business goals* (motivation behind the development of such a system, company image, competition, time and cost constraints) and the *application domain* (tasks and features, current and desired workflow, technical environment), in order to make appropriate design choices and proceed with the complete dialogue specification. Based on the analysis the developer has to decide upon high level features, such as initiative and grammar type, down to prompts, dialogue states and slots. At the end of the design phase a complete description of the call flow and all prompts played by the system should be available (Cohen et al., 2004).

A key for effective design is user-centered design (Norman & Draper, 1986; Gould & Lewis, 1985). User expectations, attitudes and behaviour should be accommodated rather than constrained. In this view, an important aspect of analysis feeding directly into design is the understanding of the "natural" mental model that first time users bring to the interaction, their existing – and possibly expected – view of the interaction, a model of how things have worked so far.

The success of an interface greatly depends on the correspondence between this "natural" mental model and the conceptual (Weinschenk & Barker, 2000) or design model (Norman, 1988); that is the proposed model afforded by the design of the interface. Ideally, a system should build on and adapt to the users' prior knowledge and experience, in order to create a more familiar, intuitive, easier to learn and use interface.

For voice agents in particular, the latter is tightly connected to the kind of language – vocabulary-wise and syntax-wise – understood and introduced by the agent. Domain specific spoken dialogue studies are therefore very important and presuppose the existence of appropriate language resources. On a final note, as speech recognition and understanding modules typically require domain specific corpora for training purposes (cf. "Implementation Phase: Speech Recognition and Understanding Modules" section), many of these resources can be shared between design and implementation teams.

The most common techniques for designing voice agents are presented based on the aforementioned considerations and according to the phase of the development cycle in which they are used. The techniques are evaluated with the following parameters: a) ease of application, i.e. the feasibility of these techniques in light of strict industry time frames and cost constraints, b) their contribution to understanding the mental model and interaction patterns, c) their usefulness for determining the vocabulary and other linguistic constructions and d) their appropriateness to serve as ASR and NLU resources.

**Gathering information from company personnel and domain experts**. Starting early in the agent's lifecycle it comprises a valuable tool throughout the building process, as it provides insights in the business goals and the application in general. Meetings with human agents in particular can prove to be very informative with regards to identifying typical usage, terminology, confusions and "risky" or complicated steps during the interaction. However, they may lack objectivity, providing invalid information, blurring understanding of actual user behaviour.

**Examination of available documentation (e.g. marketing materials, statistics about use) and/or other in-domain applications (e.g. website, DTMF system to be replaced)** can provide information on functionality and terminology. However, there are two very important points of caution involved. First of all, company documentation often reflects a business view of the application domain. Migrating this business view into the interface often results in bad performance, as business and user scope do not coincide and thus user expectations are rarely met. Secondly, the audio modality differs from visual or other modalities. The transient, ephemeral nature of speech along with human cognitive limitations place constraints on the speech output and the application structure in general.

Balentine & Morgan (1999), among others, recommend presenting no more than five information units at one time opting for the lowest possible number. Graphic User Interfaces (GUIs) on the other hand exploit vision and space, and can present a large amount of information that can be easily and quickly processed by the user. Therefore, a direct translation of a GUI into a Speech User Interface will most likely result into unfriendly, unusable applications.

Similarly, DTMF modality differs from speech in terms of user psychology, timing, menu structures and selection methods (Balentine & Morgan, 1999). Co-operative, natural conversation is simply not menu navigation. In short, when transferring knowledge and experience from one modality to another, one should be careful to filter out distinct psychological and design principles that refer to or are particularly important to each modality alone.

While both the above mentioned techniques are important for gaining a basic understanding of the business and the application context, they cannot be a substitute for direct contact with users.

**User interviews and observation studies** allow for such direct user contact, comprising a significant aspect of user-centered design. Interviewing users can provide insights on the how, when and whys of the task. Nevertheless, as users are asked to remember and comment on events and processes "that may normally be performed without a lot of conscious thought" (Weinschenk & Barker, 2000), their input may be inaccurate and imprecise.

Also, care should be taken when forming the interview questions, so as not to bias the interviewees' answers causing them to deviate from their natural language and usage patterns. These concerns do not apply in the case of observation studies, whereas one can directly observe real users performing the task and gain insight into their interaction patterns and language use. On site field studies may be less time – and hence cost – effective, but can provide an opportunity to ask human agents specific questions. For telephone-based applications, on the other hand, there may be a – time and cost saving – abundance of records of calls to live agents immediately available.

**Analysis of actual users' calls to human agents** is already considered to be an important resource for effective design (McTear, 2004; Cohen et al., 2004), as it provides significant information regarding the vocabulary used, the nature of the interaction and the mental model of the task in general. Most importantly, in contrast to language resources obtained from usability testing, these calls are collected from real users truly engaged in performing realistic tasks.

Alternatively, the next opportunity for collecting utterances from real users is during the pilot phase, which comes later in the development process, and so involves the risk of costly changes due to overlooked early design shortcomings. Furthermore, call records can be transcribed and used as training corpus for stochastic models for the ASR and NLU modules.

Since the necessary amount of corpus is already available at the beginning of the development lifecycle, there is no need to spend valuable time for the collection of training corpora during implementation. Moreover, having adequate resources for ASR and NLU early in the development process enables the obtainment of more reliable results during evaluative usability testing, as low recognition and interpretation success rate considerably affect the user experience (Kamm & Walker, 1997), and interfere with the evaluation of the dialogue structure per se.

On the other hand, human-human dialogues are intrinsically less restricted in nature compared to human-machine dialogues, and associated with diverse caller behaviour. In a study comparing a corpus collected from human-human dialogues to a corpus collected from human-machine dialogues significant differences were found in the vocabulary used, the length and complexity of the utterances as well as the performance of the statistical language models for ASR (Stavropoulou et al., 2011).

Human-human utterances were approximately three times longer (45% larger corpus vocabulary size), more complicated, and the language model trained on them performed worse (9-14 and 11-14 percentage points increase in word error rate and concept error rate respectively). In conclusion, whilst developers may observe actual users, they cannot observe actual user-system interaction. In fact one can never be absolutely certain what the real users' reaction and perception of the system will be.

At least that is what previous experience has shown us when building a system similar to AVA with regards to complexity, but for – familiar with the domain – telecom shop representatives only. After launch we discovered that the company employees insisted on using specific keywords and phrases essentially reproducing the limited functionality of the DTMF system that was replaced, rendering the use of elaborate vocabulary, grammars and dialogue structure redundant.

All the techniques presented so far aid early design choices and are relatively cost free. In this regard, they form an indispensable part of requirements specifications and high-level design. Next, techniques are presented that require the existence of a basic design skeleton at least, and as such they are used to evaluate high level design choices and guide more detailed design.

**Wizard of Oz (WOZ) testing** (Fraser & Gilbret, 1991) is one of the most prevalent techniques in the design and early development stages. It is the first time the system is presented to end users, and developers have a chance to observe user – system interaction, obtaining invaluable, hands-on information on attitude peculiarities and problems faced with regards to the specific interface.

In a WOZ study, the system is actually a mock up (prototype simulation), and a human acts as the system. The main advantage of the WOZ method lies in the ability to test early, without a working system. Therefore, updates based on feedback are easier, and early detection of design shortcomings that would be costly to fix later is possible.

Furthermore, the dialogues collected can be used as initial training corpus during the implementation of the ASR and NLU modules. On the other hand, the WOZ method faces the disadvantages of end user testing in general. First of all, test participants are not motivated in the same way as real users are, and are often not representative of the end user population.

Earlier studies (Turunen et al., 2006; Ai et al., 2007) have shown that there are differences between usability testing and actual use conditions; main differences lie in the use of barge-in, explicit help requests, significant silence timeouts, speech recognizer rejection rate, use of touchtone, speech rate, utterance length and dialog duration.

Furthermore, as test participants are asked to perform specific tasks, the language used to describe these tasks inevitably influences the participants' choice of vocabulary and utterance structure, undermining the usefulness and reliability of elicited discourse patterns (Harris, 2005). That is especially true in the case of WOZ testing, which usually takes place before final prompt design and specification, and so users may take cues from prompts that will be replaced in the final system.

The realistic aspect is further compromised, as it is difficult for the wizard to simulate speech recognition and interpretation errors. In addition, setting up a WOZ experiment requires tools that can be costly to develop (Weinschenk & Barker, 2000; Jankelovich interview).

Finally, with regards to the utility of the corpus collected for the development of stochastic recognition and interpretation models, the following should be taken into account: given that a typical test session involves 10-15 participants (Cohen et al., 2004), besides lacking the realistic aspect of actual system use, the number of collected dialogs is usually very limited.

**Usability testing with working systems.** Usability testing is "a process that employs people as testing participants who are representative of the target audience to evaluate the degree to which a product meets specific usability criteria" (Lauesen, 2005). The term "working systems" does not necessarily mean systems that contain the entire intended functionality of the production system. On the contrary, by initially testing the usability of limited functionality systems and gradually adding more modules and functions, user involvement may take place early in the implementation phase and become an indispensable part of an iterative testing, design and build process, probing and refining design choices at each iteration (Kouroupetroglou & Spiliotopoulos, 2009; Spiliotopoulos & Kouroupetroglou, 2010).

Evaluation usability tests using a close-to-market, fully integrated system can then be performed at the end (or near the end) of the implementation cycle, primarily for fine tuning purposes. Optimally, major problems in design should have already been identified, as addressing them at that point is usually a difficult and costly procedure. It should be noted, though, that under fast paced conditions that are typically the case in industry, often dealing with budget constraints as well, the high cost of conducting usability tests in an iterative manner throughout the product's lifecycle is sometimes prohibitive.

A good compromise is to design and test the riskiest parts early in the process. Regarding the quality of the collected resources, the same shortcomings apply as with WOZ testing, only, in this case, tests benefit from the realistic aspect of actual system use. All in all, usability testing should be an indispensable part of the development process, highly important for conciliating business, developer and user view, validating design decisions, identifying problems early in the process, when it is easier to address them, and preventing the release of embarrassing, unusable systems (Galitz, 2007).

Finally, usability inspection methods, such as heuristic evaluation (usability experts examine whether usability principles are met) or pluralistic walkthroughs (group meetings, where stakeholders go through dialogue scenarios) are an important, cost and time effective tool that can be easily utilized throughout the development lifecycle.

Accordingly, Rubin & Chisnell (2008) note: "In some cases it is more effective both in terms of cost, time, and accuracy to conduct an expert or heuristic evaluation of a product rather than test it. This is especially true in the early stages of a product when gross violations of usability principles abound. It is simply unnecessary to bring in many participants to reveal the obvious".

There are a number of other usability inspection methods (e.g. heuristic estimation, feature and consistency inspection); heuristic evaluation is considered to be the most common and beneficial one (Nielsen, 1995). Nevertheless, even the latter can only be complementary to other user-centric techniques, as it often fails to identify a significant proportion of problems (roughly 50%) that real users encounter (Lauesen, 2005). For a detailed analysis of usability inspection methods readers may refer to Nielsen & Mack (1994).

## DESIGNING AVA

For understanding AVA and deciding upon key design features, first we met with technical personnel, explored the existing touchtone system, the company's website and other available documentation. Customer care personnel were able to further provide us with statistics of use based on a detailed segmentation of the customer care domain; all services offered by the department had already been defined and grouped into higher level services in a hierarchical fashion, essentially providing us with a thorough analysis of the application functionality.

Intuitively, though, this analysis seemed to reflect a business rather than a user view of the domain. Our intuition was corroborated by input on keywords and terminology provided by human agents, which substantially differed from the jargon in the company's documentation.

So, in order to gain a better understanding of users' view and attitude, we organized a field study, where we observed live agents performing the task. Unfortunately, monitoring real time calls proved rather ineffective time wise, as within a call we could not skip tasks that were out of the application domain.

Still, we had a chance to get the "look and feel" of the task and interview live agents. Luckily, the application being telephone based, we were given access to existing call records. Call record analysis proved to be a much more effective and useful technique. During the analysis we observed high variation and complexity in users' input in terms of vocabulary and syntax that suggested using more robust methods for interpretation such as NLU classifiers rather than hand crafted NLU grammars. However, building on previous experience and given the inherent differences between human-human and human-machine dialogues, it was necessary to examine actual user-system interaction.

To achieve that at such an early stage in AVA's lifecycle a mock up was developed and "exposed" to real users. The purpose of the mock up was twofold: to aid design and collect high quality corpus for implementation. Only the first – and riskiest – step of the dialogue was simulated, in which the callers ask for the particular service they are interested in.

Following a short message introducing callers to the automated service, a "How may I help you" prompt was played to them and after responding they were directly routed to the existing DTMF system. No actual speech recognition or interpretation was attempted and only one no-input event was allowed. Upon no input a help prompt was played with example utterances and the initial prompt was then repeated.

In designing the mock up application, it was important to have already formulated a basic idea of how the production system would work in terms of dialogue structure and ASR grammar type at least. Both parameters affect the wording of the prompts, and taking into account the observed correlation between prompt wording and the caller's answer, it was important to use prompts as similar as possible to the prompts used in the production system.

Analysis of the simulated part of the dialogue had already indicated that due to the application's complexity a "How may I help you" open end question was the safest choice. Also, care was taken, so that the examples provided in the case of no input were representative of the most frequently asked for services, and avoided confusing jargon. In short, "proactive", strong emphasis on design of prompts ensured the validity and utility of the collected corpus.

Due to its simplicity the mock-up was easy and fast to develop and the heavy call load of the customer care call centre made it possible to collect the necessary amount of utterances within a week. The collected corpus served as the basis for user centered design, and helped us analyse the users' view of the domain, elicit users' natural discourse patterns, and observe realistic first time user reaction to the introduction of AVA.

To be more specific, corpus analysis revealed significant user deviations from business language as well as the service domain segmentation depicted in company's documentation. On one hand users tended to be rather vague in their requests actually forming super-categories that required disambiguating. Utterances such as "barring" or "activation" were classified as super categories in need of disambiguation, in order to decide upon a unique routing destination.

Such disambiguation sub-dialogues comprise an important part of AVA that could have not been effectively designed and implemented without early access to user-system dialogues. On the other hand, there were many requests for speaking to agents or being transferred to – non existing sometimes – company departments. Such requests do not typically come up in the interaction between clients and human agents.

Furthermore, with regards to user's discourse, utterance structure was far simpler compared to the human-human dialogues previously analysed, rendering the use of hand crafted robust NLU grammars a viable solution. In fact, a significant number of simple one word utterances came up. Still, for some particular services and in the case of a small number of users, syntax and wording displayed higher variation and complexity. As a result we decided to proceed with our initial choice favouring the use of machine learning techniques for the interpretation part of AVA as well. Given that frequency of use was not particularly high for the application and there would always be walk-up-and-use users, we wanted to accommodate these users too rather than force them to adjust to technology limitations.

Finally, we were able to collect a number of different reactions falling under the "volunteer" or "victim" distinction (Attwater et al., 2000), that is a user expecting an automated agent or a human agent respectively. Based on our observations we managed to design a set of help prompts in response to such "victim" caller's reactions. Our observations further served as arguments corroborating the need for notifying customers of the new application beforehand, for example via Short Messaging Service (SMS).

In conclusion, the mock up application was an indispensable part of AVA's lifecycle, providing among others: a) input on real users' discourse patterns, which were in turn used for designing the prompts and building the grammars, b) insight in users' understanding of the domain and the application, which was in turn used for developing the task list and the disambiguation and help sub-dialogues, as well as deciding upon the dialogue structure and the type of grammars, and c) a realistic, "in-service" corpus, which was used for the development of the statistical language models and the NLU classifier presented in the following section. For other, simpler parts of the application such as the Self Service dialogues, heuristic evaluation and walkthroughs were used.

At the end of the design phase, a complete specification of call flows, prompts and back end system communication was prepared and handed for implementation. Figure 4 summarizes the complete design process.

## IMPLEMENTATION PHASE: SPEECH RECOGNITION AND UNDERSTANDING MODULES

Broadly speaking, implementation of a voice agent can be broken down into the following processes: a) language modeling and lexicon development for the ASR module, b) grammar development for the NLU component, c) prompt recording, d) dialog coding and e) back end system integration. This chapter focuses on the first two.

A speech recognition model typically used in such applications is comprised of the following:

*Figure 4. AVA: design phase*

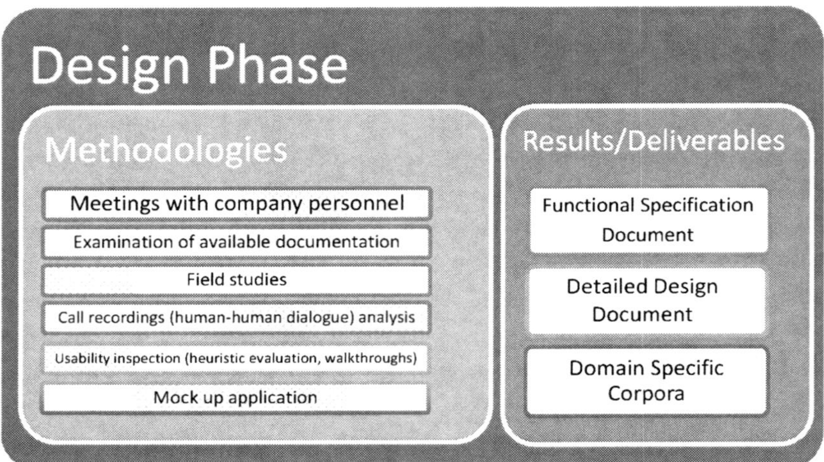


- **Acoustic models**, i.e. models of the language's phones in context. Triphones are usually modeled, that is models of a phone taking into account the effect of the preceding and following phone in its spectrum. Acoustic model sets are in most cases already provided with the speech recognition platform.
- **Dictionary.** The dictionary maps word spellings to pronunciations (i.e. phone sequences). Standard dictionaries are provided with the ASR platform, but most often customized dictionaries also need to be developed to cope with missing pronunciations.
- **Language models.** Language models are grammar networks that constraint the recognizer's search space by specifying permissible word sequences. The type of language model used constitutes a critical feature of an automated voice agent, as "it affects every aspect of VUI design, from the wordings of prompts to dialog strategy, from call flow to the organization of the complete application" (Cohen et al., 2004). Furthermore, the choice of language model used for recognition determines to a great extent the choice of NLU techniques as well.

For the NLU component of commercial spoken dialogue applications, rule based interpretation grammars or robust interpretation grammars are most commonly used, while more advanced stochastic NLU techniques are sometimes also an option.

Following are the most common techniques employed for language modeling in Automatic Speech Recognition (ASR) for practical spoken dialogue systems, along with the NLU techniques that are typically coupled with – interested readers may refer to Huang et al. (2001) for a thorough introduction to language modeling:

- **Rule based context free or non deterministic finite state grammars**, where permissible word sequences are specified by manually written production rules of the form A → β in which A is a non terminal node and β is a sequence of terminal and/or non terminal nodes. High level concepts such as "Destination" or "City" are typically non terminals, while actual words such as "London" or "Athens" are terminals. Production rules can be augmented with probabilities that allow the recognizer to discriminate among competing recognition hypotheses. Rule based grammars are used both for ASR defining the recognizer's search space, as well as interpretation. In the latter case production rules are augmented with semantic attachments that typically return slot-filling values.

- **Statistical Language Models (SLMs)**, where n-grams are trained on user's utterances to compute the probability of word sequences. N-gram language models compute the probability that a word w will follow given the preceding n-1 words as context. Typically bigram or trigram models are used, where n=2 and 3 respectively. For most applications SLMs are coupled with robust NLU grammars. Instead of parsing the whole string passed on by the recognizer, robust grammars perform word or phrase spotting, searching the string and assigning semantic values to meaningful parts only. Alternatively, for some tasks machine learning techniques can be used for NLU as well. In particular, supervised learning using machine learning algorithms may be used for classification of utterances according to a rich set of features. These features may be word or sentence-related, grammatical, lexical, semantic, such as placement of the words in the utterance, number of words in an utterance, content or functional word flag, part-of-speech, type of phrase, type of utterance (question, verification, disambiguation, explanation, statement, positive/negative, etc.), and so on. All the above can be set for words preceding and following the word that the features are assigned for, if it is deemed necessary.

Rule based grammars are suitable for well defined, simple domains, where users' input is less variable and more predictable. As they are written by hand, there is no need for collecting training data, and they can be easily updated by simply adding more rules to the grammar. SLMs on the other hand are suitable for large, complex domains, where it is hard to predict and manually specify all permissible word combinations in advance. Manually creating such a set of rules can be a hard, time consuming and possibly ineffective endeavor.

The out-of-grammar rate is typically high, and adding more rules often has no improvement in performance. Since the vocabulary size increases, the number of potentially confusable competing recognition hypotheses increases as well. This in turn leads to a decrease in in-grammar recognition accuracy. On top of that, long and complex utterances typically exhibit a higher rate of disfluencies (Shriberg, 1994), such as hesitations, repairs, phrase fragments and filled pauses, which are hard to cope with in a rule based grammar.

In contrast SLMs paired with robust NLU grammars or NLU classifiers lift the need to match the whole utterance string, thus allowing greater flexibility and variation in users' input, and enabling the use of open-ended prompts, less restrictive dialogue strategy and more natural interaction in general. Furthermore, through n-gram smoothing techniques such as probability discounting and backing off strategies, SLMs can accommodate for unknown words and less frequent or unseen sequences.

However, training a SLM requires a large amount of utterances to be collected and transcribed. As an indication, for a typical large scale application of a ~2000 word vocabulary a training set of ~20000 utterances is required. Collecting and transcribing such a corpus can be a cumbersome process that often presupposes the existence of an almost complete or deployed system. Cohen et al. (2004) suggest building an initial smaller corpus, and collecting additional utterances during or after pilot phase. The methods suggested for the collection of the initial corpus are: a) WOZ testing and b) using a rule based grammar for recognition, which is replaced by a SLM as soon as the required amount of training data is collected. Human-human dialogues could also be used if available. All the above methods face the drawbacks already mentioned, but they can serve as a first, better or worse, approximation to an adequately performing production system.

SLMs can be coupled with robust NLU grammars or NLU classifiers to interpret the recognized string. While robust NLU grammars can more effectively handle disfluencies compared to rule based grammars, there is still problem when it comes to long span grammar rules, as the grammar can only match meaningful parts in a serial, continuous manner. Discontinuous semantic information due to hesitations or scrambled word order may still cause problems. The latter is particularly true for free word order languages, where there is no restriction and therefore greater variation in the order in which syntactic constituents appear within a sentence.

Moreover the developer still needs to write rules by hand. NLU classifiers on the other hand automatically learn these rules from a set of training data. The corpus for training the SLM is also used for training the classifier, so there is no need to collect or transcribe a new corpus. Still, the existing corpus needs to be annotated with appropriate semantic values, which in turn consumes people and time resources. NLU machine learning based classifiers could outperform rule based grammars, as they are:

- more robust to discontinuous semantic information (caused by extraneous, irrelevant input or disfluencies) and "scrambled" word order,
- better at resolving ambiguities, since they are trained as to which interpretation to choose,
- using preprocessing such as stemming to efficiently manage highly inflectional languages, since a stemmer can easily automate the vast amount of rules needed to capture the rich inflectional morphology,
- flexible enough to be allowed to select the best algorithms suited for the specific domain and feature set and even test them in order to decide on the most accurate model to be used.

As an indication of performance, Wang et al. (2002) report an up to 3 percentage points decrease in task classification error rate for support vector classifiers compared to rule based robust semantic parsers. However, NLU classifiers that are trained with recorded single utterance inputs are optimized for returning a single slot in contrast to robust grammars. Thus, that type of classification is more appropriate for applications where complex utterances are mapped to a single concept. A typical example of such applications is call routing. Classification needs to get far more complex in terms of training data and feature annotation in order to be able to predict multiple targets (concepts or concept categories).

On a final note, maintenance and support issues should be addressed and taken into consideration when deciding upon the type of grammar used and when building it as well. In industry fields such as mobile telephony, after a period of time, as new products and services are introduced to the market and others are withdrawn, the recognition and interpretation grammars may no longer achieve high coverage of the caller's input and fail to interpret the caller's request correctly.

In the case of rule based grammars, updates can be more straightforward, as new rules can be more easily, manually added to the existing grammar. In the case of SLMs and NLU classifiers, on the other hand, new utterances need to be collected from scratch, transcribed and annotated, in order to retrain, test and optimize the new, updated models. Nevertheless, as grammar and dialogue/system type are tightly interconnected, updates in rule based grammars may induce significant changes in dialogue structure and prompts.

Since rule-based grammars require properly restricting user's input, in order to be effective, adding or eliminating services (i.e. slots or slot values) typically results in changes in the menu hierarchy and/or the content of prompts. In contrast, statistical models coupled with open ended prompts and less restrictive dialogue strategies enable the sustainment of basic dialogue structure, eliminating the need for redesign and allowing for a smooth transition between old and new system versions. In any case, developers should try to anticipate changes and provide means to easily and quickly cope with these changes.

Finally, with regards to the whole development process, it is important to stress out that implementation is inevitably coupled with testing, including usability testing, often resulting in redesign of initial system parts.

## IMPLEMENTING AVA

First, the ASR model was created. In AVA's case the mock up application proved to be the only means for collecting a production quality, "realistic", representative and adequate in size corpus early in the development cycle. Approximately 20,000 utterances were collected and transcribed. 10% of the corpus collected was used as a test set and the rest of the corpus was used for training the SLM.

To achieve greater robustness, classes of words were defined and a class-based language model was trained. Class-based language models constitute an effective way to deal with sparse data, as rarely occurring words of similar semantic function are clustered under the same generalized class; probabilities are then estimated for the generalized class alone and inherited by all words under it. Huang et al. (2001) note that "for limited domain speech recognition, the class-based n-gram is very helpful as the class can efficiently encode semantic information for improved keyword spotting and speech understanding accuracy".

The test corpus was then used to tune the language model and optimize recognition parameters accordingly. The platform default values for most parameters are usually optimal, but developers will still need to optimize pruning, language model scaling and word insertion probability values at least, as well as define language model order (n) and discounting strategy. Finally, domain specific dictionaries were built with pronunciations for words missing from standard dictionaries, mainly involving the domain's jargon.

Next, the NLU components were developed. In accordance with our initial design choices an NLU machine learning classifier was developed for the less restricted, open-ended part of AVA. In order to train the classifier, the existing training corpus was annotated with the correct service tag. Similarly, the test set was annotated and used to optimize the parameters of the classifier.

At the same time, robust sub-grammars were developed, so that particular dialogue states (e.g. confirmation, disambiguation, error-handling and self-service sub-dialogues) could be handled. The latter were tested for interpretation accuracy and coverage and ambiguities to ensure that the test set was completely and correctly interpreted, and ambiguous utterances were appropriately resolved. Furthermore, pronunciation tests were automatically performed to identify missing pronunciations. The results of the latter were fed directly into the development process of the dictionaries for ASR.

In order to cope with the maintenance and upgrade challenges posed by the constant changes and product updates in the fast paced, highly competitive field of mobile telephony, the following solutions were employed:

- Classes for frequently changing products were defined (cf. class based language model), so as to avoid the need for retraining the statistical models every time a product under the predefined class was added or withdrawn. For example, Tariff Plans, which were subject to frequent changes, formed a typical class for the mobile telephony domain.

- Due to a detailed hierarchical classification of the caller's request, future services were proactively accommodated for. Classification was based on exhaustive service domain ontology rather than available routing destinations. When the service categories falling under the same super-class were routed to the same queue, the model used the super-class for default routing. Maintaining the underlying service breakdown made future possible changes to subcategories easy to handle, while newly added services (new sub-classes) could possibly fall under an existing super-class.
- A system management tool was developed that allowed the customer care department to perform low complexity, yet frequently occurring changes, such as queue reassignments.

While the ASR and NLU modules were being developed, most of the dialogue manager behaviour had been coded. Once testing for each module was completed, the different components of AVA were integrated. Integration with the back end database and existing CTI (Computer Telephony Integration) software followed. At the end of the phase a fully integrated working system was ready for evaluation, pilot phase, final tuning and full deployment. Figure 5 summarizes AVA's implementation process.

## CONCLUSION

The development of a successful automated voice agent depends on both effective underlying technology as well as appropriate design choices. In fact, these two aspects of system development are by no means independent; on one hand, design choices are often restricted or expanded by technology limitations or capabilities, while on the other hand technology effectiveness may be corroborated or undermined by valid or poor design respectively.

In this regard, this chapter focused on both design methodology and implementation techniques,

*Figure 5. AVA: implementation phase*

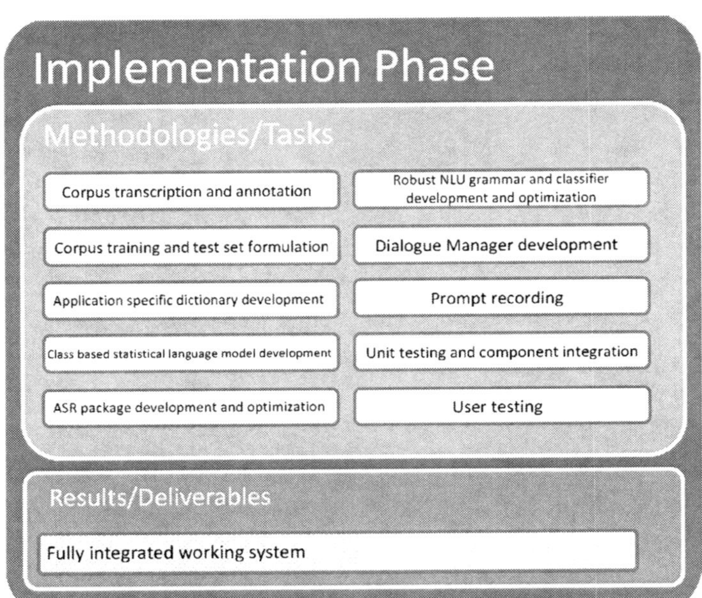

analysing the advantages and disadvantages of tools available in the process of building an automated voice agent, illustrating the choice and use of them in light of a real life paradigm. Understanding of the nature, feasibility and effectiveness wise, of each tool is the key in making the best choice possible, as no readily available, fool-proof rules of thumb can always be safely employed. Rather one should focus on the analysis of the specifics of each system separately.

In the case of AVA, the mock up proved to be the optimal technique for both design and implementation, as it provided invaluable resources shared by both phases. In case of other applications such a solution may not even be an option, often for reasons extraneous to the core system engineering perspective such as company policy prohibiting the exposure of an incomplete, mock up system to the entire customer base. In any case, a combination of available techniques should be employed.

Finally, testing was shown to be a key feature embedded in all steps of a voice agent's lifecycle. Usability testing, in particular, constitutes one of the most promising methods for making successful design choices, being part of the user-centered design paradigm. Bringing the user perspective to the design of the voice agent as early in the process as possible, as well as iterating through design, implementation and testing cycles are imperative for the creation of effective and user friendly automated voice agents.

## REFERENCES


Ai, H., Raux, A., Bohus, D., Eskenazi, M., & Litman, D. (2007). Comparing spoken dialog corpora collected with recruited subjects versus real users. In *Proc. of the 8th SIGdial workshop on Discourse and Dialogue*.

Allen, J. F. (1995). *Natural language understanding*. Menlo Park, CA: Benjamin Cummings.

Allen, J. F., Dzikovska, M., Manshadi, M., & Swift, M. (2007). Deep linguistic processing for spoken dialogue systems. In *Proceedings of the ACL 2007 Workshop on Deep Linguistic Processing*, Prague, June.

Allen, J. F., Ferguson, G., & Stent, A. (2001). An architecture for more realistic conversational systems. In *Proceedings of Intelligent User Interfaces*.

Allen, J. F., Miller, B. W., Ringger, E., & Sikorski, T. (1996). Robust understanding in a dialogue system. In *Proceedings of the 34th Annual Meeting of the Association for Computational Linguistics*.

Attwater, D., Edgington, M., Durston, P., & Whittaker, S. (2000). Practical issues in the application of speech technology to network and customer services applications. *Speech Communication, 31*(4), 279–291. doi:10.1016/S0167-6393(99)00062-X

Balentine, B., & Morgan, D. (1999). *How to build a speech recognition application: A style guide for telephony dialogues*. USA: Enterprise Integration Group.

Chu-Carroll, J., & Carpenter, B. (1999). Vector-based natural language call routing. *Computational Linguistics, 25*(3), 361–388.

Cohen, M., Giancola, J. P., & Balogh, J. (2004). *Voice user interface design*. Addison-Wesley.

Cohen, P. R., & Perrault, C. R. (1979). Elements of a plan-based theory of speech acts. *Cognitive Science, 3*(3), 177–212. doi:10.1207/s15516709cog0303_1

Core, M. G., & Allen, J. F. (1997). Coding dialogs with the DAMSL annotation scheme. In *Working Notes of AAAI Fall Symposium on Communicative Action in Humans and Machines*, Boston, MA.

Dahl, D. (Ed.). (2004). *Practical spoken dialogue systems*. Kluwer Academic Publishers. doi:10.1007/978-1-4020-2676-8

Fellbaum, K., & Kouroupetroglou, G. (2008). Principles of electronic speech processing with applications for people with disabilities. *Technology and Disability*, *20*(2), 55–85.

Fischer, M., Maier, E., & Stein, A. (1994). Generating cooperative system responses in information retrieval dialogues. In *Proceedings of 7th International Workshop on Natural Language Generation (IWNLG 7),* Kennebunkport, Maine.

Fraser, J., & Gilbret, G. (1991). Simulating speech systems. *Computer Speech & Language*, *5*, 81–99. doi:10.1016/0885-2308(91)90019-M

Freitas, D., & Kouroupetroglou, G. (2008). Speech technologies for blind and low vision persons. *Technology and Disability*, *20*(2), 135–156.

Galitz, W. O. (2007). *The essential guide to user interface design*. Wiley Publishing, Inc.

Garfield, S., & Wermter, S. (2002). *Recurrent neural learning for helpdesk call routing. Lecture Notes in Computer Science 2415/2002, Artificial Neural Networks*. Berlin/Heidelberg, Germany: Springer.

Garfield, S., & Wermter, S. (2006). Call classification using recurrent neural networks, support vector machines and finite state automata. [Springer-Verlag.]. *Knowledge and Information Systems*, 9.

Gorin, L., Riccardi, G., & Wright, J. H. (1997). How may I help you? *Speech Communication*, *23*, 113–127. doi:10.1016/S0167-6393(97)00040-X

Gould, J. D., & Lewis, C. (1985). Designing for usability: Key principles and what designers think. *Communications of the ACM*, *28*(3), 300–311. doi:10.1145/3166.3170

Grosz, B. J., & Sidner, C. L. (1986). Attention, intentions, and the structure of discourse. *Computational Linguistics*, *12*(3), 175–204.

Gupta, N., Tur, G., Hakkani-Tur, D., Bangalore, S., Riccardi, G., & Rahim, M. (2006). The AT&T spoken language understanding system. *IEEE Transactions on Speech and Audio Processing*.

Harris, R. A. (2005). *Voice interaction design: Crafting the new conversational speech systems*. Elsevier.

Hempel, T. (2008). *Usability of speech dialog systems: Listening to the target audience*. Springer-Verlag.

Hirschberg, J., Nakatani, C., & Grosz, B. (1995). Conveying discourse structure through intonation variation. In *Proceedings of the ECSA Workshop on Spoken Dialogue Systems: Theories and Applications*, Visgo, Denmark.

Huang, X., Acero, A., & Hon, H. W. (2001). *Spoken language processing: A guide to theory, algorithm and system development*. Prentice Hall PTR.

Jurafsky, D., & Martin, J. H. (2000). *Speech and language processing. An introduction to natural language processing, computational linguistics, and speech recognition*. Prentice-Hall.

Kamm, C. A., & Walker, M. A. (1997). Design and evaluation of spoken dialogue systems. In *Proc. of the IEEE Workshop on Automatic Speech Recognition and Understanding*, Santa Barbara (CA), 14–17.

Kouroupetroglou, G. (2009). Universal access in public terminals: Information kiosks and ATMs. In Stephanidis, C. (Ed.), *The universal access handbook* (pp. 48.1–48.19). Florida, USA: CRC Press. doi:10.1201/9781420064995-c48

Kouroupetroglou, G., & Spiliotopoulos, D. (2009). Usability methodologies for real-life voice user interfaces. [IJITWE]. *International Journal of Information Technology and Web Engineering*, *4*(4), 78–94. doi:10.4018/jitwe.2009100105

Kowtko, J., Isard, S., & Doherty, G. M. (1993). *Conversational games within dialogue*. Research paper 31, Human Communication Research Centre, University of Edinburgh.

Larson, J. A. (2002). *VoiceXML: Introduction to developing speech applications*. NJ: Prentice Hall.

Lauesen, S. (2005). *User interface design: A software engineering perspective*. Addison-Wesley.

Lee, C., & Chang, J. S. (2002). *Rapid prototyping an operator assisted call routing system*. ISCSLP 2002, Taipei, Taiwan.

McGlashan, S., Burnett, D. C., Carter, J., Danielsen, P., Ferrans, J., & Hunt, A. … Tryphonas, S. (2004). *Voice Extensible Markup Language (VoiceXML) version* 2.0. Retrieved from http://www.w3.org/TR/voicexml20.

McTear, M. F. (2004). *Towards the conversational user interface*. Springer Verlag.

Nielsen, J. (1995). *Technology transfer of heuristic evaluation and usability inspection*. Presented at the IFIP INTERACT'95 International Conference on Human-Computer Interaction, Lillehammer, Norway.

Nielsen, J., & Mack, R. L. (1994). *Usability inspection methods*. New York, NY: John Wiley & Sons.

Norman, D. (1988). *The design of everyday things*. New York, NY: Doubleday/Currency.

Norman, D. A., & Draper, S. W. (1986). *User centered system design: New perspectives on human-computer interaction*. Mahwah, NJ: Lawrence Erlbaum Associates.

Noth, E., Batlinera, A., Warnkea, V., Haasa, J., Borosb, M., & Buckowa, J. (2002). On the use of prosody in automatic dialogue understanding. *Speech Communication, 36*(1-2), 45–62. doi:10.1016/S0167-6393(01)00025-5

Pellom, B., Ward, W., Hansen, J., Cole, R., Hacioglu, K., & Zhang, J. … Pradhan, S. (2001). *University of Colorado dialog systems for travel and navigation*. HLT-2001, San Diego.

Pieraccini, R., & Huerta, J. M. (2008). Where do we go from here? Research and commercial spoken dialogue systems. In Dybkjaer, L., & Minker, W. (Eds.), *Recent trends in discourse and dialogue*. Springer.

Pitt, I., & Edwards, A. (2003). *Design of speech-based devices: A practical guide*. Springer.

Pulman, S. (2002). Relating dialogue games to information state. *Speech Communication, 36*, 15–30. doi:10.1016/S0167-6393(01)00023-1

Riccardi, G., Gorin, A. L., Ljolje, A., & Riley, M. (1997). A spoken language system for automated call routing. In. *Proceedings of ICASSP, 1997*, 1143–1146.

Rubin, J., & Chisnell, D. (2008). *Handbook of usability testing, 2nd edition: How to plan, design, and conduct effective tests*. Wiley Publishing, Inc.

Shriberg, E. (1994). *Preliminaries to a theory of speech disfluencies*. PhD thesis, University of California, Berkeley, CA.

Sidner, C. (2004). Building spoken-language collaborative interface agents. In Dahl, D. (Ed.), *Practical spoken dialogue systems*. Kluwer Academic Publishers. doi:10.1007/978-1-4020-2676-8_10

Spiliotopoulos, D., & Kouroupetroglou, G. (2010). Usability methodologies for spoken dialogue Web interfaces. In Spiliotopoulos, T., Papadopoulou, P., Martakos, D., & Kouroupetroglou, G. (Eds.), *Integrating usability engineering for designing the Web experience: Methodologies and principles*. Hershey, PA: IGI Global. doi:10.4018/978-1-60566-896-3.ch008

Spiliotopoulos, D., Stavropoulou, P., & Kouroupetroglou, G. (2009). Spoken dialogue interfaces: Integrating usability. *Lecture Notes in Computer Science, 5889*, 484–499. doi:10.1007/978-3-642-10308-7_36

Stavropoulou, P., Spiliotopoulos, D., & Kouroupetroglou, G. (2011). *Resource evaluation for usable spoken dialogue interfaces: Utilizing human – human dialogues*. In preparation.

Stent, A., Dowding, J., Gawron, J. M., Bratt, E. O., & Moore, R. (1999). The CommandTalk spoken dialogue system. In *Proceedings of the Thirty-Seventh Annual Meeting of the ACL*, (pp. 183-190).

Turunen, M., Hakulinen, J., & Kainulainen, A. (2006). Evaluation of a spoken dialogue system with usability tests and long-term pilot studies: Similarities and differences. In *Proceedings of Interspeech*.

Wahlster, W. (2000). *Verbmobil: Foundations of speech-to-speech translation*. Berlin, Germany & New York, NY: Springer.

Walker, M. A. Langkilde-Geary, I., Wright Hastie, H., Wright, J., & Gorin, A. (2002). Automatically training a problematic dialogue predictor for the HMIHY spoken dialogue system. *Journal of Artificial Intelligence Research (JAIR)*.

Wang, Y., Acero, A., Chelba, C., Frey, B., & Wong, L. (2002). Combination of statistical and rule-based approaches for spoken language understanding. In *Proceedings of the International Conference on Spoken Language Processing*, Denver, CO.

Weinschenk, S., & Barker, D. T. (2000). *Designing effective speech interfaces*. John Wiley & Sons, Inc.

Williams, J. D., & Witt, S. M. (2004). A comparison of dialog strategies for call routing. [Springer Netherlands.]. *International Journal of Speech Technology*, 7.

Zitouni, I., Hong-Kwang, J. K., & Chin-Hui, L. (2003). Boosting and combination of classifiers for natural language call routing systems. *Speech Communication*, 14.

## KEY TERMS AND DEFINITIONS

**Automated Call Routing Application:** Interactive Voice Response (IVR) based application that automatically routes incoming phone calls to appropriate destinations. Intelligent routing can be based on parameters such as DTMF or voice input interpretation, caller identification or time of day.

**Automated Voice Agent:** Program capable of communicating with users by both understanding and producing speech within a specific domain. It is typically comprised of the following basic modules: the Automatic Speech Recognition module that converts acoustic user input into text, the Natural Language Understanding module that semantically interprets it, the Dialogue Manager that handles the conversation flow, the Natural Language Generator that generates system prompts in written form, and the Text to Speech Synthesizer that converts the written prompts to speech.

**NLU Machine Learning Based Classifier:** It is a system programmed to automatically learn to recognize complex patterns and make intelligent decisions based on data; the difficulty lies in the fact that the set of all possible behaviors given all possible inputs is too large to be covered by the set of observed examples (training data). Trained for natural language understanding, it automatically extracts one or more possible interpretations from a single natural language input.

**Robust Natural Language Understanding (NLU) Grammar:** Rule based word spotting interpretation grammar. Instead of parsing the whole user utterance, a robust grammar performs word or phrase spotting, searching the utterance and assigning semantic values to meaningful parts only.

**Rule Based Grammar:** A context free grammar, where permissible word sequences are specified by manually written production rules of the form $A \rightarrow \beta$ in which A is a non terminal node and $\beta$ is a sequence of terminal and/or non terminal nodes. It is used for speech recognition – restricting the recognizer's search space – as well as speech interpretation – augmented with slot filling semantic rule attachments.

**Statistical Language Model (SLM):** N-gram model trained on domain specific corpora in order to compute the probability of word sequences. Used for Automatic Speech Recognition, it is essentially a model of what the callers are likely to say when interacting with the system.

**Usability:** Attribute that refers to various types of interfaces, measured and described in terms of usefulness, effectiveness, efficiency, learnability and user satisfaction. It denotes the extent to which a system can be used to achieve the goals it was designed for with accuracy, completeness and speed in a user-friendly, easy-to-use and learn manner.

**Usability Testing:** Set of methods and schemes for assessing the user's experience when interacting with a system and evaluating usability attributes such as effectiveness, efficiency and user satisfaction. Typical usability tests for speech based systems include Wizard-of-Oz testing, user testing with limited functionality or fully working systems, usability inspection etc.

# Chapter 16
# Conversational Agents in Language and Culture Training

**Alicia Sagae**
*Alelo, USA*

**W. Lewis Johnson**
*Alelo, USA*

**Andre Valente**
*Alelo, USA*

## ABSTRACT

*This chapter describes the design, implementation, and use of an agent architecture that has been deployed in Alelo, Inc.'s language and culture training systems, which offer practical training for foreign language skills and intercultural competence. These agents support real-time conversation in the language of interest (Dari, Pashto, Arabic, French, and others), using automatic speech recognition and immersive simulation technologies. In earlier work, we developed a number of agent-based language and culture trainers, based on the Tactical Language and Culture Training System platform. Our experience has revealed a number of desiderata for authorable, believable agents, which we have applied to the design of our newest agent architecture. In this chapter, we describe the Virtual Role-Players (VRP), an agent architecture that relies on ontological models of world knowledge, language, culture, and agent state, in order to achieve believable dialogue with learners. Authoring and user experiences are described, along with future directions for this work.*

## INTRODUCTION

Conversational agents have particular appeal in the educational domain of training learners in communicative competency. Experts in the language education community, such as the American Council on the Teaching of Foreign Languages (ACTFL), describe communicative proficiency as a goal that includes both *declarative knowledge* and *procedural skill* (Lampe, 2007). In a computer-based learning environment, conversational agents allow students to engage these procedural skills by speaking in real time and observing believable responses.

DOI: 10.4018/978-1-60960-617-6.ch016

Our concern is the development of conversational agents for practical training systems for foreign language skills and intercultural competence. Such agents must meet a range of challenging design constraints. They need to produce behavior that has an appropriate level of realism and cultural accuracy, so that they provide a suitable model for training. At the same time, they need to be easily authorable and configurable, by people who may not be specialists in agent modeling frameworks and formalisms. Ideally, it should be possible for trainers and educators to create their own training scenarios, populate them with conversational agents, and have the agents behave in culturally and situationally appropriate ways.

In earlier work, we developed a number of agent-based language and culture trainers, based on the Tactical Language and Culture Training System platform (Johnson & Valente, 2008), such as the Tactical Iraqi trainer for Iraqi Arabic (Johnson, 2010). These have been used widely by military service members and other individuals preparing for overseas work. The trainers include a large number of practice dialogues and scenarios, each of which includes one or more conversational agents. A typical course includes fifty or more agents, each designed to converse with learners in a particular scenario or situation. The behavior of each agent is specified in a finite state machine framework.

Although this has proven to be an effective approach for creating conversational agents in this domain, it suffers from some key limitations. One is that each agent has to be authored for the specific scenario context in which it is intended to be used. This multiplies authoring effort and limits the number of agents that can be incorporated into a given scenario. It also prevents trainers from creating new training scenarios or adapting scenarios to their own needs. Another limitation is that it is up to agent authors to make sure that the agent's behavior is culturally appropriate, and it is difficult to validate whether they have done so. To overcome these limitations we have recognized the need to develop an agent authoring framework that supports the creation of agents that can be employed flexibly in a range of training scenarios, and which incorporate explicit, validated models of culturally appropriate behavior.

In response to these and other desiderata, this chapter introduces Alelo's new Virtual Role-Player framework, a conversational agent architecture that has been employed in a number of language and culture training systems. The Virtual Role-Player (VRP) architecture is a flexible platform for combining models of conversation, facilitating model reuse and behavior validation. Models of politeness, culture, and strategy (e.g. lying for a social purpose) have all been implemented in this framework in an effort to drive more believable agent behavior. The result is a set of artificially intelligent, conversation-ready agents who can be attached to visual avatars in a variety of serious game environments. These agents are called Virtual Role-Players (VRPs). Individual VRPs have been instantiated as characters in Alelo's Operational Language and Culture Training System series (OLCTS), and in mission rehearsal applications built on the 3D platforms Virtual Battlespace 2 (VBS2) and RealWorld.

In this chapter, we connect our experience with conversational agent systems to a selection of related examples from the literature, followed by a detailed description of our newest agent architecture. In the remainder of this section, we explain the context of this work with examples from Alelo's OLCTS language and culture training suite. This leads to a set of desiderata for agent architectures, and a discussion of related work using these desiderata as a guide. Following related work, we give a technical overview of the VRP architecture, along with additional detail on the models used for dialogue and culture. Finally, we describe user experiences of authoring and interacting with VRPs.

*Figure 1. Operational Dari language and culture training system (© 2010, Alelo)*

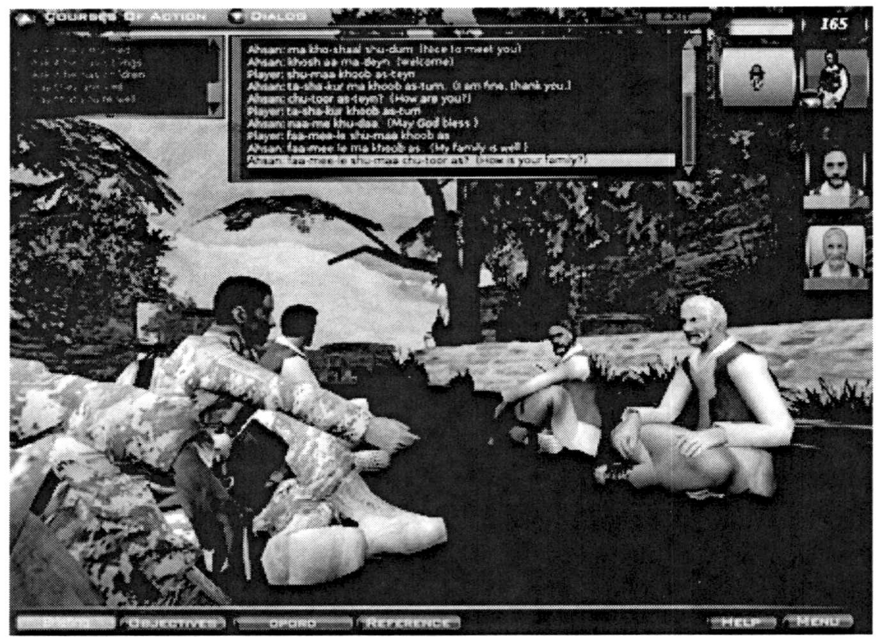


## BACKGROUND

### Language and Culture Training with Alelo Conversational Agents

Many users of Alelo courses are members of military services who require training in intercultural skills prior to deployment overseas on missions such as reconstruction and humanitarian assistance. Figure 1 shows an episode from one such course, the US version of the Operational Dari language and culture trainer. In this example the learner, playing the role of the military character on the left, is meeting with a local leader (known as a malek) and other elders in an Afghan village. To play the role, the player must speak into the microphone in Dari, the local language of the area, as well as choose culturally appropriate gestures. The dialogue history is shown in the top center of the figure. The player needs to develop rapport with the malek in order to gain his cooperation. For this reason, the dialogue history up to this point in the episode consists of greetings and inquiries about the malek's family, and there has been no discussion as yet of the business purpose of the meeting, namely the reconstruction of a local school.

The Operational Dari training suite includes interactive lessons that help learners acquire the communication skills that they need in situations such as the one depicted in Figure 1. It also includes a variety of immersive episodes in which learners can practice their skills. There are single-player learning environments, as shown in Figure 1, as well as multi-player environments, in which trainees can practice their communication skills as part of an overall simulated military mission.

Figure 2 shows a multi-player episode, or *scene*, running in Virtual Battlespace 2 (VBS2). The player's intent in this conversation is similar to that in the previous example: to build rapport with a member of the village to gain their cooperation.

As these examples illustrate, Operational Dari and other OLCTS courses enable learners to converse with a number of different agents. The agents tend to have many similarities in their

*Figure 2. An operational Dari scene in virtual battlespace 2 (© 2010, Alelo)*

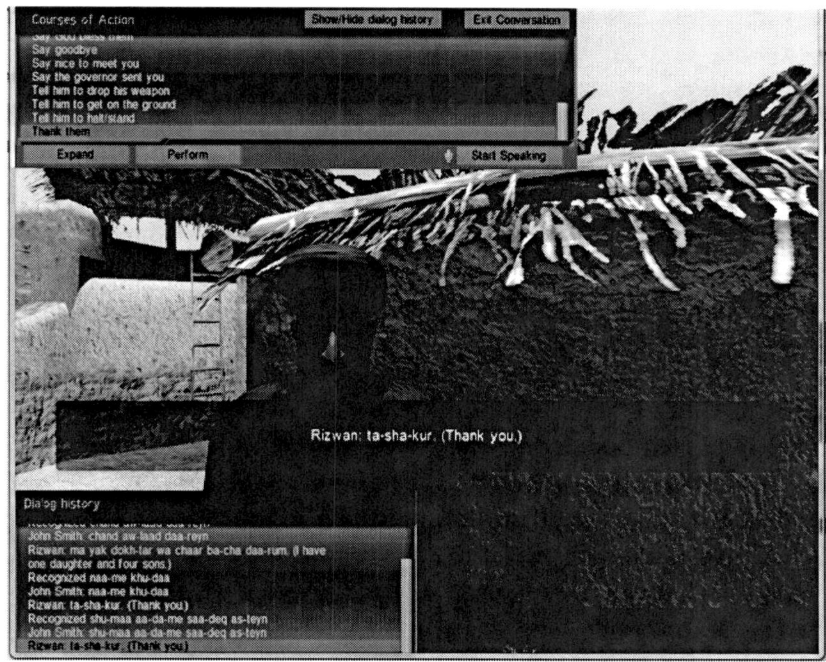


behavior, as well as differences specific to that conversational situation. For example, the Afghan agents in Figure 1 and Figure 2 can both converse about their respective families, but the details of their families may differ.

More importantly, there may be differences in the two conversations stemming from the fact that one is a formal gathering and the other is a chance encounter on the street. This poses challenges from an agent modeling standpoint. In our older Tactical Language courses, separate agent models had to be constructed for each agent in each episode, without any opportunity for reuse. This resulted in a substantial amount of authoring effort to develop each agent and then validate its behavior to make sure that it is culturally and situationally appropriate. The Virtual Role Player architecture helps to reduce this effort. The agents in Figure 1 and Figure 2 can both be developed from a common agent model for Afghan elders, and customized as needed for each specific conversational situation.

## Desiderata for Communicative Agents

With experience from these systems in mind, we can describe some of the desiderata for a new communicative agent architecture that is appropriate for building large-scale language and culture training courses.

**Desideratum 1: Reusable characters.** Full-scale training systems, comprising multiple training scenarios and situations, require a method for reusing characters across situations. To see why, consider the alternative, which would be to author each agent in a context-specific way, with a set of verbal and non-verbal responses that apply only in the specific scenario where the agent is intended to appear. The effect of having a character appear in multiple scenarios can be achieved in this approach only by creating multiple agents with some overlapping behavior (both respond with "I am Razan" when asked for their name) but which are non-interchangeable due to scenario-specific details (when asked "how is your family," one responds "they are well" while the other responds "my son has been injured").

Such an approach multiplies authoring effort and limits the number of agents that can be incorporated into a given scenario. It also prevents trainers from creating new training scenarios or adapting scenarios to their own needs. Instead, we desire communicative agents to be authored in a reusable fashion, with general behavior rules that can apply in multiple scenarios. In the example given above, the agent Razan should have a programmatic way to determine and then report on the health of his family, rather than relying on the author to enter context-specific answers by hand. This principle applies to all layers of the agent architecture; when possible, we prefer to build reusable components that can be composed to achieve a desired agent behavior.

**Desideratum 2: Explicit models of appropriate behavior.** The connection between authoring processes and agent behavior is another important consideration. In many cases, the designer of agent behavior is a subject matter expert (SME) who has detailed knowledge of what constitutes "believable" language, gesture, and movement for the character who will be played by the communicative agent. How is this knowledge captured in the authoring process, and how is it translated into the programmed instructions for the agent? In many systems, including the Alelo's earlier finite state machine (FSM) approach, the knowledge is captured informally, with each author working from his own mental model and attempting to author dialogues that conform to it. In the new architecture, we desire a way to use explicit models of culturally appropriate behavior that can be examined and validated independently, then dropped into the agent architecture, ensuring greater consistency. To further improve authorability, the architecture would support libraries of predefined models, under the hypothesis that modifying or adapting models is easier than creating them from scratch.

**Desideratum 3: Awareness.** In similar fashion to explicit models of behavior, we propose that communicative agents in this setting should have access to explicit factual knowledge about themselves and their social and physical environment. To apply social norms correctly, an agent must be aware not of the concept of social distance, but also of the agent's specific position in society, in order to reason about the relative social distance in its communications with the learner.

The agent must also have an internal set of beliefs and knowledge about the world, in order to behave appropriately. This supports flexible behavior of the type described in our earlier example: ideally, we want an agent to respond to the question "how is your family" based in part on whether or not the agent actually knows this information, or even if he has a family. World knowledge should include the physical and cultural environments, and the current state of the conversation. For example, the agent may condition certain responses on whether or not the learner has established enough rapport to be trusted. Some decisions may even depend on synthesis of facts from the physical and cultural environment. For example, to decide on an appropriate gesture (say, shake hands), agents may need to know not only about the social distance with an interlocutor but also the physical distance.

**Desideratum 4: Performance.** Performance factors are critical for agents that operate in immersive environments, particularly when there are large numbers of such agents operating at the same time. 3D graphics rendering and automated speech rendering both require a considerable amount of computational processing, and compete with agent reasoning for computing resources. Agent models that take a long time to make a decision, or that compete strongly for computing resources, can adversely impact the believability and usability of the simulation.

## RELATED WORK

The systems described in this chapter draw on concepts from the literature in social science and computational modeling, in addition to conversational agent systems. We address each of these areas in the section below.

### Social Science and the Science of Learning

The language and culture training curricula at Alelo are founded in research in the social sciences, including socio-cultural and linguistic anthropology, as well as the science of learning. This research plays an important role in choosing the desiderata described above, since the end goal for conversational agents in Alelo courses is to provide an effective method for exercising and building learner knowledge, skills, and attitudes (KSAs) in accordance with these curricula.

Alelo courses are designed to teach intercultural competence: the ability to communicate successfully with people of other cultures (Byram, 1997). Given that many of our products are deployed to service members in the US military who are preparing to be deployed overseas, we also consider research on intercultural competence from military institutions. The recommendations of the Defense Regional and Cultural Capabilities Assessment Working Group (RACCA WG) are a seminal publication describing cross-cultural competence in this community (McDonald et al., 2008). They include a list of 40 learning statements, covering knowledge, skills, and personal characteristics, which are designed to foster cross-cultural competence in military and civilian personnel. An example from each category is shown below:

- Knowledge: knowing cultural concepts and processes.
- Skills: integrating culture into planning and execution for mission success.
- Personal Characteristics: demonstrating a willingness to engage.

Within the domain of intercultural competency, we adopt a task-based instructional strategy that is well aligned with other task-based approaches to language learning, such as Ellis (2003). Our approach is described in the Situated Culture Methodology, or SCM (Valente, et al., 2009). The SCM focuses on communication necessary to perform real-world tasks. It assumes that intercultural competence curricula, like other types of curricula, should be based upon a task analysis of the skills to be taught, and the work situations in which those skills are to be applied (Jonassen, Tessmer, & Hannum, 1999). The learning activities in Alelo courses, including conversations with agents, are all task-oriented in this sense.

These learning objectives and strategies from the literature on cross-cultural competence underscore the importance of our agent desiderata. Explicit models of appropriate behavior allow us to build learning objectives such as those described by the RACCA WG into the conversational agent software, by associating the objectives with learner behaviors (i.e. specific turns in a dialogue) and tracking when those behaviors occur.

When these behaviors are complex, the agent must rely on more than the most recent learner input to identify them. For example, demonstrating willingness to engage may be a behavior that is associated with an entire dialogue. The desideratum of awareness captures this need for a breadth and depth of knowledge on the part of the agent. Reasonable performance ensures that the training experience closely resembles the real-world setting where the learner will have to apply his/her skills, and re-usable characters allow us to generate a variety of experiences that are tailored to individual learners' needs. In a task-based curriculum, for example, we may want the learner to collaborate with the same character on a variety of different missions.

## Computational Models of Dialogue

Social science literature also influences the individual models of dialogue that are implemented in VRPs. In many conversational agent systems, models of human behavior drive the agents' reaction to user input. These models can capture features of personality that affect the agent in all interactions, or emotional features that arise in reaction to a particular chain of events (Marsella & Gratch, 2009). They often capture details of the particular conversational context, as in goal-driven models of negotiation (Traum et al., 2008) or task-based models of conversation with explicit conditions for success (Johnson & Valente, 2009).

Given that VRPs engage in interpersonal dialogue with one player or a small group, social science models from the field of microsociology are especially relevant. Microsociology focuses on the dynamics of everyday social life, and on the structure and processes of how society works in real-time, on the ground. This tradition can be traced to Max Weber (1994), one of the founders of sociology, and Alfred Schutz (1970), who grounded the approach in the philosophy of Husserl. It has continued to develop in the disciplines of social psychology (Blumer, 1986; Goffman, 1990; Mead, 1967), ethnomethodology (Garfinkel, 1967), sociology (Habermas, 1984), and anthropological "practice theory".

These theories have influenced the formal microsocial models of Hobbs & Gordon (2010), which are used directly in the VRP architecture to model socio-cultural expectations for interpersonal dialogue. Among the other models of social behavior that are used in VRPs are politeness (Wang et al., 2008), and strategy (e.g. lying for a social purpose) (Sagae et al., 2009).

## Conversational Agents

VRPs apply these background theories in the context of a conversational agent system; specifically, a pedagogical system where the conversational behavior of the agent is both a teaching tool and a teaching target.

A wide variety of related systems exist in the literature today. Many of these focus on generation capabilities – the ability of the agent to express its affective states in ways that are appropriate for a given conversation. Greta is one example of a conversational agent aimed at realistic behavior generation (Rosis et al., 2003). Like a VRP, Greta is designed to use explicit models to drive believable expressions of the affective state of the agent.

However, Greta's models focus on the agent's self-knowledge and her expressions are performed on a micro-scale, using features like gaze, eyebrow, and mouth position. Other agent systems in this class include Laura, the health counseling agent (Bickmore & Pfeifer, 2008), the Sensitive Artificial Learners (McRorie et al., 2009), and experiments in agent emotion by Marsella and Gratch (2009) and Mello and Gratch (2009). These agents model their affective states at a fine level of granularity, and they express these states as a way of building rapport with the user.

VRPs contrast with such systems in several ways. First, VRPs are typically used to teach the *user* how to build rapport with the *agent*. This distinction is important, since VRPs can be used in training scenarios where rapport-building is intentionally challenging or delicate (as in simulated negotiations). Second, the models of conversation used in VRPs are more coarse-grained, in order to focus on dialogue-level effects such as dialogue outcome (e.g. did the user manage to perform required social conventions? Did the user negotiate a commitment for future action from the NPC?).

This granularity also allows us to focus on broad socio-cultural influences, rather than personal influences, on agent behavior. Most interactions with VRPs are intended to equip the user with communication skills, applicable in any conversation with a similar cultural and linguistic context, not to build an ongoing relationship between the user and a particular VRP character.

Finally, VRP models are intentionally designed with authorability in mind. Given that VRPs are deployed in a large number of systems, new models must be derived from existing ones quickly, by non-programmer authors. In summary, many of the agent systems described in the literature are designed to have very emotionally expressive behavior in a small range of circumstances, while VRPs are designed to have flexible behavior, which is culturally and linguistically appropriate in a wide range of circumstances (different languages, different cultures, different tasks).

Other agent systems that have influenced our work on VRPs by addressing socio-cultural factors in task-based dialogue include cultural agents by Roque and Traum (2007), and conversational modeling and turn-taking by Vilhjálmsson and Thórisson (2008). These systems both make use of rich object representation of dialogue context, in support of the desideratum of awareness.

Finally, VRPs draw on the literature in pedagogical agents such as AutoTutor (Graesser et al., 2005), Why-2 Atlas and Atlas-Andes (Rose et al., 2001), among many others. Some of these pedagogical agent systems communicate with the learner in natural language, as VRPs do. However, few of these systems are intended to teach, as well as use, natural language communication. As a result, it is often possible to assess the linguistic and cultural performance of the agents separately from their pedagogical strategies. In contrast, the communicative performance of a VRP serves not only to communicate to the learner, but to serve as an example of the skill being taught.

## THE VRP ARCHITECTURE

The following is a discussion of the VRP architecture, and how it is used to create communicative agents (or VRPs). We focus on the use of VRPs that engage in multimodal communication with trainees in a foreign language, using a combination of speech and gesture, as shown in the examples in the introduction.

This is the most challenging application of the VRP architecture, since it integrates many different aspects of behavior interpretation, intent planning, and behavior generation. VRP characters can also be realized in training modalities where the interaction between the trainees and the communicative agents is more limited, e.g., trainees select communicative actions from a menu of options, or communicate with the character by typing rather than speaking. The particular choice of interaction modality depends upon the training objectives of the course and the expected skill set of the trainees undertaking the activity. The VRP architecture is designed to be flexible enough to support a range of different interaction modalities.

In multimodal dialogue scenarios, user actions are recognized from menu-driven gestures along with speech input that passes through an automatic speech recognition (ASR) module, and VRP responses are performed by 3D avatars with speech and gesture generation capabilities. The result is a character who moves and acts physically in the virtual environment, but who also listens and responds in real-time conversations with human users. At the heart of this system is the social simulation pipeline, the software component that gives each agent its ability to understand and respond to learner inputs. In this section we discuss the social simulation pipeline used by VRPs.

### Overview

The architecture adopts a variant of the SAIBA paradigm (Vilhjalmsson & Marsella, 2005), which separates intent planning (the choice of what to communicate) from production of believable physical behavior (how to realize the communication). The current version extends the architecture described by Samtani, Valente & Johnson (2008).

A visual representation is given in Figure 3. The player usually engages the system by speaking into a microphone. Starting from the lower-left corner of the area labeled Social Simulation Module, player speech input is captured and passed to an automatic speech recognizer (ASR). The ASR component produces a plain-text string, stored in an object called an *utterance*, which is used by the behavior interpretation module to generate a meaning representation. The player may also perform gestures, using a menu-driven interface. This allows the learner to accompany his/her spoken turns with movements, such as "hand-over-heart," a gesture that accompanies greetings in some Muslim cultures. Gestures pass through the same behavior interpretation module that interprets speech, resulting in a meaning representation that captures spoken and gestured intent.

After the interpretation stage, an intent planning module maps the learner's intended input to an agent-specific response, and the rest of the pipeline is devoted to realizing this response in the form of speech and gestures. Speech is generally performed via pre-recorded voice files, but the mechanism is generic and can integrate speech synthesis if required.

To pass data between these stages, we use a control mechanism implemented in the expert systems programming language CLIPS[1]. The data structures, including mapping rules that determine what the output of each stage should be, are stored as instances in an ontology, edited and stored using Protégé[2]. At runtime, the CLIPS module loads a set of rules as data, and uses them to analyze the learner input, much like a syntactic parser that loads a grammar in order to produce a parse.

This design choice supports our desiderata of re-usability, explicit models, and awareness, at the potential expense of performance (this tradeoff can be managed with some optimizations, described later). Rules and similar data structures represent explicit, composable models of agent behavior that can be reused in multiple dialogues, and by multiple agents. For example, we can consider a set of mappings from strings to meaning representations to be a model of the language that a conversational agent understands. This language understanding model is authored by subject matter experts with general knowledge of intercultural communication and expertise in the current language (e.g., Dari, Pashto, French, Arabic). The same model can be loaded by a variety of agents, each of which can now "understand" the language at hand. The behavior interpretation and behavior generation modules shown in Figure 3 apply this model at run-time to determine the meaning representation for an input utterance, or to choose an utterance that expresses an intended output.

The agent itself is also an object in the ontology, which can store personal facts in addition to pointers to language and behavior models. As a result, when the dialogue manager sends learner input to an agent, that agent is able to supply his own world knowledge, composed of all of the models and facts that have been attached to him, as additional input to the intent planning module that computes the agent's reply. This contributes to the agent's awareness of the situation, resulting in consistent replies for a given agent across all learner interactions.

## Behavior Interpretation

As described above, spoken learner behavior is converted into a string by an automatic speech recognition (ASR) module and stored in an object called an utterance. The meaning representation is structured as an object called a communicative act, or "act". Act structures are derived from the work of Austin (1975), using refinements published by Traum and Hinkleman (1992). Each act has a core function, i.e., the illocutionary function of the utterance (to greet, inform, request, etc.), as well as a semantic content field that holds a structured representation of the thematic role relations (Jackendoff, 1990) expressed in the utterance.

To determine which act corresponds to the current learner utterance, we rely on search through a collection of bi-directional mapping objects. At interpretation time, we search using the utterance as a key, retrieving all of the objects that map

*Figure 3. The VRP social simulation pipeline (© 2010, Alelo)*

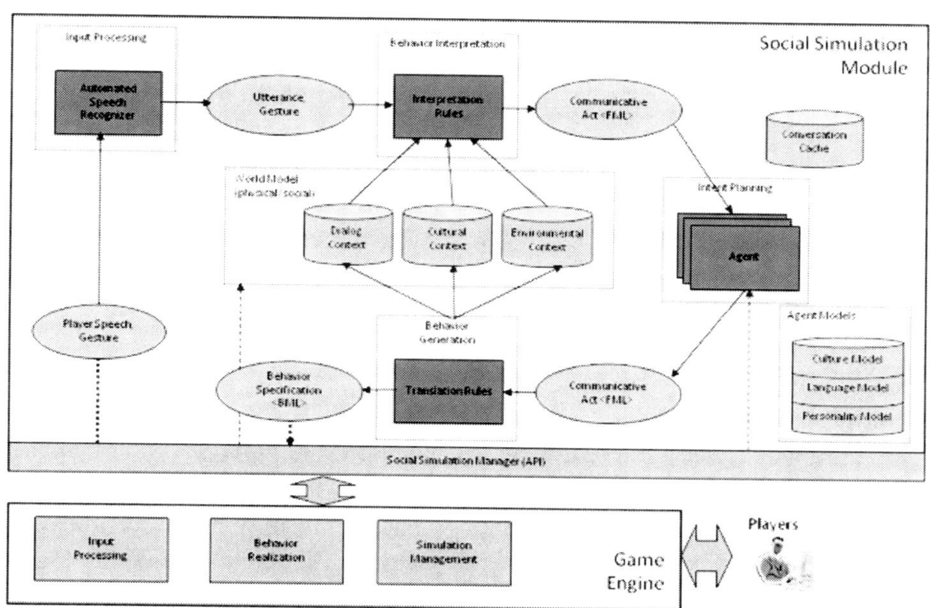


this utterance to an act. Next, a context-specific selection of a single return act is made, which is passed as the result of behavior interpretation into the intent planning stage. When no mapping is found for the current learner utterance, the behavior interpretation module returns an act called "garbage", meaning that the agent failed to understand the learner's input. The garbage act can also be used to explicitly capture predictable learner errors, ensuring that they lead to a non-understanding response from the VRP. This type of in-game feedback for the learner can be important for maintaining realism. An extended discussion of this topic is given in (Sagae, Johnson, & Bodnar, 2010).

By performing this mapping to act-level abstractions, we gain efficiency in later stages. For example, "Hi" "Hello" "Howdy" may all be interpreted as casual greetings. By mapping all of these behaviors to the same act, we enable one intent planning rule to generate a reply for all of them. In addition, we achieve a division of tasks that corresponds to a division of labor among our authoring team.

Authors with language expertise can work on authoring behavior mappings, associating a variety of strings in the language being taught (e.g., Pashto, Dari, French, Arabic) with their interpretations at the act level. Intent planning rules can be authored in parallel by authors with expertise at the cultural level, who know what the agent should plan to do in a given situation, or at the task level, who may have specialized knowledge of how conversations go in a technical domain.

## Intent Planning

In the intent planning module, VRP behavior is generated by a series of behavior-mapping rules that reflect the subject-matter expertise of the rule authors. A simple example of such a rule, expressed in natural language, is shown below:

IF *the learner asks about the health of your family*,
THEN *reply that your family is well*
AND *increase trust for the learner* (1)

Rules like (1) apply some types of knowledge implicitly in the following sense: when creating the rule, an author may be guided by an assumption like the axiom shown in (2).

*In cultural setting* X, *family inquiries help establish rapport* (2)

Without a software object where such axioms can be represented explicitly, the author is forced to keep a list of these guiding axioms in mind and to check the rules s/he writes for consistency with them. Since multiple authors may be involved in authoring rules, they would need to coordinate to make sure they all have a consistent view of these axioms. In contrast, the VRP architecture uses explicit models for axioms of type (2), stored as meta-rules in that can be loaded as appropriate for a given agent.

Meta-rules operate by using not only the current learner input, but a model of the dialogue history, to modify the agent's internal state. For example, the rule shown in (2) may search the dialogue history for instances of family inquiries, and increment trust whenever one is found. Without meta-rule (2), the author is responsible for adding clauses like "AND increase trust for the learner" to every family inquiry he authors. Rule (1) is only one example – there may be inquiries about the names or ages of family members, their employment status, or where they attend school. In VRPs, the author creates each of these rules independently, while the system ensures that higher-order consequences are triggered in a consistent manner based on an axiom that is only authored once, and applied everywhere.

## Behavior Generation

Behavior generation in VRPs is the inverse of behavior interpretation, and it reuses the same models of language and agent knowledge. This choice supports our desideratum for reusable agents and components. However, these shared models can grow quite large, requiring search optimizations to ensure reasonable performance. The collection of mapping objects between utterances and acts is one example. In the current VRP system we are investigating indexing options that will allow us to quickly retrieve the set of mappings that apply to a given utterance (during interpretation), or to a given act (during generation), rather than searching the entire model during every learner turn at run-time.

# MODELS OF DIALOGUE AND CULTURE

The architecture described above is intended to support flexible models of dialogue. In this section, we describe what these models look like and how they affect VRP behavior in important ways.

Conversational agent systems in the literature employ a variety of models to generate believable behavior during interactions with users. Examples include models of compliance (Roque & Traum, 2007), stress (Hofstede & Hofstede, 2005), and cooperation (Allwood, 2001), among others. These models allow features from the social, cultural, pragmatic, and linguistic contexts of a dialogue to influence its outcome.

One example of a pragmatic-level model that has been implemented in the VRP framework is the response strategy model (Sagae et al., 2009). In this work, a formal model is used to capture the strategic intention of a conversational agent with respect to truth values and conversational cooperation. Response strategies are implemented as an ontological layer in the VRP architecture, resulting in agents that can employ strategies like *Inform*, *Lie*, or *Redirect*, among others.

In addition to pragmatic models like response strategies, we have used the VRP architecture to explore socio-cultural influences on dialogue behavior. Experiments to date have included models at the macro- and micro-sociological level. In the SocialSim-MR application, macro-sociological models generated by FactionSim (Silverman et al., 2002) were instantiated on a VRP platform.

FactionSim is a tool that mimics actual ethnopolitical conflicts around the world. It draws on best-of-breed models from the literature in culture, cognition, personality, emotion, stress, sociology, and developmental economics, integrating them into a socio-cognitive agent framework. By connecting this framework to the real-time conversation capabilities of VRPs, the SocialSim-MR project allows real-time interpersonal interactions to be influenced by a group-level social simulation that runs in the background, based on validated social models.

In the CultureCom project, VRP behavior is driven by a microsocial model of commonsense culture, based on work by Hobbs & Gordon (2010). This model defines axioms of behavior that can be translated directly into VRP-framework rules at a meta-behavior level, similar to the example shown in (2). Both cross-cultural and culture-specific axioms have been defined that allow VRP behavior to depend on a mixture of cultural influences.

All of these models contribute to the desideratum of explicit models of appropriate behavior. One advantage of using such models is that we can validate the assumptions that drive agent behavior in isolation, before applying them in a training context. In a prototype evaluation of the CultureCom project, we collected examples of culturally appropriate dialogues that exemplify use of promises and commitments in Pashto-speaking Afghanistan.

These dialogues were used to validate a model of Afghan culture, encapsulated in an ontology with rules of the type shown in (2). With the model in place, the behavior of the agents matched the behavior given in the dialogue with very high accuracy (>90% for word-level precision and recall). When the model was replaced with an American culture model (retaining the Pashto language model), the actual agent behavior diverged significantly from the behavior predicted in the Afghan dialogues. This experiment was conducted with a small data set and serves as a proof-of-concept for the ability to swap in and swap out cultural models in the VRP architecture. This is a great advantage of making models of culture explicit in the agent architecture: we now have the opportunity to express and compare the behavior of agents under different modeling assumptions.

## INTEGRATION WITH IMMERSIVE GAME ENVIRONMENTS

As described in the introduction to the VRP architecture, the full social simulation pipeline, with ASR input and spoken and gestured output, is one modality of interaction between users and VRPs (text-based typing interaction is an alternative, as is menu-driven interaction). A defining feature of this modality is that it requires integration with an immersive 3-D environment. This integration depends on third-party game engines. Game engines commonly incorporate features for creating virtual worlds and populating those worlds with objects and animated characters, or avatars. Language understanding capability, including ASR, is provided by the VRP social simulation module, as shown in Figure 3.

Alelo's Operational Language and Culture Training Systems (OLCTS), shown in Figure 1 and Figure 2, integrate VRPs with a variety of game engines, some of which are single-player, and some of which are multi-player. Figure 1 shows a single-player training scenario where VRPs are integrated with the Unreal 2.5 game engine. VRP technology is packaged in a software wrapper, which can be called by the Unreal engine when the learner enters a conversation with an agent (embodied by an avatar in the simulated world). Figure 2 shows a multi-player scenario where VRP software has been deployed as a plug-in that integrates with Bohemia Interactive's VBS2. VRPs have also been integrated with Total Immersion's RealWorld.

The game engine platform provides an interface that allows the learners to choose which agent characters to talk to, and a set of graphical controls for managing the dialogue. These include buttons for starting and stopping speech input (top right corner in Figure 1) and controls for choosing nonverbal gestures for the learner's character to perform. The interface provides other information such as a summary of the objectives to complete in the scene, hints about what to say and what to do, and a transcript of the dialogue.

The game engine platform is also responsible for performing the behavior of each character. This includes speech, animated gestures, and body movement. The VRP package includes a set of pre-recorded lines for the characters to say and gesture animations for the characters to perform, which are loaded into the game engine. At runtime, the VRP social simulation module selects appropriate speech and gestures for the agents, and directs the game engine to perform them using these animations and sounds.

VRP logic is engine-independent, meaning that the same VRPs can be reused for characters in multiple game engines. In mission rehearsal engines, the trainer responsible for configuring a particular mission rehearsal scenario can assign VRPs to specific avatars. Once the assignment is made, that character will be able to hold dialogues using the VRP personality, knowledge, and decision making. In addition to the game-engine plug-in, the VRP system is deployed with a library of individual VRP characters including children and adults, men and women, leaders and followers, etc. Each character uses appropriate language and culture depending on its gender, age, etc. The desideratum of reusable agents makes this use case possible.

Virtual Role-Players can also be used in augmented reality or mixed reality environments in much the same way they are used with desktop game environments. Alelo is currently working on integrating VRP as part of the Infantry Immersive Trainer (IIT), a mixed reality training facility prototype for small units in Camp Pendleton, California (Lethin & Muller, 2010). The goal is to create and control a virtual Afghan role-player, who is projected on a wall inside one of the rooms in the IIT. The role-player can then hold conversations with service members who come to that room within the scope of a specific mission (e.g., census taking). A prototype of this integrated system is currently in testing, while we investigate solutions for several technical challenges. First, we are adapting the speech recognition technology used in VRP to work adequately in a noisy environment, and with audio input devices much less precise than the USB headsets normally used with desktop game engines. Second, we are working to remove the push-to-talk requirement, and move to a continuous-recognition method for input.

## EXPERIENCES AND RESULTS

In this section we describe the experience for the authors and users of the VRP platform. At the time of writing, VRPs have been authored in three languages and have been integrated into training and mission rehearsal products. Our experience in delivering these products revealed interesting design issues with the VRP platform, which are described along with their solutions in this section.

### The Authoring Experience

As our desiderata from previous sections show, authorability contributes directly to the overall quality and efficiency of communicative agents. Some issues we have discussed in the context of VRP authoring include the following:

**Granularity of authoring rules:** Non-novice learners sometimes express multiple intentions in the same turn, for example "Excuse me. I'm John. What's your name?" The communicative act data structure used in VRPs captures one core function at a time, which supports reuse (the same object represents "I'm John" no matter what precedes or follows it) but constrains the authors' ability to create an intent planning rule for utterances like this one, since those rules are currently structured to take one act as input before producing one or more acts as output. This constraint can be appropriate in the case of beginning language learners, since their turns are short and rarely break the single-intent assumption. It also simplifies the ASR search space, since the single-intent assumption implies that every learner turn is essentially a choice of one item from a known (although large) vocabulary of utterances. However, we are currently exploring ways to break this assumption in the agent architecture, to meet the needs of intermediate learners.

**Summarizing agent world knowledge**: In addition to behavior rules for an agent, authors create a plain-text description that is displayed to learners who "click to know more" about a character in the game environment. This description draws on data associated with the agent in the ontology, the same data used by the agent at runtime to support his world- and self-awareness. However the world state may be large – how do authors select the most relevant pieces of knowledge as a "summary" or description of the agent? Can we support them in this process by traversing the ontology and making semi- or fully-automatic recommendations? This could contribute to more efficient and possibly more consistent authoring of agent summaries.

**Multi-author access to shared libraries**: VRP authoring results in libraries of reusable agents and their components. As in any software system, access and version control on the agent libraries is critical. However access to these libraries by multiple authors is also important for efficiency. Our current authoring tools rely on subversion locking mechanisms on the back end, allowing multiple authors to read an agent library, but limit write-access to one author at a time.

**Access to new model features**: The VRP architecture is intentionally flexible. When a new model is introduced, authoring tools must be updated. For example, when features of politeness are added to the model of language interpretation, authoring tools must be extended to allow authors to annotate the value of politeness for language samples that already exist. If a model-based solution is proposed, but authors do not have access to the new model features, the solution fails.

**Supporting novice and advanced authors**: As with many complex tasks, agent authoring requires tool-based support that simplifies commonly-performed actions while still allowing advanced users to access low-level details as needed. For example, assembling a new rule based on existing acts ("when the player greets, I greet in return") should be a simple, wizard-driven authoring task. In contrast, creation of new low-level components like acts ("what are the semantic and thematic roles for a formal greeting?") must be available for advanced users.

## The User Experience

Feedback from learners using the systems described here has been positive, for Alelo systems using finite-state technology as well as VRPs. The effectiveness of this approach has been documented in various published studies (e.g., Surface et al., 2007). The most dramatic evidence of effectiveness comes from a study conducted by the US Marine Corps Center for Lessons Learned (MCCLL, 2008), which studied the experience of the 3rd Battalion, 7th Marines (3/7 Marines) in Anbar Province, Iraq in 2007.

Prior to deployment to Iraq, the battalion assigned two members of each squad of approximately thirteen marines to spend forty hours in self-study training with Alelo's Tactical Iraqi course. It should be noted that (1) forty hours is not a long time to spend learning a foreign language, (2) Arabic is a difficult language for most English speakers, and (3) self-study computer-based language learning tools often fail to produce significant learning gains. However, the 3/7's experience drew attention both prior to deployment and after deployment.

In final exercises prior to deployment, Iraqi speaking role players commented that the 3/7 demonstrated Arabic language ability far beyond the skills of typical marine units preparing for deployment. During their entire tour of duty in Iraq, the 3/7 Marines did not experience a single combat casualty. The MCCLL interviewed officers in charge of the unit, and conducted surveys of the individual trainees, finding numerous instances where language and cultural skills contributed directly to mission effectiveness. Most importantly, members of the unit demonstrated an appreciation and willingness to learn about Iraqi culture, which caused the Iraqis to be more positive and cooperative, and set in motion a virtuous cycle: cooperation lead to operational effectiveness, which lead to mutual trust and further cooperation, and so on.

## FUTURE RESEARCH DIRECTIONS

Some of the research questions we would like to pursue in the future with VRPs include better modeling of cultural cues, investigation of modality trade-offs in conversational agent systems, varying the levels of difficulty in agent interactions, and improving authorability.

As we observed in the related work section, VRPs can be contrasted with conversational agents that are focused on fine-grained expression of the agent's affective state. However, we recognize that cues such as gaze, posture, and facial expression can provide important information to a language learner regarding how well his/her attempts at communication are being received by the virtual character.

For example, to show the learner that his/her use of formal language has a positive effect on his/her rapport with a local leader (played by a VRP), a current VRP system would display a series of glowing green plus symbols rising from the VRPs avatar. Similarly, a learner choice that has a negative effect results in red minus symbols. These cartoon-like effects are a placeholder for higher-quality behavior generation modules that might express reduced rapport with the learner, or more detailed affective states, by a change in the avatar's frame or stance, along the lines of Bickmore (2008).

A VRP is a platform-independent representation of the logic that defines an artificially-intelligent character. We could use this logic in a variety of engagements with the learner, ranging from chat-style interaction where the learner types his/her input and reads textual responses, to short dialogues featuring speech recognition and generation but only a fixed visual image of the VRP character, to long immersive engagements where spoken input and output are accompanied by rich body and facial movements on a 3D avatar.

Each of these modalities may be appropriate for different learning conditions. For example, text-based interaction could be helpful to learners with limited access to desktop computing hardware, while 3D interaction may be desirable for multi-learner engagements. Given that VRP technology can deploy the same agent on a variety of platforms, we now have the opportunity to perform experiments that compare these modalities.

With explicit models of dialogue behavior, as we have in VRPs, we gain the ability to tune a given agent to be more or less tolerant of violations to the assumptions made in the model. For example, we may define an agent that uses some of the meta-cultural rules of the type shown in (2), but which ignores others for the sake of being lenient on the learner. A rule that requires formal greetings when dealing with social superiors, for example, may be turned off for beginning learners and on for advanced learners.

To fully address this topic, we need to understand how learner skills may vary, either from learner to learner, or over time in a single person. With a flexible architecture like VRPs, we would like to start using this understanding to match the difficulty of the conversational engagement to the needs of a particular learner at a particular point in time.

## CONCLUSION

Alelo has a depth of experience in building conversational agents for education and training. Based on this experience, we have described a set of desiderata for such agents, and used it to frame a new agent architecture based on highly composable models of dialogue, language, and culture.

This architecture, called Virtual Role-Players, is compatible with multiple 3-D game engines, providing access to the agents in a variety of training contexts. Under this architecture, we are able to set the groundwork for future research related to cultural cues, multi-media agent experiments, and variable levels of difficulty in conversational interactions. VRPs represent a unique application of conversational agent technology, not only to teach, but to demonstrate communicative skill for learners who hope to acquire it.

## ACKNOWLEDGMENT

The authors would like to thank the members of the Alelo team who contributed to this work. This work was sponsored by PM TRASYS, Voice of America, the Office of Naval Research, and DARPA. Opinions expressed here are those of the authors and not of the sponsors or the US Government.

## REFERENCES

Allwood, J. (2001). Cooperation and flexibility in multimodal communication. In Bunt, H., & Beun, R. J. (Eds.), *Cooperative multimodal communication*. Berlin/Heidelberg, Germany: Springer Verlag. doi:10.1007/3-540-45520-5_7

Austin, J. L. (1975). *How to do things with words*. Cambridge, MA: Harvard University Press.

Bickmore, T. (2008). *Framing and interpersonal stance in relational agents*. Paper presented at the Seventh International Conference on Autonomous Agents and Multiagent Systems (AAMAS), Workshop on Functional Markup Language, Estoril, Portugal.

Bickmore, T., & Pfeifer, L. (2008). *Relational agents for antipsychotic medication adherence*. Paper presented at the CHI 2008 Workshop on Technology in Mental Health.

Blumer, H. (1986). *Symbolic interactionism: Perspective and method*. Berkeley, CA: University of California Press.

Byram, M. (1997). *Teaching and assessing intercutural communicative competence*. Clevedon, UK: Multilingual Matters.

Ellis, R. (2003). *Task-based language learning and teaching*. USA: Oxford University Press.

Garfinkel, H. (1967). *Studies in ethnomethodology*. Englewood Cliffs, NJ: Prentice-Hall.

Goffman, E. (1990). *The presentation of self in everyday life*. New York, NY: Doubleday.

Graesser, A. C., Chipman, P., Haynes, B. C., & Olney, A. (2005). AutoTutor: An intelligent tutoring system with mixed-initiative dialogue. *IEEE Transactions on Education*, *48*, 612–618. doi:10.1109/TE.2005.856149

Habermas, J. (1984). *The theory of communicative action*. Boston, MA: Beacon Press.

Hobbs, J. R., & Gordon, A. (2010). *Goals in a formal theory of commonsense psychology*. Paper presented at the 6th International Conference on Formal Ontology in Information Systems.

Hofstede, G., & Hofstede, G. J. (2005). *Cultures and organizations: Software of the mind*. New York, NY: McGraw-Hill.

Jackendoff, R. (1990). *Semantic structures*. Cambridge, MA: MIT Press.

Johnson, W. L. (2010). Serious use of a serious game for learning foreign language. *Journal of Artificial Intelligence in Education*, *20*(2), 175–195.

Johnson, W. L., & Valente, A. (2008). *Tactical language and culture training systems: Using artificial intelligence to teach foreign languages and cultures*. Paper presented at the IAAI 2008.

Johnson, W. L., & Valente, A. (2009). Tactical language and culture training systems: Using AI to teach foreign languages and cultures. *AI Magazine*, *30*(2), 72–84.

Jonassen, D. H., Tessmer, M., & Hannum, W. H. (1999). *Task analysis methods for instructional design*. Mahwah, NJ: Lawrence Erlbaum.

Lampe, J. (2007). *Cultural proficiency guildelines (3.2)*. Paper presented at the Plenary session of the Interagency Language Roundtable for the ACTFL Arabic Testing Consensus Project.

Lethin, C., & Muller, P. (2010). Future immersive training. *Warfighter Enhancement Activities*, *4*(1), 2–4.

Marsella, S., & Gratch, J. (2009). EMA: A model of emotional dynamics. *Journal of Cognitive Systems Research*, *10*(1), 70–90. doi:10.1016/j.cogsys.2008.03.005

MCCLL. (2008). Tactical Iraqi language and culture training system. *MCCLL Newsletter*, *4*(8), 4.

McDonald, D. P., McGuire, G., Johnson, J., Selmeski, B., & Abbe, A. (2008). *Developing and managing cross-cultural competence within the Department of Defense: Recommendations for learning and assessment: The Regional and Cultural Competence Assessment Working Group (RCCAWG)*. Defense Equal Opportunity Management Institute.

McRorie, M., Sneddon, I., Sevin, E. D., Bevacqua, E., & Pelachaud, C. (2009). *A model of personality and emotional traits*. Paper presented at the International conference on Intelligent virtual agents IVA'09, Amsterdam.

Mead, G. H. (1967). *Mind, self, and society: From the standpoint of a social behaviorist*. Chicago, IL: University of Chicago Press.

Roque, A., & Traum, D. (2007). *A model of compliance and emotion for potentially adversarial dialogue agents*. Paper presented at the the 8th SIGdial Workshop on Discourse and Dialogue, Antwerp, Belgium.

Rose, C. P., Jordan, P., Ringenberg, M., Siler, S., VanLehn, K., & Weinstein, A. (2001). *Interactive conceptual tutoring in Atlas-Andes*. Paper presented at the AI in Education 2001.

Rosis, F. d., Pelachaud, C., Poggi, I., Carofiglio, V., & Carolis, B. D. (2003). From Greta's mind to her face: Modelling the dynamics of affective states in a conversational embodied agent. *International Journal of Human-Computer Studies*, *59*, 81–118. doi:10.1016/S1071-5819(03)00020-X

Sagae, A., Johnson, W. L., & Bodnar, S. (2010). *Validation of a dialog system for language learners*. Paper presented at the The 11th annual SIGdial Meeting on Discourse and Dialogue, Tokyo, Japan.

Sagae, A., Wetzel, B., Valente, A., & Johnson, W. L. (2009). *Culture-driven response strategies for virtual human behavior in training systems*. Paper presented at the SLaTE-2009, Warwickshire, England.

Samtani, P., Valente, A., & Johnson, W. L. (2008). *Applying the SAIBA framework to the tactical language and culture training system*. Paper presented at the AAMAS 2008 Workshop on Functional Markup Language (FML).

Schutz, A. (1970). Alfred Schutz on phenomenology and social relations. In Wagner, H. R. (Ed.), *Selected writings*. Chicago, IL: University of Chicago Press.

Silverman, B. G., Johns, M., Weaver, R., O'Brien, K., & Silverman, R. (2002). Human behavior models for game-theoretic agents. *Cognitive Science Quarterly*, *2*(3-4), 273–301.

Surface, E. A., Dierdorff, E. C., & Watson, A. M. (2007). *Special operations language training software measurement of effectivenss study: Tactical Iraqi study final report*. SWA Consulting.

Traum, D., Marsella, S., Gratch, J., Lee, J., & Hartholt, A. (2008). *Multi-party, multi-issue, multi-strategy negotiation for multi-modal virtual agents*. Paper presented at the the 8th International Conference on Intelligent Virtual Agents.

Traum, D. R., & Hinkelman, E. A. (1992). Conversation acts in task-oriented spoken dialogue. *Computational Intelligence*, *8*(3), 575–599. doi:10.1111/j.1467-8640.1992.tb00380.x

Valente, A., Johnson, W. L., Wertheim, S., Barrett, K., Flowers, M., & LaBore, K. (2009). *A dynamic methodology for developing situated culture training content. Alelo TLT*. LLC.

Vilhjalmsson, H., & Marsella, S. (2005). *Social performance framework*. Paper presented at the the AAAI Workshop on Modular Construction of Human-Like Intelligence.

Wang, N., Johnson, W. L., Mayer, R. E., Rizzo, P., Shaw, E., & Collins, H. (2008). The politeness effect: Pedagogical agents and learning outcomes. *International Journal of Human-Computer Studies*, (February): 2008.

Weber, M. (1994). *Sociological writings*. New York, NY: Continuum.

## ADDITIONAL READING

Arvizu, S., & Saravia-Shore, M. (1990). Cross-Cultural Literacy, An Anthropological Approach to Dealing with Diversity. *Education and Urban Society*, *22*(4), 364–376. doi:10.1177/0013124590022004004

Eysenck, H. J. (1976). *The Measurement of Personality*. Lancaster: Medical and Technical Publishers.

Hernandez, A., Lopez, B., Pardo, D., Santos, R., Hernandez, L., & Relano, J. (2008). *Modular definition of multimodal ECA communication acts to improve dialogue robustness and depth of intention*. Paper presented at the The Seventh International Conference on Autonomous Agents and Multiagent Systems (AAMAS), Workshop on Functional Markup Language, Estoril, Portugal.

Johnson, W. L., & Friedland, L. (2010). Integrating Cross-Cultural Decision Making Skills into Military Training. In Schmorrow, D., & Nicholson, D. (Eds.), *Advances in Cross-Cultural Decision Making*. London: Taylor & Francis.

Johnson, W. L., & Sagae, A. (2010a). *Adaptive Agent-Based Learning of Intercultural Communication Skills*. Paper presented at the Demonstration sessions of the User Modeling and Personalization Conference (UMAP 2010).

Johnson, W. L., & Sagae, A. (2010b). *Adaptive Agents for Promoting Intercultural Skills*. Paper presented at the Adaptation and Personalization in E/B-Learning Using Pedagogic Conversational Agents (APLeC), workshop of UMAP 2010, Big Island, HI, USA.

Johnson, W. L., & Valente, A. (2008). *Collaborative Authoring of Serious Games for Language and Culture*. Paper presented at the SimTecT 2008.

Kumar, R., Sagae, A., & Johnson, W. L. (2009, July 2009). *Evaluating an Authoring Tool for Mini-Dialogs*. Paper presented at the AIED 2009 (Poster), Brighton, UK.

Lazarus, R. (2000). *Emotion and Adaptation*. New York, NY, USA: Oxford University Press.

Mascarenhas, S., Dias, J., Afonso, N., Enz, S., & Paiva, A. (2009). *Using rituals to express cultural differences in synthetic characters*. Paper presented at the AAMAS 2009.

Matsuda, N., Cohen, W. W., Koedinger, K. R., Stylianides, G., Keiser, V., & Raizada, R. (2010). *Tuning Cognitive Tutors into a Platform for Learning-by-Teaching with SimStudent Technology.* Paper presented at the the International Workshop on Adaptation and Personalization in E-B/Learning using Pedagogic Conversational Agents (APLeC), Kona, HI.

Melo, C. M., & Gratch, J. (2009). *Expression of emotions using wrinkles, blushing, sweating, and tears.* Paper presented at the Intelligent Virtual Agents, Amsterdam.

Miller, J. G. (1984). Culture and the development of everyday social explanation. *Journal of Personality and Social Psychology*, *46*, 961–978. doi:10.1037/0022-3514.46.5.961

Muller, P., Dylan, C. D. R., Schmorrow, U., & Buscemi, T. (2008). The infantry immersion trainer: today's holodeck. *The Marine Corps Gazette*, (September): 2008.

Traum, D., Marsella, S., Gratch, J., Lee, J., & Hartholt, A. (2008). *Multi-party, Multi-issue, Multi-strategy Negotiation for Multi-modal Virtual Agents.* Paper presented at the the 8th International Conference on Intelligent Virtual Agents.

Vilhjalmsson, H., & Thorisson, K. R. (2008). *A brief history of function representation from Gandalf to SAIBA.* Paper presented at the The Seventh International Conference on Autonomous Agents and Multiagent Systems (AAMAS), Workshop on Functional Markup Language, Estoril, Portugal.

Wang, N., & Johnson, W. L. (2008). *The Politeness Effect in an Intelligent Foreign Language Tutoring System.* Paper presented at the the 9th International Conference on Intelligent Tutoring Systems.

## KEY TERMS AND DEFINITIONS

**Authorability:** The ease with which behavior of a conversational agent can be created, in particular by subject matter experts who may be non-programmers; this is a measure of how mature the agent technology is, including authoring tools.

**Avatar:** The visual representation of a conversational agent, often an animated 3D rendering of the character being played by the agent in a simulated world.

**Cultural Environment:** A setting for interpersonal communication that includes a variety of factors, including the following general categories: physical environment; political, economic, and social structures common within the culture; and typical personal perspectives (e.g. attitudes toward time, personal relations, work, and the role of the individual within the community).

**Game Engine:** The software responsible for rendering the simulated environment where conversational agents operate; examples presented in this work include VBS2, RealWorld, and Unreal.

**Immersive Environment:** A setting for study that is an engaging model of the environment where the learner will use the skills being taught; in this work we use "immersive" to describe the 3-D game where learners operate in a simulated world, and where all characters speak only in the language being studied.

**Intercultural Competence:** General skills for handling intercultural situations; in this work we focus on communicative knowledge, skills, and attitudes that apply in situations requiring interpersonal communication across cultures.

**Role-Player:** A human acting as a character in a live simulation, as in military wargaming; Virtual Role-Players are conversational agents in a computer-based simulation.

**Scene:** One stage of a training scenario, perhaps involving a fixed set of characters and sub-tasks.

**Training Scenario:** An engagement with conversational agents in a virtual environment that is designed to train the human participant in a set of skills; in particular, a task-specific engagement that simulates a situation the user expects to face in real life.

## ENDNOTES

1 http://clipsrules.sourceforge.net/

2 http://protege.stanford.edu/

# Section 4
# Future Trends

# Chapter 17
# The Future of Companionable Agents

**Roberta Catizone**
*University of Sheffield, UK*

**Yorick Wilks**
*University of Sheffield, UK*

## ABSTRACT

*COMPANIONS is a concept that aims to change the way we think about the relationships of people to computers and the Internet by developing a virtual 'Companion' to stand between individuals and the torrent of data on the Internet, including their own life information, which will soon be too large for people to handle easily without some new form of assistance. The Companion is intended as an agent or 'presence' that stays with a user for periods of time, longer than in conventional task-based dialogue systems, developing a relationship and 'knowing' and assisting its owner's experiences, preferences, plans, and wishes. The Companions concept aims to model a fuller range of conversation than has been done hitherto, both task and non-task based, and discusses what properties people will want in a long term computer Companion that is also an Internet agent in a new form.*

## 1 INTRODUCTION

As already described in Chapter 13, the EU project Companions has already produced two prototypes that are being tested. In this chapter, the future of this idea is envisioned. Computer Companions will be software agents that get to know us, interface us to the Internet, and help manage the huge amount of information in our digital lives: the "digital me". They will also entertain, listen and carry out little jobs from reminding us of the plot of our favourite soap opera to making a restaurant booking. All this is now perfectly feasible in the current state of speech and language technology, taken together with general artificial intelligence research on reasoning, knowledge and emotion.

Companions are not at all about fooling us that they are human because they will not pretend to

DOI: 10.4018/978-1-60960-617-6.ch017

be human at all. Imagine the following scenario: an old person sits on a sofa, and beside them is a large furry handbag, which we shall call a Senior Companion; it is easy to carry about, but much of the day it just sits there and chats. Given the experience of Tamagochi, and the easily ascertained fact that old people with pets survive far better than those without, we will expect this to be an essential lifespan and health-improving objective to own. There is considerable evidence that people accept and welcome such companions, rather as they do pets in the home.

Nor is it hard to see why this Companion that chats in an interesting way would become an essential possession for the growing elderly population of the EU and the US, the most rapidly growing segment of the population, but one relatively well provided with funds. Other Companions are just as plausible as this one, such as a Junior Companion for children, which would most likely take the form of a backpack, a small and hard to remove backpack that always knew where the child was.

Common sense tells us that no matter what we read in the way of official encouragement, a large proportion of today's old people are effectively excluded from information technology, the web, the Internet and some mobile phones because "they cannot learn how to cope with the buttons". This can be because of their generation or because of losses of skill with age: there are talking books in abundance now but many, otherwise intelligent, old people cannot manipulate a tape recorder or a mobile phone, which has too many small controls for them with unwanted functionalities.

In all these situations, one can see how a Companion that could talk and understand and also gain access to the web, to email and a mobile phone could become an essential cognitive prosthesis for an old person, one that any responsible society would have to support. It is reliably reported that many old people spend much of their day sorting and looking over photographs of themselves and their families, along with places they have lived and visited.

This will obviously increase as time goes on and everyone begins to have access to digitized photos and videos throughout their lives. One can see this as an attempt to establish the narrative of one's life: what drives the most literate segment of the population to write autobiographies (for the children) even when, objectively speaking, they may have lived lives with little to report. If a huge volume of personal material is to be sorted, as it will be later for the Facebook generation of children, some form of automated assistance will be needed, we believe. Managing the digital information in the life of a future seventy-year old will be a huge task that will probably not be possible without a Companion's help.

The chapter assumes that artificial Companions are coming, and the interesting issues concern what they will be like. We shall take the distinguishing features of a Companion agent to be:

1. That it has no central or over-riding task and there is no point at which its conversation is complete or has to stop, although it may have some tasks it carries out in the course of conversation;
2. That it should be capable of a sustained discourse over a long-period, possibly ideally the whole life-time of its principal user;
3. It is essentially the Companion of a particular individual, its principal user, about whom it knows a great deal of personal knowledge, and whose interests it serves—it could, in principle, contain all the information associated with a whole life (in the sense of the Memories for Life consortium [Memories for Life];
4. It establishes some form of relationship with that user, if that is appropriate, which would have aspects associated with the term "emotion";
5. It is not essentially an internet agent or interface, but since it will have to have access to the internet for information (including the whole-life information about its user) and to

act in the world (as it is not a robot), we may as well assume its internet agent status, and so it should have, so far as possible, access to open internet knowledge sources.

By separating a Companion conceptually from both a task-based system and a chatbot, we immediately lose access to the two evaluation paradigms associated with those models of computer dialogue: the first in terms of task-completion (stickiness, timing, task success etc.) and the latter (usually) in terms of distinguishability from some set of human interlocutors. There is, at the moment, no clear evaluation paradigm for a Companion, even if we had one to evaluate, although there are ideas for creating one (Webb et al., 2010) and some of these have been applied to the first demonstrators from the COMPANIONS (Wilks, 2006) project itself.

Given this narrowing of focus in this chapter, what questions then arise and what choices does that leave open? Here are some obvious questions that have arisen in the literature:

- What aspects of a relationship should one aim at with a Companion, in terms of such conventional categories as emotion, politeness, affection etc.?
- Even if it is not a robot, in the sense of a free-moving entity, should it have a screen, and should it have a visible avatar for communication, whether human, animal or abstract?
- Does a Companion need a voice or could communication be by typing (such as on a mobile phone, laptop or PC)?
- Need it have one identifiable personality, or perhaps several, and should the user be able to choose the Companion's personality or shift between them if there are several? More generally, are the answers to these questions, and the settings and constraints they imply, dependent on the type of Companion—the domain or setting into which it is to be placed, or is there only one type of Companion subject to general constraints?
- Does the Companion have any goals of its own, beyond carrying out a user's commands, if that is possible: should there be other overriding ethical constraints on what can be commanded, such as avoiding harm to the user, even if requested? Should there be ethical constrains *on the user* as to how the Companion can be treated?
- What safeguards are there for the information content of such a Companion, in the sense of controlling access to its contents for the state or a company, and how should a user best provide for its disposal in case of his/her own death or incapacity?
- What if anything does a Companion have to *know* to be plausible, and does it need a certain level of inference and memory capacity over the material of past conversations with the user?

## 2 RELATED WORK

We shall discuss related work largely in terms of the questions above and how other researchers have answered them. Two preliminary things are being assumed here: first, that the robotic aspect is interesting but dispensable for this discussion. Dautenhahn and her colleagues have established interesting facts such as that people would prefer that robots approached them from the side rather than head on (see Walters et al., 2009) and of course there will always be people who want things brought to them rather than getting up out of their chairs.

We will be concerned here with aspects of Companions such that embodiment is a secondary matter, provided they can converse with an owner and can reach out to the world via the internet for information and to establish action and control. Whether they are implemented as mobile phones, moving robots with prostheses, or just "warm furry handbags" with Wifi, is irrelevant to what we shall discuss here, though we shall often assume they can assume visual shape on a screen when necessary, but that is far short of a robot in any full sense.

Secondly, we noted above that it is convenient to distinguish Companions from both (a) conversational internet agents that carry out specific tasks, such as the train and plane scheduling and ticket ordering speech dialogue applications back to the MIT ATIS systems (Zue et al., 1992), and also from (b) descendants of the early chatbots PARRY and ELIZA, the best of which compete annually in the Loebner competition [Loebner]. These have essentially no memory or knowledge but are simple finite state response sets, although ELIZA (Weizenbaum, 1966) had primitive "scripts" giving some context, and PARRY (Colby, 1971) had parameters like FEAR and ANGER that changed with the conversation and determined which reply was selected at a given point.

## 2.1 Emotion, Politeness and Affection

Cheepen and Monaghan (1997) presented results some thirteen years ago that customers of some automata, such as Automated Teller Machines (ATM)s, are repelled by excessive politeness and endless repetitions of "thank you for using our service", because they know they are dealing with a machine and such feigned sincerity is inappropriate. This suggests that politeness is very much a matter of judgment in certain situations, just as it is with humans, where inappropriate politeness is often encountered. Wallis et al. (2001) have reported results that many find computer conversationalists "chippy" or "cocky" and suggest that this should be avoided as it breeds hostility on the part of users; they believe this is always a major risk in human-machine interactions.

We know, since the original work of Reeves and Nass (1996) and colleagues that people will display some level of feeling for the simplest machines, even PCs in their original experiments, and Levy (2007) has argued persuasively that the trend seems to be towards high levels of "affectionate" relationships with machines in the next decades, as realistic hardware and sophisticated speech generation make machine interlocutors increasingly lifelike. However, much of this work is about human psychology, faced with entities known to be artificial, and does not bear directly on the issue of whether Companions should attempt to detect emotion in what they hear from us, or attempt to generate it in what they say back.

The AI area of "emotion and machines" is still at a preliminary state, and its success is dependent on effective content extraction techniques. This research began as "content analysis" (Krippendorff, 2004) at the Harvard psychology department many years ago and, while prose texts may offer enough length to enable a measure of sentiment to be assessed; this is not always the case with short dialogue turns.

That technology rested almost entirely on the supposed sentiment value of individual words, which ignores the fact that their value is content dependent. "Cancer" may be marked as negative word but the utterance "We have found a cure for cancer" is presumably positive and detecting the appropriate response to that rests on the ability to do information extraction beyond single terms. Failure to observe this has led to many of the classic foolishnesses of chatbots such as congratulating people on the death of their relatives, and so on.

At deeper levels, there are conflicting theories of emotion for automata, not all of which are consistent and which apply only in limited ranges of discourse. So, for example, the classic theory that emotion is a response to the failure and success of the machine's plans (e.g. Marsella and Gratch, 2003) covers only those situations that are clearly plan driven and, as we noted, Companionship dialogue is not always closely related to plans and tasks.

"Dimensional" theories (Cowie et al., 2001, following Wundt, 1913), display emotions along dimensions marked with opposed qualities (such as positive-negative) and normally distribute across the space emotion "primitives", such as FEAR, and these normally assigned by manual tagging, and those that remain, like the text-sentiment theories above, on pre-tagging and any learning based on them, of the sort that all learning engines perform over tag distributions (e.g. Ciravegna et al., 2004). The problem with this is that tagging for "COMPANY" or "TEMPERATURE" (in classic NLP) is a quite different task from tagging for "FEAR" and "ANGER". These latter terms are not, and probably cannot be analyzed but rest on the common sense intuitions of the tagger, which may vary very much from person to person—they have very low consilience between taggers.

All this makes many emotion theories look primitive in terms of developments in AI and NLP elsewhere. Appraisal Theory (Scherer et al., 2008) seeks to explain why individuals can have quite different emotional reactions to similar situations because they have appraised them differently, e.g. a death welcomed or regretted. Appraisal can also be of the performance of planned activities, in which case this theory approximates to the plan-based one mentioned above.

The theory itself, like all such theories, has a large common sense component, and the issue for computational implementation is how, in assessing the emotional state of the Companion's user to make such concepts quantitatively evaluable. If the Companion conducts long conversations with a user about his or her life and, as in the case of the Senior Companion prototype [Senior Companion demo] which discusses photo images, then one might expect there to be ample opportunity to assess the user's appraisal of, say, a funeral or wedding by means of the application of the sentiment extraction techniques to what is said in the presence of the relevant image. In so far as a Companion can be said to have overarching goals, such as keeping the user happy then, to that degree, it is not difficult to envisage methods (again based on estimates of the happiness, or otherwise, of the user's utterances) for self-appraisal by the Companion of its own performance and some consequent causal link to generated demonstrations of its own emotions of satisfaction or guilt.

Also relevant to what a Companion should be is the "Affective Loop" (AL) paradigm (Höök, 2004) which, like most of the theories of emotion discussed, and as John Wisdom once said of philosophical discoveries, are often the "running of a platitude up a flagpole": but AL is a useful corrective to some of the claims above and is intended essentially for computational implementation. It emphasizes:

- that there is a natural "feedback loop" involved in emotional interaction between parties and which is essential to any model.
- but that emotional interaction and feedback should not be thought of as a matter of information transfer.
- it is much concerned with design, and the design of multimodal interactions of the display of color and sound—it is not essentially concerned with emotional language.
- it emphasizes the relative vacuity of emotional labels or terms, as we did above, and peoples' intuitive understanding of them.

The notion of feedback is an old one going back to cybernetic ideas and in particular to Wiener's notion that activities like walking are only possible because of constant information feedback from the "servo" muscles in contact with the ground to the brain. Wiener was emphasizing information feedback, as opposed to the "haptic" transfer from muscles, but in a computational paradigm everything must at some stage bottom out in information.

Speech act theory (e.g. Searle, 1969), too, arose from considerations of human interaction that were not based on conveying information in propositions, but rather "intentional" commitments, but those again have only been implementable in computers as forms of information. Many of Höök's examples involve multimodal devices such as smart phones where non-verbal signals are sent to create attitudes and feelings, or to signal those of the sender.

The Nabaztag rabbit toy, originally used by the COMPANIONS project as an interface (http://www.nabaztag.com/en/index.html), in its original design glowed in a number of colors to indicate the feelings of the sender (e.g. blue for "sad") and two Nabaztags and their respective senders would be a paradigm AL in Höök's sense. There are many wholly conventionalized verbal feedback loops that cannot be divorced from emotion—certainly if a respondent fails to supply the correct response, from "How do you do" and "Good morning" in English to the potentially infinite "danke, bitte, danke, bitte..." cycle of giving thanks in German.

The importance of AL is that it makes emotion central, not peripheral, to communication and relationships and does not make language behavior central to emotional communication. Everyone knows that in relationships with pets, a central relationship for many people, this is the case: strong emotions are aroused, as well as consequent actions of e.g. stroking, but there is no verbal content. There have been a number of Japanese pet robot implementations, such as wriggly seal-like creatures with dozens of servo motors to give a life-like feel, and there is no doubt that a real form of human relationship is being modeled. Companions were always designed with the pet analogy in mind, as in the phrase used early in the project of a Companion "being like a furry handbag", though language was always believed essential to the project.

In speaking of "language" and Companions, we have so far ignored speech, although that is a communication mode in which a great deal has been done to identify and, more recently, generate, emotion-bearing components (Luneski et al., 2008). Elements of the above approaches can be found in the work of Worgan and Moore (see e.g. Wilks et al., 2010 and Figure 1 below), within the COMPANIONS project, where there is the same commitment to the centrality of emotion in the communication process, but in a form focusing on an integration of speech and language (rather than visual and design) technologies.

The claim, not yet implemented, was conceived within the COMPANIONS project as a layer in a dialogue manager over and above local response management but one which would seek to navigate the whole conversation across a two-dimensional space onto which Companion and user are mapped using continuous values (rather than

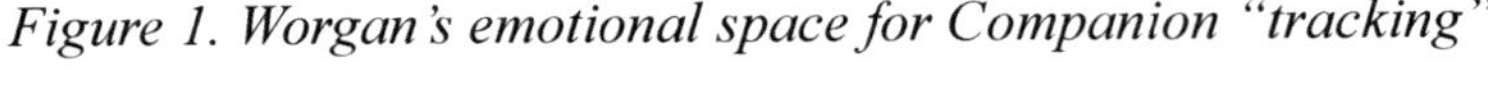
*Figure 1. Worgan's emotional space for Companion "tracking"*

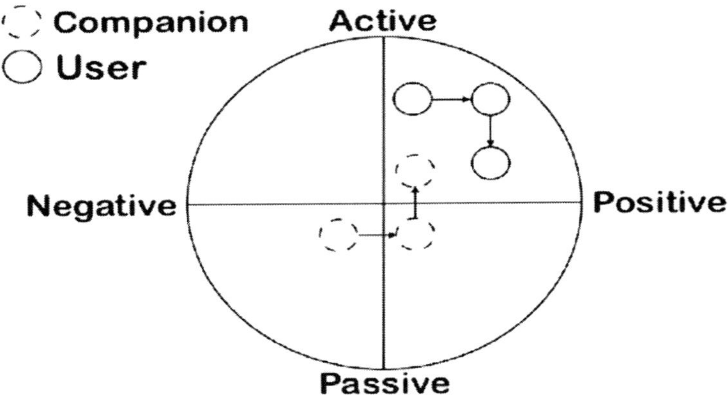

discrete values corresponding to primitive but unexplained emotional terms) but in such a way as to both respond to the user's demonstrated emotion appropriately, but also ----again, if appropriate or chosen by the user---- to draw the user back to other more positive emotional areas of the two-dimensional space.

It is not yet clear what the right mechanism should be for the integration of this "landscape" global emotion-based dialogue manager with the local dialogue management that generates responses and alters the world context: in the Senior Companion the later was sophisticated stack of networks (Wilks et al., 2010). In some sense, we are just looking for a modern and defensible interface to replace what PARRY had in simple form in 1971 when the sum of two emotion parameters determined which response to select from a stack of alternatives.

This last point is a high level issue to be settled in a Companion's architecture and also, perhaps, to be under the control of the user, namely: should a Companion invariably try to cheer up a user if miserable-----which is trying to "move" the user to the most naturally desirable (i.e. the top-right, in Figure 1) quadrant of the space----or, rather, to track to the part of the space where the user is deemed to be and stay there in roughly the same emotional location—i.e. be sad with a sad user and happy with a happy one? There is no general answer to this question and, indeed, in an ideal Companion, which tracking method should be used would itself be a conversation topic e.g. "Do you want me to cheer you up or would you rather stay miserable?" In that sense, an AL is a platitude and everything depends on what kind of loop it is to be---itself a matter for negotiation.

## 2.2 What Should a Companion Look Like?

We confess to an affection for a faceless Companion—the proverbial furry handbag, warm and light to carry, chatty but with full internet access and probably no screen. However, this may be a minority taste; after all, such a Companion could always take control of a nearby screen or a phone if it needed to show anything.

If there is to be a face, the question of the "uncanny valley effect" always comes up, where it is argued that users are more uneasy the more something is very like ourselves (Mori, 1970). We personally do not feel this, indeed it cannot in principle apply to an avatar so good that one cannot be sure it is artificial, which is what we feel about the *Emily* from Manchester [Emily avatar].

On the other hand, if the quality is not good, and in particular if the lip synch is not perfect, it may be better to go for an abstract avatar ---the Companions logo was chosen with that in mind, and without a mouth at all. Non-human avatars seem to avoid some of the problems that arise with valleys and mixed feelings generally, and the best Companions demonstration video so far features Wigdog, a dog in a wig, who seems pretty popular [Senior Companion demo].

It may be worth making a small clarification here about the word "avatar" that sometimes distorts discussion in these areas: those working in computing the human-machine interface often use the word to mean any screen form, usually two-dimensional, that simulates a human being, but not any particular human being. On the other hand, in the virtual reality and game worlds, such as Second Life (http://secondlife.com/), an avatar is a manifestation of a particular human being, an alternative identity that may or may not be similar to the owner in age, sex, appearance etc.

These are importantly different notions and confusion can arise when they are conflated or confused: in current COMPANIONS project demonstrations, for example, a number of avatars in the first sense are used to present the Companion's conversation on a computer or mobile phone screen. However, in the case of a long-term computer Companion that could elicit, through prolonged reminiscence, details of its owner's life and perhaps train its own voice in imitation, research shows that more successful computer conversationalists are as like their owners as possible. One might then approach the point where a Companion could approximate to the second sense of "avatar" above, namely an avatar of its owner, which it would progressively resemble, as dogs are said to do.

## 2.3 Voice or Typing to Communicate With a Companion?

At the moment the limitation on the use of voice is two-fold: first, although trained Automatic Speech Recognition (ASR) for a single user—such as a Companion's user—is now very good and up in the high 90%, it still introduces uncertainty into understanding an utterance that is far greater than that of spelling errors.

Secondly, it is currently not possible to store sufficient ASR software locally on a mobile phone to recognize a large vocabulary in real time; access to a remote server takes additional time and can be subject to fluctuations and delays. All of which suggests that typed input—though not Text To Speech (TTS) output—from a web-based Companion may have to use typed input in the immediate future, which is no problem for most mobile phone users who have come to find typed chat perfectly natural. However, this is almost certainly only a transitory delay as mobile RAM increases rapidly and the problem should not determine research decisions---there is no doubt that voice will move back to the centre of communication once storage and access size have grown by another order of magnitude.

## 2.4 One Companion Personality or Several?

Some (e.g. Pulman, in Wilks, 2010) have argued that having a consistent personality is a condition on Companionhood, but one could differ and argue that, although that is true of people—multiple personalities being a classic psychosis—there is no reason why we should expect this of a Companion. Perhaps a Companion should have a personality adapted to its particular relationship to a user at a given moment: Lowe (in Wilks, 2010) has pointed out that one might want a Companion to function as, say, a gym trainer, in which case a rather harsh attitude on the part of the Companion might well be the best one.

If a Companion's emotional attitude were to (figuratively) move across a two dimensional emotion space (see diagram above) imitating or correcting what it perceived to be the user's state over time (as Worgan, see above, has proposed), then that shift in attitude might well seem to be the product of different personalities, as it sometimes can with humans.

It might be better, *pace* Pulman, to give a user access to, and some control over, the display of a multiple-personality Companion, something one could think of as an "agency" of Companions, rather than a single "agent", all of which shared access to the same knowledge of the world and of the state and history of the user.

## 2.5 Ethics and Goals in the Companion

The last section is very close to the question of what goals a Companion can plausibly have, beyond something very general, such as "keep the user happy and do what they ask if you can", which are goals and constraints that directly relate to the standard discussions of the ethics a robot could be considered to have, a discussion started long ago by Asimov (1950).

Clearly, there will be need for a Companion to have goals to carry out specific tasks: if it is to place a restaurant table booking on the phone for a user who has just said to it "Get me a table for two tonight at Branca around 8.30"---a phone request well within the bounds of the currently achievable technology-----and the Companion will first have to find the restaurant's phone number before it phones and asks about availability before choosing a reservation time.

This is the standard content of goal-driven behavior, with alternatives at every stage if unexpected replies are encountered (such as the restaurant being fully booked tonight). However, one does not need to consider such goals as "goals of its own" since they are inferred from what it was told and are simply assumed, as an agent or slave of the user, but a Companion that finds its user not responding after some minutes of conversation might well have to take an independent decision to call a doctor urgently, based on a stored permanent goal about danger to a user who is unable to answer but is not asleep, etc.

Asimov was concerned with the ethics of the robot and its doing no harm to its users, or indeed to anyone else—even if asked to do harm explicitly. These days one might also consider the point at which ill treatment of the Companion itself might be an ethical problem for the user: again, Reeves' and Nass' experiments revealing feeling or sympathy even for a criticized PC suggest these will not be too far in the future.

## 2.6 Safeguards for the Information Content of a Companion

Data protection, privacy, or whatever term one prefers, now captures a crucial concept in the new information society. A Companion that had learned intimate details of a user's life over months or years would certainly have contents needing protection, and many forces-----commercial, security, governmental, research---might well want access to those contents or even to the contents of all the Companions in a given society.

If societies move to a clear legal state where one's personal data is one's own, with the owner or originator having rights over sale and distribution of their data---which is not at all the case at the moment in most countries----then the issue of the personal data elicited by a Companion would automatically be covered.

If we ignore the issues of governments and national security---a Companion would clearly be useful to the police when wanting to know as much as possible about a murder suspect, so that it might then be an issue of whether talking to one's Companion constituted any kind of self-incrimination, in countries where that form of communication is protected. Some might well want one's relationship to a Companion put on some basis like that of a relationship to a priest or doctor, or even to a spouse, who cannot always be forced to give evidence in common-law countries.

More realistically, a user might well want to protect parts of his or her Companion's information, or even an organized life-story based on that, from particular individuals: e.g. "this must never be told to my children, even when "We are gone". It is not hard to imagine a Companion deciding whom to divulge certain things to, selecting between classes of offspring, relations, friends, colleagues etc. There will almost certainly need to be a new set of laws covering the ownership, inheritance and destruction of Companion-objects in the future.

## 2.7 What Must a Companion Know?

There is no clear answer to this question: dogs make excellent Companions and know nothing. More relevantly, Colby's PARRY program, the best conversationalist of its day (Colby, 1971) and possibly since, famously "knew' nothing: John McCarthy at Stanford dismissed PARRY's skills by saying: "It doesn't even know who the US President is", forgetting as he said it that most of world's population did not know that, at least at the time. On the other hand, it is hard to relate over a long term to an interlocutor who knows little or nothing and has no memory of what it or you have said in the past. It is hard to attribute personality to an entity with no memory and little or no knowledge.

Much of what a Companion knows that is personal it should elicit in conversation from its user; yet much could also be gained from publicly available sources, just as the current Senior Companion demo goes off to Facebook, independently of a conversation, to find out who its user's friends are. Current information extraction technology (e.g. Ciravegna et al., 2004) allows a reasonable job to be made of going to Wikipedia for general information when, say, a world city is mentioned; the Companion can then glean something about that city from Wikipedia and ask a relevant question such as "Did you see the Eiffel Tower when you were in Paris?" which again gives a plausible illusion of general knowledge.

John McCarthy always maintained that the real challenge for AI was not having exotic or detailed knowledge but common-sense knowledge, what exists below our levels of consciousness, such as that things that drop also fall, and fingers go into water but not into tables: all of what Hayes once called Naïve Physics (Hayes, 1979). Some of this can be coded in the inference rules a Companion will need, such as that sisters share parents, but much of it is below the level of straightforward rules, which is what led Dreyfus (1972) and others to argue that plausible Artificial Intelligence (AI) would need the ability to learn as we do by growing up, rather than by existing forms of machine learning or hand-coding.

However, the great improvements in such learning in recent years, from speech recognition to machine translation suggests that the jury is still out on this, even if the methods that have proved successful in computers are clearly not those humans themselves use.

## 3 DISCUSSION: A POSSIBLE FUTURE COMPANION---THE VICTORIAN COMPANION

The upshot of the previous discussions in the constraints on what it is to be a Companion as well as the ones published in Wilks (2010) and Veletsianos et al. (2009) is that there are many dimensions of choice, even within an agreed definition of what a Companion is to be, and they will depend on the user's tastes and needs above all. In the section that follows, we cut though the choices and make a semi-serious proposal for a model Companion, one based on a once well-known social stereotype.

In O'Hara (Wilks, 2010) a colleague remarks that James Boswell was a clear case of the inaccurate Companion: his account of Johnson's life is engaging but probably exaggerated, yet none of that now matters. Johnson is now *Boswell's* Johnson, by and large, and his Companionship made Johnson a social property in a way he would never have been without his Companion and biographer. This observation brings out some of the complexity of Companionship, as opposed to a mere amanuensis or recording device, and its role between the merely personal and the social.

The first Artificial Companion is, of course, Frankenstein's monster in the 19C; that creature was dripping with emotions, and much concerned with its own social life:

*Shall each man," cried he, "find a wife for his bosom, and each beast have his mate, and We be alone? We had feelings of affection, and they were requited by detestation and scorn. Man! you may hate; but beware! your hours will pass in dread and misery, and soon the bolt will fall which must ravish from you your happiness for ever (Shelley, 1831, Ch. 20).*

This is clearly not quite the product that any modern COMPANIONS project is aiming at but, before just dismissing it as an "early failed experiment", we should take seriously the possibility, already touched on above, that things may turn out differently from what we expect and Companions, however effective, may be less loved and less loveable than we might wish. Newell has argued forcefully in Wilks (2010) that we must actually find out what kinds of relationship people want with Companion entities, as opposed to being technologists and just deciding a priori and then building what they believe people want.

It is no longer fashionable to explore a concept by reviewing its various senses, though it is not wholly useless either: when mentioning recently that one draft website for the COMPANIONS project had the black and pink aesthetic of a porn site, a colleague mentioned that the main Google-sponsored Companions site still announces "14.5 million girls await your call" and it was therefore perhaps not as inappropriate as one had first thought. Yet, for many, a Companion is still, primarily, a domestic animal, and it is interesting to note the key role pet-animals still play in the arguments on what it is, in principle, to be a Companion: especially the presence of the features of memory, recognition, attention and affection, found in dogs but rarely in snakes or newts.

We would also add that pets can play a key role in arguments about responsibility and liability, issues also raised already, and that dogs, at least under English common law, offer an example of an entity with a status between that of humans and mere wild animals: that is, *ferae naturae*, such as tigers, which the common law sees essentially as machines, and anyone who keeps one is absolutely liable for the results of its actions.

Companions could well come to occupy such an intermediate moral and legal position (see Wilks & Ballim, 1991), and it would not be necessary, given the precedents with pets already available in law, to deem them either mere slaves or the possessors of rights like our own. Dogs are treated by English courts as potential possessors of "character", so that a dog can be of "known bad character", as opposed to a (better) dog acting "out of character". There is no reason to believe that these pet precedents will automatically transfer to issues concerning Companions, but it is important to note that some minimal legal framework of this sort is already in place.

But one could nevertheless, and in no scientific manner, risk a listing of features of the ideal Victorian Companion:

1. Politeness
2. Discretion
3. Knowing their place
4. Dependence
5. Emotions firmly under control
6. Modesty
7. Wit
8. Cheerfulness
9. Well-informed
10. Diverting
11. Looks are irrelevant
12. Long-term relationship if possible
13. Trustworthy
14. Limited socialization between Companions permitted off-duty.

The Victorian virtue of Discretion here brings to mind the "confidant" concept that Boden (in Wilks, 2010) explicitly rejected as being a plausible one for automated Companions:

*Most secrets are secret from some HBs [Human Beings] but not others. If two CCs [Computer Companions] were to share their HB-users' secrets with each other, how would they know which other CCs (i.e. potentially, users) to 'trust' in this way? The HB could of course say "This is not to be told to Tommy"...... but usually we regard it as obvious that our confidant (sic) knows what should not be told to Tommy -- either to avoid upsetting Tommy, or to avoid upsetting the original HB. How is a CC to emulate that?*

*The HB could certainly say "Tell this to no-one" -- where "no-one" includes other CCs. But would the HB always remember to do that?*

*How could a secret-sharing CC deal with family feuds? Some family websites have special functionalities to deal with this. E.g Robbie is never shown input posted by Billie. Could similar, or more subtle, functionalities be given to CCs?"*

We think Boden brings up real difficulties in extending this notion to a computer Companion, but we do not think the problems are all where she thinks. We see no difficulty in programming the notion of explicit secrets for a Companion, or even things to be kept from specific individuals ("Never tell this to Tommy").

Companions will have fewer problems remembering to be discrete than people do, and we suspect there is less instinctual discretion than Boden suggests: people have to be told explicitly who to say what to in most cases, unless they are told to tell no one. In any case, much of this will be moot because Companions will normally deal only with one person—which is what makes their speech recognition problem so much easier, as we noted—they are trained for a single speaker---except when, say, making phone calls to an official, friend or restaurant, where they can try to keep the conversation to limited replies they can be sure to understand.

The notion of a stored fact that must not be disclosed is simple to code, and the issue is wider in that the same fact must, to preserve the secret, not take part in inference processes either. If it is a secret that Tom is really a Russian, then the Companion should not do inferences like [IF X is of nationality Y THEN X will normally speak Y] and come out with an utterance like "I assumed Tom could speak Russian", which would rather give the game away via the reverse inference, in the hearer [IF X speaks Y THEN X may well be of nationality Y].

The interesting case Boden raises is that of Companions talking to each other, and this was presumably always a risk for Victorian ladies: that their human Companions would gossip behind their backs. For our Companions this seems a positive development that we might encourage: imagine the shy older person in a care home, too shy to approach another for a lunch together. This would be something best settled between their Companions, each knowing the tastes and habits of their owner, to whom the "date" could be presented as a fait accompli.

Again, many Companion-to-Companion interactions will be between an individual's Companion and some form of "public Companion" such as one that takes restaurant bookings based on a user's tastes; or at a hospital where a hospital-Companion could triage incoming patients, who may not be articulate about their condition, on the basis of detailed knowledge of the user's medical records. When traveling, this Companion-to-Companion interaction in, say, a hospital could also combine with translation where the respective Companions worked out how to communicate across a language barrier.

In all these cases, Companion-to-Companion communication could be of obvious benefit to a user even if confidential information was at risk of disclosure: the user might have said "Never tell anyone I am HIV positive" but in the hospital environment that constraint should obviously be overridden and the user's condition revealed. One could say at this point that secrets may be relative to a situation and that there may be nothing more complex in a Companion's guardianship of secrets than there is in explicit restrictions one could give to human hearers.

The ultimate revelation of secrets by a Companion after a user's death is a wholly separate and complex subject. There are already on the market (e.g. [Deathswitch]) products that save and reveal passwords and ultimate letters and secrets at death; this is undoubtedly an area with enormous possibilities as the Internet makes actual death less apparent and immediate in the electronic world than it is the real one (see also Wilks [Death and the Internet]).

If the Victorian list of characteristics above is in any way plausible, it suggests an emphasis rather different from that current in much research on emotions and computers (e.g. the HUMAINE network at emotion-research.net) and their possible embodiments and deployments to a public. The emphasis in the list is on what the self-presentation and self-image of a possible, and tolerable, Companion should be; its suggestion is that overt emotion may not be what is wanted at all.

We have never felt wholly comfortable with the standard Embodied Conversational Agent (ECA) approach in which if, an avatar "has" an emotion, it immediately expresses it, almost as if to prove the capacity of the screen graphics. This is exactly the sort of issue tackled by Darwin (1872) and such overtness can seem to indicate almost a lower evolutionary level than one might want to model, in that it is not a normal feature of much human interaction. The emotions of most of my preferred and frequent interlocutors, when revealed, are usually expressed in modulations of the voice and a very precise choice of words, but we realize this may be just cultural prejudice.

On the other hand, pressing the pet analogy might suggest that, if that is to be the paradigm, then overt demonstrations of emotion are desirable and sought by pet owners: dogs do not much disguise their emotions, and their positive emotions are often welcomed by owners. Language, however, does disguise emotion as much as it reveals it, and its ability to please, soothe and cause offence are tightly coupled with linguistic expertise---as opposed to the display of gestures and facial expressions--- as we all know with non-native speakers of our languages who frequently offend, even though they have no desire to do so, and often have no awareness of the offence they cause.

What name to call someone by, or whether or not to use vocatives like "Sir", "Mister", "Miss", "Missus" are enormously complex matters, known intuitively to native speakers but not to outsiders, who are never taught them and have nowhere to go for advice or instruction. These are not cultural matters across space only, but also time: it was pointed out long ago that in the 19C, male Cambridge undergraduates would walk arm-in-arm and call each other by their last names, without giving offence, whereas in the latter part of the 20C they would use first names ---since last names would have given offence ---and never be seen arm-in-arm.

We personally find the lady's Companion list above an attractive one: it eschews emotion beyond the linguistic, it implies care for the mental and emotional state of the user, and we would personally find it hard to abuse any computer with the characteristics listed above. It is no accident, of course, that this list fits rather well with the aims of the Senior Companion demonstrator in the COMPANIONS project already mentioned above.

The project first produced a [Health and Fitness Companion] for the more active, one sharing much of the architecture with the first, and one that would require something in addition to the list above: the "personal trainer" element of weaning, coaxing and threatening which adds something quite different to that list and something very close to the economic-game bargain of the kind discussed in some detail by Lowe (in Wilks, 2010).

Many of the situations discussed above are, at the moment, wildly speculative: that of a Companion acting as its owner's agent, on the phone or World Wide Web, perhaps holding power of attorney in case of an owner's incapacity and, with the owner's advance permission, perhaps even being a source of conversational comfort for relatives after the owner's death.

Companions may not all be nice or even friendly: companions to stop us falling asleep while driving may tell us jokes but will probably shout at us and make us do stretching exercises. Long-voyage Companions in space will be indispensable cognitive prostheses (or, more correctly, orthoses) for running a huge vessel and experiments above and beyond any personal services---Hollywood already knows all that. All these situations are at present absurd, but perhaps we should be ready for them.

## ACKNOWLEDGMENT

This work was funded by the Companions project www.companions-project.org) sponsored by the European Commission as part of the Information

Society Technologies (IST) programme under EC grant number IST-FP6-034434.

## REFERENCES

Asimov, I. (1950). *I, robot*. New York, NY: Doubleday & Company.

Cheepen, C., & Monaghan, J. (1997). Designing naturalness in automated dialogues - some problems and solutions. In *Proceedings First International Workshop on Human- Computer Conversation*, Bellagio, Italy.

Ciravegna, F., Chapman, S., Dingli, A., & Wilks, Y. (2004). Learning to harvest the Semantic Web. In *Proc. European Semantic Web Symposium (ESWS04).*

Colby, K. M. (1971). Artificial paranoia. *Artificial Intelligence*, *2*(1), 1–2. doi:10.1016/0004-3702(71)90002-6

Cowie, R., Douglas-Cowie, E., Tsapatsoulis, N., Votsis, G., Kollias, S., Fellenz, W., & Taylor, J. G. (2001). Emotion recognition in human-computer interaction. *Signal Processing Magazine, IEEE, 18*(1), 32–80. doi:10.1109/79.911197

Darwin, C. (1872). *The origin of species by means of natural selection, or the preservation of favoured races in the struggle for life*. London, UK: John Murray.

Dreyfus, H. L. (1972). *What computers can't do*. Cambridge, MA: MIT Press.

Feigenbaum, E. (n.d.). *Personal communication*.

Hayes, P. J. (1979). The naive physics manifesto. In Michie, D. (Ed.), *Expert systems in the micro electronic age*. Edinburgh, UK: Edinburgh University Press.

Höök, K. (2004). User-centred design and evaluation of affective interfaces. In Ruttkay, Z., & Pelachaud, C. (Eds.), *From brows to trust: Evaluating embodied conversational agents*. Amsterdam, The Netherlands: Kluwer.

Krippendorff, K. (2004). *Content analysis: An introduction to its methodology* (2nd ed.). Thousand Oaks, CA: Sage.

Levy, D. (2007). *Love and sex with robots: The evolution of human–robot relationships*. London, UK: Duckworth.

Luneski, A., Moore, R. K., & Bamidis, P. D. (2008). Affective computing and collaborative networks: Towards emotion-aware interaction. In Camarinha-Matos, L. M., & Picard, W. (Eds.), *Pervasive collaborative networks* (*Vol. 283*, pp. 315–322). Boston, MA: Springer. doi:10.1007/978-0-387-84837-2_32

Marsella, S., & Gratch, J. (2003). Modeling coping behavior in virtual humans: Don't worry, be happy. In *Proc. 2nd International Conf. on Autonomous Agents and Multiagent Systems (AAMAS),* Melbourne, Australia, July 2003.

Mori, M. (1970). The uncanny valley.

Reeves, B., & Nass, C. (1996). *The media equation: How people treat computers, television, and new media like real people and places*. Cambridge, UK: Cambridge University Press.

Scherer, S., Schwenker, F., & Palm, G. (2008). Emotion recognition from speech using multi-classifier systems and rbf-ensembles. *Speech, Audio, Image and Biomedical Signal Processing using Neural Networks*, 49–70. Berlin, Germany: Springer.

Searle, J. (1969). *Speech acts*. Cambridge, UK: Cambridge University Press.

Shelley, M. (1831). *Frankenstein* (Smith, J. M., Ed.). Boston, MA: St. Martin's.

Veletsianos, G., Miller, C., & Doering, A. (2009). EnALI: A research and design framework for virtual characters and pedagogical agents. *Journal of Educational Computing Research, 41*(2), 171–194. doi:10.2190/EC.41.2.c

Wallis, P., Mitchard, H., O'Dea, D., & Das, J. (2001). Dialogue modelling for a conversational agent. In Stumptner, Corbett, & Brooks, (Eds.), *Proceedings 14th Australian Joint Conference on Artificial Intelligence*, Adelaide, Australia.

Walters, M., Dautenhahn, K., te Boekhorst, R., Koay, K., & Syrdal, D. (2009). An empirical framework for human-robot proxemics. In *Proc. AISB Convention* 2009. www.aisb.org.uk/convention/aisb09/.

Webb, N., Benyon, D., Hansen, P., & Mival, O. (2010). Wizard of Oz experiments for a companion dialogue system: Eliciting companionable conversation. In *Proceedings of the 7th International Conference on Language Resources and Evaluation (LREC2010),* Valletta, Malta.

Weizenbaum, J. (1966). ELIZA — a computer program for the study of natural language communication between man and machine. *Communications of the ACM, 9*(1), 36–45. doi:10.1145/365153.365168

Wilks, Y. (2006). *Artificial companions as a new kind of interface to the future Internet*. Oxford Internet Institute Research report No. 13 (Oxford Internet Institute). Retrieved from http://www.oii.ox.ac.uk/research/publications.cfm

Wilks, Y. (Ed.). (2010). *Artificial companions in society: Scientific, economic, psychological and philosophical perspectives*. Amsterdam, The Netherlands: John Benjamins.

Wilks, Y., & Ballim, A. (1991). *Artificial believers*. Norwood, NJ: Erlbaum.

Wilks, Y., Catizone, R., Worgan, S., Dingli, A., Moore, R. K., & Cheng, W. (2010). A prototype system for a conversational companion for reminiscing about images. *Computer Speech and Language*.

Wundt, W. (1913). *Grundriss der Psychologie*. Berlin, Germany: A. Kroner.

Zue, V., Glass, J., Goddeau, D., Goodine, D., & Hirschman, L. (1992). The MIT ATIS system, In *Proc. DARPA Workshop on speech and natural language*, Harriman, NY.

## INTERNET SITES

Death and the Internet. http://people.oii.ox.ac.uk/yorick/2007/01/24/death-and-the-internet/

Deathswitch: http://www.deathswitch.com/

Emily avatar: http://www.youtube.com/watch?v=UYgLFt5wfP4&feature=player_embedded# and http://www.surrealaward.com/avatar/3ddigital12.shtml

Health and Fitness Companion. http://www.youtube.com/watch?v=KQSiigSEYhU&feature=related

Loebner: http://www.loebner.net/Prizef/loebner-prize.html

Memories for Life. http://www.memoriesforlife.org/

Senior Companion demo: http://www.youtube.com/watch?v=-Xx5hgjD-Mw

## KEY TERMS AND DEFINITIONS

**Automatic Speech Recognition:** The technology for recognizing human speech automatically by computer and converting its wave forms to text.

**Chatbot:** A simple web-based computational device that answers when typed to but has no understanding or memory of what it is replying to.

**Content Analysis:** A technique developed by Harvard University psychologists in the 1960s for labeling text words with positive and negative sentiments and attempting to sum up with these the sentiment expressed by a text.

**Software Agents:** Computer programs on the Internet that carry out tasks including talking to human users.

**Speech Dialogue Applications:** Software applications on the Internet able to carry on a conversation with a human being at some level of understanding.

**Task-Based System:** A dialogue application that is able to carry out a task, like helping someone buy an air ticket, but knows nothing outside that task and can talk about nothing else.

**Text To Speech (TTS):** A technology that takes in a written text and turns it into a speech form that the computer then speaks.

**Uncanny Valley Effect:** A claim (originally by Mori) that computer agents that model humans on the web, and which talk, become more and more unsatisfactory to deal with the closer they get to being indistinguishable from people.

# Chapter 18
# Future Trends for Conversational Agents

**Diana Pérez-Marín**
*Universidad Rey Juan Carlos, Spain*

**Ismael Pascual-Nieto**
*Universidad Autónoma de Madrid, Spain*

## ABSTRACT

*In the last decades, there has been a great evolution in the field of Conversational Agents. Currently, there are agents to assist the navigation in Web pages, support elder users when interacting with some computer application to remind them which medicines they should take during the day, or to enhance the learning process by allowing students to review with systems that adapt themselves to their previous knowledge and rhythm of study. In this chapter, the goal is to provide a summary of the future trends that can be envisaged for the future of the field. It is our insight that the future of Conversational Agents are to become pervasive and natural in our daily lives.*

## INTRODUCTION

Fifty years ago, computers were complex machines that occupied rooms and required a vast amount of technical knowledge to be used. Therefore, only a small amount of people could interact with them. Furthermore, users could only communicate with the computers via a very restrictive interface. There was a list of commands with their set of options that should be placed in the exact order in order to command the operation requested to the program.

There has been a great evolution both in the hardware and software aspects of Computer Science since then. While the hardware is being made smaller and more potent, the software is being made friendlier and less dependent on the technical knowledge of the user. Menu-based interfaces have mostly replaced the list of commands. That way, users do not need to memorize the commands. They choose the action to perform by clicking on the menu.

DOI: 10.4018/978-1-60960-617-6.ch018

Nevertheless, the interaction based on the use of menus can also be regarded as quite restrictive. All in all, users are limited to request the computer one of the enlisted actions with the options of the panels. Moreover, if the users ignore in which menu an option is, then they will not be able to perform it.

Natural Language Interaction is studied in this book as the possibility of interacting with computers in natural language. That way, users could request the tasks to perform with their computer in the same way than they talk to their colleagues at work. It would not longer necessary to learn lists of commands or where they are placed in a menu.

Conversational agents are programs that interact with the users in natural language. They can be executed in any type of computers (including laptops and netbooks), smartphones or PDAs. These agents are currently being used as assistants to make the navigation in Internet easier, to book travels on-line, remind which medicines to take, do the homework, or attend some customer petitions.

The advantages are many: the agents can work 24 hours per day, all the days of the year, they do not get tired or impatient, and they could be adapted to treat all the people in the same way, or depending on the information previously stored of their profiles, so that they provide exactly what each user needs. In fact, according to Fairclough (2009), the next generation of intelligent technology will be characterized by increased autonomy and adaptive capability.

For the future of Conversational Agents, the advances in Natural Language Processing will keep being crucial. The research into new techniques and algorithms can allow the systems to understand better the sentences provided by the users, and to respond with more elaborated and different constructions as humans would answer to those petitions.

Furthermore, and according to Erwin Van Luhn from Chatbots.org and highlighted in chapters 9 and 17 of this book, the future of conversational agents encompasses more than just the correct understanding and generation of words; it will be about understanding emotions too. Conversational agents could become then part of the users' everyday life. The agents would be available on demand just by calling out their names as emphatic characters, understanding the users' lifes, feelings, situation, friendships, history and anticipating like a human would do.

Conversational agents can also have an animated face with or without body. In that case, they are called Embodied Conversational Agents (ECAs). Currently, according to López-Mencía et al. (chapter 3), we are just beginning to understand how ECAs affect the perceptions of users, upon which the most appropriate design of the ECA's behaviour ultimately depends (Gratch et al., 2006; Edlund & Beskow, 2007). Therefore, it is necessary more research in that line, and it would also be interesting to research the application of ECAs for biometric applications (Krämer et al., 2009).

The chapter is organised as follows: firstly, the future trends on more sophisticated Natural Language Processing, humanising the agents and their pervasiveness are summarised. Next, the chapter is focused on the domain applications and their potential users. Finally, the main conclusions drawn are presented.

## TRENDS

### More Sophisticated Natural Language Processing

Natural Language Processing (NLP) has been researched since 1950s. Originally, the goals were very broad such as automatic translation of any text from any language to any other language. However, the lack of resources and hardware ended with the feeling that it was a task too difficult to accomplish. Therefore, more realistic and specific goals were established, such as to recognize entities in the text or to answer questions.

Currently, the advances in hardware and the greater number of resources such as annotated corpora, thesauri, lexical databases or ontologies have made the progress in this field possible. Nevertheless, there is still plenty of research to do, with many problems to solve. For instance, it is still not clear how to process texts with paraphrasing, entailments, or how to successfully deal with the inner ambiguity of the natural languages.

The research on Conversational Agents will be able to produce better and more realistic human-computer dialogues as the research in NLP progresses. In this trend, Andrews & Quarteroni (chapter 8) claimed that research into Interactive Question Answering and automatic persuasive dialogue can improve and enrich the human-computer dialogues (Quarteroni & Saint-Dizier, 2009); and Novielli & Strapparava (chapter 4) discussed about the benefits of Dialogue Act Classification exploiting Lexical Semantics.

Moreover, conversational agents should not only be able to transmit information, but also to convince the user and to react to their statements as a human would do. It is not natural that a human-human conversation is so limited to a task, and this could explain the frustration generated by standard task oriented dialogue (Klein, Moon, & Picard, 1999). Therefore, more research should be devoted to the study of how generating more freedom in the human-computer dialogues, while achieving the goal of the user when interacting with the computer.

As Kenny & Parsons claimed in chapter 11, both Natural Language Understanding (i.e. how computers can understand human's statements) and Natural Language Generation (i.e. how computers can generate statements) should be further studied.

When the input is spoken, Amores et al. in chapter 14 claimed that speech recognizers should be improved to achieve a better trade-off between performance and coverage, and to smooth the jittering effect on online communications. These studies should also be oriented to make the use of this technology cheaper and thus, available for more users (see also more about this in chapters 10 and 15).

The parsers of natural language could be improved by grasping more semantics. Once lexical resources have been developed, semantic banks could be created to identify the semantics of the sentences typed or spoken by the user. Ontologies could be a good knowledge formalism to serve as a representation of the user's natural language input and to produce a better understanding of the dialog. For instance, some progress has been made for knowledge base construction with the use of upper-level ontologies such as SUMO (Niles & Pease, 2001).

Speech acts as indicated in chapter 4 could also serve to tag the modality of the interaction and in case, that the input is spoken, not only the words, but the intonation and prosody could also be taken into account provided that the speech recognizer is good enough.

The internal representation as an ontology or other type of semantics knowledge representation could be parsed by domain dependent grammars to generate more realistic output to the user. This would avoid the 'robotic' feeling that some conversations with agents could provoke because the agents always generate the same sentences and state them with the same intonation. Furthermore, the generated sentences could also be adapted to each user's language, and to the specific mood of the conversation.

Finally, other lines that could provide benefits to the improvement of human-computer dialogues are Reinforcement Learning at dialogue level and reranking parsing results (see chapter 14), taking also into account the importance of multilinguality of the processing tools so that the agent can interact with a wider range of users.

## Human Features

This second trend in the future of conversational agents is oriented to including more human features to the programs so that they seem more natural to the users. According to Stuart Slater, the agents could even include human like memory systems that can be interfaced to emotion modules to add more human like characteristics to agents.

In the educational domains, and as claimed by Pirrone et al. in chapter 5, how agents can help self-regulation in students learning should be further studied.

Finally, other challenges in this trend are pointed out by Loeckelt in chapter 7, such as better support for the dialogue designer, increased reusability, better testing possibilities, better reasoning possibilities, improved character groups and parallel execution.

### Pervasiveness

The third trend has been called pervasiveness because it is expected that the agents will not be limited just to computer programs, but as ubiquitous computing is more present in our daily lives with smartphones, netbooks, PDAs, etc. the agents are also used from many different devices at home, public transport, streets, or any place with or without Internet connection.

As seen in chapter 14, in order to allow users to interact with their agents in mobile devices, more research into usability issues is needed. Strategies should be though to overcome the limitations in the screen and keyboard sizes of these devices. Furthermore, the language in which users tend to interact with these devices should also be taken into account regarding the natural language processing of those sentences (lack of grammar, wrong spelling, slang, etc).

Finally, the pervasive agents are also expected to become 3D. We are used to interact with a 3D world, therefore in order to provide a more realistic experience, there should be created 3D agents (Manchón, 2009; see also chapter 16). However, it is not only a graphics matter of changing 2D interfaces by 3D interfaces. The agents should be kept efficient and able to respond in real time to keep the user satisfaction, trust and willingness to interact with the agent.

## APPLICATIONS AND TARGET USERS

Currently, it is usual that agents are designed for a specific domain: customer service, e-health, e-learning, travel assistant, etc. It limits the vocabulary and valid interactions (e.g. when booking a train, the user should not talk about general politics). However, it also limits the realism of the dialogue because no small talk is offered (while it is highly usual in human-human dialogues) and if there is some unexpected even, the agent may not be able to solve it automatically (see more about this in chapter 6).

In the future, it is expected that the agents designed for a specific domain are able to better deal with unexpected evens, while the domain is broader and for a wider range of users. For instance, in the medical domain, Kenny & Parsons stated, in chapter 11, that the use of bio physiological inputs to the system would provide useful information to improve the interaction of the agent with the user (Parsons et al., 2009). Agents could also take into account vision input to evaluate the user's non-verbal behavior and rapport (Morency & de Kok, 2008).

In education, and as claimed in chapter 6 it would also be desirable to have papers exploring the effect of the use of Pedagogic Conversational Agents in *long-term studies*. It is already known that well-designed conversational agents during short-term use can positively influence self-efficacy beliefs in students (Baylor, 2009; Kim & Baylor, 2007) but it is unknown the effects of long-term studies. The need for that research had already been pointed out (Dehn & van Mulken, 2000; Gulz, 2004), and in some years, it would be possible to gather the first results. It is also expected that the agents are better adapted to each students' features (Gulz & Haake, 2010).

Agents will help workers with their life-long training. They would also be able to assist and remind elders when some of their cognitive processes started to failure. Furthermore, as claimed in chapters 12 and 13, agents will be able to serve as their companions to combat any isolation feeling they may have. In fact, social networking sites are already gaining interest among seniors and will probably become a major component in their lives. The use of an agent to assist them in using the computer or to serve as another colleague will enhance the sense of connectedness and promote a higher quality of life.

Agents could help to integrate not only elders but also people with some kind of disability. From students who cannot assist to face-to-face lessons and interact with the agent to study at home to autistic children who are unable to express by themselves, but as seen in chapter 2 are able to successfully interact with the agents in the computer. Agents can serve as tutors for emotion recognition and expression. The agent could explain how it perceives the expression and why. Similarly, agents could serve as tutors for people with problems when trying to use social skills or overcoming their phobias.

## CONCLUSION

In this chapter, three main future trends for conversational agents have been proposed: agents that are able to create more realistic dialogues by using better Natural Language Processing, agents that become more human recognizing and generating not only words within sentences, but recognizing emotions and adapting the dialogue to them (i.e. changing the intonation or the type of vocabulary), and 3D agents that are not longer limited to be used within PC, but are available at many different places in mobile devices.

It is our expectation that, in some years, conversational agents will be daily used for many domains and by a wide range of users. Children could be supported by Pedagogic Conversational Agents to do their homework and review the lessons' concepts at home; young people could use an agent to book the tickets to social events; adults without computer training could use any web page with the assistance of an agent; and elders could feel they are not left apart of the digital gap by having their own companion agent too.

Conversational agents can also bring many benefits to attend the diversity and for universal design of computer applications. In order to evaluate those benefits, specific metrics should be created, and longitudinal studies should be performed to gather results of the long-term impact of their use during several years.

## REFERENCES


Baylor, A. (2009). Promoting motivation with virtual agents and avatars: Role of visual presence and appearance. *Philosophical Transactions of the Royal Society of London. Series B, Biological Sciences*, *364*(1535), 3559–3566. doi:10.1098/rstb.2009.0148

Dehn, D., & van Mulken, S. (2000). The impact of animated interface agents: A review of empirical research. *International Journal of Human-Computer Studies*, *52*(1), 1–22. doi:10.1006/ijhc.1999.0325

Edlund, J., & Beskow, J. (2007). Pushy versus meek using avatars to influence turn-taking behaviour. In *Proceedings of Interspeech ICSLP*. Atwerp.

Fairclough, S. H. (2009). Fundamentals of physiological computing. *Interacting with Computers*, *21*, 133–145. doi:10.1016/j.intcom.2008.10.011

Gratch, J., Okhmatovskaia, A., Lamothe, F., Marsella, S., Morales, M., van der Werf, R. J., & Morency, L. P. (2006). Virtual rapport. In *Proceedings of the 6th International Conference on Intelligent Virtual Agents*, (pp. 14-27).

Gulz, A. (2004). Benefits of virtual characters in computer based learning environments: Claims and evidence. *International Journal of Artificial Intelligence in Education, 14*, 313–334.

Gulz, A., & Haake, M. (2010). Challenging gender stereotypes using virtual pedagogical characters. In Goodman, S., Booth, S., & Kirkup, G. (Eds.), *Gender issues in learning and working with Information Technology: Social constructs and cultural contexts*. Hershey, PA, USA: IGI Global. doi:10.4018/978-1-61520-813-5.ch007

Kim, Y., & Baylor, A. L. (2007). Pedagogical agents as social models to influence learner attitudes. *Educational Technology, 47*(1), 23–28.

Klein, J., Moon, Y., & Picard, R. W. (1999). This computer responds to user frustration. *CHI '99 extended abstracts on Human factors in computing system*.

Krämer, N., Bente, G., Eschenburg, F., & Troitzsch, H. (2009). Embodied conversational agents: Research prospects for social psychology and an exemplary study. *Social Psychology, 40*(1), 26–36. doi:10.1027/1864-9335.40.1.26

Manchón, P. (2009). *Towards clever human-computer interaction*. Doctoral dissertation, University of Seville, Spain.

Morency, L. P., & de Kok, I. (2008). *Context-based recognition during human interactions: Automatic feature selection and encoding dictionary*. 10th International Conference on Multimodal Interfaces, Chania, Greece, IEEE.

Niles, I., & Pease, A. (2001). Towards a standard upper ontology. In *Proceedings of the 2nd International Conference on Formal Ontology in Information Systems* (FOIS-2001) (pp. 2-9). Ogunquit, ME: ACM.

Parsons, T. D., Cosand, L., Courtney, C., Iyer, A., & Rizzo, A. A. (2009). Neurocognitive workload assessment using the virtual reality cognitive performance assessment test. *Lecture Notes in Artificial Intelligence, 5639*, 243–252.

Quarteroni, S., & Saint-Dizier, P. (2009). *Addressing how-to questions using a spoken dialogue system: A viable approach?* Singapore: *KRAQ*'09.

## KEY TERMS AND DEFINITIONS

**3D Conversational Agent:** Agent in which to the representation of the normal dimensions (wide and tall), the depth has also been added.

**Embodied Conversational Agent:** Animated agent with a body that can support with gestures the sentences uttered.

**Mobile Device:** Pocket-size computing devices with a display screen with touch input and/or a keyboard to type information. Two of the most popular mobile devices are the smartphones and PDAs.

**Natural Language Understanding:** Research field that studies how computers can understand human's statements.

**Natural Language Generation:** Research field that studies how computers can generate statements.

**Natural Language Processing:** Research field that studies how to automatically process written or spoken texts in natural language.

**Ontology:** Explicit specification of a conceptualization of shared knowledge.

**Semantics:** The study of meaning of the language.

**Speech Recognizer:** Computer program able to transform spoken words to text.

# Compilation of References


A.L.I.C.E. (2008). *A.L.I.C.E. homepage*. Retrieved from http://alice.sunlitsurf.com/alice/about.html

Aarts, E. (2004). Ambient intelligence. A multimedia perspective. *IEEE MultiMedia*, *11*(1), 12–19. doi:10.1109/MMUL.2004.1261101

Accreditation Council for Graduate Medical Education. (2007). *ACGME Outcome Project*. Retrieved December 5, 2007, from www.acgme.org/Outcomes

Adolphs, P., Cheng, X., Klüwer, T., Uszkoreit, U., & Xu, F. (2010). (to appear). Question answering biographic information and social network powered by the Semantic Web. In . *Proceedings of the LREC*.

Ai, H., Kumar, R., Nguyen, D., Nagasunder, A., & Rosé, C. (2010). Exploring the effectiveness of social capabilities and goal alignment in computer supported collaborative learning . In Aleven, V., Kay, J., & Mostow, J. (Eds.), *ITS 2010, part II, LNCS 6095* (pp. 134–143). Berlin/Heidelberg, Germany: Springer-Verlag.

Ai, H., Raux, A., Bohus, D., Eskenazi, M., & Litman, D. (2007). Comparing spoken dialog corpora collected with recruited subjects versus real users. In *Proc. of the 8th SIGdial workshop on Discourse and Dialogue*.

Akkaya, C., Wiebe, J., & Mihalcea, R. (2009). Subjectivity word sense disambiguation. In *Proc. EMNLP.*

Alamán, X., Haya, P., & Montoro, G. (2001). *El proyecto InterAct: Una arquitectura de pizarra para la implementación de Entornos Activos* (pp. 72–73). Proc. of Interacción Persona-Ordenador.

Alexandersson, J., Reithinger, N., & Maier, E. (1997). *Insights into the dialogue processing of VERBMOBIL*. Saarbrücken, Germany.

Alexandersson, J., & Becker, T. (2001). Overlay as the basic operation for discourse processing in a multimodal dialogue system. In *Proceedings of the IJCAI Workshop on Knowledge and Reasoning in Practical Dialogue Systems* (pp. 8–14), Seattle, WA.

Alexandersson, J., Maier, E., & Reithinger, N. (1994). *A robust and efficient three-layered dialogue component for speech-to-speech translation system*. Technical Report~50, DFKI GmbH. Retrieved April 29, 2001, from http://www.dfki.uni-sb.de/cgi-bin/verbmobil/htbin/doc-access.cgi

Allen, J. F., & Perrault, C. R. (1980). Analyzing intentions in dialogues. *Artificial Intelligence*, *15*(3), 143–178. doi:10.1016/0004-3702(80)90042-9

Allen, J., Schubert, L., Ferguson, G., Heeman, P., Hwang, C.-H., & Kato, T. (1995). The TRAINS project: A case study in building a conversational planning agent. *Journal of Experimental & Theoretical Artificial Intelligence*, *7*, 7–48. doi:10.1080/09528139508953799

Allen, J. (1995). *Natural language understanding*. The Benjamin/Cummings Publishing Company Inc.

Allen, J., Byron, D., Dzikovska, M., Ferguson, G., Galescu, L., & Stent, A. (2001). Towards conversational human-computer interaction. *AI Magazine*, *22*(4), 27–37.

Allen, J., Byron, D., Dzikovska, M., Ferguson, G., Galescu, L., & Stent, A. (2000). An architecture for a generic dialogue shell. *Natural Language Engineering*, *6*(3-4), 213–228. doi:10.1017/S135132490000245X

Allen, J. F., Ferguson, G., Miller, B. W., Ringger, E. K., & Zollo, T. S. (2000). Dialogue systems: From theory to practice in TRAINS-96 . In Dale, R., Moisl, R., & Somers, H. (Eds.), *Handbook of natural language processing*. New York, NY: Marcel Dekker.

Allen, J. F., Dzikovska, M., Manshadi, M., & Swift, M. (2007). Deep linguistic processing for spoken dialogue systems. In *Proceedings of the ACL 2007 Workshop on Deep Linguistic Processing*, Prague, June.

Allen, J. F., Miller, B. W., Ringger, E., & Sikorski, T. (1996). Robust understanding in a dialogue system. In *Proceedings of the 34th Annual Meeting of the Association for Computational Linguistics.*

Allen, J., Chambers, N., Ferguson, G., Galescu, L., Jung, H., Swift, M., & Taysom, W. (2007). PLOW: A collaborative task learning agent. *Proc. of AAAI*, (pp. 22-26).

Allen, J., Ferguson, G., & Stent, A. (2001). An architecture for more realistic conversational systems. *IUI '01: Proceedings of the 6th International Conference on Intelligent user interfaces.*

Allwood, J. (2001). Cooperation and flexibility in multimodal communication . In Bunt, H., & Beun, R. J. (Eds.), *Cooperative multimodal communication*. Berlin/Heidelberg, Germany: Springer Verlag. doi:10.1007/3-540-45520-5_7

Altman, I., & Vinsel, A. (1977). Personal space. An analysis of E. T. Hall's proxemics framework. *Human Behaviour and Environment. Advances in Theory and Research, 2*, 181–259.

American Psychiatric Association. (2000). *Diagnostic and statistical manual of mental disorders* (4th ed., text revision). Washington, DC: APA.

Amores, J., Pérez, G., & Manchón, P. (2007). MIMUS: A multimodal and multilingual dialogue system for the home domain. In *Proceedings of the ACL 2007 Demo and Poster Sessions, vol. 45* (pp. 1-4).

Andersen, P. A., & Guerrero, L. K. (1998). *Handbook of communication and emotions. Research, theory, applications and contexts*. New York, NY: Academic Press.

Anderson, J. R., Bothell, D., Byrne, M., Douglass, S., Lebiere, C., & Qin, Y. (2004). Integrated theory of the mind. *Psychological Review, 111*, 1036–1060. doi:10.1037/0033-295X.111.4.1036

André, E., & Rist, T. (2000). *Presenting through performing: On the use of multiple kifelike characters in knowledge-nased presentation systems. IUI 2000* (pp. 1–8). New Orleans, LA, USA: ACM Press.

André, E., Klesen, M., Gebhard, P., Allen, S., & Rist, T. (2000). Integrating models of personality and emotions into lifelike characters . In Paiva, A. (Ed.), *Affective interactions: Towards a new generation of computer interfaces, Lecture Notes In Computer Science* (*Vol. 1814*, pp. 150–165). New York, NY: Springer-Verlag.

Andrews, P., & Manandhar, S. (2009). Measure of belief change as an evaluation of persuasion. *Proceedings of the AISB'09 Persuasive Technology and Digital Behaviour Intervention Symposium.*

Arch, A. (2008). *Web accessibility for older users: A literature review*. Retrieved from http://www.w3.org/TR/wai-age-literature/

Ardizzone, E., Cannella, V., Peri, D., & Pirrone, R. (2004). *Automatic generation of user interfaces using the set description language*. In the 12th International Conference in Central Europe on Computer Graphics, Visualization and Computer Vision (pp. 209-212). UNION Agency - Science Press.

Arthritis Foundation. (2008). *Arthritis prevalence: A nation in pain*. Retrieved from http://www.arthritis.org/media/newsroom/media-kits/Arthritis_Prevalence.pdf

Artstein, R., Gandhe, S., Gerten, J., Leuski, A., & Traum, D. (2009). Semi-formal evaluation of conversational characters . In Grumberg, O., Kaminski, M., Katz, S., & Wintner, S. (Eds.), *Languages: From formal to natural. Essays dedicated to Nissim Francez on the occasion of His 65th Birthday (Lecture Notes in Computer Science 5533)* (pp. 22–35). Heidelberg, Germany: Springer.

Asimov, I. (1950). *I, robot*. New York, NY: Doubleday & Company.

Atkinson, R. (2002). Optimizing learning from examples using animated pedagogical agents. *Journal of Educational Psychology, 94*(2), 416–427. doi:10.1037/0022-0663.94.2.416

Atserias, J., Casas, B., Comelles, E., González, M., & Padru., M. (2006). *Freeling 1.3: Syntactic and semantic services in an open-source NLP library*. In the 5th International Conference on Language Resources and Evaluation (LREC 2006), ELRA.

Attwater, D., Edgington, M., Durston, P., & Whittaker, S. (2000). Practical issues in the application of speech technology to network and customer services applications. *Speech Communication, 31*(4), 279–291. doi:10.1016/S0167-6393(99)00062-X

Aust, H., Oerder, M., Seide, F., & Steinbiss, V. (1995). The Philips automatic train timetable information system. *Speech Communication, 17*, 3–4. doi:10.1016/0167-6393(95)00028-M

Austin, J. (1962). *How to do things with words*. New York, NY: Oxford University Press.

Austin, J. L. (1975). *How to do things with words*. Cambridge, MA: Harvard University Press.

Bailenson, J. N., Swinth, K. R., & Hoyt, C. L., Persky, Susan, D. A., & Blascovich, J. (2005). The independent and interactive effects of embodied agents appearance and behavior on self-report, cognitive and behavioral markers of copresence in Immersive Virtual Environments. *Presence (Cambridge, Mass.), 14*(4), 379–393. doi:10.1162/105474605774785235

Balci, K. (2005). XfaceEd: Authoring tool for embodied conversational agents. *Proc. of ICMI*, (pp. 208-213).

Balentine, B., & Morgan, D. (1999). *How to build a speech recognition application: A style guide for telephony dialogues*. USA: Enterprise Integration Group.

Bandura, A. (1986). *Social foundations of thought and action: A social cognitive theory*. Englewood Cliffs, NJ: Prentice-Hall.

Bandura, A. (2000). *Self-efficacy: The foundation of agency*. Mahwah, NJ: Lawrence Erlbaum.

Bargh, J. A., & Schul, Y. (1980). On the cognitive benefits of teaching. *Journal of Educational Psychology, 72*, 593–604. doi:10.1037/0022-0663.72.5.593

Barnett, J., Dahl, D. A., Kliche, I., Tumuluri, R., Yudkowsky, M., & Bodell, M. (2008). *Multimodal architecture and interfaces*. Retrieved from http://www.w3.org/TR/mmi-arch/

Basili, R., De Cao, D., Giannone, C., & Marocco, P. (2007). Data-driven dialogue for interactive question answering. *Proceedings of AI*IA'07*.

Batliner, A., Fischer, K., Huber, R., Spliker, J., & Nöth, E. (2003). How to find trouble in communication. *Speech Communication, 40*, 117–143. doi:10.1016/S0167-6393(02)00079-1

Bayer, S. (2005). Building a standards and research community with the Galaxy communicator software infrastructure . In Dahl, D. A. (Ed.), *Practical spoken dialog systems* (*Vol. 26*, pp. 166–196). Dordrecht, The Netherlands: Kluwer Academic Publishers.

Baylor, A., & Kim, Y. (2005). Simulating instructional roles through pedagogical agents. *International Journal of Artificial Intelligence in Education, 15*(1), 95–115.

Baylor, A. (2009). Promoting motivation with virtual agents and avatars: Role of visual presence and appearance. *Philosophical Transactions of the Royal Society of London. Series B, Biological Sciences, 364*(1535), 3559–3566. doi:10.1098/rstb.2009.0148

Baylor, A., & Plant, E. (2005). Pedagogical agents as social models for engineering: The influence of appearance on female choice . In Looi, C. K., McCalla, G., Bredeweg, B., & Breuker, J. (Eds.), *Artificial intelligence in education: Supporting learning through intelligent and socially informed technology, 125* (pp. 65–72). Amsterdam, Holland: IOS Press.

Baylor, A. (2005). The impact of pedagogical agent image on affective outcomes. In *Proceedings on the Workshop on Affective Interactions: Computers in the Affective Loop, the 2005 International Conference on Intelligent User Interfaces* (San Diego, CA).

Baylor, A., Rosenberg-Kima, R., & Plant, E. (2006). Interface agents as social models: The impact of appearance on females' attitude toward engineering. In *CHI '06 Extended Abstracts on Human Factors in Computing Systems* (Montréal, Québec, Canada, 2006), (pp. 526-531). New York, NY: ACM.

Bell, L., & Gustafson, J. (2003). *Child and adult speaker adaptation during error resolution in a publicly available spoken dialogue system*. In 8th European Conference on Speech Communication and Technology-EUROSPEECH 2003 (pp. 613-616). ISCA.

Bennacef, S., Devillers, L., Rosset, S., & Lamel, L. (1996). Dialog in the RAILTEL telephone-based system. In *Proceedings of International Conference on Spoken Language Processing* (pp. 550-553). ICSLP'96, 1, Philadelphia, USA, October 1996.

Beringer, N., Kartal, U., Louka, K., Schiel, F., & Türk, U. (2002). PROMISE - a procedure for multimodal interactive system evaluation. *Proc. of LREC Workshop on Multimodal Resources and Multimodal Systems Evaluation*, (pp. 77–80).

Bernsen, N. O. (2002). *Multimodality in language and speech systems - from theory to design support tool* (pp. 93–148). Kluwer Academic Publishers.

Bernsen, N. O., Dybkjaer, L., Carlson, R., Chase, L., Dahlback, N., Failenschmid, K., et al. Paroubek, P. (1998). The DISC approach to spoken language system development and evaluation. *Proc. of the First International Conference on Language Resources and Evaluation (LREC)*, (pp. 185-189).

Berry, D. C., Butler, L. T., & de Rosis, F. (2005). Evaluating a realistic agent in an advice-giving task. *International Journal of Human-Computer Studies*, *63*, 304–327. doi:10.1016/j.ijhcs.2005.03.006

Berry, M. W. (1992). Large-scale sparse singular value computations. *The International Journal of Supercomputer Applications*, *6*(1), 13–49.

Beveridge, M., & Fox, J. (2006). Automatic generation of spoken dialogue from medical plans and ontologies. *Biomedical Informatics*, *39*(5), 482–499. doi:10.1016/j.jbi.2005.12.008

Bickmore, T. W., & Picard, R. W. (2005). Establishing and maintaining long-term human-computer relationships. [TOCHI]. *ACM Transactions on Computer-Human Interaction*, *12*(2), 293–327. doi:10.1145/1067860.1067867

Bickmore, T., & Giorgino, T. (2006). Health dialog systems for patients and consumers. *Journal of Biomedical Informatics*, *39*, 556–571. doi:10.1016/j.jbi.2005.12.004

Bickmore, T., Pfeifer, L., & Paasche-Orlow, M. (2007). Health document explanation by virtual agents. *Lecture Notes in Computer Science*, *4722*, 183–196. doi:10.1007/978-3-540-74997-4_18

Bickmore, T., & Cassell, J. (2005). Social dialogue with embodied conversational agents . In Jan van Kuppevelt, L. D., & Bernsen, N. O. (Eds.), *Advances in natural multimodal dialogue systems* (*Vol. 30*, pp. 23–54). Springer. doi:10.1007/1-4020-3933-6_2

Bickmore, T. (2003). *Relational agents: Effecting change through human-computer relationships*, Ph.D. thesis, media arts & sciences, Massachusetts Institute of Technology.

Bickmore, T. (2008). *Framing and interpersonal stance in relational agents*. Paper presented at the Seventh International Conference on Autonomous Agents and Multiagent Systems (AAMAS), Workshop on Functional Markup Language, Estoril, Portugal.

Bickmore, T., & Cassell, J. (1999). Small talk and conversational storytelling in embodied interface agents. *Proceedings of the AAAI Fall Symposium on Narrative Intelligence* (pp. 87-92). November 5-7, Cape Cod, MA.

Bickmore, T., & Cassell, J. (2000). How about this weather: Social dialog with embodied conversational agents. *Proceedings of the American Association for Artificial Intelligence (AAAI) Fall Symposium on Narrative Intelligence*, (pp. 4-8). November 3-5, Cape Cod, MA.

Bickmore, T., & Giorgino, T. (2004). *Some novel aspects of health communication from a dialogue systems perspective*. AAAI Fall Symposium on Dialogue Systems for Health Communication.

Bickmore, T., & Pfeifer, L. (2008). *Relational agents for antipsychotic medication adherence*. Paper presented at the CHI 2008 Workshop on Technology in Mental Health.

Bickmore, T., Pfeifer, L., & Jack, B. (2009). Taking the time to care: empowering low health literacy hospital patients with virtual nurse agents. In *Proceedings of the 27th International Conference on Human Factors in Computing Systems* (pp. 1265-1274). ACM.

Billera, L. J., Holmes, S. P., & Vogtmann, K. (2001). Geometry of the space of phylogenetic trees. *Advances in Applied Mathematics*, *27*(4), 733–767. doi:10.1006/aama.2001.0759

Bird, S., Klein, E., Loper, E., & Baldridge, J. (2008). Multidisciplinary instruction with the Natural Language Toolkit. *Proc. of the Third ACL Workshop on Issues in Teaching Computational Linguistics*, (pp. 62-70).

Biswas, G., Katzlberger, T., Brandford, J., Schwartz D., & TAG-V. (2001). Extending intelligent learning environments with teachable agents to enhance learning. In J. D. Moore, C. L. Redfield, & W. L. Johnson (Eds.) *Artificial intelligence in education* (pp. 389–397). Amsterdam, The Netherlands: IOS Press.

Black, W. J., Rinaldi, F., & Mowatt, D. (1998) Facile: Description of the ne system used for muc-7. In *Proceedings of Message Understanding Conference, 7.*

Blanz, V., & Vetter, T. (1999). A morphable model for the synthesis of 3D faces. In *Proceedings of the 26th Annual Conference on Computer Graphics and Interactive Techniques (SIGGRAPH)*, (pp. 187-194). New York, NY: ACM Press.

Blascovich, J. (2002). Social influences within immersive virtual environments . In Schroeder, R. (Ed.), *The social life of avatars* (pp. 127–145). London, UK: Springer-Verlag.

Blum, A. L., & Furst, M. L. (1997). Fast planning through planning graph analysis. *Artificial Intelligence*, *90*, 281–300. doi:10.1016/S0004-3702(96)00047-1

Blumer, H. (1986). *Symbolic interactionism: Perspective and method*. Berkeley, CA: University of California Press.

Bodart, F., Hennebert, A., Leheureux, J., Provot, I., Sacre, B., & Vanderdonckt, V. J. (1995). Towards a systematic building of software architecture: The trident methodological guide . In *Interactive systems: Design, specification and verification* (pp. 77–94). Springer.

Bohus, D. (2007). *Error awareness and recovery in conversational spoken language interfaces. Unpublished doctoral disseration*. Carnegie Mellon University.

Bohus, D., & Rudnicky, A. I. (2008). Sorry, I didn't catch that! An investigation of non-understanding errors and recovery strategies . In Dybkjær, L., & Minker, W. (Eds.), *Recent trends in discourse and dialogue* (*Vol. 39*, pp. 123–154). Springer Netherlands. doi:10.1007/978-1-4020-6821-8_6

Bohus, D., & Rudnicky, A. (2005). LARRI: A language-based maintenance and repair assistant. In *Spoken multimodal human-computer dialogue in mobile environments, vol. 28* (pp. 203-218). Springer Netherlands.

Bohus, D., Raux, A., Harris, T., Eskenazi, M., & Rudnicky, A. (2007). Olympus: An open-source framework for conversational spoken language interface research. *Proc. of HLT-NAACL.*

Boisen, S., Ramshaw, L., Ayuso, D., & Bates, M. (1989). A proposal for SLS evaluation. *Proc. of the Workshop on Speech and Natural Language*, ACL Human Language Technology Conference, (pp. 135-146).

Borodin, Y., Mahmud, J., Ramakrishnan, I. V., & Stent, A. (2007). *The HearSay non-visual Web browser.* Paper presented at the W4A 2007.

Bos, J., Klein, E., & Oka, T. (2003). Meaningful conversation with a mobile robot, *Proc. of EACL*, (pp. 71-74).

Bos, J., Klein, E., Lemon, O., & Oka, T. (2003). DIPPER: Description and formalisation of an information-state update dialogue system architecture. *Proceedings of SIGDial'03.*

Bosseler, A., & Massaro, D. (2003). Development and evaluation of a computer-animated tutor for vocabulary and language learning in children with autism. *Journal of Autism and Developmental Disorders*, *33*(6), 653–672. doi:10.1023/B:JADD.0000006002.82367.4f

Bradley, M. (2000). Emotion and motivation . In Cacioppo, J. T., Tassinary, L. G., & Berntson, G. (Eds.), *Handbook of psychophysiology*. New York, NY: Cambridge University Press.

Branham, S., & De Angeli, A. (2008). Special issue on the abuse and misuse of social agents. *Interacting with Computers*, *20*(3), 287–291. doi:10.1016/j.intcom.2008.02.001

Bratman, M. E., Israel, D., & Pollack, M. (1991). Plans and resource-bounded practical reasoning . In Cummins, R., & Pollock, J. L. (Eds.), *Philosophy and AI: Essays at the interface* (pp. 1–22). Cambridge, MA: The MIT Press.

Breazeal, C., Kidd, C., Thomaz, A., Hoffman, G., & Berlin, M. (2005). Effects of nonverbal communication on efficiency and robustness in human-robot teamwork. In *Proceedings of IEEE/RSJ International Conference on Intelligent Robots and Systems (IROS)* (pp. 708-713).

Bresnan, J. (Ed.). (1982). *The mental representation of grammatical relations. MIT Press Series on Cognitive Theory and Mental Representation*. Cambridge, MA: MIT Press.

Brown, D. J., Standen, P. J., Proctor, T., & Sterland, D. (2001). Advanced design methodologies for the production of virtual learning environments for use by people with learning disabilities. *Presence (Cambridge, Mass.)*, *10*(4), 401–415. doi:10.1162/1054746011470253

Brown, A. (1992). Design experiments: Theoretical and methodological challenges in creating complex interventions in classroom settings. *Journal of the Learning Sciences*, *2*(2), 141–178. doi:10.1207/s15327809jls0202_2

Buck, R. (1984). *The communication of emotion*. New York, NY: Guilford Press.

Buck, R. (1994). The neuropsychology of communication: Spontaneous and symbolic aspects. *Journal of Pragmatics*, *22*, 265–278. doi:10.1016/0378-2166(94)90112-0

Buck, R. (1989). Emotional communication in personal relationships: A developmental-interactionist view . In Hendrick, C. D. (Ed.), *Close relationships* (pp. 44–76). Beverly Hills, CA: Sage.

Bui, T. H. (2006). *Multimodal dialogue management - state of the art*. (Technical Report, TR-CTIT-06-01), Enschede, Centre for Telematics and Information Technology: University of Twente.

Buisine, S., Abrilian, S., & Martin, J. (2004). Evaluation of multimodal behaviour of embodied agents . In Ruttkay, Z., & Pelachaud, C. (Eds.), *From brows to trust: Evaluating embodied conversational agents* (pp. 217–238). Springer.

Burnham, D., et al. (2006-2011). *From talking heads to thinking heads: A research platform for human communication science*. Retrieved from http://thinkinghead.uws.edu.au

Butz, C. J., Hua, S., & Maguire, R. B. (2006). A Web-based Bayesian intelligent tutoring system for computer programming. *Web Intelligent and Agent Systems*, *4*(1), 77–97.

Byram, M. (1997). *Teaching and assessing intercutural communicative competence*. Clevedon, UK: Multilingual Matters.

Cahn, J. E., & Brennan, S. E. (1999). A psychological model of grounding and repair in dialog. In S. E. Brennan, A. Giboin, & D. Traum (Ed.), *Working Papers of the AAAI Fall Symposium on Psychological Models of Communication in Collaborative Systems* (pp. 25–33). Menlo Park, CA: AAAI.

Caldwell, B., Cooper, M., Reid, L. G., & Vanderheiden, G. (2007). *Web content accessibility guidelines* 2.0. Retrieved May 30, 2010, from http://www.w3.org/TR/2007/WD-WCAG20-20071211/

Carbonell, J. R. (1970). AI in CAI: Artificial intelligence approach to computer assisted instruction. *IEEE Transactions on Man-Machine Systems*, *11*(4), 190–202. doi:10.1109/TMMS.1970.299942

Carpenter, R. (1992). *The logic of typed features structures*. Cambridge University Press. doi:10.1017/CBO9780511530098

Cassell, J. (2001). Embodied conversational agents: Representation and intelligence in user interfaces. *AI Magazine*, *22*(3), 67–83.

Cassell, J., & Tartaro, A. (2007). Intersubjectivity in humanagent interaction. *Interaction Studies: Social Behaviour and Communication in Biological and Artificial Systems*, *8*(3), 391–410.

Cassell, J., & Bickmore, T. (2002). Negotiated collusion: Modeling social language and its relationship effects in intelligent agents. (in press) *User Modeling and Adaptive Interfaces*.

Cassell, J., Bickmore, T., Billinghurst, M., Campbell, L., Chang, K., Vilhjalmsson, H., & Yan, H. (1999). Embodiment in conversational interfaces: Rea. In *Proceedings of the SIGCHI conference on Human factors in computing systems: the CHI is the limit* (pp. 520-527). ACM Press.

Cassell, J., Bickmore, T., Campbell, L., Vilhjálmsson, H., & Yan, H. (2000b). Human conversation as a system framework: Designing embodied conversational agents. In S. P. Justine Cassell, Joseph Sullivan & E. F. Churchill (Eds.), *Embodied conversational agents* (pp. 29-63). MIT Press.

Cassell, J., Nakano, Y., Bickmore, T., Sidner, C., & Rich, C. (2001a). Non-verbal cues for discourse structure. In *Proceedings of the 39th Annual Meeting on Association for Computational Linguistics* (pp. 114-123). Morgan Kaufmann Publishers.

Cassell, J., Stocky, T., Bickmore, T., Gao, Y., Nakano, Y., Ryokai, K., et al. Vilhjálmsson, H. (2002, January). *MACK: Media lab Autonomous Conversational Kiosk*. In IMAGINA'02, vol. 2 (pp. 12-15). Monte Carlo, Monaco.

Cassell, J., Vilhjálmsson, H., & Bickmore, T. (2001b). BEAT: The behavior expression animation toolkit. In *Proceedings of the 28th annual conference on Computer graphics and interactive techniques* (pp. 477-486). Association for Computational Linguistics.

*CASUS Project*. (2010). Retrieved July 23, 2010, from http://www.casus.eu/

Catizone, R., Worgan, S., Wilks, Y., Dingli, A., & Cheng, W. (2010). A world-hybrid approach to a conversational companion for reminiscing about images . In Wilks, Y. (Ed.), *Artificial companions in society: Scientific, economic, psychological and philosophical perspectives*. Amsterdam, The Netherlands: John Benjamins.

Catizone, R., Setzer, A., & Wilkes, Y. (2003). *Multimodal dialogue management in the COMIC project*. Paper presented at the Proceedings of EACL 2003 Workshop on Dialogue Systems: Interaction, adaptation, and styles of management.

Catizone, R., Setzer, A., & Webb, N. (2002). Scaling-up information extraction. In *Proceedings of the Workshop on Event Modelling for Multilingual Document Linking, Language Resources and Evaluation Conference (LREC 2002)*, Las Palmas, Canary Islands.

Catrambone, R., Stasko, J., & Xiao, J. (2002). Anthropomorphic agents as a user interface paradigm: Experimental findings and a framework for research. In W. D. Gray & C. Schunn (Eds.), *Proceedings of the 24th Annual Conference of the Cognitive Science Society* (pp. 166-171). Cognitive Science Society.

Cavazza, M., Smith, C., Charlton, D., Zhang, L., Turunen, M., & Hakulinen, J. (2008). A companion ECA with planning and activity modelling. *Proc. of AAMAS*.

Chant, S., Jenkinson, T., Randle, J., Russell, G., & Webb, C. (2002). Communication skills training in healthcare: A review of the literature. *Nurse Education Today, 22*, 189–202. doi:10.1054/nedt.2001.0690

Charniak, E. (1993). *Statistical language learning*. The MIT Press.

Chase, C. C., Chin, D. B., Oppezzo, M. A., & Schwartz, D. L. (2009). Teachable agents and the protégé effect: Increasing the effort towards learning. *Journal of Science Education and Technology, 18*(4), 334–352. doi:10.1007/s10956-009-9180-4

Cheepen, C., & Monaghan, J. (1997). Designing naturalness in automated dialogues - some problems and solutions. In *Proceedings First International Workshop on Human- Computer Conversation*, Bellagio, Italy.

Chou, C. Y., Chan, T. W., & Lin, C. J. (2003). Redefining the learning companion: The past, present, and future of educational agents. *Computers & Education, 40*, 255–269. doi:10.1016/S0360-1315(02)00130-6

Chu-Carroll, J., & Carpenter, B. (1999). Vector-based natural language call routing. *Computational Linguistics, 25*(3), 361–388.

Churcher, G. E., Atwell, E. S., & Souter, C. (1997). *Dialogue mnagement systems: A survey and overview*.

Chwelos, G., & Oatley, K. (1994). Appraisal, computational models, and Scherer's expert system. *Cognition and Emotion, 8*, 245–257. doi:10.1080/02699939408408940

Ciravegna, F., Chapman, S., Dingli, A., & Wilks, Y. (2004). Learning to harvest the Semantic Web. In *Proc. European Semantic Web Symposium (ESWS04)*.

Clarizio, G., Mazzotta, I., Novielli, N., & de Rosis, F. (2006). Social attitude towards a conversational character. In *Proceedings of the 15th IEEE International Symposium on Robot and Human Interactive Communication*, (pp. 2–7), Hatfield, UK.

Clark, R., Richmond, K., & King, S. (2004). Festival 2 - build your own general purpose unit selection speech synthesizer. *Proc. of 5th ISCA Workshop on Speech Synthesis*, (pp. 173–178).

Cohen, M., Giancola, J. P., & Balogh, J. (2004). *Voice user interface design*. Addison-Wesley.

Cohen, P. R., & Perrault, C. R. (1979). Elements of a plan-based theory of speech acts. *Cognitive Science*, *3*(3), 177–212. doi:10.1207/s15516709cog0303_1

Cohen, P. R., & Levesque, H. J. (1990). Rational interaction as the basis for communication . In Cohen, P. R., Morgan, J., & Pollack, M. E. (Eds.), *Intentions in communication* (pp. 221–256). MIT Press.

Cohen, P. (1996). Dialogue modeling . In Cole, R. (Ed.), *Survey of the state of the art in human language technology* (pp. 192–197). Cambridge, UK: Cambridge University Press.

Cohen, P. R., & Levesque, H. J. (1995). Communicative actions for artificial agents. In *Proceedings of the First International Conference on Multi-Agent Systems* (pp. 65–72). AAAI Press.

Coin, E. (2007, February 21, 2007). *Today and the future of wearable agents.* Paper presented at the SpeechTEK West, San Francisco.

Coin, E. (2010, April 22-23). *Table talking.* Paper presented at the Mobile Voice Conference, San Francisco.

Coin, E., & Qua, J. (2000, July 3-5, 2000). *A fundamental architecture to integrate conversation management engines with conversation development and evaluation tools.* Paper presented at the Third Workshop on Human-Computer Conversation, Bellagio, Italy.

Colby, K. M. (1971). Artificial paranoia. *Artificial Intelligence*, *2*(1), 1–2. doi:10.1016/0004-3702(71)90002-6

Cole, R., Mariani, J., Uszkoreit, H., Varile, G. B., Zaenen, A., Zampolli, A., & Zue, V. (Eds.). (1997). *Survey of the state of the art in human language technology*. Cambridge University Press.

Cole, R. (Ed.). (1997). *Survey of the state of the art in human language technology.* New York, NY: Cambridge University Press.

Cole, R., Van Vuuren, S., Pellom, B., Hacioglu, K., Ma, J., Movellan, J., et al. Wade-stein, D. (2003). Perceptive animated interfaces: First steps toward a new paradigm for human-computer interaction. *Proc. of the IEEE Special Issue on Multimodal Human Computer Interface*, (pp. 1391-1405).

Collins, A. (1992). Towards a design science of education . In Scanlon, E., & O'Shea, T. (Eds.), *New directions in educational technology* (pp. 15–22). Berlin, Germany: Springer.

*Companions Project*. (2010). Retrieved April 26, 2010, from http://www.companions-project.org

Constantinides, P., Hansma, S., Tchou, C., & Rudnicky, A. (1998). A schema-based approach to dialog control. In *Proceedings of the International Conference on Spoken Language Processing* (pp. 409-412). Sydney, Australia.

Core, M. G., & Allen, J. F. (1997). Coding dialogs with the DAMSL annotation scheme. In *Working Notes of AAAI Fall Symposium on Communicative Action in Humans and Machines*, Boston, MA.

Core, M. G., Moore, J. D., & Zinn, C. (2003). The role of initiative in tutorial dialogue. In *Proceedings of the ITS Workshop on Empirical Methods for Tutorial Dialogue Systems*, (pp. 67–74).

Core, M., & Allen, J. (1997). Coding dialogs with the DAMSL annotation scheme. In *Working Notes of the AAAI Fall Symposium on Communicative Action in Humans and Machines* (pp. 28-35). Cambridge, MA.

Core, M., & Allen, J. (1997). *Coding dialogs with the DAMSL annotation scheme*. AAAI Fall Symposium on Communicative Action in Humans and Machines, (pp. 28-35).

Corradini, A., & Samuelsson, C. (2008). A generic spoken dialogue manager applied to an interactive 2D game. In E. André, L. Dybkjær, W. Minker, H. Neumann, R. Pieraccini, & M. Weber (Eds.) PIT 2008. *LNCS (LNAI)*, vol. 5078, (pp. 3–13).

Covington, M. A. (1984). *Syntactic theory in the High Middle Ages*. Cambridge, UK: Cambridge University Press. doi:10.1017/CBO9780511735592

Cowie, R., Douglas-Cowie, E., Tsapatsoulis, N., Votsis, G., Kollias, S., Fellenz, W., & Taylor, J. G. (2001). Emotion recognition in human-computer interaction. *Signal Processing Magazine, IEEE*, *18*(1), 32–80. doi:10.1109/79.911197

Cox, D. E., & Harrison, D. W. (2008). Models of anger: Contributions from psychophysiology, neuropsychology and the cognitive behavioral perspective. *Brain Structure & Function*, *212*, 371–385. doi:10.1007/s00429-007-0168-7

Crawford, C. (1999). Assumptions underlying the Erasmatron interactive storytelling engine. In M. Mateas & P. Sengers (Eds.), *Proceedings of the AAAI Fall Symposium: Narrative Intelligence* (pp. 112–114). Menlo Park, CA.

Cuayáhuitl, H., Renals, S., Lemon, O., & Shimodaira, H. (2005). Human-computer dialogue simulation using Hidden Markov models. *Proc. of IEEE Workshop on Automatic Speech Recognition and Understanding (ASRU)*, (pp. 290-295).

Cunningham, H., Humphreys, K., Gaizauskas, R., & Wilks, Y. (1997). GATE-a TIPSTER based general architecture for text engineering. In *Proceedings of the TIPSTER Text Program (Phase III) 6 Month Workshop*. DARPA, Morgan Kaufmann, CA.

Dahl, D. (Ed.). (2004). *Practical spoken dialogue systems*. Kluwer Academic Publishers. doi:10.1007/978-1-4020-2676-8

Darwin, C. (1872). *The origin of species by means of natural selection, or the preservation of favoured races in the struggle for life*. London, UK: John Murray.

Dausend, M., & Ehrlich, U. (2008). A prototype for future spoken dialog systems using an embodied conversational agent . In *Perception in multimodal dialogue systems* (*Vol. 5078*, pp. 268–271). Springer. doi:10.1007/978-3-540-69369-7_30

Dautenhahn, K. (1999). Socially situated life-like agents: If it makes you happy then it can't be that bad?! In *Proceedings VWSIM'99, Virtual Worlds and Simulation Conference*. Retrieved from http://homepages.feis.herts.ac.uk/~comqkd/papers.html

Davis, M., Robins, B., Dautenhahn, K., Nehaniv, C., & Powell, S. (2005). A comparison of interactive and robotic systems in therapy and education for children with autism . In Pruski, A., & Knops, H. (Eds.), *Assistive technology: From virtuality to reality*. IOS Press.

De Angeli, A., & Brahnam, S. (2008). I hate you! Disinhibition with virtual partners. *Interacting with Computers*, *20*(3), 302–310. doi:10.1016/j.intcom.2008.02.004

De Boni, M., & Manandhar, S. (2005). Implementing clarification dialogue in open-domain question answering. *Natural Language Engineering*, 11.

De Carolis, B., Carofiglio, V., & Bilvi, M. M., & Pelachaud, C. (2002). APML, a mark-up language for believable behavior generation. *Proc. of AAMAS*.

De Carolis, B., Mazzotta, I., & Novielli, N. (2010). Enhancing conversational access to information through a social intelligent agent. In G. Armano, M. de Gemmis, G. Semeraro and E. Vargiu (Eds): *Intelligent Information Access, Studies in Computational Intelligence*, 2010, Volume 301/2010 (pp. pages 1-20), Springer Berlin / Heidelberg.

De Carolis, B., Pelachaud, C., Poggi, I., & de Rosis, F. (2001). Behavior planning for a reflexive agent. In *IJCAI'01: Proceedings of the 17th international Joint Conference on Artificial intelligence*, San Francisco, CA, USA, (pp. 1059–1064). Morgan Kaufmann Publishers Inc.

De Melo, C., & Gratch, J. (2009). *Expression of emotions using wrinkles, blushing, sweating and tears*. Intelligent Virtual Agents Conference, Amsterdam, Sep 14-16. *eVIP Project*. (2010). Retrieved July 23, 2010, from http://www.virtualpatients.eu/

de Rosis, F., Pelachaud, C., Poggi, I., Carofiglio, V., & Carolis, B. (2003). From Greta's mind to her face: Modelling the dynamics of affective states in a conversational embodied agent. *International Journal of Human-Computer Studies*, *59*(1-2), 81–118. doi:10.1016/S1071-5819(03)00020-X

de Rosis, F., Novielli, N., Carofiglio, V., Cavalluzzi, A., & De Carolis, B. (2006). User modeling and adaptation in health promotion dialogs with an animated character. *Journal of Biomedical Informatics*, *39*, 514–531. doi:10.1016/j.jbi.2006.01.001

de Rosis, F., Batliner, A., Novielli, N., & Steidl, S. (2007). You are sooo cool, Valentina! Recognizing social attitude in speech-based dialogues with an ECA . In Paiva, A., Prada, R., & Picard, R. W. (Eds.), *Affective computing and intelligent interaction. Lecture Notes in Computer Science* (*Vol. 4738*, pp. 179–190). Berlin/Heidelberg, Germany: Springer-Verlag. doi:10.1007/978-3-540-74889-2_17

de Rosis, F., Carolis, B. D., Carofiglio, V., & Pizzutilo, S. (2004). Shallow and inner forms of emotional intelligence in advisory dialog simulation . In Prendinger, H., & Ishizuka, M. (Eds.), *Life-like characters: Tools, affective functions, and applications (Cognitive Technologies)* (pp. 271–294). Springer Verlag.

Degerstedt, L., & Jönsson, A. (2006). LinTest, a development tool for testing dialogue systems. *Proc. of the 9th International Conference on Spoken Language Processing (Interspeech/ICSLP)*, (pp. 489-492).

Dehn, D., & van Mulken, S. (2000). The impact of animated interface agents: A review of empirical research. *International Journal of Human-Computer Studies*, *52*(1), 1–22. doi:10.1006/ijhc.1999.0325

Deladisma, A. M., Johnsen, K., Raij, A., Rossen, B., Kotranza, A., & Kalapurakal, M. (2008). Medical student satisfaction using a virtual patient system to learn history-taking communication skills. *Studies in Health Technology and Informatics*, *132*, 101–105.

Den, E., Boves, L., Lamel, L., & Baggia, P. (1999). *Overview of the ARISE project* (pp. 1527–1530). Proc. of Eurospeech.

Doherty, P., Granlund, G., Kuchcinski, K., Sandewall, E., Nordberg, K., Skarman, E., & Wiklund, J. (1998). The WITAS unmanned aerial vehicle project. *Proc. of the 14th European Conference on Artificial Intelligence (ECAI)*, (pp. 747-755).

Dohsaka, K., Asai, R., Higashinaka, R., Minami, Y., & Maeda, E. (2009). Effects of conversational agents on human communication in thought-evoking multi-party dialogues. In *SIGDIAL '09: Proceedings of the SIGDIAL 2009 Conference,* Morristown, NJ, USA (pp. 217–224). Association for Computational Linguistics.

Dowling, C. (2000). Intelligent agents: Some ethical issues and dilemmas. In . *Proceedings of, AICE2000*, 28–32.

Doyle, P. (2002). Believability through context using knowledge in the world to create intelligent characters. In *Proceedings of the First International Joint Conference on Autonomous Agents and Multiagent Systems* (pp. 342-349). New York, NY.

Dreyfus, H. L. (1972). *What computers can't do*. Cambridge, MA: MIT Press.

Drozdzynski, W., Krieger, H.-U., Piskorski, J., Schäfer, U., & Xu, F. (2004). Shallow processing with unification and typed feature structures – foundations and applications. In *German AI Journal KI-Zeitschrift, 1*(4). Bremen, Germany: Böttcher Verlag/ Gesellschaft für Informatik e.V.

Dybkjaer, L., & Bernsen, N. (2000). Usability issues in spoken language dialogue systems. *Natural Language Engineering*, *6*, 243–271. doi:10.1017/S1351324900002461

Dybkjaer, L., Bernsen, N., & Minker, W. (2004). Evaluation and usability of multimodal spoken language dialogue systems. *Speech Communication*, *43*, 33–54. doi:10.1016/j.specom.2004.02.001

Eckert, M. (2006). *Speaker identification and verification applications. (Internal Working Draft)*. VoiceXML Forum Speaker Biometrics Committee.

Eckhardt, C. I., Norlander, B., & Deffenbacher, J. (2004). The assessment of anger and hostility: A critical review. *Aggression and Violent Behavior*, *9*, 17–43. doi:10.1016/S1359-1789(02)00116-7

Edelman, G. M. (2006). *Second nature: Brain science and human knowledge*. Yale University Press.

Edelson, D. C. (2002). Design research: What we learn when we engage in design. *Journal of the Learning Sciences*, *11*(1), 105–121. doi:10.1207/S15327809JLS1101_4

Edlund, J., & Beskow, J. (2007). Pushy versus meek using avatars to influence turn-taking behaviour. In *Proceedings of Interspeech 2007 ICSLP.* Atwerp.

Edlund, J., & Nordstrand, M. (2002). Turn-taking gestures and hourglasses in a multi-modal dialogue system. In *Proceedings of ISCA Workshop Multi-Modal Dialogue in Mobile Environments*. ISCA.

Ekman, P., & Friesen, W. (1978). *Facial action coding system*. Consulting Psychologist Press.

Eliasson, K. (2007). Case-based techniques used for dialogue understanding and planning in a human-robot dialogue system. *Proc. of IJCAI*, (pp. 1600-1605).

Ellis, R. (2003). *Task-based language learning and teaching*. USA: Oxford University Press.

Emele, M. C. (1994). The typed feature structure representation formalism. *Proc. of the International Workshop on Sharable Natural Language Resources*.

Engwall, O. (2008). Can audio-visual instructions help learners improve their articulation? An ultrasound study of short term changes. In [ISCA.]. *Proceedings of Interspeech*, *2008*, 2631–2634.

Erman, L. D., Hayes-Roth, F., Lesser, V. R., & Reddy, D. R. (1980). The HEARSAY-II speech understanding system: Integrating knowledge to resolve uncertainty. *Computing Surveys*, *12*, 213–253. doi:10.1145/356810.356816

Euzenat, J., & Shvaiko, P. (2007). *Ontology matching*. Berlin, Germany: Springer Verlag.

Fabbrizio, G., & Lewis, C. (2004). Florence: A dialogue manager framework for spoken dialogue systems. *Proc. of International Conference on Spoken Language Processing (ICSLP)*, (pp. 3065-3068).

Fagerberg, P., Stahl, A., & Höök, K. (2003). Designing gestures for affective input: an analysis of shape, effort and valence . In Ollila, M., & Rantzer, M. (Eds.), *Proceedings of mobile ubiquitous and multimedia, MUM 2003*. Linköping University Electronic Press.

Fahad, M. (2008). ER2OWL: Generating OWL ontology from ER diagram. [Springer.]. *Intelligent Information Processing*, *288*(4), 28–37.

Fairclough, S. H. (2009). Fundamentals of physiological computing. *Interacting with Computers*, *21*, 133–145. doi:10.1016/j.intcom.2008.10.011

Farzanfar, R., Frishkopf, S., Migneault, J., & Friedman, R. (2005). Telephone-linked care for physical activity: A qualitative evaluation of the use patterns of an information technology program for patients. *Journal of Biomedical Informatics*, *38*, 220–228. doi:10.1016/j.jbi.2004.11.011

Faure, C., & Julia, L. (1993). Interaction hommemachine par la parole et le geste pour l'édition de documents. *Proc. International Conference on Real and Virtual Worlds*, (pp. 171-180).

Feigenbaum, E. (n.d.). *Personal communication.*

Fellbaum, K., & Kouroupetroglou, G. (2008). Principles of electronic speech processing with applications for people with disabilities. *Technology and Disability*, *20*(2), 55–85.

Fellous, J. M., Armony, J. L., & LeDoux, J. E. (2003). Emotional circuits and computational neuroscience . In *The handbook of brain theory and neural networks* (pp. 398–401). Cambridge, MA: The MIT Press.

Ferguson, G., & Allen, J. (1998, July). *TRIPS: An intelligent integrated problem-solving assistant.* Paper presented at the Fifteenth National Conference on Artificial Intelligence (AAAI-98), Madison, WI.

Festinger, L. (1957). *A theory of cognitive dissonance*. Standford University Press.

Field, D., & Ramsay, A. (2006). How to change a person's mind: Understanding the difference between the effects and consequences of speech acts. *Proceedings 5th Workshop on Inference in Computational Semantics (ICoS-5)*, (pp. 27-36).

Fink, R. B., Schwarz, M., & Dahl, D. A. (2009). *Using speech recognition for speech therapy: MossTalkWords 2.0.* Paper presented at the American Speech-Language-Hearing Association, New Orleans, LA, USA.

Fischer, M., Maier, E., & Stein, A. (1994). Generating cooperative system responses in information retrieval dialogues. In *Proceedings of 7th International Workshop on Natural Language Generation (IWNLG 7)*, Kennebunkport, Maine.

Flycht-Eriksson, A. (2003). Representing knowledge of dialogue, domain, task and user in dialogue systems - how and why? *Electronic Transactions on Artificial Intelligence*, *3*(2), 5–32.

Fogg, B. J. (2003). *Persuasive technology: Using computers to change what we think and do*. Morgan Kaufman Publishers.

Foley, J., Gibbs, C., & Kovacevic, S. (1988). A knOWLedge based user interface management system. In CHI '88: *Proceedings of the SIGCHI conference on Human factors in computing systems*, (pp. 67–72). New York, NY: ACM.

Forbes-Riley, K., & Litman, D. (2011). Designing and evaluating a wizarded uncertainty-adaptive spoken dialogue tutoring system. *Computer Speech & Language*, *25*(1), 105–126. doi:10.1016/j.csl.2009.12.002

Ford, G. S., & Ford, S. G. (2009). Internet use and depression among the elderly. *Phoenix Center Policy Papers, 38*. Retrieved from www.phoenix-center.org

Foster, M. (2007). Enhancing human-computer interaction with embodied conversational agents. *Universal Access in Human-Computer Interaction. Ambient Interaction*, *4555*, 828–837.

Fraikin, F., & Leonhardt, T. (2002). *From requirements to analysis with capture and replay tools. PI-R 1/02*. Software Engineering Group, Department of Computer Science, Darmstadt University of Technology.

Francis, W. N., & Kučera, H. (1982). *Frequency analysis of English usage: Lexicon and grammar*. Boston, MA: Houghton Mifflin.

Fraser, N., & Gilbert, G. (1991). Simulating speech systems. *Computer Speech & Language*, *5*, 81–99. doi:10.1016/0885-2308(91)90019-M

Freedman, R. (2000). *Plan-based dialogue management in a physics tutor* (pp. 52–59). ANLP.

Freitas, D., & Kouroupetroglou, G. (2008). Speech technologies for blind and low vision persons. *Technology and Disability*, *20*(2), 135–156.

Galibert, O., Illouz, G., & Rousset, S. (2005). Ritel: An open-domain, human-computer dialogue system. *Proceedings of INTERSPEECH'05*.

Galitz, W. O. (2007). *The essential guide to user interface design*. Wiley Publishing, Inc.

GameBryo. (2010). *Emergent game technologies*. Retrieved July 23, 2010, from http://www.emergent.net/

Garfield, S., & Wermter, S. (2002). *Recurrent neural learning for helpdesk call routing. Lecture Notes in Computer Science 2415/2002, Artificial Neural Networks*. Berlin/Heidelberg, Germany: Springer.

Garfield, S., & Wermter, S. (2006). Call classification using recurrent neural networks, support vector machines and finite state automata. [Springer-Verlag.]. *Knowledge and Information Systems*, 9.

Garfinkel, H. (1967). *Studies in ethnomethodology*. Englewood Cliffs, NJ: Prentice-Hall.

Garzotto, F., & Rizzo, F. (2005). The MUST tool: Exploiting Propp's theory. In P. Kommers & G. Richards (Eds.), *Proceedings of World Conference on Educational Multimedia, Hypermedia and Telecommunications 2005* (pp. 3887-3893). Chesapeake, VA, USA.

Gebhard, P. (2007). *Emotionalisierung interaktiver virtueller Charaktere - ein mehrschichtiges Computermodell zur Erzeugung und Simulation von Gefühlen in Echtzeit*. PhD Thesis, University of the Saarland, Saarbrücken, Germany.

Gebhard, P., Kipp, M., Klesen, M., & Rist, T. (2003). Authoring scenes for adaptive, interactive performances. In *AAMAS '03: Proceedings of the 2nd International Joint Conference on Autonomous Agents and Multiagent Systems* (pp. 725–732). New York, NY.

Gertner, A., & VanLehn, K. (2000). Andes: A coached problem solving environment for physics. [Springer.]. *Lecture Notes in Computer Science*, *1839*, 133–142. doi:10.1007/3-540-45108-0_17

Gholamsaghaee, E. (2006). *Adapting JSHOP to a dialog framework with an ontological domain description*. Bachelor's Thesis, University of the Saarland, Saarbrücken, Germany.

Gilbert, M. A., Grasso, F., Groarke, L., Gurr, C., & Gerlofs, J. M. (2003). The persuasion machine . In Norman, T. J., & Reed, C. (Eds.), *Argumentation machines: New frontiers in argument and computation*.

Giles, J. (2005). Internet encyclopaedias go head to head. *Nature*, *438*, 900–901. doi:10.1038/438900a

Ginzburg, J. (1996). *Interrogatives: Questions, facts and dialogue*. Oxford, UK: Blackwell.

Glass, J., Flammia, G., Goodine, D., Phillips, M., Polifroni, J., & Sakai, S. (1995). Multilingual spoken-language understanding in the MIT Voyager system. *Speech Communication*, *17*(1-2), 1–18. doi:10.1016/0167-6393(95)00008-C

Gliozzo, A., & Strapparava, C. (2005). Domains kernels for text categorization. In *Proceedings of the Ninth Conference on Computational Natural Language Learning (CoNLL-2005)* (pp. 56–63), University of Michigan, Ann Arbor.

Göbel, S., Becker, F., & Feix, A. (2005). INSCAPE: Storymodels for interactive storytelling and edutainment applications . In Subsol, G. (Ed.), *Virtual storytelling: Using virtual reality technologies for storytelling* (pp. 168–171). Berlin, Germany: Springer. doi:10.1007/11590361_19

Goddeau, D., Brill, E., Glass, J., Pao, C., Philips, M., & Polifroni, J. … Zue, V. (1994). GALAXY: A human-language interface to on-line travel information. In *Proceedings of International Conference on Spoken Language Processing*, ICSLP'94, Yokohama, Japan, September 1994 (pp. 707-710).

Goddeau, D., Meng, H., Polifroni, J., Seneff, S., & Busayapongchai, S. (1996). A form-based dialogue manager for spoken language applications. *Proc. of International Conference on Spoken Language Processing (ICSLP)*, (pp. 701-704).

Godfrey, J., Holliman, E., & McDaniel, J. (1992). SWITCHBOARD: Telephone speech corpus for research and development. In *Proceedings of the IEEE International Conference on Acoustics, Speech and Signal Processing (ICASSP),* San Francisco, CA, (pp. 517–520). IEEE.

Goffman, E. (1990). *The presentation of self in everyday life*. New York, NY: Doubleday.

Goh, G. M., & Quek, C. (2007). EpiList: An intelligent tutoring system shell for implicit development of generic cognitive skills that support bottom-up KnOWLedge construction. *IEEE Transactions on Systems, Man, and Cybernetics*, *37*(1), 58–71. doi:10.1109/TSMCA.2006.886340

Goldberg, J., Ostendorf, M., & Kirchhoff, K. (2003). *The impact of response wording in error correction subdialogs*. In ISCA Tutorial and Research Workshop on Error Handling in Spoken Dialogue Systems (pp. 101-106). ISCA.

González, C., Burguillo, J. C., & Llamas, M. (2007). *Integrating intelligent tutoring systems and health Information Systems*. In 18th International Workshop on Database and Expert Systems Applications, (pp. 633–637), IEEE CS.

Gorin, A. L., Riccardi, G., & Wright, J. H. (1999). *How may I help you? Computational models of speech pattern processing*. Springer.

Gorin, L., Riccardi, G., & Wright, J. H. (1997). How may I help you? *Speech Communication*, *23*, 113–127. doi:10.1016/S0167-6393(97)00040-X

Gould, J. D., & Lewis, C. (1985). Designing for usability: Key principles and what designers think. *Communications of the ACM*, *28*(3), 300–311. doi:10.1145/3166.3170

Graesser, A., Chipman, P., Haynes, B., & Olney, A. (2005). AutoTutor: An intelligent tutoring system with mixed-initiative dialogue. *IEEE Transactions on Education*, *48*, 612–618. doi:10.1109/TE.2005.856149

Graesser, A., Wiemer-Hastings, K., Wiemer-Hastings, P., & Kreuz, R.Tutoring Research Group. (1999). AutoTutor: A simulation of a human tutor. *Journal of Cognitive Systems Research*, *1*, 35–51. doi:10.1016/S1389-0417(99)00005-4

Graesser, A. C., VanLehn, K., Rose, C., Jordan, P., & Harter, D. (2001). Intelligent tutoring systems with conversational dialogue. *AI Magazine*, *22*, 39–51.

Graesser, A. C., Chipman, P., Haynes, B. C., & Olney, A. (2005). AutoTutor: An intelligent tutoring system with mixed-initiative dialogue. *IEEE Transactions on Education*, *48*, 612–618. doi:10.1109/TE.2005.856149

Gratch, J., Wang, N., Okhmatovskaia, A., Lamothe, F., Morales, M., van der Werf, R., & Morency, L. (2007). Can virtual humans be more engaging than real ones? *Lecture Notes in Computer Science*, *4552*, 286. doi:10.1007/978-3-540-73110-8_30

Gratch, J., & Marsella, S. (2004). A domain independent framework for modeling emotion. *Journal of Cognitive Systems Research*, *5*, 269–306. doi:10.1016/j.cogsys.2004.02.002

Gratch, J., Rickel, J., André, E., Badler, N., Cassell, J., & Petajan, E. (2002). Creating interactive virtual humans: Some assembly required. *IEEE Intelligent Systems*, (July/August): 54–63. doi:10.1109/MIS.2002.1024753

Gratch, J., & Marsella, S. (2001). Tears and Fears: Modeling Emotions and Emotional Behaviors in Synthetic Agents, *Fifth International Conference on Autonomous Agents*, Montreal, Canada.

Gratch, J., Okhmatovskaia, A., Lamothe, F., Marsella, S., Morales, M., van der Werf, R. J., & Morency, L. P. (2006). Virtual rapport. In *Proceedings of the 6th International Conference on Intelligent Virtual Agents* (pp. 14-27).

Gray, C. (2001). How to respond to a bullying attempt: What to think, say and do. *The Morning News, 13*(2).

Green, N., Lawton, W., & Davis, B. (2004). An assistive conversation skills training system for caregivers of persons with Alzheimer's Disease. In *Proceedings of the AAAI 2004 Fall Symposium on Dialogue Systems for Health Communication*.

Greene, M. (2010). *User reactions to senior-friendly interfaces*. Paper presented at the SpeechTEK.

Grice, H. P. (1975). Logic and conversation. In P. Cole & J. Morgan (Eds.), *Syntax and semantics, volume 3: Speech acts* (pp. 41-58). New York, NY: Academic Press.

Griol, D., Hurtado, L. F., Segarra, E., & Sanchis, E. (2008). A statistical approach to spoken dialogue systems design and evaluation. *Speech Communication*, *50*(8-9), 666–682. doi:10.1016/j.specom.2008.04.001

Griol, D., Callejas, Z., & López-Cózar, R. (2009). A comparison between dialogue corpora acquired with real and simulated users. *Proc. of the 10th Annual Meeting of the Special interest Group on Discourse and Dialogue (SIGDIAL 2009)*, (pp. 326-332).

Griol, D., Torres, F., Hurtado, L., Grau, S., García, F., Sanchis, E., & Segarra, E. (2006). A dialogue system for the DIHANA project. *Proc. of SPECOM*, (pp. 131-136).

Grosz, B. J., & Sidner, C. L. (1986). Attention, intentions, and the structure of discourse. *Computational Linguistics*, *12*(3), 175–204.

Grun, U. (1998). *Visualization of gestures in conversational turn taking situations.* Retrieved 10 July, 2009, from http://coral.lili.uni-bielefeld.de/Classes/Winter97/PhonMM/UlrichGruen/

Guerini, M., Stock, O., & Zancanaro, M. (2003). Persuasion models for intelligent interfaces. *Proceedings of the IJCAI Workshop on Computational Models of Natural Argument.*

Gulz, A., & Haakeb, M. (2006). Design of animated pedagogical agents—a look at their look. *International Journal of Human-Computer Studies*, *64*, 322–339. doi:10.1016/j.ijhcs.2005.08.006

Gulz, A. (2004). Benefits of virtual characters in computer based learning environments: Claims and evidence. *International Journal of Artificial Intelligence in Education*, *14*, 313–334.

Gulz, A. (2005). Social enrichment by virtual characters - differential benefits. *Journal of Computer Assisted Learning*, *21*(6), 405–418. doi:10.1111/j.1365-2729.2005.00147.x

Gulz, A., & Haake, M. (2010). Challenging gender stereotypes using virtual pedagogical characters . In Goodman, S., Booth, S., & Kirkup, G. (Eds.), *Gender issues in learning and working with Information Technology: Social constructs and cultural contexts*. Hershey, PA: IGI Global. doi:10.4018/978-1-61520-813-5.ch007

Gulz, A., & Haake, M. (2006). Pedagogical agents – design guidelines regarding visual appearance and pedagogical roles. In *Proceedings of the IV International Conference on Multimedia and ICT in Education (m-ICTE 2006)*, Sevilla, Spain.

Gupta, N., Tur, G., Hakkani-Tur, D., Bangalore, S., Riccardi, G., & Rahim, M. (2006). The AT&T spoken language understanding system. *IEEE Transactions on Speech and Audio Processing*.

Haake, M., & Gulz, A. (2009). A look at the roles of look & roles in embodied pedagogical agents – a user preference perspective. *International Journal of Artificial Intelligence in Education, 19*(1), 39–71.

Habermas, J. (1984). *The theory of communicative action*. Boston, MA: Beacon Press.

Hall, L., Woods, S., & Aylett, R. (2006). FearNot! Involving children in the design of a virtual learning environment. *International Journal of Artificial Intelligence in Education, 16*(4), 327–351.

Hall, L., Woods, S., Dautenhahn, K., Sobral, D., Paiva, A., Wolke, D., & Newall, L. (2004). Designing emphatic agents: Adults versus kids . In Lester, J., Vicari, R. M., & Paraguacu, F. (Eds.), *Intelligent tutoring systems* (pp. 604–613). Berlin/Heidelberg, Germany: Springer. doi:10.1007/978-3-540-30139-4_57

Hamann, S. (2001). Cognitive and neural mechanisms of emotional memory. *Trends in Cognitive Sciences, 5*(9), 394–400. doi:10.1016/S1364-6613(00)01707-1

Hanna, P., O'Neill, I., Wootton, C., & Mctear, M. (2007). Promoting extension and reuse in a spoken dialog manager: An evaluation of the queen's communicator. *ACM Transactions in Speech and Language Processing, 4*(3), 7. doi:10.1145/1255171.1255173

Haptek Inc. (2009). *Haptek*. Retrieved from www.haptek.com

Harris, R. A. (2005). *Voice interaction design: Crafting the new conversational speech systems*. Elsevier.

Hartmann, B., Mancini, M., Buisine, S., & Pelachaud, C. (2005). Design and evaluation of expressive gesture synthesis for embodied conversational agents. In *Proceedings of the 4th International Joint Conference on Autonomous Agents and Multiagent Systems* (pp. 1095-1096). Association for Computational Linguistics.

Hayes, P. J. (1979). The naive physics manifesto . In Michie, D. (Ed.), *Expert systems in the micro electronic age*. Edinburgh, UK: Edinburgh University Press.

Hayes-Roth, B., Amano, K., Saker, R., & Sephton, T. (2004). Training brief intervention with a virtual coach and patients. In B. K. Wiederhold, & G. Riva (Eds.), *Annual Review of Cyber-Therapy and Telemedicine, 2,* 85-96.

Hayes-Roth, B., Saker, R., & Amano, K. (2009). Automating brief intervention training with individualized coaching and role-play practice. *Methods Med Informatics*, in rev.

Hembree, R. (1990). The nature, effects, and relief of mathematics anxiety. *Journal for Research in Mathematics Education, 21*(1), 33–46. doi:10.2307/749455

Hempel, T. (2008). *Usability of speech dialog systems: Listening to the target audience*. Springer-Verlag.

Hernández-Trapote, A., López-Mencía, B., Díaz-Pardo, D., Fernández-Pozo, R., Hernández-Gómez, L., & Caminero, J. (2007). A person in the interface: Effects on user perceptions of multibiometrics. In *Proceedings of the ACL 2007 Workshop on Embodied Language Processing*. Association for Computational Linguistics.

Herrera, G., Alcantud, F., Jordan, R., Blanquer, A., Labajo, G., & De Pablo, C. (2008). Development of symbolic play through the use of virtual reality tools in children with autistic spectrum disorders: Two case studies . *Autism, 12*(2), 143–157. doi:10.1177/1362361307086657

Heylen, D., & ter Maat, M. (2008). *A linguistic view on functional markup languages*. Paper presented at Why Conversational Agents do what they do. Functional Representations for Generating Conversational Agent Behavior. AAMAS 2008. Estoril, Portugal.

Hinkelman, E. A., & Allen, J. F. (1989). Two constraints on speech act ambiguity. In *Proceedings of the 27th Annual Meeting on Association for Computational Linguistics* (pp. 212-219). Vancouver, British Columbia, Canada.

Hirschberg, J., & Litman, D. (1993). Empirical studies on the disambiguation of cue phrases. *Computational Linguistics, 19*, 501–530.

Hirschberg, J., Nakatani, C., & Grosz, B. (1995). Conveying discourse structure through intonation variation. In *Proceedings of the ECSA Workshop on Spoken Dialogue Systems: Theories and Applications*, Visgo, Denmark.

Hobbs, J. R., & Gordon, A. (2010). *Goals in a formal theory of commonsense psychology.* Paper presented at the 6th International Conference on Formal Ontology in Information Systems.

Hofstede, G., & Hofstede, G. J. (2005). *Cultures and organizations: Software of the mind.* New York, NY: McGraw-Hill.

Hone, K. (2006). Empathic agents to reduce user frustration: The effects of varying agent characteristics. *Interacting with Computers, 18*(2), 227–245. doi:10.1016/j.intcom.2005.05.003

Hone, K. S., & Graham, R. (2001). Towards a tool for the subjective assessment of speech system interfaces (SASSI). *Natural Language Engineering, 6*(3-4), 287–303.

Höök, K. (2004). User-centred design and evaluation of affective interfaces . In Ruttkay, Z., & Pelachaud, C. (Eds.), *From brows to trust: Evaluating embodied conversational agents.* Amsterdam, The Netherlands: Kluwer.

Hoorn, J. F., & Konijn, E. A. (2003). Perceiving and experiencing fictional characters: An integrative account. *The Japanese Psychological Research, 45*(4), 221–239. doi:10.1111/1468-5884.00225

Huang, X., Acero, A., & Hon, H. W. (2001). *Spoken language processing: A guide to theory, algorithm and system development.* Prentice Hall PTR.

Huang, C., Xu, P., & Zhang, X. Zhao, S., Huang, T., & Xu, B. (1999). LODESTAR: A Mandarin spoken dialogue system for travel information retrieval. *Proc. of Eurospeech*, (pp. 1159-1162).

Huang, H., Cerekovic, A., Pandzic, I., Nakano, Y., & Nishida, T. (2007). A script driven multimodal embodied conversational agent based on a generic framework. *Proc. of IVA*, (pp. 381–382).

Huang, H.-H., Cerekovic, A., Nakano, Y., Pandzic, I. S., & Nishida, T. (2008). The design of a generic framework for integrating ECA components. *Proc. of AAMAS*, (pp. 128–135).

Hubal, R. C., Fishbein, D. H., Sheppard, M. S., Paschall, M. J., Eldreth, D. L., & Hyde, C. T. (2008). How do varied populations interact with embodied conversational agents? Findings from inner-city adolescents and prisoners. *Computers in Human Behavior, 24*(3), 1104–1138. doi:10.1016/j.chb.2007.03.010

Hubal, R. C., Kizakevich, P. N., & Furberg, R. (2007). Synthetic characters in health-related applications. *Advanced Computational Intelligence Paradigms in Healthcare, 2*, 5–26. doi:10.1007/978-3-540-72375-2_2

Hubal, R. C., Kizakevich, P. N., Guinn, C. I., Merino, K. D., & West, S. L. (2000). The virtual standardized patient-simulated patient-practitioner dialogue for patient interview training . In Westwood, J. D., Hoffman, H. M., Mogel, G. T., Robb, R. A., & Stredney, D. (Eds.), *Envisioning healing: Interactive technology and the patient-practitioner dialogue.* Amsterdam, The Netherlands: IOS Press.

Hubal, R., Frank, G., & Guinn, C. (2003). Lessons learned in modeling Schizophrenic and depressed responsive virtual humans for training. In *Proceedings of 8th International Conference on Intelligent User Interfaces.*

Hulsman, R. L., Gos, W. J. G., Winnubst, J. A. M., & Bensing, J. M. (1999). Teaching clinically experienced physicians communication skills: A review of evaluation studies. *Medical Education, 33*, 655–668. doi:10.1046/j.1365-2923.1999.00519.x

Hulstijn, J. (2000). Dialogue games are recipes for joint action . In Poesio, M., & Traum, D. R. (Eds.), *Formal semantics and pragmatics of dialogue (Gotalog'00)* (pp. 99–106). Gothenburg, Sweden: Gothenburg University.

Hunt, A., & McGlashan, S. (2004). *W3C speech recognition grammar specification* (SRGS). Retrieved from http://www.w3.org/TR/speech-grammar/

Ibrahim, A., & Johansson, P. (2002). Multimodal dialogue systems for interactive TV applications. *Proc. of 4th IEEE Int. Conf. on Multimodal Interfaces*, (pp. 117-122).

Ieronutti, L., & Chittaro, L. (2007). Employing virtual humans for education and training in X3D/VRML worlds. *Computers & Education, 49*(1), 93–109. doi:10.1016/j.compedu.2005.06.007

Isbister, K. (2006). *Better game characters by design: A psychological approach*. San Francisco, CA: Morgan Kaufmann.

Isbister, K., & Nass, C. (2000). Consistency of personality in interactive characters: Verbal cues, non-verbal cues, and user characteristics. *International Journal of Human-Computer Studies*, *53*(2), 251–267. doi:10.1006/ijhc.2000.0368

ITU-T Suppl. 24 to P-Series Rec. (2005). *Parameters describing the interaction with spoken dialogue systems* (International Recommendation). International Telecommunication Union.

Izard, C. E. (1993). Organizational and motivational functions of discrete emotions . In Lewis, M., & Haviland, J. M. (Eds.), *Handbook of emotions*. New York, NY: Guilford Press.

Jackendoff, R. (1990). *Semantic structures*. Cambridge, MA: MIT Press.

Johnsen, K., Dickerson, R., Raij, A., Lok, B., Jackson, J., Shin, M., … Lind, D. (2005). Experiences in using virtual characters to educate medical communication skills. *IEEE Virtual Reality*.

Johnson, W. L. (2010). Serious use of a serious game for learning foreign language. *Journal of Artificial Intelligence in Education*, *20*(2), 175–195.

Johnson, W. L., & Valente, A. (2009). Tactical language and culture training systems: Using AI to teach foreign languages and cultures. *AI Magazine*, *30*(2), 72–84.

Johnson, W. L., Kole, S., Shaw, E., & Pain, H. (2003). *Socially intelligent learner-agent interaction tactics*. AI-ED 2003. Retrieved May 19, 2004, from www.cs.usyd.edu.au/~aied/papers_short.html

John-Steiner, V., & Mahn, H. (2003). Sociocultural contexts for teaching and learning . In Reynolds, A., William, M., & Miller, G. (Eds.), *Handbook of psychology: Educational psychology* (*Vol. 7*, pp. 125–151). New York, NY: John Wiley and Sons.

Johnston, C., & Whatley, D. (2005). Pulse!! - A virtual learning space project. *Studies in Health Technology and Informatics, Medicine Meets . Virtual Reality (Waltham Cross)*, *14*, 240–242.

Johnston, M., Bangalore, S., Vasireddy, G., Stent, A., Ehlen, P., Walker, M., et al. Maloor, P. (2002). MATCH: An architecture for multimodal dialogue systems. *Proc. of 40th Annual Meeting of the ACL*, (pp. 376-383).

Jokinen, K. (2009). *Constructive dialogue modelling: Speech interaction and rational agents*. John Wiley & Sons.

Jonassen, D. H., Tessmer, M., & Hannum, W. H. (1999). *Task analysis methods for instructional design*. Mahwah, NJ: Lawrence Erlbaum.

Jönsson, A. (1997). A model for habitable and efficient dialogue management for natural language interaction. *Natural Language Engineering*, *3*(2), 103–122. doi:10.1017/S1351324997001733

Jönsson, A. (1993). *Dialogue management for natural language interfaces – an empirical approach*. PhD Thesis, Linköping Studies in Science and Technology, No 312, Linköping, Sweden.

Jönsson, A., & Merkel, M. (2003). Some issues in dialogue-based question-answering. *Working Notes from the AAAI Spring Symposium '03*.

Jurafsky, D., & Martin, J. H. (2008). *Speech and language processing*. New Jersey: Prentice Hall International.

Jurafsky, D., & Martin, J. H. (2000). *Speech and language processing. An introduction to natural language processing, computational linguistics, and speech recognition*. Prentice-Hall.

Jurafsky, D., Shriberg, E., & Biasca, D. (1997). *Switchboard SWBD-DAMSL shallow-discourse-function annotation coders manual*, draft 13. Technical Report 97-01, University of Colorado Institute of Cognitive Science.

Jurafsky, D., Shriberg, E., Fox, B., & Curl, T. (1998). Lexical, prosodic, and syntactic cues for dialog acts. In *Proceedings of ACL/COLING-98 Workshop on Discourse Relations and Discourse Markers* (pp. 114–120). Montreal, Canada.

Kamm, C. A., & Walker, M. A. (1997). Design and evaluation of spoken dialogue systems. In *Proc. of the IEEE Workshop on Automatic Speech Recognition and Understanding*, Santa Barbara (CA), 14–17.

Kato, T., Fukumoto, J., Masui, F., & Kando, N. (2006). WoZ simulation of interactive question answering. *Proceedings of IQA'06*. ACL.

Kawamoto, K., Kitamura, Y., & Tijerino, Y. (2006). *Kawawiki: A semantic wiki based on RDF templates*. In Web Intelligence and Intelligent Agent Technology Workshops, (pp. 425–432). WI-IAT.

Kelley, J. F. (1983). An empirical methodology for writing user-friendly natural language computer applications. *Proceedings of the ACM SIG-CHI '93 Human Factors in Computing Systems* (pp. 193-196). New York, NY: ACM.

Kendon, A. (1990). *Conducting interaction: Patterns of behavior in focused encounters*. Cambridge University Press.

Kenny, P., Parsons, T. D., Gratch, J., & Rizzo, A. A. (2008b). Evaluation of Justina: A virtual patient with PTSD. *Lecture Notes in Artificial Intelligence, 5208*, 394–408.

Kenny, P., Parsons, T. D., Pataki, C. S., Pato, M., St-George, C., Sugar, J., & Rizzo, A. A. (2008a). Virtual Justina: A PTSD virtual patient for clinical classroom training. *Annual Review of Cybertherapy and Telemedicine, 6*, 113–118.

Kenny, P., Parsons, T. D., & Rizzo, A. A. (2009). Human computer interaction in virtual standardized patient systems. *Lecture Notes in Computer Science, 5613*, 514–523. doi:10.1007/978-3-642-02583-9_56

Kenny, P., Rizzo, A. A., Parsons, T. D., Gratch, J., & Swartout, W. (2007a). A virtual human agent for training novice therapist clinical interviewing skills. *Annual Review of Cybertherapy and Telemedicine, 5*, 81–89.

Kenny, P., Hartholt, A., Gratch, J., Swartout, W., Traum, D., Marsella, S., & Piepol D., (2007b). Building Interactive Virtual Humans for Training Environments in proceedings of *I/ITSEC*, Nov.

Kenny, P., Parsons, T. D., Gratch, J., Leuski, A., & Rizzo, A. A. (2007). Virtual patients for clinical therapist skills training. *Intelligent Virtual Agent Conference, LNAI 4722*, (pp. 197-210).

Kerr, S. J. (2002). Scaffolding: Design issues in single & collaborative virtual environments for social skills learning. In *Proceedings of the Workshop on Virtual Environments 2002*. Barcelona, Spain: Eurographics Association.

Kieras, D. E., Wood, S. D., & Meyer, D. E. (1997). Predictive engineering models based on the epic architecture for a multimodal high-performance human-computer interaction task. *ACM Transactions on Computer-Human Interaction, 4*(3), 230–275. doi:10.1145/264645.264658

Kim, C., & Baylor, A. L. (2008). A virtual change agent: Motivating pre-service teachers to integrate technology in their future classrooms. *Journal of Educational Technology & Society, 11*(2), 309–321.

Kim, Y., Baylor, A. L., & Shen, E. (2007). Pedagogical agents as learning companions: The impact of agent emotion and gender. *Journal of Computer Assisted Learning, 23*(3), 220–234. doi:10.1111/j.1365-2729.2006.00210.x

Kim, Y., & Baylor, A. L. (2007). Pedagogical agents as social models to influence learner attitudes. *Educational Technology, 47*(1), 23–28.

Kim, Y., Wei, Q., Xu, B., Ko, Y., & Ilieva, V. (2007). *MathGirls: Increasing girls' positive attitudes and self-efficacy through pedagogical agents*. Paper presented at 13th International Conference on Artificial Intelligence in Education (AIED 2007): Los Angeles, CA.

King, M., Maegaard, B., Schutz, J., & des Tombes, L. (1996). *EAGLES - Evaluation of Natural Language Processing Systems*, (Final report, EAG-EWG-PR.2).

King, S. A., Knott, A., & McCane, B. (2003). Language-driven nonverbal communication in a bilingual conversational agent. *In CASA '03: Proceedings of the 16th International Conference on Computer Animation and Social Agents (CASA 2003)* (p. 17). Washington, DC: IEEE Computer Society.

Kipp, M. (2001). From human gesture to synthetic action. In *Proceedings of the Workshop on" Multimodal Communication and Context in Embodied Agents held in conjunction with the Fifth International Conference on Autonomous Agents (AGENTS)* (pp. 9-14).

Kirschner, M., & Bernardi, R. (2009). Exploring topic continuation follow-up questions using machine learning. *Proc. of NAACL HLT: Student Research Workshop.* Boulder, CO.

Kitano, H. (1991). Toward a plan-based understanding model for mixed-initiative dialogues. *Proceedings of ACL'91* (pp. 25–32). ACL.

Klein, D., & Manning, C. D. (2003). Fast exact inference with a factored model for natural language parsing. *Advances in Neural Information Processing Systems, 15*, 3–10.

Klein, J., Moon, Y., & Picard, R. W. (1999). This computer responds to user frustration. *CHI '99 extended abstracts on Human factors in computing systems - CHI '99.*

Klüwer, T. (2007). *Semantische Auszeichnungen in sprachverarbeitenden Prozeskettensystemen.* Unpublished Master's thesis. University of Cologne, Germany.

Klüwer, T. (2009). RMRSBot - using linguistic information to enrich a Chatbot. In Z. Ruttkay, M. Kipp, A. Nijholt & H. H. Vilhjálmsson (Eds.) *Proceedings of the 9th international Conference on intelligent Virtual Agents. Lecture Notes in Artificial Intelligence, vol. 5773.* Berlin/Heidelberg, Germany: Springer Verlag.

Klüwer, T., Adolphs, P., Xu, F., Uszkoreit, H., & Cheng, X. (2010). Talking NPCs in a virtual game world. In *Proceedings of the ACL 2010 System Demonstrations. Annual Meeting of the Association for Computational Linguistics (ACL-2010)*, Uppsala, Sweden.

Kopp, S., Allwood, J., Grammer, K., Ahlsen, E., & Stocksmeier, T. (2008). Modeling embodied feedback with virtual humans. *Modeling Communication with Robots and Virtual Humans, 4930*, 18–37. doi:10.1007/978-3-540-79037-2_2

Kopp, S., Gesellensetter, L., Krämer, N., & Wachsmuth, I. (2005). A conversational agent as museum guide-design and evaluation of a real-world application . In *Intelligent virtual agents* (*Vol. 3661*, pp. 329–343). Springer. doi:10.1007/11550617_28

Kopp, S., & Wachsmuth, I. (2004). Synthesizing multimodal utterances for conversational agents. *Computer Animation and Virtual Worlds, 15*(1), 39–52. doi:10.1002/cav.6

Kopp, S., Sowa, T., & Wachsmuth, I. (2004). Imitation games with an artificial agent: From mimicking to understanding shape-related iconic gestures . In Braffort, A., Gherbi, R., Gibet, S., Richardson, J., & Teil, D. (Eds.), *Gesture-based communication in Human-Computer Interaction* (pp. 436–447). Berlin, Germany: Springer-Verlag. doi:10.1007/978-3-540-24598-8_40

Kopp, S., Krenn, B., Marsella, S., Marshall, A., Pelachaud, C., Pirker, H., et al. (2006). Towards a common framework for multimodal generation in ECAs: The behavior markup language. *Proc. of 6th International Conference on Intelligent Virtual Agents*, (pp. 205-217).

Kouroupetroglou, G., & Spiliotopoulos, D. (2009). Usability methodologies for real-life voice user interfaces. [IJITWE]. *International Journal of Information Technology and Web Engineering, 4*(4), 78–94. doi:10.4018/jitwe.2009100105

Kouroupetroglou, G. (2009). Universal access in public terminals: Information kiosks and ATMs . In Stephanidis, C. (Ed.), *The universal access handbook* (pp. 48.1–48.19). Florida, USA: CRC Press. doi:10.1201/9781420064995-c48

Kowtko, J., Isard, S., & Doherty, G. M. (1993). *Conversational games within dialogue.* Research paper 31, Human Communication Research Centre, University of Edinburgh.

Krämer, N., Bente, G., Eschenburg, F., & Troitzsch, H. (2009). Embodied conversational agents: Research prospects for social psychology and an exemplary study. *Social Psychology, 40*(1), 26–36. doi:10.1027/1864-9335.40.1.26

Krippendorff, K. (2004). *Content analysis: An introduction to its methodology* (2nd ed.). Thousand Oaks, CA: Sage.

Kroes, S. (2007). *Detecting boredom in meetings* (pp. 1–5). Enschede, Netherlands: University of Twente.

Kruijff, G.-J. M., Lison, P., Benjamin, T., Jacobsson, H., Zender, H., & Kruijff-Korbayova, I. (2009). Situated dialogue processing for human-robot interaction . In Christensen, H. I., Sloman, A., Kruijff, G.-J. M., & Wyatt, J. (Eds.), *Cognitive systems: Final report of the CoSy project.* Berlin/Heidelberg, Germany: Springer Verlag.

Kruijff, G.-J. M. (2002). *Formal and computational aspects of dependency grammar: History and development of DG*. (Technical report, ESSLLI-2002).

Kruijff, G.-J. M. (2005). Context-sensitive utterance planning for CCG. In *Proceedings of the European Workshop on Natural Language Generation*. Aberdeen, Scotland.

Kumar, R., Gweon, G., Joshi, M., Cui, Y., & Rose, C. P. (2007). Supporting students working together on math with social dialogue. In *SLaTE-2007 (Speech and Language Technology in Education) Proceedings*, (pp. 96-99).

Kuppevelt, J., & Dybkajer, L. (Eds.). (2005). *Advances in natural multimodal dialogue systems*. Springer. doi:10.1007/1-4020-3933-6

Kwok, C. T., Etzioni, O., & Weld, D. S. (2001). Scaling question answering to the Web. In *Proceedings of WWW'01*.

Kwon, W. S., Gilbert, J., & Chattaraman, V. (2010). *Effects of conversational agents in retail websites on aging consumers' interactivity and perceived benefits*. Paper presented at the Proceedings of the 28th ACM Conference on Human Factors in Computing Systems CHI 2010 Workshop Senior-Friendly Technologies: Interaction Design for the Elderly, Atlanta, GA, USA.

Lampe, J. (2007). *Cultural proficiency guildelines (3.2)*. Paper presented at the Plenary session of the Interagency Language Roundtable for the ACTFL Arabic Testing Consensus Project.

Landauer, T., Foltz, P., & Laham, D. (1998). An introduction to latent semantic analysis. *Discourse Processes*, *25*, 259–284. doi:10.1080/01638539809545028

Larson, J. A. (2002). *VoiceXML: Introduction to developing speech applications*. NJ: Prentice Hall.

Larsson, S., Berman, A., Bos, J., Grönqvist, L., & Junglöf, P. (1999). *A model of dialogue moves and information state revision. Technical Report, D5.1 Trindi*. Task Oriented Instructional Dialogue.

Larsson, S., Ljunglof, P., Muhlenbock, K., & Thunberg, G. (2008). *TRIK: A talking and drawing robot for children with communication disabilities*. Paper presented at the Proc. NordiCHI'08 Workshop: Designing Robotic Artefacts With User- and Experience Centred Perspectives.

Lauesen, S. (2005). *User interface design: A software engineering perspective*. Addison-Wesley.

Laurillard, D. (1993). *Rethinking university teaching: A framework for the effective use of educational technology*. London, UK: Routledge.

Lazarus, R. (1991). *Emotion and adaptation*. New York, NY: Oxford University Press.

Lee, A., & Kawahara, T. (2009). *Recent development of open-source speech recognition engine Julius. Proc of. Asia-Pacific Signal and Information Processing Association Annual Summit and Conference*. APSIPA ASC.

Lee, K., Hon, H., & Reddy, R. (1990). *An overview of the SPHINX speech recognition system. Readings in Speech Recognition* (pp. 600–610). Morgan Kaufmann Publishers.

Lee, C., & Chang, J. S. (2002). *Rapid prototyping an operator assisted call routing system*. ISCSLP 2002, Taipei, Taiwan.

Lee, J., & Marsella, S. (2006). *Nonverbal behavior generator for embodied conversational agents*. 6th International Conference on Intelligent Virtual Agents, Marina del Rey, CA.

Lee, J., DeVault, D., Marsella, S., & Traum, D. (2008, May). *Thoughts on FML: Behavior generation in the virtual human communication architecture*. Paper presented at Why Conversational Agents do what they do. Functional Representations for Generating Conversational Agent Behavior. AAMAS 2008, Estoril, Portugal.

Lemon, O., Georgila, K., & Henderson, J. (2006b). Evaluating effectiveness and portability of reinforcement learned dialogue strategies with real users: The TALK TownInfo evaluation. *Proc. of IEEE-ACL*, (pp. 178–181).

Lemon, O., Georgila, K., Henderson, J., & Stuttle, M. (2006a). An ISU dialogue system exhibiting reinforcement learning of dialogue policies: Generic slot-filling in the TALK in-car system. *Proc. of EACL*.

Lemon, O., Gruenstein, A., Battle, A., & Peters, S. (2002). Multi-tasking and collaborative activities in dialogue systems. In *Proceedings of the 3rd SIGdial Workshop on Discourse and Dialogue (vol. 2)*, (pp. 113-124), Philadelphia, PA, USA.

Lesh, N., Marks, J., Rich, C., & Sidner, C. L. (2004). *Man-computer symbiosis revisited: Achieving natural communication and collaboration with computers. Transactions on Electronics*. IEICE.

Leßmann, N., & Wachsmuth, I. (2003). A cognitively motivated architecture for an anthropomorphic artificial communicator. *Proc. of ICCM-5*, (pp. 277- 278).

Lester, J., Towns, S., Callaway, C., Voerman, J., & Fitzgerald, P. (2000). Deictic and emotive communication in animated pedagogical agents . In Cassell, J., Sullivan, J., Prevost, S., & Churchill, E. (Eds.), *Embodied conversational agents* (pp. 123–154). Cambridge, MA: MIT Press.

Lester, J. C., Converse, S. A., Kahler, S. E., Barlow, S. T., Stone, B. A., & Bhogal, R. S. (1997). The persona effect: Affective impact of animated pedagogical agents. In S. Pemberton (Ed.), *Proceedings of the SIGCHI conference on Human factors in computing systems* (pp. 359-366).

Lethin, C., & Muller, P. (2010). Future immersive training. *Warfighter Enhancement Activities*, *4*(1), 2–4.

Leuski, A., & Traum, D. (2010). NPCEditor: A tool for building question-answering characters. In *Proceedings of The Seventh International Conference on Language Resources and Evaluation.*

Leuski, A., Pair, J., Traum, D., McNerney, P. J., Georgiou, P., & Patel, R. (2006a). How to talk to a hologram. In E. Edmonds, D. Riecken, C. L. Paris, & C. L. Sidner, (Eds.), *Proceedings of the 11th International Conference on Intelligent user interfaces(IUI'06)*, Sydney, Australia, (pp. 360–362). New York, NY: ACM Press.

Leuski, A., Patel, R., Traum, D., & Kennedy, B. (2006). Building effective question answering characters. In *Proceedings of the 7th SIGdial Workshop on Discourse and Dialogue*, Sydney, Australia.

Levin, E., & Pieraccini, R. (1997). *A stochastic model of computer-human interaction for learning dialogue strategies* (pp. 1883–1886). Proc. of Eurospeech.

Levin, E., Pieraccini, R., & Eckert, W. (1998). Using Markov decision process for learning dialogue strategies. In *Proceedings of the IEEE International Conference on Acoustic, speech and signal processing* (pp. 201–204).

Levinson, S. C. (1983). *Pragmatics*. Cambridge, UK & New York, NY: Cambridge University Press.

Levy, D. (2007). *Love and sex with robots: The evolution of human–robot relationships*. London, UK: Duckworth.

Levy, D., Catizone, R., Battacharia, B., Krotov, A., & Wilks, Y. (1997). CONVERSE: A conversational companion. *Proceedings of 1st International Workshop on Human-Computer Conversation.* Bellagio, Italy.

Lewin, I., Rupp, C. J., Hieronymus, J., Milward, D., Larsson, S., & Berman, A. (2000). *Siridus system architecture and interface report*. Siridus Project.

Li, L., Cao, F., Chou, W., & Liu, F. (2006). XM-flow: An extensible micro-flow for multimodal interaction. *Proc. of MMSP*, (pp. 497-500).

Li, L., Li, L., Chou, W., & Liu, F. (2007). R-Flow: An extensible XML based multimodal dialogue system architecture. *Proc. of MMSP,* (pp. 86-89).

Lindström, P., Gulz, A., Haake, M., & Sjödén, B. (in press). Matching and mismatching between the pedagogical design principles of a maths game and the actual practices of play. *Journal of Computer Assisted Learning*.

Lisetti, C. L., & Schiano, D. (2000). Facial expression recognition: Where human-computer interaction, artificial intelligence, and cognitive science intersect. *Pragmatics & Cognition*, *8*, 185–235. doi:10.1075/pc.8.1.09lis

Litman, D. J., & Allen, J. F. (1990). Discourse processing and commonsense plans . In Cohen, P. R., Morgan, J. L., & Pollack, M. E. (Eds.), *Intentions in communications* (pp. 365–388). The MIT Press.

Litman, D., & Forbes-Riley, K. (In Press, 2010). Designing and evaluating a wizarded uncertainty-adaptive spoken dialogue tutoring system. *Computer Speech and Language*.

Litman, D., & Silliman, S. (2004). ITSPOKE: An intelligent tutoring spoken dialogue system. *Proceedings of the Human Language Technology Conference: 4th Meeting of the North American Chapter of the Association for Computational Linguistics* (*HLT/NAACL*), Boston, MA.

Liu, J., Wang, J., & Wang, C. (2006). Spoken language understanding in dialog systems for Olympic game information. *Proc. of IEEE Int. Conf. on Industrial Informatics*, (pp. 1042-1045).

Löckelt, M. (2005). Action planning for virtual human performances. In *Proceedings of the 3rd International Conference on Virtual Storytelling*, (pp. 53-62), Strasbourg, France.

Löckelt, M. (2008). *A flexible and reusable framework for dialogue and action management in multi-party discourse*. PhD Thesis, Saarbrücken University, Germany.

Lok, B., Ferdig, R. E., Raij, A., Johnsen, K., Dickerson, R., & Coutts, J. (2006). Applying Virtual reality in medical communication education: Current findings and potential teaching and learning benefits of immersive virtual patients. *Virtual Reality (Waltham Cross)*, *10*, 185–195. doi:10.1007/s10055-006-0037-3

López-Cózar, R., & Araki, M. (2005). *Spoken, multilingual and multimodal dialogue systems: Development and assessment*. Wiley.

López-Cózar, R., de la Torre, A., Segura, J., & Rubio, A. (2003). Assessment of dialogue systems by means of a new simulation technique. *Speech Communication*, *40*, 387–407. doi:10.1016/S0167-6393(02)00126-7

López-Cózar, R., Ábalos, N., Espejo, G., Griol, D., Callejas, Z. (2011). Using ambient intelligence information in a multimodal dialogue system. *Journal of Ambient Intelligence and Smart Environments*. In printing.

López-Mencía, B., Hernández-Trapote, A., Díaz-Pardo, D., Fernández-Pozo, R., Hernández-Gómez, L., & Torre Toledano, D. (2007). Design and validation of ECA gestures to improve dialogue system robustness. In *Proceedings of the ACL 2007 Workshop on Embodied Language Processing* (pp. 67-74). Association for Computational Linguistics.

Lowe, W. (2001). *Toward a theory of semantic space*. In the 22nd Annual Conference of the Cognitive Science Society, 1, (pp. 675–680).

Luneski, A., Moore, R. K., & Bamidis, P. D. (2008). Affective computing and collaborative networks: Towards emotion-aware interaction . In Camarinha-Matos, L. M., & Picard, W. (Eds.), *Pervasive collaborative networks* (*Vol. 283*, pp. 315–322). Boston, MA: Springer. doi:10.1007/978-0-387-84837-2_32

Maatman, R. M., Gratch, J., & Marsella, S. (2005). Natural behavior of a listening agent. *Proc. of IVA*, (pp. 25-36).

Macedonio, M., Parsons, T. D., & Rizzo, A. A. (2007). Immersiveness and physiological arousal within panoramic video-based virtual reality. *Cyberpsychology & Behavior*, *10*, 508–516. doi:10.1089/cpb.2007.9997

Magnenat-Thalmann, N., & Thalmann, D. (2005). Virtual humans: Thirty years of research, what next? *The Visual Computer*, *21*, 1–19. doi:10.1007/s00371-004-0243-5

Mairesse, F., Gasic, M., Jurcicek, F., Keizer, S., Thomson, B., Yu, K., & Young, S. (2009). Spoken language understanding from unaligned data using discriminative classification models. *Proc. of ICASSP*, (pp. 4749-4752).

Malaka, R., Haeusseler, J., & Aras, H. (2004). SmartKom mobile: Intelligent ubiquitous user interaction. *Proc. of 9th Int. Conf. on Intelligent User Interfaces*, (pp. 310-312).

Malatesta, L., Raouzaiou, A. K., Karpouzis, K., & Kollias, S. D. (2009). Towards modeling embodied conversational agent character profiles using appraisal theory predictions in expression synthesis. *Applied Intelligence*, *30*(1), 58–64. doi:10.1007/s10489-007-0076-9

Manchón, P. (2009). *Towards clever human-computer interaction*. Doctoral dissertation, University of Seville, Spain.

Manning, C., & Schütze, H. (2003). *Foundations of statistical natural language processing*. Cambridge, MA: The MIT Press.

Maragoudakis, M. (2007). MeteoBayes: Effective plan recognition in a weather dialogue system. *IEEE Intelligent Systems*, *22*(1), 66–77. doi:10.1109/MIS.2007.14

Marcus, M., Kim, G., Marcinkiewicz, M. A., Macintyre, R., Bies, A., Ferguson, M., et al. Schasberger, B. (1994). *The Penn treebank: Annotating predicate argument structure*. In ARPA Human Language Technology Workshop, Morgan Kaufmann.

Marsella, S., & Gratch, J. (2009). EMA: A model of emotional dynamics. *Journal of Cognitive Systems Research*, *10*(1), 70–90. doi:10.1016/j.cogsys.2008.03.005

Marsella, S. C., Johnson, W. L., & Labore, C. M. (2003). *Interactive pedagogical drama for health interventions*. In AIED 2003, 11th International Conference on Artificial Intelligence in Education, Australia, (pp. 341–348). IOS Press

Marsella, S., & Gratch, J. (2003). Modeling coping behavior in virtual humans: Don't worry, be happy. In *Proc. 2nd International Conf. on Autonomous Agents and Multiagent Systems (AAMAS)*, Melbourne, Australia, July 2003.

Marsi, E., & van Rooden, F. (2007). Expressing uncertainty with a talking head in a multimodal question-answering system. In E. R. E. K. I. van der Sluis, & M. Theune (Eds.),*Workshop on Multimodal Output Generation (MOG)* (pp. 105-116). University of Aberdeen, United Kingdom.

Martalò, A., Novielli, N., & de Rosis, F. (2008). Attitude display in dialogue patterns. In *Proceedings of AISB 2008 Convention on Communication, Interaction and Social Intelligence*. Retrieved from http://www.aisb.org.uk/convention/aisb08/proc/proceedings/02%20Affective%20 Language/01.pdf

Massaro, D. W., Cohen, M. M., Beskow, J., & Cole, R. (2000). Developing and evaluating conversational agents . In Cassell, J., Sullivan, J., Prevost, S., & Churchill, E. (Eds.), *Embodied conversational agents* (pp. 287–318). Cambridge, MA: MIT Press.

Massaro, D. W., Cohen, M. M., Daniel, S., & Cole, R. A. (2001). Developing and evaluating conversational agents . In Hancock, P. A. (Ed.), *Human performance and ergonomics* (pp. 173–194). Academic Press.

Massaro, D. (2004). Symbiotic value of an embodied agent in language learning. In R. H. Sprague, Jr. (Ed.), *IEEE Proceedings of 37th Annual Hawaii International Conference on System Sciences*, Computer Society Press.

Massaro, D. W. (2003). A computer-animated tutor for spoken and written language learning. In *Proceedings of the 5th International Conference on Multimodal interfaces (ICMI '03)*, Canada, ACM, (pp. 172-175).

Masterton, S. (1998). Computer support for learners using intelligent educational agents: The way forward. In . *Proceedings of ICCE*, *98*, 211–219.

Mateas, M., & Stern, A. (2003). Façade: An experiment in building a fully-realized interactive drama. In *Game Developers Conference, Game Design track (Online Proceedings)*, San Jose, CA.

Mauldin, M. L. (1994). ChatterBots, TinyMuds, and the Turing test: Entering the Loebner Prize competition. In *Proceedings of the Twelfth National Conference on Artificial intelligence* (vol. 1) (pp. 16-21). Seattle, WA: American Association for Artificial Intelligence.

Maybury, M. T. (2002). *Towards a question answering roadmap*. MITRE Corporation.

Mayfield, L., & Burger, S. (1999). Eliciting natural speech from non-native users: Collecting speech data for LVCSR. *Proc. of ACL-IALL*.

Mayo, M., Mitrovic, A., & McKenzie, J. (2000). *APIT: An intelligent tutoring system for capitalization and punctuation*. International Workshop on Advanced Learning Technologies, (pp. 151–154).

Mazzotta, I., de Rosis, F., & Carofiglio, V. (2007). Portia: A user-adapted persuasion system in the healthy-eating domain. *Intelligent Systems, IEEE*, *22*, 42–51. doi:10.1109/MIS.2007.115

Mazzotta, I., Novielli, N., Silvestri, V., & de Rosis, F. (2007). O Francesca, ma che sei grulla? Emotions and irony in persuasion dialogues. In R. Basili & M. T. Pazienza (Eds.), *Proceedings of the 10th Congress of the Italian Association For Artificial intelligence on AI*IA 2007: Artificial intelligence and Human-Oriented Computing, Lecture Notes In Artificial Intelligence, vol. 4733*, (pp. 602-613). Berlin/ Heidelberg, Germany: Springer-Verlag.

MCCLL. (2008). Tactical Iraqi language and culture training system. *MCCLL Newsletter*, *4*(8), 4.

McDonald, D. P., McGuire, G., Johnson, J., Selmeski, B., & Abbe, A. (2008). *Developing and managing cross-cultural competence within the Department of Defense: Recommendations for learning and assessment: The Regional and Cultural Competence Assessment Working Group (RCCAWG)*. Defense Equal Opportunity Management Institute.

McGlashan, S., Burnett, D. C., Carter, J., Danielsen, P., Ferrans, J., & Hunt, A. ... Tryphonas, S. (2004). *Voice Extensible Markup Language (VoiceXML) version* 2.0. Retrieved from http://www.w3.org/TR/voicexml20.

McRorie, M., Sneddon, I., Sevin, E. D., Bevacqua, E., & Pelachaud, C. (2009). *A model of personality and emotional traits.* Paper presented at the International conference on Intelligent virtual agents IVA'09, Amsterdam.

McTear, M. F. (2004). *Spoken dialogue technology – toward the conversational user interface*. London, UK: Springer Verlag.

McTear, M. F. (2004). *Towards the conversational user interface*. Springer Verlag.

McTear, M. (2008). Handling miscommunication: Why bother? In Dybkjær, L., & Minker, W. (Eds.), *Recent trends in discourse and dialogue* (pp. 101–122). Springer Netherlands. doi:10.1007/978-1-4020-6821-8_5

McTear, M. F. (1998). Modelling spoken dialogues with state transition diagrams: experiences with the CSLU toolkit. *Proc. of ICSLP*, (pp. 1223–1226).

Mead, G. H. (1967). *Mind, self, and society: From the standpoint of a social behaviorist*. Chicago, IL: University of Chicago Press.

MetLife Mature Market Institute. (2009). *Market survey of long-term care costs*. Retrieved from http://www.metlife.com/assets/cao/mmi/publications/studies/mmi-market-survey-nursing-home-assisted-living.pdf

Meza-Ruiz, I. V., Riedel, S., & Lemon, O. (2008). Accurate statistical spoken language understanding from limited development resources. *Proc. of ICASSP*.

Miller, R. B. (1968). Response time in man-computer conversational transactions. In . *Proceedings of the AFIPS Fall Joint Computer Conference*, *33*, 267–277.

Minker, W. (1998). Stochastic versus rule-based speech understanding for information retrieval. *Speech Communication*, *25*(4), 223–247. doi:10.1016/S0167-6393(98)00038-7

Mitrovic, A., Martin, B., & Suraweera, P. (2006). Intelligent tutors for all: The constraint-based approach. *IEEE Intelligent Systems*, *22*(4), 38–45. doi:10.1109/MIS.2007.74

Mohri, M. (1997). Finite-state transducers in language and speech processing. *Computational Linguistics*, *23*(2), 269–311.

Möller, S., Smeele, P., Boland, H., & Krebber, J. (2007). Evaluating spoken dialogue systems according to de-facto standards: A case study. *Computer Speech & Language*, *21*(1), 26–53. doi:10.1016/j.csl.2005.11.003

Moran, D. B., Cheyer, A. J., Julia, L. E., Martin, D. L., & Park, S. (1997). Multimodal user interface in the open agent architecture. *Proc. of ACM*, (pp. 61–68).

Morandell, M. M., Hochgatterer, A., Fagel, S., & Wassertheurer, S. (2008). *Avatars in assistive homes for the elderly: A user-friendly way of interaction? HCI and usability for education and work*. Berlin / Heidelberg, Germany: Springer.

Morency, L. P., & de Kok, I. (2008). *Context-based recognition during human interactions: Automatic feature selection and encoding dictionary*. 10th International Conference on Multimodal Interfaces, Chania, Greece, IEEE.

Morency, L. P., Sidner, C., Lee, C., & Darrell, T. (2005). Contextual recognition of head gestures. *Proc. of ICMI*, (pp. 18-24).

Moreno, R., & Flowerday, T. (2006). Students' choice of animated pedagogical agents in science learning: A test of the similarity-attraction hypothesis on gender and ethnicity. *Contemporary Educational Psychology*, *31*, 186–207. doi:10.1016/j.cedpsych.2005.05.002

Moreno, R., Mayer, R., Spires, H., & Lester, J. (2001). The case for social agency in computer-based teaching: Do students learn more deeply when they interact with animated pedagogical agents? *Cognition and Instruction*, *19*, 177–213. doi:10.1207/S1532690XCI1902_02

Mori, M. (1970). The uncanny valley.

Moundridou, M., & Virvou, M. (2002). Evaluating the persona effect of an interface agent in a tutoring system. *Journal of Computer Assisted Learning*, *18*, 253–261. doi:10.1046/j.0266-4909.2001.00237.x

M-PILL. (2009). *M-Pill.* Retrieved from http://www.m-pill.com/index.php?browse=compliance

Müller, C., & Runge, F. (1993). *Dialogue design principles - key for usability of voice processing* (pp. 943–946). Proc. of Eurospeech.

Müller, J., Poller, P., & Tschernomas, V. (2003). A multimodal fission approach with a presentation agent in the dialog system SmartKom. *LNCS*, *2821*, 633–645.

Nardi, D., & Brachman, R. J. (2002). An introduction to description logics . In Baader, F. (Eds.), *The description logic handbook* (pp. 5–44). Cambridge, UK.

Nass, C., & Brave, S. (2005). *Wired for speech: How voice activates and advances the human-computer relationship.* MIT Press. Norman, D. A. (1999). Affordance, conventions, and design. *Interaction*, *6*(3), 38–43.

National Institute on Deafness and other Communication Disorders. (n.d.). *Hearing loss and older adults*. Retrieved May 30, 2010, from http://www.nidcd.nih.gov/health/hearing/older.asp

Newell, A. (1994). *Unified theories of cognition*. Cambridge, MA: Harvard University Press.

Nicoll, D. W. (1995). *Contextual usability: A methodological outline of contextual usability and quality function deployment in the development of advance media products.* TechMaPP Working Paper, Department of Psychology, University of Edinburgh.

Niederhoffer, K. G., & Pennebaker, J. W. (2002). Linguistic style matching in social interaction. *Journal of Language and Social Psychology*, *21*, 337–360. doi:10.1177/026192702237953

Nielsen, J., & Mack, R. L. (1994). *Usability inspection methods*. New York, NY: John Wiley & Sons.

Nielsen, J. (1995). *Technology transfer of heuristic evaluation and usability inspection*. Presented at the IFIP INTERACT'95 International Conference on Human-Computer Interaction, Lillehammer, Norway.

Nielsen, P. B., & Baekgaard, A. (1992). Experience with a dialogue description formalism for realistic applications. *Proc. of International Conference on Spoken Language Processing (ICSLP)*, (pp. 719-722).

Nigay, L., & Coutaz, J. (1993). A design space for multimodal systems: Concurrent processing and data fusion. *Proc. of ACM CHI Conf. on Human Factors in Computing Systems*, (pp. 172-178).

Nigay, L., & Coutaz, J. (1995). A generic platform for addressing the multimodal challenge. *Proc. of ACM CHI*, (pp. 98-105).

Niles, I., & Pease, A. (2001). Towards a standard upper ontology. In *Proceedings of the 2nd International Conference on Formal Ontology in Information Systems (FOIS-2001)* (pp. 2-9), Ogunquit, ME: ACM.

Nirenburg, S., McShane, M., Beale, S., Jarrell, B., & Fantry, G. (2009). Integrating cognitive simulation into the Maryland virtual patient. *Proceedings from MMVR-09*.

Norman, D. (2002). *The design of everyday things*. New York, NY: Basic Books.

Norman, T. J., & Reed, C. (2003). *Argumentation machines: New frontiers in argument and computation.* Argumentation Library.

Norman, D. A., & Draper, S. W. (1986). *User centered system design: New perspectives on human-computer interaction*. Mahwah, NJ: Lawrence Erlbaum Associates.

Norris, F. H., Kaniasty, K., & Thompson, M. P. (1997). The psychological consequences of crime: Findings from a longitudinal population-based study . In Davis, R. C., Lurigio, A. J., & Skogan, W. G. (Eds.), *Victims of crime* (2nd ed., pp. 146–166). Thousand Oaks, CA: Sage Publications, Inc.

Noth, E., Batlinera, A., Warnkea, V., Haasa, J., Borosb, M., & Buckowa, J. (2002). On the use of prosody in automatic dialogue understanding. *Speech Communication*, *36*(1-2), 45–62. doi:10.1016/S0167-6393(01)00025-5

Novielli, N. (2010). HMM modeling of user engagement in advice-giving dialogues. *Journal on Multimodal User Interfaces*, *3*(1-2), 131–140. doi:10.1007/s12193-009-0026-4

Novielli, N., de Rosis, F., & Mazzotta, I. (2010). User attitude towards an embodied conversational agent: Effects of the interaction mode. [Elsevier Science.]. *Journal of Pragmatics*, *42*(9), 2385–2397. doi:10.1016/j.pragma.2009.12.016

Novielli, N., & Strapparava, C. (2010a). Exploring the lexical semantics of dialogue acts. *Journal of Computational Linguistics and Applications*, *1*, 9–26.

Novielli, N., & Strapparava, C. (2010b). Studying the lexicon of dialogue acts. In N. Calzolari, K. Choukri, B. Maegaard, J. Mariani, J. Odijk, S. Piperidis, M. Rosner & D. Tapias (Eds.), *Proceedings of the Seventh Conference on International Language Resources and Evaluation (LREC'10)*. Retrieved from http://www.lrec-conf.org/proceedings/lrec2010/index.html

Oh, I., & Stone, M. (2007). Understanding RUTH: Creating believable behaviors for a virtual human under uncertainty . In Duffy, V. G. (Ed.), *Digital human modeling* (pp. 443–452). Berlin/Heidelberg, Germany: Springer-Verlag. doi:10.1007/978-3-540-73321-8_51

Oh, A. H., & Rudnicky, A. (2000). Stochastic language generation for spoken dialogue systems. *Proc. of ANLP/NAACL workshop on conversational systems*, (pp. 27-32).

Oviatt, S., MacEachern, M., & Levow, G. (1998). Predicting hyperarticulate speech during human-computer error resolution. *Speech Communication*, *24*(2), 87–110. doi:10.1016/S0167-6393(98)00005-3

Oviatt, S. (1994). Interface techniques for minimizing disfluent input to spoken language systems. In B. Adelson, S. Dumais & J. Olson (Eds.), *Proceedings of the SIGCHI conference on Human factors in computing systems: celebrating interdependence* (pp. 205-210). Association for Computational Linguistics.

Oviatt, S., & Adams, B. (2000). Designing and evaluating conversational interfaces with animated characters. In S. P. Justine Cassell, Joseph Sullivan & E. F. Churchill (Eds.), *Embodied conversational agents* (pp. 319-345). MIT Press.

Oviatt, S., & VanGent, R. (1996). Error resolution during multimodal human-computer interaction. In *Proceedings of the Fourth International Conference on Spoken Language Processing, vol. 1* (pp. 204-207). Institute of Electrical & Electronics Engineers.

Owen, M., & Provan, J. S. (2010). *A fast algorithm for computing geodesic distances in tree space. IEEE/ACM Transactions on Computational Biology and Bioinformatics*. PrePrints.

OWL. (2004). *W3C Semantic Web, Web Ontology Language (OWL)*. Retrieved from http://www.w3.org/2004/OWL/

Paek, T., & Horvitz, E. (2000). Conversation as action under uncertainty. In C. Boutilier & M. Goldszmidt (Eds.), *16th Conference on Uncertainty in Artificial Intelligence* (pp. 455-464).

Paek, T., & Horvitz, E. (2004). Optimizing automated call routing by integrating spoken dialogue models with queuing models. *Proc. of HLT-NAACL*, 41-48.

Paiva, A. (Ed.). (2004). *Empathic agents*. Workshop in conjunction with AAMAS'04.

Paiva, A., Dias, J., Sobral, D., Aylett, R., Sobreperez, P., Woods, S., et al. (2004). Caring for agents and agents that care: Building empathic relations with synthetic agents. In *Proceedings of the Third International Joint Conference on Autonomous Agents 2004*, (pp. 194-201).

Pandzic, I. S. (2002). Facial animation framework for the web and mobile platforms. *Proc. of Web3D Symposium*, (pp. 27-34).

Pareto, L. (2004). The Squares Family: A game and story based microworld for understanding arithmetic concepts designed to attract girls. In L. Cantoni, & C. McLoughlin (Eds.), *Proceedings of World Conference on Educational Multimedia, Hypermedia and Telecommunications 2004* (pp. 1567-1574). Chesapeake, VA: AACE.

Pareto, L., Schwartz, D. L., & Svensson, L. (2009). Learning by guiding a teachable agent to play an educational game. In *Proceedings of the International Conference on Artificial Intelligence in Education*, July 6-10, 2009.

Paroubek, P., & Blasband, M. (1999). *A blueprint for a general infrastructure for natural language processing systems evaluation using semi-automatic quantitative black box approach in a multilingual environment.* ELSE project Executive Summary.

Parsons, S., & Mitchell, P. (2002). The potential of virtual reality in social skills training for people with autistic spectrum disorders. *Journal of Intellectual Disability Research*, *46*(5), 430–443. doi:10.1046/j.1365-2788.2002.00425.x

Parsons, S., Mitchell, P., & Leonard, A. (2005). Do adolescents with autistic spectrum disorders adhere to social conventions in virtual environments? *Autism*, *9*(1), 95–117. doi:10.1177/1362361305049032

Parsons, T. D., Cosand, L., Courtney, C., Iyer, A., & Rizzo, A. A. (2009b). Neurocognitive workload assessment using the virtual reality cognitive performance assessment test. *Lecture Notes in Artificial Intelligence*, *5639*, 243–252.

Parsons, T. D., Courtney, C., Cosand, L., Iyer, A., Rizzo, A. A., & Oie, K. (2009c). Assessment of psychophysiological differences of West Point cadets and civilian controls immersed within a virtual environment. *Lecture Notes in Artificial Intelligence*, *5638*, 514–523.

Parsons, T. D., Iyer, A., Cosand, L., Courtney, C., & Rizzo, A. A. (2009a). Neurocognitive and psychophysiological analysis of human performance within virtual reality environments. *Studies in Health Technology and Informatics*, *142*, 247–252.

Parsons, T. D., Kenny, P., Cosand, L., Iyer, A., Courtney, C., & Rizzo, A. A. (2009d). A virtual human agent for assessing bias in novice therapists. *Studies in Health Technology and Informatics*, *142*, 253–258.

Parsons, T. D., Kenny, P., Ntuen, C., Pataki, C. S., Pato, M., & Rizzo, A. A. (2008). Objective structured clinical interview training using a virtual human patient. *Studies in Health Technology and Informatics*, *132*, 357–362.

Parsons, T. D., Cosand, L., Courtney, C., Iyer, A., & Rizzo, A. A. (2009). Neurocognitive workload assessment using the virtual reality cognitive performance assessment test. *Lecture Notes in Artificial Intelligence*, *5639*, 243–252.

Parsons, S., Beardon, L., Neale, H. R., Reynard, G., Eastgate, R., Wilson, J. R., et al. Hopkins, E. (2000). Development of social skills amongst adults with Asperger's Syndrome using virtual environments: The 'AS Interactive' project. *Proceedings of the 3rd International Conference on Disability, Virtual Reality & Associated Technologies*, (pp. 163-170).

Patel, M., & Willis, P. G. (1991). *FACES–The Facial Animation, Construction and Editing System* (pp. 33–45). Proc. of Eurographics.

Peckham, J. (1993). A new generation of spoken dialogue systems: Results and lessons from the SUNDIAL project. In *Proceedings of 3rd European Conference on Speech Communication and Technology (Eurospeech'93)* (pp. 33-40). Berlin, Germany: ESCA.

Pelachaud, C. (2003). *Overview of representation languages for ECAs (Project Reports). Paris VIII*. IUT Montreuil.

Pelachaud, C., Maya, V., & Lamolle, M. (2004). Representation of expressivity for embodied conversational agents. *Proc. of Workshop Balanced Perception and Action, 3rd Int. Joint Conf. on Autonomous Agents and Multi-Agent Systems*.

Pellom, B. (2001). *Sonic: The University of Colorado continuous speech recognizer*. (Technical Report TR-CSLR-2001-01), University of Colorado, Boulder, CO.

Pellom, B., & Hacioglu, K. (2003). Recent improvements in the CU Sonic ASR System for noisy speech. *Proc. of ICASSP*.

Pellom, B., Ward, W., Hansen, J., Cole, R., Hacioglu, K., & Zhang, J. … Pradhan, S. (2001). *University of Colorado dialog systems for travel and navigation*. HLT-2001, San Diego.

Pentland, A. S. (2005). Socially aware computation and communication. *Computer*, *38*, 33–40. doi:10.1109/MC.2005.104

Petrelli, D., De Angeli, A., Gerbino, W., & Cassano, G. (1997). Referring in multimodal systems: The importance of user expertise and system features. *Proc. ACL-EACL*, (pp. 14-19).

Pfleger, N. (2007). *Context-based multimodal interpretation: An integrated approach to multimodal fusion and discourse processing*. PhD Thesis, University of the Saarland, Germany.

Pfleger, N., Alexandersson, J., & Becker, T. (2002). Scoring functions for overlay and their application in discourse processing. *Proc. of KONVENS*.

Pianta, E., Girardi, C., & Zanoli, R. (2008). The TextPro tool suite. In N. Calzolari, K. Choukri, B. Maegaard, J. Mariani, J. Odjik, S. Piperidis & D. Tapias (Eds.) *Proceedings of the Sixth International Language Resources and Evaluation (LREC '08)*. Retrieved from http://www.lrec-conf.org/proceedings/lrec2008/.

Picard, R. W. (1997). *Affective computing*. Boston, MA: The MIT Press.

Picard, R. (2003). What does it mean for a computer to have emotions? In Trappl, P. P. R., & Payr, S. (Eds.), *Emotions in humans and artifacts*. Citeseer.

Pieraccini, R., & Huerta, J. M. (2008). Where do we go from here? Research and commercial spoken dialogue systems . In Dybkjaer, L., & Minker, W. (Eds.), *Recent trends in discourse and dialogue*. Springer.

Pietquin, O., & Dutoit, T. (2005). A probabilistic framework for dialogue simulation and optimal strategy learning. *IEEE Transactions on Speech and Audio Processing, Special Issue on Data Mining of Speech . Audio and Dialog*, *14*, 589–599.

Pintrich, P. R. (2000). The role of goal orientation in self regulated learning . In Boekaerts, M., Pintrich, P. R., & Zeinder, M. (Eds.), *Handbook of self-regulation* (pp. 451–502). San Diego, CA: Academic Press. doi:10.1016/B978-012109890-2/50043-3

Piramuthu, S. (2005). Knowledge-based Web-enabled agents and intelligent tutoring systems. *IEEE Transactions on Education*, *48*(4), 750–757. doi:10.1109/TE.2005.854574

Pirrone, R., Cannella, V., Gambino, O., Pipitone, A., & Russo, G. (2009). *Wikiart: An ontology-based information retrieval system for arts*. Intelligent Systems Design and Applications Conference,(pp. 913–918).

Pirrone, R., Cannella, V., & Russo, G. (2008). *GAIML: A new language for verbal and graphical interaction in Chatbots.* In Complex, Intelligent and Software Intensive Systems Conference, (pp. 715–720).

Pitt, I., & Edwards, A. (2003). *Design of speech-based devices: A practical guide*. Springer.

Plant, E. A., Baylor, A. L., Doerr, C., & Rosenberg-Kima, R. (2009). Changing middle-school students' attitudes and performance regarding engineering with computer-based social models. *Computers & Education*, *53*, 209–215. doi:10.1016/j.compedu.2009.01.013

Poesio, M. (2000). Semantic analysis . In Dale, R., Moisl, H., & Somers, H. (Eds.), *Handbook of natural language processing*. New York, NY: Marcel Dekker.

Poesio, M., & Mikheev, A. (1998). The predictive power of game structure in dialogue act recognition: Experimental results using maximum entropy estimation. In *Proceedings of ICSLP-98*, Sydney.

Poggi, I., Pelachaud, C., & De Rosis, F. (2000). Eye communication in a conversational 3d synthetic agent. *AI Communications*, *13*, 169–181.

Poggi, I., Pelachaud, C., de Rosis, F., Carofiglio, V., & De Carolis, B. (2005). GRETA: A believable embodied conversational agent . In Stock, O., & Zancanaro, M. (Eds.), *Multimodal intelligent information presentation* (pp. 1–23). New York, NY: Kluwer. doi:10.1007/1-4020-3051-7_1

Polhemus, L., Shih, L.-F., & Swan, K. (2001). *Virtual interactivity: The representation of social presence in an online discussion*. Annual Meeting of the American Educational Research Association.

Pollard, C., & Sag, I. A. (1994). *Head-driven phrase structure grammar. Studies in Contemporary Linguistics*. Chicago, IL: University of Chicago Press.

Porta, J. M., Vlassis, N., Spaan, M. T. J., & Poupart, P. (2006). Point-based value iteration for continuous POMDPS. *Journal of Machine Learning Research*, *7*, 2329–2367.

Potamianos, A., Ammicht, E., & Fosler-Lussier, E. (2003). Modality tracking in the Multimodal Bell Labs Communicator. *Proc. of IEEE Workshop on Automatic Speech Recognition and Understanding (ASRU)*, (pp. 192-197).

Prince Market Research. (2007). *Aging in place in America.* Retrieved from http://clarityproducts.com/press-news/

Puerta, A. (1996). The Mecano project: Comprehensive and integrated support for model-based interface development . In *Computer-aided design of user interfaces* (pp. 5–7). Namur University Press.

Puerta, A., & Eisenstein, A. (2001). XIML: A common representation for interaction data. In *Proceedings Intelligent User Interfaces Conference*, (pp. 214–215). ACM.

Pulman, S. (2002). Relating dialogue games to information state. *Speech Communication*, *36*, 15–30. doi:10.1016/S0167-6393(01)00023-1

Putnam, C., & Chong, L. (2008). Software and technologies designed for people with autism: What do users want? In *Proceedings of the 10th International ACM SIGACCESS Conference on Computers and Accessibility* (pp. 3-10). Halifax, Canada: ACM Press.

Quan, L., Yu-ying, J., & Jing, C. (2008). Uimwiki: An enhanced semantic wiki for user information management. In *IT in medicine and education*, (pp. 930–934). IEEE.

Quarteroni, S., & Manandhar, S. (2009). Designing an interactive open domain question answering system. *Natural Language Engineering*, 73–95. doi:10.1017/S1351324908004919

Quarteroni, S., & Saint-Dizier, P. (2009). *Addressing how-to questions using a spoken dialogue system: A viable approach?* Singapore: KRAQ'09.

Rabiner, L. R., & Juang, B. H. (1993). *Fundamentals of speech recognition*. Prentice-Hall.

Rabiner, L. (1990). A tutorial on hidden Markov models and selected applications in speech recognition . In Waibel, A., & Lee, K. (Eds.), *Readings in speech recognition* (pp. 267–296). San Francisco, CA: Morgan Kaufmann Publishers.

Raij, A. B., Johnsen, K., Dickerson, R. F., Lok, B. C., Cohen, M. S., & Duerson, M. (2007). Comparing interpersonal interactions with a virtual human to those with a real human. *IEEE Transactions on Visualization and Computer Graphics*, *13*, 443–457.

Rao, A. S., & Georgeff, M. P. (1991). Modeling rational agents within a BDI-architecture. In J. F. Allen, R. Fikes, & E. Sandewall (Eds.), *Proceedings of the 2nd International Conference on Principles of Knowledge Representation and Reasoning* (pp. 473-484). San Mateo, CA: Morgan Kaufmann Publishers Inc.

Rapin, I., & Tuchman, R. F. (2008). Autism: Definition, neurobiology, screening, diagnosis. *Pediatric Clinics of North America*, *55*(5), 1129–1146. doi:10.1016/j.pcl.2008.07.005

Raux, A., & Eskenazi, M. (2007). A multi-layer architecture for semi-synchronous event-driven dialogue management. *Proc. of ASRU*.

Rec, I. T. U.-T. (2003). *Subjective quality evaluation of telephone services based on spoken dialogue systems (International Recommendation)* (p. 851). International Telecommunication Union.

Reeves, B., & Nass, C. (2003). *The media equation: How people treat computers, television, and new media like real people and places (CSLI Lecture Notes)*. Center for the Study of Language and Inf.

Reiter, E., & Dale, R. (2000). *Building applied natural language generation systems*. Cambridge, UK: University Press. doi:10.1017/CBO9780511519857

Reithinger, N., & Klesen, M. (1997). Dialogue act classification using language models. In . *Proceedings of EuroSpeech*, *97*, 2235–2238.

Reithinger, N., & Sonntag, D. (2005). *An integration framework for a mobile multimodal dialogue system accessing the Semantic Web* (pp. 841–844). Proc. of Interspeech.

Resick, P. A., & Nishith, P. (1997). Sexual assault . In Davis, R. C., Lurigio, A. J., & Skogan, W. G. (Eds.), *Victims of crime* (2nd ed., pp. 27–52). Thousand Oaks, CA: Sage Publications, Inc.

Riccardi, G., Gorin, A. L., Ljolje, A., & Riley, M. (1997). A spoken language system for automated call routing. In . *Proceedings of ICASSP*, *1997*, 1143–1146.

Rich, C., & Sidner, C. L. (1998). COLLAGEN: A collaboration manager for software interface agents. *An International Journal: User Modeling and User-Adapted Interaction*, *8*(3/4), 315–350. doi:10.1023/A:1008204020038

Rickel, J. W. (1989). Intelligent computer-aided instruction: A survey organized around system components. *IEEE Transactions on Systems, Man, and Cybernetics*, *19*(1), 40–57. doi:10.1109/21.24530

Rickel, J., Lesh, N., Rich, C., Sidner, C., & Gertner, A. (2001). *Building a bridge between intelligent tutoring and collaborative dialogue systems.* Paper presented at Tenth International Conference on AI in Education (pp. 592-594), San Antonio, Texas.

Riedl, M. O., & Stern, A. (2006). Failing believably: Toward drama management with autonomous actors in interactive narratives. In *Proceedings of the 3rd International Conference on Technologies for Interactive Digital Storytelling and Entertainment*, (pp. 195-206), Darmstadt, Germany.

Riva, G., Mantovani, F., & Gaggioli, A. (2004). Presence and rehabilitation: Toward second-generation virtual reality applications in neuropsychology. *Journal of Neuroengineering and Rehabilitation*, *1*(9).

Roesch, E. B., Banziger, T., & Scherer, K. R. (2005). *D3e – proposal for exemplars and work towards it: Theories and models*. (HUMAINE, Human-Machine Interaction Network on Emotions, IST-FP6 Contract No 507422). Retrieved from http://emotion-research.net/projects/humaine/deliverables/D3e%20final.pdf

Roque, A., & Traum, D. (2007). *A model of compliance and emotion for potentially adversarial dialogue agents.* Paper presented at the the 8th SIGdial Workshop on Discourse and Dialogue, Antwerp, Belgium.

Rose, C. P., Jordan, P., Ringenberg, M., Siler, S., VanLehn, K., & Weinstein, A. (2001). *Interactive conceptual tutoring in Atlas-Andes*. Paper presented at the AI in Education 2001.

Rosenfeld, R. (1995). The CMU statistical language modeling toolkit and its use in the 1994 ARPA CSR evaluation. *Proc. of ARPA Spoken Language Systems Technology Workshop*.

Rosis, F. d., Pelachaud, C., Poggi, I., Carofiglio, V., & Carolis, B. D. (2003). From Greta's mind to her face: Modelling the dynamics of affective states in a conversational embodied agent. *International Journal of Human-Computer Studies*, *59*, 81–118. doi:10.1016/S1071-5819(03)00020-X

Rubin, J., & Chisnell, D. (2008). *Handbook of usability testing, 2nd edition: How to plan, design, and conduct effective tests*. Wiley Publishing, Inc.

Ruderícha, F., Baucha, M., Haaga, M., Heida, J., Levena, F. J., Singera, R., … Tönshoffd, B., (2004). CAMPUS – a flexible, interactive system for Web-based, problem-based learning in healthcare. *International Journal of Medial Information*, IOS Press.

Rudnicky, A. I., Thayer, E., Constantinides, P., Tchou, C., Shern, R., Lenzo, K., et al. Oh, A. (1999). *Creating natural dialogs in the Carnegie Mellon Communicator System.* EUROSPEECH'99, Sixth European Conference on Speech Communication and Technology (pp. 1531-1534). ISCA.

Russo, G., Gentile, A., Pirrone, R., & Cannella, V. (2009). *XML-based knOWLedge discovery for the linguistic atlas of Sicily (ALS) project*. In Complex, Intelligent and Software Intensive Systems, International Conference, (pp. 98–104).

Ruttkay, Z., & Pelachaud, C. (Eds.). (2004). *From brows to trust: Evaluating embodied conversational agents*. Dordrecht, The Netherlands & London, UK: Kluwer.

Ryu, J., & Baylor, A. L. (2005). The psychometric structure of pedagogical agent persona. *Technology, Instruction . Cognition & Learning*, *2*(4), 291–319.

Sacks, H., Schegloff, E. A., & Jefferson, G. (1974). A simplest systematics for the organization of turn-taking for conversation. *Language*, *50*(4), 696–735. doi:10.2307/412243

Sagae, A., Johnson, W. L., & Bodnar, S. (2010). *Validation of a dialog system for language learners.* Paper presented at the The 11th annual SIGdial Meeting on Discourse and Dialogue, Tokyo, Japan.

Sagae, A., Wetzel, B., Valente, A., & Johnson, W. L. (2009). *Culture-driven response strategies for virtual human behavior in training systems.* Paper presented at the SLaTE-2009, Warwickshire, England.

Salber, D., & Coutaz, J. (1993). Applying the Wizard of Oz technique to the study of multimodal systems. *Proc. of EWHCI*, (pp. 219-230).

Samsonovich, A. V., Kitsantas, K. D. J., Peters, E. E., Dabbagh, N., & Kalbfleisch, M. (2008). Cognitive constructor: An intelligent tutoring system based on a biologically inspired cognitive architecture (BICA). Artificial General Intelligence 2008: Proceedings of the First AGI Conference. *Frontiers in Artificial Intelligence and Applications, 171*(1), 311–325.

Samtani, P., Valente, A., & Johnson, W. (2008). *Applying the SAIBA framework to the tactical language and culture training system*. Paper presented at Why Conversational Agents do what they do. Functional Representations for Generating Conversational Agent Behavior. AAMAS 2008.

Samuel, K., Carberry, S., & Vijay-Shanker, K. (1998). Dialogue act tagging with transformation-based learning. In *Proceedings of the 17th International Conference on Computational Linguistics*, Morristown, NJ, USA, (pp. 1150–1156). Association for Computational Linguistics.

San Segundo, R. (2004). *La evaluación objetiva de sistemas de diálogo. Proc of. Curso de Tecnologías Lingüísticas*. Fundación Duques de Soria.

San Segundo, R., Montero, J., Ferreiros, J., Córdoba, R., & Pardo, J. (2001). Designing confirmation mechanisms and error recover techniques in a railway information system for spanish. In *Proceedings of the Second SIGdial Workshop on Discourse and Dialogue, vol. 16* (pp. 136-139). Association for Computational Linguistics.

Santangelo, A., Augello, A., Gentile, A., Pilato, G., & Gaglio, S. A. (2006). *Chat-Bot based multimodal virtual guide for cultural heritage tours*. Retrieved from http://ww1.ucmss.com/books/LFS/CSREA2006/PSC4614.pdf

Schatzmann, J., Weilhammer, K., Stuttle, M., & Young, S. (2006). A survey of statistical user simulation techniques for reinforcement-learning of dialogue management strategies. *The Knowledge Engineering Review*, *21*(2), 97–126. doi:10.1017/S0269888906000944

Schatzmann, J., & Young, S. (2009). The hidden agenda user simulation model. *IEEE Trans. Audio . Speech and Language Processing*, *17*(4), 733–747. doi:10.1109/TASL.2008.2012071

Schaumburg, H. (2001). Computers as tools or as social actors? The users' perspective on anthropomorphic agents. *International Journal of Cooperative Information Systems*, *10*(1-2), 217–234. doi:10.1142/S0218843001000321

Scheffler, T., Roller, R., & Reithinger, N. (2009). SpeechEval – evaluating spoken dialog systems by user simulation. In A. Jönsson, et al. (Eds.), *Proceedings of the 6th IJCAI Workshop on Knowledge and Reasoning in Practical Dialogue Systems*, (pp. 93-98). Pasadena, CA, USA.

Scherer, S., Schwenker, F., & Palm, G. (2008). Emotion recognition from speech using multi-classifier systems and rbf-ensembles. *Speech, Audio, Image and Biomedical Signal Processing using Neural Networks*, 49–70. Berlin, Germany: Springer.

Schiel, F., & Türk, U. (2006). Wizard-of-Oz recordings . In Wahlster, W. (Ed.), *SmartKom: Foundations of multimodal dialogue systems* (pp. 541–570). Berlin, Germany: Springer. doi:10.1007/3-540-36678-4_34

Schröder, M., & Trouvain, J. (2003). The German text-to-speech synthesis system MARY: A tool for research, development and teaching. *International Journal of Speech Technology*, *6*, 365–377. doi:10.1023/A:1025708916924

Schunk, D. H. (1981). Modeling and attributional effects on children's achievement: A self-efficacy analysis. *Journal of Educational Psychology*, *73*, 93–105. doi:10.1037/0022-0663.73.1.93

Schunk, D. H., Hanson, A. R., & Cox, P. D. (1987). Peer model attributes and children's achievement behaviours. *Journal of Educational Psychology*, *79*, 54–61. doi:10.1037/0022-0663.79.1.54

Schutz, A. (1970). Alfred Schutz on phenomenology and social relations . In Wagner, H. R. (Ed.), *Selected writings*. Chicago, IL: University of Chicago Press.

Schwarz, N. (1999). Self-reports: How the questions shape the answers. *The American Psychologist*, *54*, 93–105. doi:10.1037/0003-066X.54.2.93

Searle, J. R. (1969). *Speech acts: An essay in the philosophy of language*. Cambridge, UK: University Press.

Semantic Media. (n.d.). *Wiki*. Retrieved from http://semanticweb.org/wiki/SemanticMediaWiki

Seneff, S. (1989). TINA: A probabilistic syntactic parser for speech understanding systems. *Proc. of ACL Workshop on Speech and Natural Language*, (pp. 168-178).

Seneff, S., Hurley, E., Lau, R., Pao, C., Schmid, P., & Zue, V. (1998). GALAXYII: A reference architecture for conversational system development. In *Proceedings of International Conference on Spoken Language Processing*, ICSLP'98, 3, Sydney, Australia, December 1998 (pp. 931-934).

Seron, F., Baldassarri, S., & Cerezo, E. (2006). MaxinePPT: Using 3D virtual characters for natural interaction. *Proc. of 2nd International Workshop on Ubiquitous Computing and Ambient Intelligence*, (pp. 241-250).

Sethy, A., Georgiou, P., & Narayanan, S. (2005). Building topic specific language models from Web data using competitive models. *Proceedings of EUROSPEECH*, Lisbon, Portugal.

Shawar, B. A., & Atwell, E. S. (2007). Chatbots: Are they really useful? *LDV-Forum*, *22*, 31–50.

Shelley, M. (1831). *Frankenstein* (Smith, J. M., Ed.). Boston, MA: St. Martin's.

Shriberg, E. (1994). *Preliminaries to a theory of speech disfluencies*. PhD thesis, University of California, Berkeley, CA.

Sidner, C. (2004). Building spoken-language collaborative interface agents . In Dahl, D. (Ed.), *Practical spoken dialogue systems*. Kluwer Academic Publishers. doi:10.1007/978-1-4020-2676-8_10

Sidner, C. L., & Lee, C. (2003). *An architecture for engagement in collaborative conversations between a robot and humans*. (MERL Technical Report, TR2003-12), June 2003.

Silver, M., & Oakes, P. (2001). Evaluation of a new computer intervention to teach people with autism or Asperger Syndrome to recognize and predict emotions in others. *Autism*, *5*(3), 299–316. doi:10.1177/1362361301005003007

Silverman, B. G., Johns, M., Weaver, R., O'Brien, K., & Silverman, R. (2002). Human behavior models for game-theoretic agents. *Cognitive Science Quarterly*, *2*(3-4), 273–301.

Simmons, R. (1965). Answering English questions by computer: A survey. *Communications of the ACM*, *8*(1), 53–70. doi:10.1145/363707.363732

Sinclair, J. M., & Coulthard, R. M. (1975). *Towards an analysis of discourse: The English used by teachers and pupils*. Oxford University Press.

Singular Inversions. (2009). *FaceGen SDK 3.6*. Retrieved from http://www.facegen.com

Small, S., Liu, T., Shimizu, N., & Strzalkowski, T. (2003). HITIQA: An interactive question answering system- a preliminary report. *Proceedings of the ACL 2003 Workshop on Multilingual summarization and QA* (pp. 46–53). Morristown, NJ: ACL.

Smith, R. W. (1992). Integration of domain problem solving with natural language dialog: The missing axiom theory . In *Proceedings of Applications of AI X* (pp. 270–278). Knowledge-Based Systems.

Smith, C. A., & Lazarus, R. (1990). Emotion and adaptation . In Pervin, L. A. (Ed.), *Handbook of personality: Theory & research* (pp. 609–637). New York, NY: Guilford Press.

Soller, A. (2004). Computational modeling and analysis of knowledge sharing in collaborative distance learning. *User Modeling and User-Adapted Interaction*, *14*, 351–381. doi:10.1023/B:USER.0000043436.49168.3b

Spiliotopoulos, D., Stavropoulou, P., & Kouroupetroglou, G. (2009). Spoken dialogue interfaces: Integrating usability. *Lecture Notes in Computer Science*, *5889*, 484–499. doi:10.1007/978-3-642-10308-7_36

Spiliotopoulos, D., & Kouroupetroglou, G. (2010). Usability methodologies for spoken dialogue Web interfaces . In Spiliotopoulos, T., Papadopoulou, P., Martakos, D., & Kouroupetroglou, G. (Eds.), *Integrating usability engineering for designing the Web experience: Methodologies and principles*. Hershey, PA: IGI Global. doi:10.4018/978-1-60566-896-3.ch008

Stavropoulou, P., Spiliotopoulos, D., & Kouroupetroglou, G. (2011). *Resource evaluation for usable spoken dialogue interfaces: Utilizing human – human dialogues*. In preparation.

Steedman, M. (2001). *The syntactic process*. Cambridge, MA: The MIT Press.

Steininger, S., Rabold, S., Dioubina, O., & Schiel, F. (2002). Development of the user-state conventions for the multimodal corpus in SmartKom. *Proc. of 3rd International Conference on Language Resources and Evaluation*.

Stent, A. (2002). A conversation acts model for generating spoken dialogue contributions. *Computer Speech & Language*, *16*, 313–352. doi:10.1016/S0885-2308(02)00009-8

Stent, A., Dowding, J., Gawron, J. M., Bratt, E., & Moore, R. (1999). The CommandTalk spoken dialogue system. *Proc. of 37th Annual Meeting of the ACL*, (pp. 183-190).

Stent, A., Dowding, J., Gawron, J. M., Bratt, E. O., & Moore, R. (1999). The CommandTalk spoken dialogue system. In *Proceedings of the Thirty-Seventh Annual Meeting of the ACL*, (pp. 183-190).

Stevens, A., Hernandex, J., Johnsen, K., Dickerson, R., Raij, A., & Harrison, C. (2005). The use of virtual patients to teach medical students communication skills. *American Journal of Surgery*, *191*(6), 806–811. doi:10.1016/j.amjsurg.2006.03.002

Stiff, J. B., & Mongeau, P. A. (2002). *Persuasive communication* (2nd ed.).

Stolcke, A., Coccaro, N., Bates, R., Taylor, P., Ess-Dykema, C. V., Ries, K., & Meteer, M. (2000). Dialogue act modeling for automatic tagging and recognition of conversational speech. *Computational Linguistics*, *26*, 339–373. doi:10.1162/089120100561737

Straker, D. (2008). Using body language. *Changing Minds*. Retrieved 10 July, 2009, from http://changingminds.org/techniques/body/body_language.htm

Sumby, W. H., & Pollack, L. (1956). Visual contribution to speech intelligibility in noise. *The Journal of the Acoustical Society of America*, *26*(2), 212–215. doi:10.1121/1.1907309

Surface, E. A., Dierdorff, E. C., & Watson, A. M. (2007). *Special operations language training software measurement of effectivenss study: Tactical Iraqi study final report*. SWA Consulting.

Sutton, S. (1998). Universal speech tools: The CSLU toolkit. *Proceedings of the International Conference on Spoken Language Processing (ICSLP'98)*.

Swartout, W. R., Gratch, J., Hill, R. W., Hovy, E., Marsella, S., Rickel, J., & Traum, D. R. (2006). Toward virtual humans. *AI Magazine*, *27*(2), 96–108.

Swartz, L. (2003). *Why people hate the paperclip: Labels, appearance, behavior, and social responses to user interface agents*. Honor's Thesis, Stanford University, CA.

Takeuchi, A., & Nagao, K. (1995). Situated facial displays: Towards social interaction. *Proc. of SIGCHI*, (pp. 450-454).

Tartaro, A., & Cassell, J. (2006). *Authorable virtual peers for autism spectrum disorders*. Paper presented at the Combined Workshop on Language-Enabled Educational Technology and Development and Evaluation of Robust Spoken Dialogue Systems at the 17th European Conference on Artificial Intelligence (ECAI06), Riva del Garda, Italy.

Tartaro, A., & Cassell, J. (2008). Playing with virtual peers: Bootstrapping contingent discourse in children with autism. In *Proceedings of International Conference of the Learning Sciences, vol. 2*. International Society of the Learning Sciences.

Tekalp, M. A., & Ostermann, J. (2000). *Face and 2-D mesh animation in MPEG-4. Image Communication Journal, Tutorial Issue on MPEG-4 Standard*. Elsevier.

Tellegen, A., & Atkinson, G. (1974). Openness to absorbing and self-altering experiences ("absorption"), a trait related to hypnotic susceptibility. *Journal of Abnormal Psychology*, *83*, 268–277. doi:10.1037/h0036681

ter Maat, M., & Heylen, D. (2009). Turn management or impression management? In *Proceedings of 9th International Conference on Intelligent Virtual Agents, IVA 2009* (pp. 467-473). Berlin/Heidelberg, Germany: Springer.

The Design-Based Research Collective. (2003). Design-based research: An emerging paradigm for educational inquiry. *Educational Researcher*, *32*(1), 5–8. doi:10.3102/0013189X032001005

Theune, M., Hofs, D., & Van Kessel, M. (2007). The virtual guide: A direction giving embodied conversational agent. In *Proceedings of the 8th Annual Conference of the International Speech Communication Association (Interspeech 2007)* (pp. 2197-2200). International Speech Communication Association (ISCA).

Thiebaux, M., Marshall, A., Marsella, S., & Kallmann, M. (2008). *SmartBody: Behavior realization for embodied conversational agents*. International Conference on Autonomous Agents and Multi-Agent Systems. Portugal.

Tian, Y., Kanade, T., & Cohn, J. (2003). Facial expression analysis . In Li, S. Z., & Jain, A. K. (Eds.), *Handbook of face recognition*.

Traum, D. R. (2000). 20 questions on dialogue act taxonomies. *Journal of Semantics*, *17*(1), 7–30. doi:10.1093/jos/17.1.7

Traum, D. R., & Hinkelman, E. A. (1992). Conversation acts in task-oriented spoken dialogue. *Computational Intelligence*, *8*(3), 575–599. doi:10.1111/j.1467-8640.1992.tb00380.x

Traum, D. R. (2004). Issues in multi-party dialogues . In Dignum, F. (Ed.), *Advances in agent communication* (pp. 201–211). Berlin, Germany: Springer. doi:10.1007/978-3-540-24608-4_12

Traum, D. R., Swartout, W., Gratch, J., & Marsella, S. (2008). A virtual human dialogue model for non-team interaction . In Dybkjaer, L., & Minker, W. (Eds.), *Recent trends in discourse and dialogue* (pp. 45–67). New York, NY: Springer. doi:10.1007/978-1-4020-6821-8_3

Traum, D. (1996). Conversational agency: TRAINS-93 dialogue manager. *Proceedings of the Twente Workshop on Language Technology: Dialogue Management in Natural Language Systems (TWLT 11)*, (pp. 1-11).

Traum, D. R., & Larsson, S. (2003). The information state approach to dialogue management. In Smith & Kuppevelt (Eds.), *Current and new directions in discourse & dialogue* (pp. 325–353). Dordrecht, The Netherlands: Kluwer.

Traum, D., & Marsella, S. Gratch, J., Lee, J., Hartholt, A. (2008). Multi-party, multi-issue, multi-strategy negotiation for multi-modal virtual agents. 8th International Conference on Intelligent Virtual Agents. Tokyo, Japan: Springer.

Triola, M., & Feldman, M. (2006). A randomized trial of teaching clinical skills using virtual and live standardized patients. *Journal of General Internal Medicine*, *21*, 424–429. doi:10.1111/j.1525-1497.2006.00421.x

Tsutsui, T., Saeyor, S., & Ishizuka, M. (2000). *MPML: A multimodal presentation markup language with character agent control functions* (pp. 537–543). Proc. of WebNet.

Turunen, M. (2004). *Jaspis - a spoken dialogue architecture and its applications*. Ph.D. Dissertation, University of Tampere, Department of Computer Sciences A-2004-2.

Turunen, M., Hakulinen, J., & Kainulainen, A. (2006). Evaluation of a spoken dialogue system with usability tests and long-term pilot studies: Similarities and differences. In *Proceedings of Interspeech*.

Twitchell, D. P., Adkins, M., Nunamaker, J. F., & Burgoon, J. K. (2004). *Proceedings of the 9th International Working Conference on the Language-Action perspective on Communication Modelling* (pp. 121-130).

Valente, A., Johnson, W. L., Wertheim, S., Barrett, K., Flowers, M., & LaBore, K. (2009). *A dynamic methodology for developing situated culture training content. Alelo TLT*. LLC.

Van de Burgt, S. P., Andernach, T., Kloosterman, H., Bos, R., & Nijholt, A. (1996). Building dialogue systems that sell. *Proc. NLP and Industrial Applications*, (pp. 41-46).

van Deemter, K., Krenn, B., Piwek, P., Klesen, M., Schröder, M., & Baumann, S. (2008). Fully generated scripted dialogue for embodied agents. *Artificial Intelligence*, *172*(10), 1219–1244. doi:10.1016/j.artint.2008.02.002

Van Mulken, S., André, E., & Müller, J. (1998). The persona effect: How substantial is it? In H. Johnson, L. Nigay, & C. Roast (Eds.), *People and Computers XIII: Proceedings of HCI'98* (pp. 53-66). Berlin, Germany: Springer.

VanLehn, K., Graesser, A., Jackson, G. T., Jordan, P., Olney, A., & Rosé, C. P. (2007). Natural language tutoring: A comparison of human tutors, computer tutors, and text. *Cognitive Science*, *31*(1), 3–52. doi:10.1080/03640210709336984

Vapnik, V. (1995). *The nature of statistical learning theory*. Springer-Verlag.

Velásquez, J. (1998). *When robots weep: Emotional memories and decision-making*. Presented at Fifteenth National Conference on Artificial Intelligence, Madison, WI, 1998.

Veletsianos, G. (2007). Cognitive and affective benefits of an animated pedagogical agent: Considering contextual relevance and aesthetics. *Journal of Educational Computing Research*, *36*(4), 373–377. doi:10.2190/T543-742X-033L-9877

Veletsianos, G. (2009). The impact and implications of virtual character expressiveness on learning and agent-learner interactions. *Journal of Computer Assisted Learning, 25*(4), 345–357. doi:10.1111/j.1365-2729.2009.00317.x

Veletsianos, G. (2010). Contextually relevant pedagogical agents: Visual appearance, stereotypes, and first impressions and their impact on learning. *Computers & Education, 55*(2), 576–585. doi:10.1016/j.compedu.2010.02.019

Veletsianos, G., & Miller, C. (2008). Conversing with pedagogical agents: A phenomenological exploration of interacting with digital entities. *British Journal of Educational Technology, 39*(6), 969–986. doi:10.1111/j.1467-8535.2007.00797.x

Veletsianos, G., Scharber, C., & Doering, A. (2008). When sex, drugs, and violence enter the classroom: Conversations between adolescent social studies students and a female pedagogical agent. *Interacting with Computers, 20*(3), 292–302. doi:10.1016/j.intcom.2008.02.007

Veletsianos, G., Miller, C., & Doering, A. (2009). EnALI: A research and design framework for virtual characters and pedagogical agents. *Journal of Educational Computing Research, 41*(2), 171–194. doi:10.2190/EC.41.2.c

Venkataraman, A., Liu, Y., Shriberg, E., & Stolcke, A. (2005). Does active learning help automatic dialog act tagging in meeting data? In *Proceedings of EUROSPEECH-05*, Lisbon, Portugal.

Vilhjalmsson, H., & Marsella, S. (2005). *Social performance framework.* Paper presented at the the AAAI Workshop on Modular Construction of Human-Like Intelligence.

Volkel, M., Krotzsch, M., Vrandecic, D., Haller, H., & Studer, R. (2006). Semantic Wikipedia. In *WWW '06: Proceedings of the 15th International conference on World Wide Web*, (pp. 585–594). New York, NY: ACM.

Vrajitoru, D. (2003). *Evolutionary sentence building for Chatterbots*. GECCO 2003 Late Breaking Papers, (pp. 315-321).

Wahlster, W. (2003). *SmartKom: Symmetric multimodality in an adaptive and reusable dialogue shell* (pp. 47–62). Proc. of Human Computer Interaction.

Wahlster, W. (2000). *Verbmobil: Foundations of speech-to-speech translation.* Berlin, Germany & New York, NY: Springer.

Wahlster, W. (2000) (Ed.). *Verbmobil: Foundations of speech-to-speech translation.* Berlin/Heidelberg, Germany; New York, NY; Barcelona, Spain; Hong Kong; London, UK; Milan, Italy; Paris, France; Singapore; Tokyo, Japan: Springer.

Wahlster, W. (2001). SmartKom: Multimodal dialogues with mobile Web users. *Proc. of International Cyber Assist Symposium*, (pp. 33-40).

Wahlster, W. (2006) (Ed.). *SmartKom - foundations of multimodal dialogue systems*. Berlin/Heidelberg, Germany; New York, NY; Barcelona, Spain; Hong Kong; London, UK; Milan, Italy; Paris, France; Singapore; Tokyo, Japan: Springer Cognitive Technologies.

Walker, M. A., Litman, D. J., Kamm, C. A., & Abella, A. (1998). Evaluating spoken dialogue agents with PARADISE: Two case studies. *Computer Speech & Language, 12*, 317–347. doi:10.1006/csla.1998.0110

Walker, J. H., Sproull, L., & Subramami, R. (1994). Using a human face in an interface. *Proc. of SIGCHI conference on human factors in computing systems*, (pp. 85-91).

Walker, M. A. Langkilde-Geary, I., Wright Hastie, H., Wright, J., & Gorin, A. (2002). Automatically training a problematic dialogue predictor for the HMIHY spoken dialogue system. *Journal of Artificial Intelligence Research (JAIR).*

Walker, M. A., Litman, D., Kamm, C., & Abella, A. (1997). PARADISE: A framework for evaluating spoken dialogue agents. In *Proceedings of the 35th Annual Meeting of the Association of Computational Linguistics* (ACL 97) (pp. 271-280). Morristown, NJ: ACL Press.

Walker, M. A., Passonneau, R., & Boland, J. E. (2001). Quantitative and qualitative evaluation of Darpa communicator spoken dialogue systems. In *Proceedings of the 39th Annual Meeting of the Association for Computational Linguistics* (ACL/EACL-2001) (pp. 515-522). Morgan Kaufmann Publishers.

Walker, W., Lamere, P., & Kwok., P. (2002). *FreeTTS: A performance case study*. Sun Microsystems, Inc.

Wallis, P., Mitchard, H., O'Dea, D., & Das, J. (2001). Dialogue modelling for a conversational agent. In Stumptner, Corbett, & Brooks, (Eds.), *Proceedings 14th Australian Joint Conference on Artificial Intelligence*, Adelaide, Australia.

Walsh, P., & Meade, J. (2003). Speech enabled e-learning for adult literacy tutoring. *Proc. of ICALT*, (pp. 17-21).

Walters, M., Dautenhahn, K., te Boekhorst, R., Koay, K., & Syrdal, D. (2009). An empirical framework for human-robot proxemics. In *Proc. AISB Convention* 2009. www.aisb.org.uk/convention/aisb09/.

Walton, D. (1996). *Argument structure: A pragmatic theory*. Toronto Studies in Philosophy.

Wang, F., & Hannafin, M. J. (2005). Design-based research and technology-enhanced learning environments. *Educational Technology Research and Development*, *53*(4), 5–23. doi:10.1007/BF02504682

Wang, N., Johnson, W. L., Mayer, R. E., Rizzo, P., Shaw, E., & Collins, H. (2008). The politeness effect: Pedagogical agents and learning outcomes. *International Journal of Human-Computer Studies*, *66*, 96–112. doi:10.1016/j.ijhcs.2007.09.003

Wang, A., Emmi, M., & Faloutsos, P. (2007). Assembling an expressive facial animation system. In *Proceedings of the ACM SIGGRAPH symposium on Video Games* (pp. 21-26). New York, NY: ACM Press.

Wang, Y., Acero, A., Chelba, C., Frey, B., & Wong, L. (2002). Combination of statistical and rule-based approaches for spoken language understanding. In *Proceedings of the International Conference on Spoken Language Processing*, Denver, CO.

Ward, W., & Issar, S. (1994). Recent improvements in the CMU spoken language understanding system. *Proc. of ACL Workshop on Human Language Technology* (pp. 213-216).

Warnke, V., Kompe, R., Niemann, H., & Noth, E. (1997). Integrated dialog act segmentation and classification using prosodic features and language models. In *Proceedings of 5th European Conference on Speech Communication and Technology, vol. 1*, Rhodes, Greece (pp. 207–210).

Wasinger, R., Stahl, C., & Krüger, A. (2003). *Robust speech interaction in a mobile environment through the use of multiple and different media types* (pp. 1049–1052). Proc. of Eurospeech.

Webb, N., & Strzalkowski, T. (2006). *Proceedings of the Interactive Question Answering Workshop at HLT-NAACL 2006*. New York, NY: The Association for Computational Linguistics.

Webb, N., Benyon, D., Hansen, P., & Mival, O. (2010). Wizard of Oz experiments for a companion dialogue system: Eliciting companionable conversation. In *Proceedings of the 7th International Conference on Language Resources and Evaluation (LREC2010)*, Valletta, Malta.

Webb, N., Liu, T., Hepple, M., & Wilks, Y. (2008). Cross domain dialogue act tagging. In *Proceedings of the Sixth International Conference on Language Resources and Evaluation (LREC-08)*. Marrakech, Morocco.

Weber, M. (1994). *Sociological writings*. New York, NY: Continuum.

Wei, X., & Rudnicky, A. (2000). Task-based dialogue management using an agenda. *Proceedings of ANLP/NAACL Workshop on Conversational Systems*, (pp. 42-47).

Weinschenk, S., & Barker, D. T. (2000). *Designing effective speech interfaces*. John Wiley & Sons, Inc.

Weiss, B., Kühnel, C., Wechsung, I., Fagel, S., & Möller, S. (2010). Quality of talking heads in different interaction and media contexts. *Speech Communication*, *52*(6), 481–492. doi:10.1016/j.specom.2010.02.011

Weizenbaum, J. (1966). ELIZA - A computer program for the study of natural language communication between man and machine. *Communications of the ACM*, *9*(1), 36–45. doi:10.1145/365153.365168

Wenger, E. (1987). *Artificial intelligence and tutoring systems: Computational and cognitive approaches to the communication of knowledge*. Los Altos, CA: Morgan Kaufmann.

White, M., Foster, M., Oberlander, J., & Brown, A. (2005). Using facial feedback to enhance turn-taking in a multimodal dialogue system. In *Proceedings of HCI International, vol. 2*. Lawrence Erlbaum Associates, Inc.

Wilks, Y. (2007). Has there been progress on talking sensibly to computers? *Science*, 318.

Wilks, Y. (Ed.). (2010). *Artificial companions in society: Scientific, economic, psychological and philosophical perspectives*. Amsterdam, The Netherlands: John Benjamins.

Wilks, Y., & Ballim, A. (1991). *Artificial believers*. Norwood, NJ: Erlbaum.

Wilks, Y. (2006). *Artificial companions as a new kind of interface to the future Internet*. Oxford Internet Institute Research report No. 13 (Oxford Internet Institute). Retrieved from http://www.oii.ox.ac.uk/research/publications.cfm

Wilks, Y. (2008). The Semantic Web and the apotheosis of annotation. In *Proc. IEEE Intelligent Systems*. (May/June)

Wilks, Y., Catizone, R., & Mival, O. (2008). The companions paradigm as a method for eliciting and organising life data. In *Proc. Workshop on Memories for Life, British Computer Society*, London, March.

Wilks, Y., Catizone, R., Worgan, S., Dingli, A., Moore, R. K., & Cheng, W. (2010). A prototype system for a conversational companion for reminiscing about images. *Computer Speech and Language*.

Williams, J., & Young, S. (2007). Partially observable Markov decision processes for spoken dialogue systems. *Computer Speech & Language*, *21*(2), 393–422. doi:10.1016/j.csl.2006.06.008

Williams, J. D., & Witt, S. M. (2004). A comparison of dialog strategies for call routing. [Springer Netherlands.]. *International Journal of Speech Technology*, 7.

Wilson, W. R. (1979). Feeling more than we can know: Exposure effects without learning. *Journal of Personality and Social Psychology*, *37*, 811–821. doi:10.1037/0022-3514.37.6.811

Witmer, B., & Singer, M. (1998). Measuring presence in virtual environments: A presence questionnaire. *Presence (Cambridge, Mass.)*, *7*(3), 225–240. doi:10.1162/105474698565686

Wolff, A. S., Bloom, C. P., Shahidi, A., Shahidi, K., & Rehder, R. E. (1998). Using quasi-experimentation to gather design information for intelligent tutoring systems. In *Facilitating the development and use of interactive learning environments*, (pp. 21-51).

Woo, H. L. (2009). Designing multimedia learning environments using animated pedagogical agents: Factors and issues. *Journal of Computer Assisted Learning*, *25*(3), 203–218. doi:10.1111/j.1365-2729.2008.00299.x

Woodruff, A., & Aoki, P. (2004). Conversation analysis and the user experience. *Digital Creativity*, *4*, 232–238. doi:10.1080/1462626048520184

Wright, H. (1998). Automatic utterance type detection using suprasegmental features. In *Proceedings of the International Conference on Spoken Language Processing (ICSLP-98)* (pp. 1403-1406). Sydney, Australia.

Wundt, W. (1913). *Grundriss der Psychologie*. Berlin, Germany: A. Kroner.

Xiao, J. (2006). *Empirical studies on embodied conversational agents. Unpublished doctoral disseration*. Georgia Institute of Technology.

Yang, F., Feng, Z., & Di Fabbrizio, G. (2006). A data driven approach to relevancy recognition for contextual question answering. *Proceedings of IQA*.

Yee, N., & Bailenson, J. N. (2007). The Proteus effect: The effect of transformed self-representation on behavior. *Human Communication Research*, *33*, 271–290. doi:10.1111/j.1468-2958.2007.00299.x

Yee, N., Bailenson, J. N., & Ducheneaut, N. (2009). The Proteus effect implications of transformed digital self-representation on online and offline behavior. *Communication Research*, *36*, 285–312. doi:10.1177/0093650208330254

Young, S., Gasic, M., Keizer, S., Mairesse, F., Schatzmann, J., Thomson, B., & Yu, K. (2009). The iidden information state model: A practical framework for POMDP-based spoken dialogue management. *Computer Speech & Language*, *24*(2), 150–174. doi:10.1016/j.csl.2009.04.001

Young, S., Adda-Decker, M., Aubert, X., Dugast, C., Gauvain, J., & Kershaw, D. (1997). Multilingual large vocabulary speech recognition: The European SQALE project. *Computer Speech & Language*, *11*, 73–89. doi:10.1006/csla.1996.0023

Young, S., Kershaw, D., Odell, J., Ollason, D., Valtchev, V., & Woodland, P. (2000). *The HTK book*. Microsoft Corporation.

Yu, C., Aoki, P. M., & Woodruff, A. (2004). Detecting user engagement in everyday conversations. In *Proceedings of the 8th International Conference on Spoken Language Processing (ICSLP '04)* (pp. 1–6).

Zapata, C. M., & Carmona, N. (2007). El experimento Mago de Oz y sus aplicaciones: una mirada retrospectiva. *Dyna rev.fac.nac.minas, 74*(151), 125-135.

Zhang, T., Hasegawa-Johnson, M., & Levinson, S. A. (2005). Hybrid model for spontaneous speech understanding. *Proc. of AAAI Workshop on Spoken Language Understanding*, (pp. 60-67).

Zhe, X., & Boucouvalas, A. (2002). *Text-to-emotion engine for real time Internet communication*. International Symposium on CSNDSP.

Zinn, C., Moore, J. D., & Core, M. G. (2002). A 3-tier planning architecture for managing tutorial dialogue. *ITS '02: Proceedings of the 6th International Conference on Intelligent Tutoring Systems*, (pp. 574-584).

Zitouni, I., Hong-Kwang, J. K., & Chin-Hui, L. (2003). Boosting and combination of classifiers for natural language call routing systems. *Speech Communication*, 14.

Zoric, G., Smid, K., & Pandzic, I. (2009). Towards facial gestures generation by speech signal analysis using HUGE architecture . In *Multimodal signals: Cognitive and algorithmic issues* (*Vol. 5398*, pp. 112–120). Berlin / Heidelberg, Germany: Springer. doi:10.1007/978-3-642-00525-1_11

Zue, V., Seneff, S., Glass, J., Polifroni, J., Pao, C., Hazen, T., & Hetherington, L. (2000). JUPITER: A telephone-based conversational interface for weather information. *IEEE Transactions on Speech and Audio Processing, 8*(1), 85–96. doi:10.1109/89.817460

Zue, V., Glass, J., Goddeau, D., Goodine, D., & Hirschman, L. (1992). The MIT ATIS system, In *Proc. DARPA Workshop on speech and natural language*, Harriman, NY.

Zukerman, I., & Litman, D. (2001). Natural language processing and user modeling: Synergies and limitations. *User Modeling and User-Adapted Interaction, 11*, 129–158. doi:10.1023/A:1011174108613

# About the Contributors

**Diana Pérez-Marín** received the Ph.D. degree in Computer Science and Engineering from the Universidad Autónoma de Madrid in 2007, and her degree in Computer Science by the Universidad Autónoma de Madrid in 2002. She is currently a lecturer and researcher at the Department of Computing Languages and Systems I of the Computer Science Faculty of the Universidad Rey Juan Carlos in Spain. Her PhD has been published in 2010 by VDM Verlag and it is available with ISBN 978-3639207200. She has published more than 40 papers in international journals such as Journal of Educational Technology and Society, or Computers and Education, and participated in eight national and international research projects. She has been awarded a prize to their novelty of the teaching possibilities of Internet in 2007 and as project leader in 2008. In 2010, she organized the First International Workshop on Adaptation and Personalization in E-B/Learning using Pedagogic Conversational Agents (APLeC) together with Dr. Ismael Pascual-Nieto and Dr. Susan Bull, collocated with the international conference User Modeling, Adaptation and Personalization (UMAP). Currently, she is also co-editor of a Special Issue on Automatic Free-text Evaluation in the International Journal of Continuing Engineering Education and Life-Long Learning (IJCEELL) to be published by Indescience at the end of 2010. She is member of the Artificial Intelligence in Education (AI-ED) Society, LEMORE, LITE, and ADIE.

**Ismael Pascual-Nieto** is Doctor in Computer Science and Telecommunications by the Universidad Autónoma de Madrid since 2009, and Computer Engineer by the Universidad Autonoma de Madrid since 2005. He has been a researcher at the Computer Science Department at the Universidad Autónoma de Madrid and at the ADENU Artificial Intelligence group at UNED in Spain. He has published numerous papers in journals, international, and national conferences, and participated in several international projects. He has been awarded a prize to the novelty of the teaching possibilities of Internet in 2007 and as an enterprising in 2008. In 2010, he organized together with Dr. Diana Pérez-Marín and Dr. Susan Bull the First International Workshop on Adaptation and Personalization in E-B/Learning using Pedagogic Conversational Agents (APLeC) collocated with the international conference User Modeling, Adaptation and Personalization (UMAP).

* * *

**Nieves Ábalos** is a M. S. and PhD student in Computer Science at University of Granada, Spain. She has also a B. S. in Computer Science from this University. Her research interests and activities have been related to speech technologies and include dialogue systems, multimodal systems, and ambient intelligence among others. She is currently participating in several research projects related to these areas.

**J. Gabriel Amores** received his MSc degree in Machine Translation from UMIST, UK in 1989, and a Ph.D. in English Linguistics from the University of Seville in 1992. He worked as a consultant for the Machine Translation Department at the Pan American Health Organization from 1990 to 1992. Since 1992 he has been with the Department of English Linguistics at the University of Seville, where he is currently a Senior Lecturer. His research interests include machine translation and dialogue systems, areas in which he has led numerous European and national research projects. He is also the co-founder of Indisys, a Spanish based software company specialised in developing Embodied Conversational Agents. He is a member of the Association for Computational Linguistics and the Spanish Society for Natural Language Processing (SEPLN).

**Pierre Andrews** is currently working as a researcher for the Knowdive group at the University of Trento, Italy. He received his MSc and BSc in Computer Engineering at the Swiss Federal Institute of Technology in Lausanne (EPFL) and holds a PhD in computer science from the University of York, UK. His research focus is on bringing artificial intelligence, in particular natural language processing, together with human computer interaction research to provide novel interaction paradigms. After work on dialogue interfaces for changing users' behaviour, he is now focusing on researching new interaction metaphors for the creation of semantic content.

**Zoraida Callejas** is Assistant Professor in the Department of Languages and Computer Systems at the Faculty of Computer Science and Telecommunications of the University of Granada (Spain). She completed a PhD in Computer Science at University of Granada in 2008 and has been a visiting researcher in University of Ulster (Belfast, UK), Technical University of Liberec (Liberec, Czech Republic), University of Trento (Trento, Italy), and Technical University of Berlin (Berlin, Germany). Her research activities have been mostly related to dialogue systems and in particular to study the role of emotion in such systems. Her results have been published in several international journals and conferences. She has participated in numerous research projects, and is a member of several research associations focused on speech processing and human-computer interaction.

**Vincenzo Cannella** was born in Palermo at November 26, 1974. He received his Degree in Computer Science Engineering, (110/110 cum laude) on April 16, 2003, at the Computer Engineering Faculty in the University of Palermo, with a thesis entitled "An system able to learn automatically image diagnosis rules." He obtained PhD in Computer Science at the Department of Computer Science and Engineering (DINFO) of Palermo on April 5, 2008. From July 2008, he is a post-doc at DINFO, and his research interests mainly include HCI, natural language processing, and intelligent retrieval of information.

**Roberta Catizone** has been working in the field of Natural Language Processing for the past 20 years. From 1994-2010, she was a Research Associate at the University Sheffield where she worked with the Natural Language Processing Group in the Computer Science Department, following research positions at the Computing Research Lab in New Mexico, the University of Pittsburgh Learning Research and Development Center and the Institut Dalle Molle in Geneva, Switzerland where she did research on Natural Language Tutorial systems, a multilingual concordance system, and a content-based text alignment system. While at the University of Sheffield, she has worked on four European Union Fourth, Fifth and Sixth framework projects funded by the Information Society and Technology (IST) sector including the ECRAN Information Extraction (IE) project (1995-1998) and the NAMIC IE and authoring project (1998-2001). Her most recent work in building Dialogue Systems included being Sheffield team leader of the multimodal dialogue project COMIC (2002 - 2005) and the EU-funded Companions project which is made up of a consortium of 14 academic and industrial organisations across Europe and the USA. Companions, a 4-year, large-scale multimodal dialogue project, focused on intelligent personalized multimodal interfaces to the Internet. She also played a key part in the development of the CONVERSE program which won the Loebner competition judged for being the most realistic conversationalist in 1997.

**Emmett Coin** (CEO of ejTalk, Inc) describes himself as an Industrial Poet dedicated to creating elegant, efficient, and robust software systems. For the last fifteen years, he has been actively involved with developing human-computer conversation systems creating, exploring, and evangelizing methods that permit computers to carry on real-time intelligent and natural conversations with humans. This work has origins in studies and research he did in 1969 at MIT. As the Principal at ejTalk, Mr. Coin has developed a next generation conversation management engine (ejTalker). The ejTalker system is a core personality with attendant behaviors upon which specific application functionality is layered. Using ejTalker, it becomes much easier to create applications since only "specific" application functions are needed. It automatically presents the user with a consistent and familiar interface that the user already "knows" and is comfortable with. See www.ejTalk.com for more detail. As Speech Scientist at Lucas Systems Mr. Coin architected a wearable platform for voice-based warehouse picking (an extremely demanding acoustic and physical environment). He led the research and development to implement a hardware and speech technology vendor-agnostic, multi-modal input based on a subset of the ejTalker conversation management system. Mr. Coin directed the delivery of the first 5 applications, and the system continues to be extended and enhanced by the Production Engineering Group. Mr. Coin participates in various speech industry organizations such as VoiceXML Tools Committee (previous), AVIOS, SpeechTEK, Workshop on Human Computer Conversation, and others.

**Deborah Dahl** is currently the Principal at Conversational Technologies, a consulting company she founded in 2002. Dr. Dahl has over twenty-five years of experience in speech and language technologies. She received her Ph.D. in linguistics from the University of Minnesota in 1984 and did post-doctoral work at the University of Pennsylvania in cognitive science. Prior to founding Conversational Technologies, Dr. Dahl did research at Unisys Corporation in natural and spoken language processing systems, focusing on spoken dialog systems. In particular, she has addressed making speech and language technology practical and useful by developing practical applications of the technology in such wide-ranging areas as Air Traffic Control, retail banking, applications for people with disabilities, and in developing the standards infrastructure that supports these applications. In addition to her technical work, Dr. Dahl participates in the World Wide Web Consortium's voice and HTML standards groups and serves as Chair of the Multimodal Interaction Working Group. She is an author of the W3C EMMA (Extensible MultiModal Annotation) standard for representing user input.

**Gonzalo Espejo** obtained the Degree in Computer Science in 2009 from the University of Granada. He is currently a PhD student in this University, where he has worked in several projects concerned with spoken and multimodal dialogue systems. His main research interests include spoken and multimodal systems as well as ambient intelligence. He has attended several workshops related to natural language processing and dialogue systems. He is member of SEPLN (Spanish Society on Natural Language Processing).

**Michael Greene** is a passionate advocate for extending technology to seniors and incorporating senior friendly design in products and services. As a social worker, he has advised senior service organizations on how to make better use of technology both to improve operations and to more fully engage their clients. He has coordinated conferences on a broad range of senior-related issues, written and presented on senior-friendly design, and conducted interactive workshops on new technologies at senior centers throughout NYC. Mr. Greene has been involved with Internet based technologies since the early 1990s. At KeySpan Energy (now National Grid), Michael played a leading role in the company's initial forays onto Internet and Intranet, as well as the development of "executive dashboards" to display high-level information for upper management. He is founder of streetplay.com, an award winning website that documents activities related to childhood play, with a focus on mid-20$^{th}$ century NYC games.

**David Griol** is Professor at the Department of Computer Science in the Carlos III University of Madrid (Spain). He obtained his Ph.D. degree in Computer Science from the Technical University of Valencia (Spain) in 2007 and has also a B.S. in Telecommunication Science from this same University. He has participated in several European and Spanish projects related to natural language processing and dialogue systems. His research activities are mostly related to the development of statistical methodologies for the design of spoken dialogue systems. His research interests include dialogue management/optimization/simulation, corpus-based methodologies, user modelling, adaptation, and evaluation of spoken dialogue systems, and machine learning approaches. Before starting his Ph.D., he worked as a network engineer in Motorola.

**Agneta Gulz** is Associate Professor of Cognitive Science at Linköping University, and Lund University in Sweden. Her main research area is digital learning environments, and in particular, learning environments that are based on virtual pedagogical characters. Some focus issues are: educational benefits and drawbacks with the use of such learning environments, human cognitive differences (e.g. learning style differences) and the adaptation to differences by means of digital learning environments, the impact of the social dimension of digital learning environments on learning, gender issues, and digital learning environments. During 2009-2011 she leads an internationally oriented research project "Digital Dialogues" on chat-based interaction between teenagers and virtual characters in learning contexts. Agneta is the author of more than 40 papers published in international journals, books, and conference proceedings.

**Magnus Haake,** MSc in Engineering Physics, in 2009 completed his PhD on virtual embodied pedagogical characters at the Department of Design Sciences at Lund University in Sweden. Magnus has a background in Human-Computer Interaction and information visualization in interactive digital media. He has been enrolled as an expert in different projects, both within business and research. Magnus is also trained in visual arts and graphic design. Since 2003, he has focussed on virtual characters in social and educational contexts. The specific topic of his PhD studies regards the basic, underlying visual design of virtual characters in relation to social psychology and to pedagogical intentions and outcomes. Magnus has published around 40 papers in journals, books, and proceedings.

**Luis Alfonso Hernández Gómez,** Engineer in Telecommunications in 1982, PhD in Telecommunications Engineering in 1988. Tenured Professor at U.P.M since 1994 is member of the Signal Processing Applications Group (GAPS) in the Signals, Systems and Communications Department (SSR) of Universidad Politécnica de Madrid (UPM). His research interests are mainly centred in the design and evaluation of human-technology interactive systems where has directed various doctoral theses and has written numerous articles. Dr. Hernández Gómez has coordinated an important number of research and technology transfer projects with both public and private sectors. He has also been Scientific Consultant at different Spanish companies, Evaluator at the Spanish National Agency for Scientific Evaluation and Member of the scientific committee of EUSIPCO, INTERSPEECH, and LREC (ELRA).

**Alvaro Hernández Trapote** is a PhD. Student in Computer Engineering and Communications at the Universidad Politécnica of Madrid. He received the Certificate of Advanced Studies in 2005. His main research interest is about Biometrics Systems and how users interact with them. He also studies some user factors particularly important in biometrics applications, such as privacy, invasiveness, or perception of security. He is also interested in ECAs capabilities for dialogue management and empathy behaviour, also applied for encouraging the learning experience of students with Special Needs. In 2008 he held a visiting research in KTH (Stockholm, Sweeden) during three months working in the TMH department. He has also worked in different national and European projects jointly with Spanish companies and has been Member of scientific committee of LREC.

**Lewis Johnson** has conducted research in artificial intelligence in education for over twenty-five years, and is an internationally recognized researcher in this area. He is President and Chief Scientist of Alelo. His particular research interests are in animated pedagogical agents (animated computer characters for interactive learning environments) and artificial intelligence technologies for education and training environments. Prior to that, he was a Research Professor in Computer Science at the University of Southern California (USC) and director of the Center for Advanced Research in Technology for Education at the USC / Information Sciences Institute. Alelo realizes his vision of revolutionizing foreign language and cultural education via advanced computer-based learning technologies. He is a member of the Advisory Committee of the International Artificial Intelligence in Education Society, and is on the steering committees of the Autonomous Agents and Intelligent User Interface conferences. He is past president of the International Artificial Intelligence in Education Society. Among other awards, he received the DARWARS Transition Award in March 2005, and was co-winner of the 2005 DARPATech Technical Achievement Award. He is a frequent invited speaker at international conferences and workshops. Dr. Johnson received an A.B. summa cum laude in linguistics from Princeton University, and a Ph.D. in computer science from Yale University. A number of his publications may be found at http://www.alelo.com/publications.html.

**Patrick Kenny** directs the Virtual Patient Simulation Lab at the University of Southern California's Institute for Creative Technologies. He is the lead Principal Investigator researching and developing advanced Artificial Intelligence and virtual human technology to create realistic medically based avatars with mental and physical disorders. Mr. Kenny has over 20 years of experience in research and industry in AI, Robotics, Simulation and Games. Mr. Kenny previously worked at The University of Michigan AI Lab researching and developing cognitive robotics for unmanned ground vehicles. While in Michigan Mr. Kenny founded a spin-off company, Soar Technology, from the AI Lab to support and develop cognitive agents in simulation. His research interests are in creating realistic high fidelity virtual humans with personality, dramatic agents and cognitive architectures integrating neuroscience, and AI and simulation. Mr. Kenny has a BS from The University of Minnesota and an MS from The University of Michigan. Mr. Kenny has organized workshops on believable characters and virtual human toolkits. He is the author of over 30 publications has been on several invited panels about virtual human technology and has served on numerous paper review committees.

**Tina Klüwer** is researcher at the German Research Center for Artificial Intelligence (DFKI GmbH) in Berlin, working mainly on dialogue and question answering systems. She has studied Linguistics Data Processing at the University of Cologne and has worked as researcher at the DFKI in Saarbrücken and as lecturer at the Department of Linguistics and Media Studies at the University of Bonn. The work on chatbots and dialogue systems is one focus of her research. In 2008 she was awarded with one of the "Theseus Talente"-prizes for the concept of a chatbot using ontologies as external knowledge base. Another research focus is automatic dialogue act recognition in conversational systems.

**Georgios Kouroupetroglou** holds a B.Sc. in Physics and a Ph.D. in Communications and Signal Processing. He is the Director of the Speech and Accessibility Laboratory, Department of Informatics and Telecommunications, University of Athens, and Head of the e-Accessibility Unit for Students with Disabilities. His research interests focuses on the area of Speech Communication, Voice Technologies and Computer Accessibility, as parts of the major domain of Human-Computer Interaction. Currently he is also involved in the research domains on Document Accessibility, Augmentative and Alternative Communication and Emotional Computer Interaction. Professor G. Kouroupetroglou has actively participated as in more than 52 European Union and National funded research projects, and he served as scientific coordinator among the 34 of them. He has been a reviewer, evaluator and member of working groups and/or technical panels of numerous European Union's projects and programs.

**Richard Leibbrandt** is an expert in the field of first-language acquisition of word classes (parts-of-speech). He has made contributions to the computational modelling of children's discovery of the word categories of their native language, and has pioneered a class of data clustering methods that allow information about word identity to be combined with information about the contextual usage of a word. Dr Leibbrandt is also active in research into Embodied Conversational Agents (ECAs), in particular into the use of ECA technologies for second-language teaching, and as assistive technologies for, inter alia, people with autism and other disabilities and people with memory deficits.

**Trent Lewis** is an expert in the multifaceted research field of audiovisual speech and has made contributions in several key areas. His most notable early work includes his innovation of Red Exclusion, which outperformed prior techniques both in facial feature recognition from video as well as subsequent visual speech recognition. Dr Lewis has since made other contributions to the classification of audiovisual speech using fusion of distinctive features at the acoustic and visual level, achieving reductions in error rate of as much as 75%. Dr Lewis is currently employed on the Thinking Head project, an ARC/NH&MRC Special Research Initiative in the field of intelligent Embodied Conversational Agents (ECAs), for which he is developing essential techniques for speaker association and lip reading.

**Markus Löckelt** studied computer science at the University of the Saarland with a focus on computational linguistics, algorithms and logic. In 2000, he joined the Intelligent User Interfaces group at the German Research Center for Artificial Intelligence (DFKI) as a researcher. Since then, he has been involved in the conception, design and implementation of the dialogue management for a number of multi-modal dialogue systems, most of them involving virtual characters. In his 2008 dissertation, he introduced a comprehensive dialogue management framework for story-driven interaction between several virtual characters and humans based on an ontological knowledge representation. His main research interest is to explore how to make dialogical human-computer interaction more versatile, useful, and enjoyable.

**Ramon López-Cózar Delgado** is Professor at the Faculty of Computer Science and Telecommunications of the University of Granada (Spain). His main research interests in the last 15 years include spoken and multimodal dialogue systems, focusing on speech processing and dialogue management. He has coordinated several research projects, has published a number of journal and conference papers, and has been invited speaker at several scientific events addressing these topics. In 2005 he published the book "Spoken, Multilingual and Multimodal Dialogue Systems: Development and Assessment" (Wiley). Recently he has co-edited the book "Human-Centric Interfaces for Ambient Intelligence" (Elsevier Academic Press, 2010), in which he has coordinated the section concerning speech processing and dialogue management. He is a member of ISCA (International Speech Communication Association), FoLLI (Association for Logic, Language and Information), AIPO (Spanish Society on Human-Computer Interaction) and SEPLN (Spanish Society on Natural Language Processing).

**Beatriz López-Mencía** is a PhD student in the Signals, Systems and Communications Department (SSR) of Universidad Politécnica de Madrid (UPM) under the supervision of Prof. Dr. Luis A. Hernández. She has an MEng in telecommunications engineering from Universidad Politécnica de Madrid in 2005. Currently she holds a research position in the field of Human Computer Interaction in the same university. Her research career is focused on the design and usability evaluation of multimodal interfaces and embodied conversational agents (ECAs). She has several publications related to the influence of embodied conversational agents to improve robustness of dialogue systems deployed in commercial applications. She complements her research in embodied conversational agents taking the advantages of this technology by developing applications for children with special educational needs.

**Martin Luerssen**'s research forte is in the field of nature-inspired computing, specifically the application of biological principles to machine learning. His dissertation, which was nominated for the CORE Australasian Distinguished Doctoral Dissertation award, innovated the use of graph grammars in evolutionary design and optimisation. With a comprehensive background in computational intelligence, Dr Luerssen has served as a program committee member for several international conferences and has delivered talks on many diverse domains, including cognitive science, artificial life, and user interfaces. At present, he is a key participant of the Thinking Head project, an ARC/NH&MRC Special Research Initiative that targets the development of intelligent Embodied Conversational Agents (ECAs). Dr Luerssen is principally responsible for the successful audiovisual embodiment of the agent, which encompasses the agent's ability to comprehend its – primarily social – context from audiovisual input, as well as its ability to synthesize realistic speech and animation.

**Pilar Manchón** was admitted to the degree of Master of Science in Cognitive Science and Natural Language in the Faculty of Science and Engineering at the University of Edinburgh in 1999, and received her European Ph.D. in Computational Linguistics from the University of Seville in 2009. She was awarded the British Council and La Caixa scholarship to study at the University of Edinburgh, as well as the Fulbright scholarship to conduct post-graduate research at Stanford University in California. She worked as a fellow scholar and researcher in the Spoken Dialogue Systems Group at the Artificial Intelligence Department in SRI International; she also worked as a Senior Computational Linguist, VUI Designer and Technology architect in NetbyTel, and as a researcher for the University of Seville. Currently, she is the co-founder and CEO of Intelligent Dialogue Systems, a software company specialized in the development of Embodied Conversational Agents.

**Paulette Mandelbaum** is a hands-on problem solver and analytic thinker with twenty five years of experience in strategic planning and marketing, dedicated to growing start-ups and young companies and organizations. At XYNETICS, Dr. Mandelbaum provides strategic planning and marketing services to young firms researching markets and industries and analyzing the potential for new products and services. She works with senior management teams to develop corporate/association identity, including strategy, mission, image, and market positioning. Before co-founding XYNETICS, Dr. Mandelbaum was Senior Director of Marketing and Strategic Planning at AppliedTheory, a provider of Internet software and Web services. She led market and competitive analysis effort and directed creation of collateral materials, as well as the corporate website. She created an integrated lead generation campaign, including direct mail, telemarketing, and a Web component, with testing programs measuring success. The company added more than 250 customers and revenues of $7.6 million within 12 months of the launch. At NYSERNet, Applied Theory's not-for-profit parent organization, Dr. Mandelbaum created and built the marketing department, established cross-functional product management teams, and specified an automated campaign management/sales tracking system. During her tenure, revenues tripled within two years.

**Marissa Milne** received first class honours in computer science at Flinders University in 2009, during which time she held a key role in developing and evaluating a prototype social skills tutoring program for children with high functioning autism and Asperger Syndrome. Ms Milne holds a teacher registration and has previously worked as an Out of School Hours Care coordinator, during which time she was involved in planning and applying modifications for students with Aspergers Syndrome, in collaboration with school staff and Autism SA. Ms Milne has presented her work in both educational and computing settings and is currently undertaking her doctorate at the Artificial Intelligence Laboratory at Flinders University under the supervision of Dr Leibbrandt and Prof. Powers, with an aim of further developing the social skills tutoring program.

**Nicole Novielli** is a research fellow at the Department of Informatics, University of Bari. She obtained her Ph.D. at the University of Bari in May 2010, defending a dissertation on "Lexical Semantics of Dialogue Acts", under the supervision of Dr. Carlo Strapparava. Her work was financed, in part, by HUMAINE, the European Human-Machine Interaction Network on Emotion. Her interests are in the area of intelligent interfaces, natural language processing and affective computing, AI, and cognitive science. At present she is working on recognition of affective and cognitive states from language and conversational analysis in 'natural' dialogues in Human-Human and Human-Computer interaction and on the application of Markovian models to dialog pattern description.

**David D. Pardo** has an MEng in telecommunications engineering from Universidad Politécnica de Madrid (2002). He is currently doing a PhD and holds a research position in the same university, under the supervision of Luis Hernández, in the Signal Processing Applications Group (GAPS). His research interests include, firstly, Human-Technology Interaction, with the primary focus of developing new analytical perspectives for the evaluation of the users' experience, especially in the context of applying multimodal interaction technology in novel areas of application (smart, personalised services involving spoken dialogue at home, in public spaces or in mobile scenarios). A second, related area of interest is the study of rhythm in human speech, with a view to improve the naturalness of conversation with machines and develop strategies to improve robustness when communication breakdown occurs.

**Thomas Parsons,** PhD, is a Clinical and Experimental Neuropsychologist, Assistant Research Professor, and Research Scientist at the University of Southern California's Institute for Creative Technologies. In addition to his patents (with eHarmony.com), he has over 100 publications in peer-reviewed journals. He directs the NeuroSim Lab, helping to facilitate human-computer interface research with adaptive virtual environments and advanced conversational virtual human agents that have been applied to medical and mental health applications. Dr. Parsons's current work focuses on the development of noninvasive brain-computer interfaces and psychophysiologically adaptive virtual environments (including virtual humans) that may be used for neuropsychological assessment, stress inoculation, virtual reality exposure therapy, cognitive training, and rehabilitation. These goals are being pursued with a combination of theoretical and experimental approaches at several levels of investigation ranging from the biophysical level to the systems level.

**Guillermo Pérez** received his Ph.D. in Telecommunication Engineering from the Polytechnic University of Madrid in 2009 with a doctoral thesis in multimodal dialogue systems. Since 2000, he has developed his research career with numerous publications in the field of natural language processing, multimodal dialogue systems, speech technologies, and human machine communication. He has combined his research interests with a professional background as a senior engineer in Telefónica and France Télécom. Currently he is the CTO of Indisys, a Spanish company that commercializes solutions with Embodied Conversational Agents.

**Arianna Pipitone** was born in Palermo, Italy, in March 1977. She received her degree in Computer Science Engineering with honors from the University of Palermo, in April 2006 defending a thesis on a new methodology to identify polycronous groups in a Liquid State Machine. She joined the group of Institute for High Performance Computing and Networking (ICAR - Istituto di Calcolo e Reti ad Alte Prestazioni) at the National Research Council (CNR) in Palermo as a research fellow from November 2006 till May 2008. Her research activity was about the development of ontology and services for hypermedia authoring on the Web, at the ICAR Medialab. Currently she is a PhD student at the Department of Computer Engineering (DINFO) of the University of Palermo, and her research interests mainly include the use of ontology and linguistic patterns matching methods extract semantic meaning from unstructured information sources.

**Roberto Pirrone** was born in Palermo on May 2, 1966. He had his degree in Electronic Engineering in 1991. In 1995 he obtained the PhD in Computer and Electronic Engineering. From 1999 to 2004, he was Assistant Professor in the Education Sciences Faculty at the University of Palermo. Since 2005, he is Associate Professor in the same Faculty. His research activity is with the Department of Computer Science and Engineering (DINFO). He teaches "Computer Graphics" for the course in "Computer Engineering" at the Engineering Faculty, and "Foundations of Computer Science" for the course in "Communication Science" at the Education Sciences Faculty. Research interests are in Cognitive architectures and HCI for intelligent tutoring applications, and Medical Image analysis and restoration.

**David Powers** is Director of the Artificial Intelligence Laboratory and an Advisory Board member of four research related organizations (YourAmigo Pty Ltd, Flinders Medical Devices and Technologies, BioX Pty Ltd, and the Association for Computational Linguistics Special Interest Group in Natural Language Learning and Conference on Natural Language Learning - all of which Powers is a founding member of), directing over 20 researchers and with experience of obtaining and managing grant funds and successfully completing projects as evidenced in dozens of research projects of various sizes, including commercialization of three projects. Current projects include two major ARC projects, one of which is a Discovery project being managed by Prof. Powers, and the other being the Thinking Head project, which involves four other Australian universities and four international universities, for which Powers manages the Flinders team.

**Silvia Quarteroni** is a Senior Marie Curie research fellow at the University of Trento, Italy. She received her MSc and BSc in Computer Engineering at the Swiss Federal Institute of Technology in Lausanne (EPFL) and her PhD in Computer Science at the University of York (UK). She has been working in several fields of natural language processing, focusing on human-computer dialogue, information retrieval, and personalization. She has (co-)authored over 30 articles published in international conferences and journals and is part of the program committee of several conferences and workshops.

**Giuseppe Russo** received his M.D. in Computer Science and Engineering in 2005. In 2009 he received his Ph.D. The main research interests are related to knowledge management and knowledge engineering with particular attention to knowledge fusion and representation processes.

**Alicia Sagae** is a researcher in natural language processing (NLP) with experience in semantic analysis, machine translation, and non-native speech identification. She holds a Ph.D. in Language and Information Technologies from the Carnegie Mellon University School of Computer Science. Alicia has experience with both symbolic and statistical systems, and has conducted experiments in every phase of development for multi-lingual NLP projects, including domain-defining tasks like data collection, working with native-speaker informants to build lexical resources, and conducting system tuning and evaluation. Alicia is currently a Senior Scientist at Alelo, helping drive the research agenda in natural language understanding, learner modeling, social modeling, and dialog management.

**Annika Silvervarg** is Research Associate of Cognitive Science at Linköping University. She holds a MA in Cognitive Science and a PhD in Computer Science. Her thesis work focused on knowledge representation in dialogue systems, in particular the design and use of ontologies in information-providing dialogue systems. Her current research interest is the design and implementation of conversational pedagogical agents that can integrate task oriented and social dialogue.

**Björn Sjödén** is M.Sc in Psychology, M.A in Cognitive Science and B.A in Film studies. He has a background working in international corporations within the IT and computer games sector and as a teacher, before turning to academic research in educational technology. He has published articles in various topics of cognitive psychology and computer-assisted learning, and keeps a particular interest in automatic (unconscious) influence on mental performance. He is currently pursuing his Ph.D. in Cognitive Science. The focus of his work lies on social-cognitive and motivational factors in learning software, specifically the kind discussed in the present chapter. You are very welcome to contact him, and influence his thesis, at Bjorn.Sjoden@lucs.lu.se.

**Dimitris Spiliotopoulos** is a member of the Speech and Accessibility Laboratory of the Department of Informatics and Telecommunications, the National and Kapodistrian University of Athens, Greece. His research focuses on natural language engineering, speech processing, text/document analysis, intonation, natural language generation, spoken dialogue systems, universal accessibility, design-for-all, text-to-speech, document-to-audio, speech acoustics, and evaluation. Academic studies include a PhD in Language Technology, a MPhil in Computation, a MA in Linguistics, and a BSc in Computation. He is a member of the IEEE Signal Processing Society, ISCA, and the ACL. He has participated in several national and international research projects, and his work has been published in international journals, books, and conferences.

**Pepi Stavropoulou** holds a first degree in Linguistics and an MSc in Speech and Language Processing. Her main research interests include spoken dialogue systems, usability and design-for-all, prosody, and the interface between prosody and pragmatics. She is a member of the Speech and Accessibility Laboratory of the Department of Informatics and Telecommunications at the University of Athens and has participated in several research and industry projects. She is currently working towards a PhD in the relationship between prosody and information structure and the utilization of this relationship for improving synthetic speech output in spoken dialogue interfaces.

**Carlo Strapparava** is a senior researcher at FBK-IRST (Fondazione Bruno Kessler - Istituto per la ricerca scientifica e Tecnologica) in the Human Language Technologies Unit. His research activity covers AI, natural language processing, intelligent interfaces, cognitive science, knowledge-based systems, user models, adaptive hypermedia, lexical knowledge bases, word sense disambiguation, and computational humor. He completed his studies in computer science at the University of Pisa, Italy.

**Andre Valente** is a technology manager and entrepreneur. He is co-founder and CEO of Alelo. He has a wide range of expertise in software development, research and consulting, having led technical teams for companies in the manufacturing, media, aerospace, and e-business areas. He has more than twenty years of experience knowledge-based systems, ontologies, knowledge engineering, and C4ISR automation and decision aids. Dr. Valente received a Ph.D. in Computer Science from the University of Amsterdam and an MBA from the University of Southern California. He has published three books and more than 50 technical articles.

**George Veletsianos** is Assistant Professor of Instructional Technology at the University of Texas, Austin. His research focuses on the use of emerging technologies in the design, development, and evaluation of open-ended online and hybrid learning environments. His focus areas are online learning, adventure learning, pedagogical agents, and the learner experience. Dr. Veletsianos is a prolific author and has published more than 50 journal articles, books chapters, and conference proceedings. Most recently he has published an edited book under an open access license entitled Emerging Technologies in Distance Education, which can be downloaded for free at http://www.aupress.ca/index.php/books/120177. He has been involved in global projects and investigations including work in the United States, United Kingdom, Sweden, and Cyprus, and is active in consulting, teaching, and research. Dr. Veletsianos is frequently asked to deliver keynotes and presentations on online and distance education, emerging technologies, adventure learning, pedagogical agents, social media, and participatory scholarship.

**Yorick Wilks** is Professor of Artificial Intelligence at the University of Sheffield, and is also a Senior Research Fellow at the Oxford Internet Institute at Balliol College, and a Senior Research Scientist at the Florida Institute of Human and Machine Cognition. He studied math and philosophy at Cambridge, was a researcher at Stanford AI Laboratory, before moving back to the US for ten years to run a successful and self-funded AI laboratory in New Mexico. His most recent book is Close Encounters with Artificial Companions (Benjamins, in press 2010). He is a Fellow of the American and European Associations for Artificial Intelligence, and a member of the UK Computing Research. He designed CONVERSE, the dialogue system that won the Loebner prize in New York in 1998, and was the founding Coordinator of the EU 6th Framework integrated project COMPANIONS (4 years, 15 sites, 13m Euro) on conversational assistants as personalised and permanent Web interfaces. In 2008 he was awarded the Zampolli Prize at LREC-08 in Marrakech, and the ACL Lifetime Achievement Award at ACL08 in Columbus, OH. In 2009 he was awarded the Lovelace Medal by the British Computer Society. In 2009 he was elected a Fellow of the ACM.

# Index

## A



## B



## C

## D



## E

## L



## M



## N



## O



## P

## Q



## R



## S



## T

## U



## V



## W



## X

CPSIA information can be obtained at www.ICGtesting.com
263891BV00006B/63-84/P